Cranial Osteopathy

of related interest

Cranial Osteopathy – Volume 2

Special Sense Organs, Orofacial Pain, Headache, and Cranial Nerves

Torsten Liem

ISBN 978 1 91342 669 9

eISBN 978 1 83997 615 5

Fascia in the Osteopathic Field

Edited by Torsten Liem, Paolo Tozzi and Anthony Chila

ISBN 978 1 90914 127 8

eISBN 978 1 91208 525 5

Foundations of Morphodynamics in Osteopathy

An Integrative Approach to Cranium, Nervous System, and Emotions

Edited by Torsten Liem and Patrick van den Heede

ISBN 978 1 90914 124 7

eISBN 978 1 90914 163 6

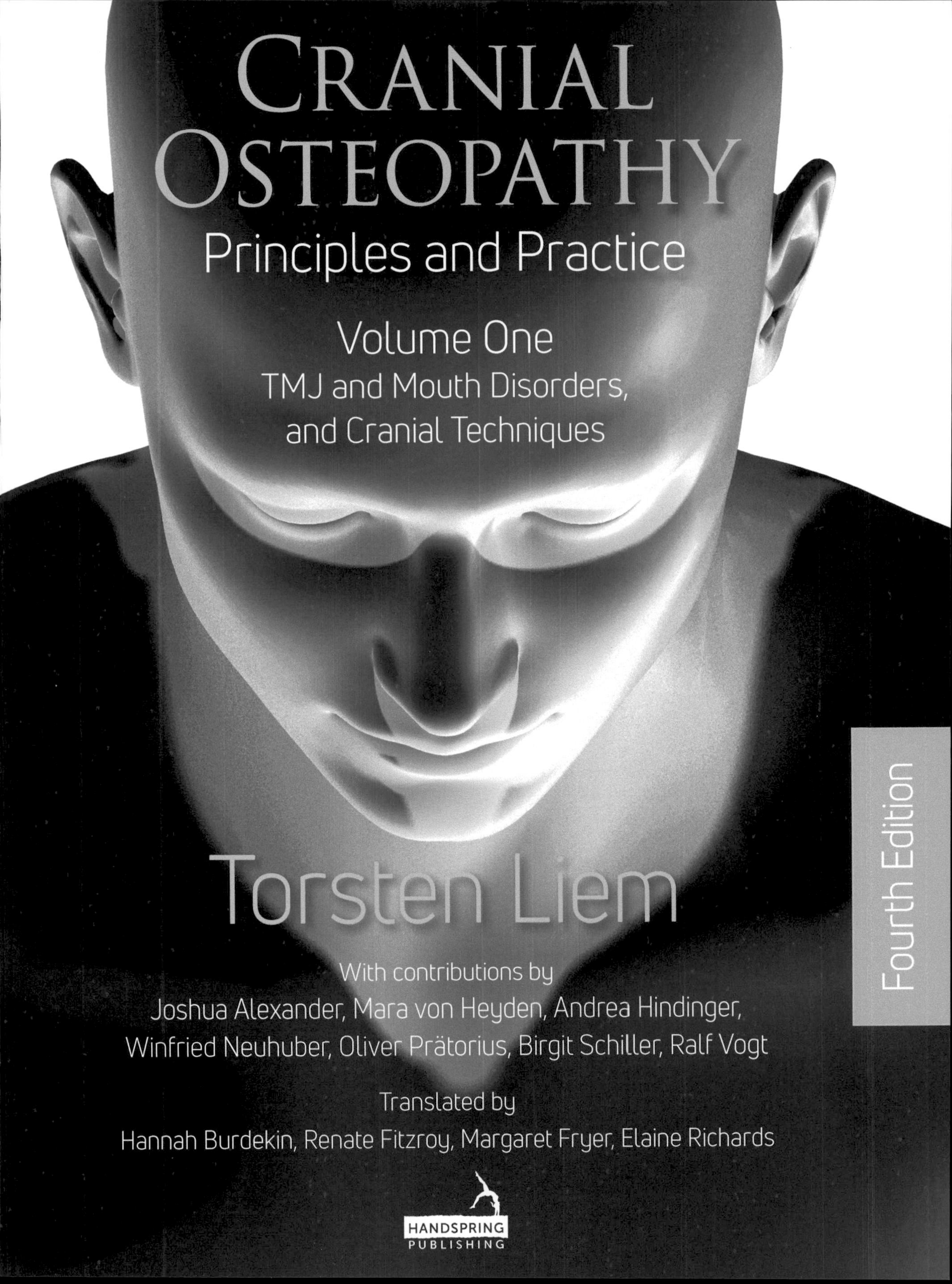

Cranial Osteopathy

Principles and Practice

Volume One

TMJ and Mouth Disorders, and Cranial Techniques

Fourth Edition

Torsten Liem

With contributions by

Joshua Alexander, Mara von Heyden, Andrea Hindinger, Winfried Neuhuber, Oliver Prätorius, Birgit Schiller, Ralf Vogt

Translated by

Hannah Burdekin, Renate Fitzroy, Margaret Fryer, Elaine Richards

HANDSPRING PUBLISHING

First edition in German published by Hippokrates Verlag in MVS Medizinverlage Stuttgart, GmbH & Co. KG, 2000
Second edition in German published by Hippokrates Verlag in MVS Medizinverlage Stuttgart, GmbH & Co. KG, 2003
Third edition in German published by Karl F. Haug Verlag in MVS Medizinverlage Stuttgart GmbH & Co. KG, 2010
Fourth edition published by Georg Thieme Verlag KG, 2020
This two-volume edition in English published in Great Britain in 2023 by Handspring Publishing, an imprint of Jessica Kingsley Publishers
Part of John Murray Press

1

A CIP catalogue record for this title is available from the British Library and the Library of Congress

ISBN 978 1 91342 671 2
eISBN 978 1 83997 612 4

Printed and bound in Great Britain by Ashford Colour Press Ltd

Jessica Kingsley Publishers' policy is to use papers that are natural, renewable and recyclable products and made from wood grown in sustainable forests. The logging and manufacturing processes are expected to conform to the environmental regulations of the country of origin.

Handspring Publishing
Carmelite House
50 Victoria Embankment
London EC4Y 0DZ

www.handspringpublishing.com

John Murray Press
Part of Hodder & Stoughton Limited
An Hachette UK Company

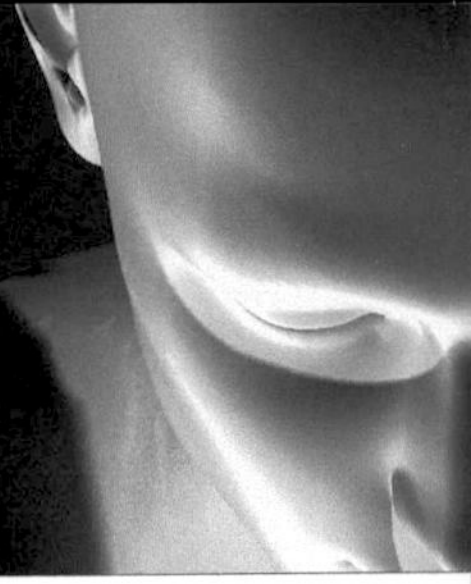

CONTENTS

Acknowledgments vi
Foreword by Jean Pierre Barral viii
Foreword by Fred L. Mitchell Jr. ix
Foreword by Richard A. Feely x
Prefaces xii
Abbreviations xv
About the Author xvii

CHAPTER 1 Methodology of Treatment: An Introduction 2

CHAPTER 2 Mandible and Temporomandibular Joint 12

CHAPTER 3 The Orofacial Structures, Pharynx, and Larynx 198

CHAPTER 4 The Occipital Bone 260

CHAPTER 5 The Sphenoid 278

CHAPTER 6 The Spheno-Occipital Synchondrosis/Synostosis (Sphenobasilar Synchondrosis) (SBS) 290

CHAPTER 7 The Ethmoid Bone 304

CHAPTER 8 The Vomer 322

CHAPTER 9 The Temporal Bones 332

CHAPTER 10 The Frontal Bone 372

CHAPTER 11 The Parietal Bones 390

CHAPTER 12 The Maxillae 406

CHAPTER 13 The Palatine Bones 424

CHAPTER 14 The Zygomatic Bones 432

CHAPTER 15 Nasal Bones, Lacrimal Bones, Inferior Nasal Concha 442

Glossary 449
Index 457

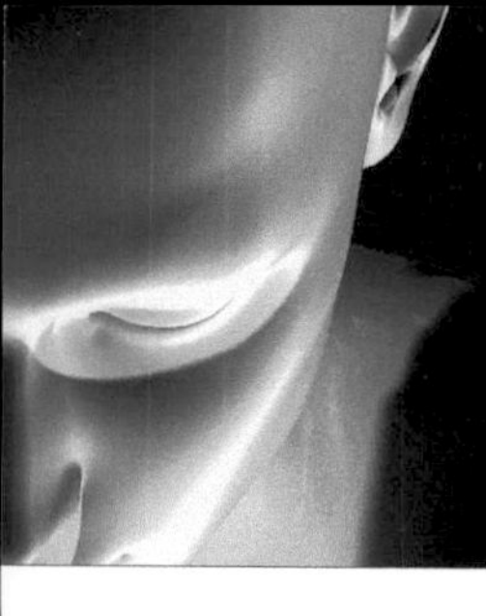

ACKNOWLEDGMENTS

I should like to thank in particular

- Alan R. Becker D.O., F.A.A.O., F.C.A. for his friendship and for introducing me to listening, open palpation. He took me to his heart as a student and taught me the simplicity of touch.
- Patrick van den Heede D.O. for his friendship and teaching. His genius and intuition inspired me deeply.
- Viola Frymann D.O., F.A.A.O., F.C.A., the "grande dame" of cranial osteopathy, on account of her sensitive and knowledgeable hands, her experience, and her sharing of it.
- Leopold Busquet D.O. for enlightening me on many aspects of biomechanical connections in the cranial system.
- Robert Fulford D.O., F.A.A.O., F.C.A., a great example to me in showing me that it is important in osteopathy too to follow one's heart and inner voice, one's conviction, even if it sometimes provokes controversy.
- When I remember Anne Wales D.O., F.A.A.O., F.C.A. I feel quite at ease about growing old as an osteopath (though I am still quite young). Even in later years she held her entire audience spellbound by her intellectual and spiritual perception. It is so good to see a person whose life is so imbued with uprightness, modesty, and devotion that they are surrounded, even in old age, by a seemingly timeless youth, beauty, and unique radiance.
- Jim Jealous D.O., F.A.A.O. for helping me to sense the phenomena of energies in palpation.
- Richard A. Feely D.O., F.A.A.O., F.C.A. for explaining the neurological aspects of cranial osteopathy.
- Herb Miller D.O., F.A.A.O., F.C.A., who gave me confidence in my own hands by his presence and sensitive hands, and Edna Lay for the knowledge of Sutherland's approach that she provided in a course.
- Thomas Schooley D.O., F.A.A.O., F.C.A. for the insights into early osteopathy and Still's lost biographical texts.
- John Upledger D.O., F.A.A.O. for the creativity and inspiration I found in meeting with him.
- Prof. Frank Willard PhD, whose outstanding lectures on anatomical and physiological relations are a constant inspiration to me.
- Harold I. Magoun Jr. D.O., F.A.A.O., F.C.A. for the experience of being treated by him.
- I am greatly inspired by the teaching of Jean Pierre Barral D.O., M.R.O. This inspiration derives not only from his unique experience, the silent accompaniment to all his lectures, but especially from the effortless manner in which he helps me, as he does others, to have confidence and find enjoyment in my palpation.
- I owe a great deal to Franz Buzet M.R.E.O., M.S.B.O. It feels so good to have someone believe in you.
- I should also like to thank Beatrice Macazaga, who inspired me many years ago as a friend and involuntary mother-substitute, in my entry into complementary medicine.
- Fred L. Mitchell Jr. D.O., F.A.A.O., F.C.A. is to me a wonderful example of a teacher who combines empathy, clarity and comprehensibility, modesty, and sheer competence, making him able to answer even the most stupid of questions with the same constant concern and attentiveness.
- Renzo Molinari D.O., M.R.O. for his great help and support. I could not imagine a more able, involved and empathetic President of the European School of Osteopathy.

- If I ever believed that osteopathy had anything to do with strength, then it was Lawrence H. Jones D.O., F.A.A.O. who convinced me of the opposite. I was impressed at the lightness and grace—like that of a dancer—of Dr. Jones (even when advanced in age) as he touched, moved, and treated me.

- My thanks go too to John Wernham D.O. In his teaching, personally and in treatment sessions, he passed on to me a wealth of information about classical osteopathy and his own experience with the principles of Littlejohn.

- I should like to thank Paul Chauffour D.O. and Eric Prat D.O. for their friendship and their inspiring instruction in the concept of osteopathic mechanical integration.

- My thanks likewise to Philip Greenman D.O., F.A.A.O., Robert C. Ward D.O., F.A.A.O., Ed Styles D.O., F.A.A.O., Michael Kuchera D.O., F.A.A.O., and the many other teachers who gave me an understanding of the other areas of osteopathy.

- I should also especially like to thank my many dear friends and colleagues, among them Alain Abehsera D.O., M.D., Alan R. Becker D.O., F.A.A.O., F.C.A. (†), Cristian Ciranna-Raab D.O., Christian Fossum D.O., Bruno Chickly M.D., D.O. (Hon.), Dr. Ganesan, Jenny Parkinson, Prof. John Glover D.O., F.A.A.O., Prof. John McPartland D.O., Prof. Dr. Paul Klein D.O., Peter Sommerfeld D.O., Steve Paulus D.O., Uwe Senger D.O., and many more.

- Thank you, Sat Hari and Robert, who inspired me to seek the way from overmuch youthful confusion to yoga. It is wonderful to feel the slowly growing trust in self-regulation.

- My heartfelt thanks to Vijayananda, a former French physician, who left France to live a life of seclusion for 14 years in the Himalayas. What his work in itself revealed to me was less a matter of profound religious teaching than of immediate experience and his interaction with me and other people. It gave me confidence that, through devotion, perseverance, and sincerity, I too can achieve a little more "lightness" and consciousness.

- I am especially grateful for all the wide-ranging interdisciplinary exchange of ideas over these last decades. This enabled me to expand my understanding of the body's regulatory processes and the way they are intimately linked with external circumstances.

- I wish to express my gratitude to all my patients, who gave me the opportunity to learn and mature and to pass on what I have learned. Thanks too to all those teachers and the other people not named here, who have assisted in the production of this book and in my own personal growth and still continue to do so.

I should also very much like to thank Dr. Walter Schöttl, Dr. Carola Pfeiffer, Dr. Michael Jaehne, Rainer Quast, Uwe Senger, Irene Özbay, Michael Kaufmann, Katja Hinz, Kerstin Herre, Philip Van Caille, Dr. Angelika Milutin-Lantzi, Dr. Hubertus von Treuenfels, Marlene Carvalho, Dr. Caroline Clauder, and especially Stefan Collier for their huge help in the work of checking the text.

Special thanks to my co-authors of this edition: Dr. Joshua Alexander, Mara von Heyden, Andrea Hindinger, Prof. Dr. Winfried Neuhuber, Dr. Oliver Prätorius, Birgit Schiller, and Ralf Vogt.

And, quite especially, I wish to thank my publishers Thieme Verlag and Frau Monika Grübener and Frau Stefanie Teichert for their support and flexibility through to the late stage of the production process.

FOREWORD by Jean Pierre Barral

Life is motion—this principle applies just as surely to osteopathy and its subdivisions. As a science, an art, and a philosophy, osteopathy is not static but continually in motion. The great challenge before us is to remain firmly rooted in the principles of osteopathy as we simultaneously open ourselves to the dynamics of life, allowing ourselves to be affected by our daily contact with patients, by new scientific insights, by the exchange of ideas among colleagues, and by the demands of the time in which we live.

Torsten Liem's previous volume in German impressed me at first sight on account of its instructional layout and uniquely comprehensive and lively presentation of craniosacral osteopathy.

The present work continues that tradition. The anatomical and physiological aspects of the visceral structures of the cranium and their associated dysfunctions and methods of treatment are presented with the utmost detail and clarity. This work serves at the same time as a speedy reference manual in the course of practice, providing a description of the techniques relating to each cranial bone and the diagnosis and treatment of the facial organs, and systematically setting out their possible dysfunctions. The author meanwhile does not lose sight of the essential: that capacity to be inwardly touched by the uniqueness of each contact and of osteopathy itself.

I am convinced that students of osteopathy and practicing osteopaths will agree in welcoming this book.

Jean Pierre Barral
Academic Director of the Collège International d'Osteopathie in St Etienne, Lecturer in the Faculty of Medicine in Paris Nord, the European School of Osteopathy (ESO) in Maidstone, and the Osteopathie Schule Deutschland (OSD, German School of Osteopathy)

FOREWORD by Fred L. Mitchell Jr.

I have for some years been aware of the need for a comprehensive textbook of craniosacral work. For many years *The Cranial Bowl* (1939) by Sutherland and Magoun's *Osteopathy in the Cranial Field* (1951) were the sole works in this field, although neither had been conceived or written as a textbook. Each of these books focused in the first instance on the clinical relevance of investigating and treating the phenomenon that Sutherland called the primary respiratory mechanism, and providing a theoretical basis for craniosacral osteopathy.

Howard and Rebecca Lippincott compiled their first handbook of craniosacral techniques from the notes they made during their period of study under William G. Sutherland and published it in 1943 through the auspices of the Academy of Applied Osteopathy. A second revised edition was published in 1946 by the Osteopathic Cranial Association. This describes about 60 techniques, many of which were later exchanged or replaced by the authors or by other students of the cranial concept. Many of these changes, however, still remain to be written down.

Since the 1930s/1940s, cranial techniques have multiplied in the minds and hearts of creative students. Many of these students, such as Charlotte Weaver, Beryl Arbuckle, and Viola Frymann, have emphasized the importance of embryology and the use of craniosacral osteopathy in practical pediatrics. Special techniques were developed for use in this field. Will Sutherland's courses must have attracted especially creative minds. Paul Kimberly, Alan R. Becker, Rollin Becker, Robert Fulford, Kenneth Little, J. Gordon Zink, Olive Stretch, Tom Schooley, Howard Lippincott, Rebecca Lippincott, Anne Wales, and Harold Magoun Sr. were some of the students of Sutherland whose ideas formed my own craniosacral concept. Each of these made their own unique contributions as to methods.

Torsten Liem has produced outstanding work in research, and presents in this edition an excellent selection of beautifully illustrated craniosacral techniques, which will provide the reader with well-balanced instruction in the basics of craniosacral work. The section on temporomandibular dysfunctions will be an inspiration to many readers with its depth and detail.

A word of caution: gentleness is the first essential to master in any course of training in craniosacral osteopathy. Clinically effective craniosacral manipulation demands gentleness and patience. Craniosacral work is often described as "non-invasive," but that is too simplistic. The art is to learn to reach down through the tissue with sympathetically attuned understanding and not just with the hands. The treatment route to be followed is decided on the basis of the clinical assessment, founded on scientific anatomical and physiological knowledge, which indicates whether particular techniques of manual medicine can helpfully be employed.

Fred L. Mitchell Jr., D.O., F.A.A.O., F.C.A.,
Professor Emeritus of the
College of Osteopathic Medicine,
Michigan State University

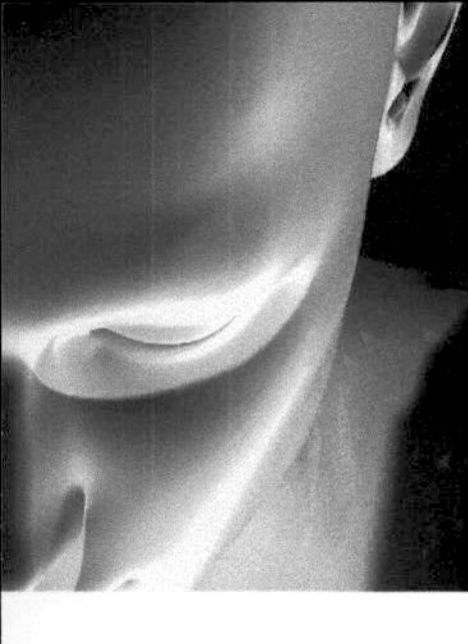

FOREWORD by Richard A. Feely

Torsten Liem's stimulating work on cranial osteopathy is designed for the osteopathic physician/student as well as the craniosacral therapist/student. In his German edition, he gave the historical background of the discoverer William Garner Sutherland D.O. DSc(Hon.). In this complete textbook, he provides a glossary in which he explains the most important concepts of cranial osteopathy, with extensive references.

Dr. W. G. Sutherland was a student of Andrew Taylor Still M.D., the founder of osteopathy. Late in his life, Dr. Sutherland had this to say: "In 75 years, in the crucible of time, not one statement made by Dr AT Still has needed revising."

The beginning of this unique, truly American school of medicine dates back to June 22, 1874, when after years of personal research and discovery, Dr. Still, on the wheat fields of Kansas, "flung the banner to the breeze—Osteopathy." The first school was founded in 1892 in Kirksville, Missouri. With the success of patient care and cures, osteopathy's fame spread and caught the attention of a young newspaper reporter from Minnesota, W. G. Sutherland. Sutherland entered the original American School of Osteopathy in Kirksville in 1898 where Dr. A. T. Still was to have said, "There's a few right thinking people here." Dr. A. T. Still taught his students to think osteopathically; that is, that the Creator designed the human body perfectly and there is a reason and purpose for each and every structure, design, relationship, and function. Reasoning from anatomy and physiology, the osteopath designs a treatment that restores the body to its maximum efficiency, wholeness, and health. In 1899, while examining an open, disarticulated cranium at the American School of Osteopathy, W. G. Sutherland was struck by the observation of how closely the squama of the temporal bones resembled the gills of a fish. The next stage in his train of thought followed logically, that the structure of the skull must be designed for some sort of motion, gills—respiration—motion. This outrageous (for the time, 1899) thought, that the skull had motion, because of its anatomical design and the laws of physics, continued to plague Dr. W. G. Sutherland for the rest of his life. Until at last, in 1938, he was able to prove to himself that the cranium does have an inherent capacity for motion, the Primary Rhythmic Impulse. He recognized the existence of the motility of the central nervous system; fluctuation in the cerebrospinal fluid; the mobility of the dura mater that acts, in this respect, as a reciprocal tension membrane; and the articular mobility of the cranial bones, backed by the mobility of the sacrum between the alae of the ilium.

Dr. A. T. Still gave the profession its concepts: the rule of the artery is supreme; the body has the inherent capacity to heal itself; and structure and function are reciprocally interrelated. Dr. W. G. Sutherland added that the rule of the artery is supreme, but the cerebrospinal fluid is in command and its fluctuation can be observed by palpation with cranial technique. In 1950, Robert E. Truhlar D.O. neatly summed it all up: "Osteopathy is divine geometry, physics, and chemistry."

The author, Torsten Liem, brings to the profession a fresh, new, and improved presentation of both well-known and recent advancements in the field of cranial osteopathy and craniosacral therapy. The author directs your attention to the intricate anatomical and physiological function that make up the dynamic cranial sacral mechanism. His direct and easy-to-read palpatory procedures for diagnosis and treatment are refreshing. Torsten Liem deals with each cranial bone in turn, describing its physiological mobility and restrictions to motion, as well as diagnostic and therapeutic methods and procedures. The reader is assisted in visualizing these methods and procedures by the magnificent photographs and illustrations that accompany the text.

The section dealing with the treatment of the bones and organs of the face is most interesting with a thorough treatment of the diagnostic and treatment procedures of the cranial structures. A selection of well-known pathologies is used to illustrate the osteopathic approach, providing guidance to the reader new to osteopathy. In this connection, the book follows the original theme in relation to diagnosis and treatment utilizing cranial osteopathy. Throughout, excellent references to the literature complete this work.

American osteopathic physicians and surgeons have long been aware of the healing and life-giving effect of the physiological phenomenon known as the Primary Rhythmic Impulse. Torsten Liem presents this effectively, while making no secret of the difficulties of the diagnostic and therapeutic methods needed to bring a favorable influence to bear on the life and health of patients. If the life and the condition of humanity are to be improved, precise understanding and correct application in the cause of restoration and wholeness of the entire person are indispensable. This art is a powerful psychomotor skill, and it is essential to use the knowledge contained in this book only in combination with personal instruction from competent masters of this skill. Personal training with validation of the development of your osteopathic skills is the only way to become sure and trustworthy practitioners, confident in diagnosis and treatment, able to rely on the desired outcome of your work.

Richard A. Feely, D.O., F.A.A.O., F.C.A.,
Former president of the Cranial Academy,
Associate Professor of the Chicago College of
Osteopathic Medicine/Midwestern University

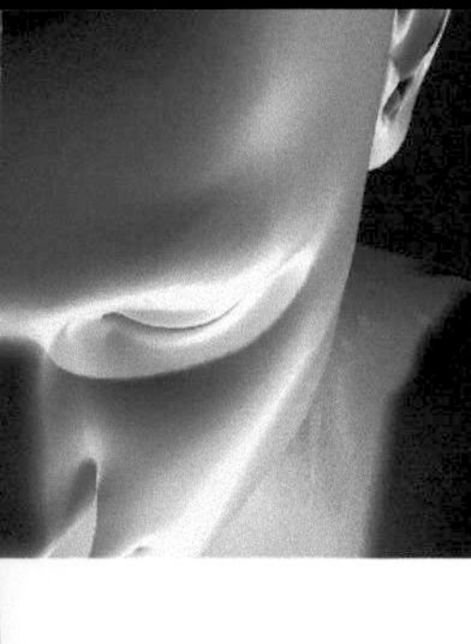

PREFACE to the present edition

A complete revision of the text has been undertaken and a new introductory chapter provided on treatment methodology. This is central to an understanding of osteopathic treatment of the organs concerned.

The chapter dealing with the mouth and jaw and the sensory organs of the head has largely been rewritten to include the relevant up-to-date scientific findings; it also presents ideas concerning formative dynamics, new diagnostic approaches relating to practice, and innovative approaches to treatment. The chapters on the treatment of the viscerocranium and of headache have been significantly extended so as to deal in sufficient depth with the complex interactions involved and with the approaches in terms of practice. A further chapter provides extensive additional information on the treatment of the cranial nerves.

As well as incorporating the current state of scientific understanding, the content of this book is distinguished by its close relevance to actual practice and by its clarity of layout. The introductory sections, treatment tips, summaries of treatment methods, and clearly organized new layout further improve the accessibility to the reader. A fresh approach has also been taken to the graphics and photographs, using color for all the photographs illustrating diagnosis and treatment and for most of the graphics.

This is to the best of my knowledge the most comprehensive work on osteopathic approaches, including as it does the organs of the mouth and jaw and sensory organs of the head. The individual chapters all offer solid information for the osteopath that is above all usefully practice-related. It is likewise helpful for interdisciplinary co-operation.

It would be a great pleasure to me if this textbook can play a part in furthering the growing recognition of osteopathic treatment in the cranial field and that of the sensory organs of the head.

Torsten Liem

PREFACE to the first edition

This book focuses primarily on those mechanisms of dysfunction and treatment techniques that belong to the more narrowly defined field of craniosacral and craniomandibular osteopathy. It also includes some material beyond this immediate field.

The reason for the somewhat mechanical presentation of the structures in this book is entirely didactic. It is by no means the intention to imply that therapeutic intervention is merely a matter of finely executed manual techniques. Intuition, caring attention, and empathy on the part of the therapist, and the sensitivity of the practitioner's hands, are just as important for the success of treatment. Listening, non-invasive attentiveness, and consciousness in palpation activates the body's inherent healing powers. It is a great gift when hands begin to see, hear, and know, and a still greater gift that this remains a constant adventure.

Practicing therapists know that each touch conveys new insights into the integrated working together of the body as a whole. Only an open spirit that has emptied itself is capable of receiving these insights. Just as much weight should therefore be placed on the approach, which must focus on the entirety, and on an open and listening touch, as on the learning and absorbing of the specific structures and their functional and anatomical relationships. It is less a question of "doing" than the capacity of "being" with the other person, and permitting the closeness and intimacy that open doors in the therapeutic encounter.

The repetition of material from the first book was inevitable; it is also practical from the instructional point of view, since it would otherwise have been necessary to make reference to the relevant parts of the first. That would make the text difficult to use, especially for quick reference.

The account of the localization, origin, and treatment of dysfunctions of the various bones has been limited to the structures directly involved.

The format of the present work is to present techniques in relation to each cranial bone and the organ systems of the viscerocranium. A large number of additional variations and possible methods of performing them do in fact exist, and can be employed with at least as much success. During the course of a career, every therapist will to some extent develop individual approaches. These stem not only from experiences during that practice and from individual characteristics, but also from the fact that every patient, every treatment, and each one of the body's structures is unique.

The basis of osteopathy according to Andrew Taylor Still was not in the first instance the teaching of particular techniques, but insight into particular principles that might give individual osteopaths the capacity to develop techniques of their own. The more a therapist internalizes the differentiation between the living tissues, their reciprocal anatomical and physiological relationships, and the osteopathic principles of diagnosis and treatment and develops manual sensitivity, the greater that capacity will be.

The intuitive, "living," and spiritual content of Sutherland's work and his concept of the "Breath of Life" were to some degree deleted from the revised standard work by Harold Ives Magoun: *Osteopathy in the Cranial Field*, 3rd edition (1976), published after Sutherland's death. The intention was to achieve greater political acceptance among the osteopaths living at that time and to make the cranial approach accessible to further research. In today's climate there is more readiness to consider these ideas too. An accompanying understanding of the historical associations and roots, as well as a common language, are important for the practice of craniosacral osteopathy, its further development, and its transmission. For this reason the Glossary explains the fundamental principles using primarily the original Sutherland sources.

PREFACE to the first edition *continued*

It simply remains for me to thank most sincerely all those who have written or sent ideas in response to the first book.

I wish you as much pleasure in reading this book, in palpation and in applying the techniques described, as I have had in writing it and experience day by day in my contact with patients.

In particular I wish you the same courageous spirit and devotion in your search and application of this living osteopathy as the founders of this unique discipline themselves possessed.

Torsten Liem

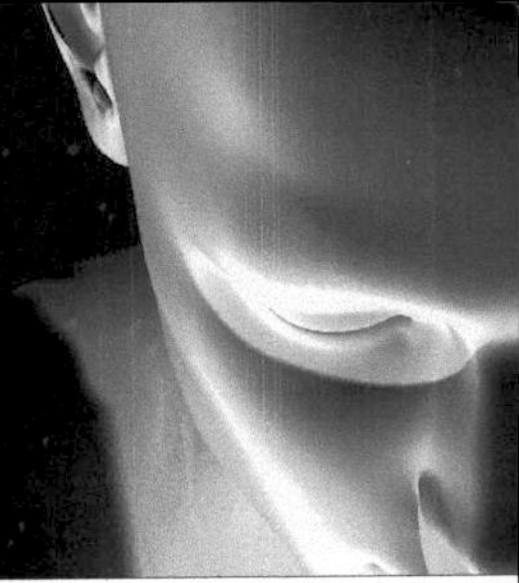

ABBREVIATIONS

Key to abbreviations and guide to landmarks on the skull

AAOP	American Academy of Orofacial Pain
ARAS	ascending reticular activation system
ASA	acetylsalicylic acid (aspirin)
BDT	basophil degranulation test
BLT	balanced ligamentous tension
BMP	bone morphogenetic protein
CCSIT	Cross-Cultural Smell Identification Test
CFMAS	craniofacial musculoaponeurotic system
CGRP	calcitonin gene-related peptide
CMD	craniomandibular dysfunction
CN	cranial nerve
CNS	central nervous system
COMT	catechol-O-methyltransferase
COPA	craniomandibular orthopedic positioning appliance
CSF	cerebrospinal fluid
CSMP	condylo-squamoso-mastoid pivot point
CT	computed tomography
DBT	dynamic balanced tension
ENT	ear, nose, and throat
ER	external rotation
FGF	fibroblast growth factor
HELLP syndrome	hemolysis, elevated liver enzymes, low platelets
HLA	human leukocyte antigen
HPA axis	hypothalamus–pituitary–adrenal axis
HVLA	high velocity, low amplitude
IHS	International Headache Society
IR	internal rotation
LTT	lymphocyte transformation test
MET	muscle energy technique
MRI	magnetic resonance imaging
MS	multiple sclerosis
NLP	neurolinguistic programming
NMDA	N-methyl-D-aspartate
OAA	occiput-atlas-axis
OPG	orthopantomogram
PAG	periaqueductal gray
PBET	point of balanced electrodynamic tension
PBFT	point of balanced fluid tension
PBLT	point of balanced ligamentous tension
PBMT	point of balanced membranous tension
PBT	point of balanced tension
PRM	primary respiratory mechanism/movement
RDC/TMD	Research Diagnostic Criteria for Temporomandibular Disorders
SBS	sphenobasilar synchondrosis
SHH	sonic hedgehog
SMAS	superficial musculoaponeurotic system
SSP	sphenosquamous pivot
SUNA syndrome	short-lasting unilateral neuralgiform headache attacks with cranial autonomic symptoms
SUNCT syndrome	short-lasting unilateral neuralgiform headache attacks with conjunctival injection and tearing
TFI	Tinnitus Functional Index
TGF	transforming growth factor

ABBREVIATIONS *continued*

TMJ	temporomandibular joint
TNF	tumor necrosis factor (e.g., anti-TNF-α)
TRP	transient receptor potential
VAS	visual analog scale
VHI	Voice Handicap Index

Guide to landmarks:

- Nasion—Median point of frontonasal suture
- Glabella—Level region between eyebrows, located on the lower part of the metopic suture
- Ophryon—Above glabella
- Bregma—Point at which sagittal suture and coronal suture meet
- Vertex—Highest point of skull
- Lambda—Point at which sagittal suture and lambdoid suture meet
- Inion—External occipital protuberance
- Pterion—Point at which frontal bone, sphenoid, temporal bone, and parietal bone join
- Asterion—Point at which parietal, occipital, and temporal bones join
- Basion—Middle of the anterior border of the foramen magnum
- Opisthion—Middle of the posterior border of the foramen magnum
- Gnathion—Inferiormost, centrally located point on the tip of the chin, on the mandible

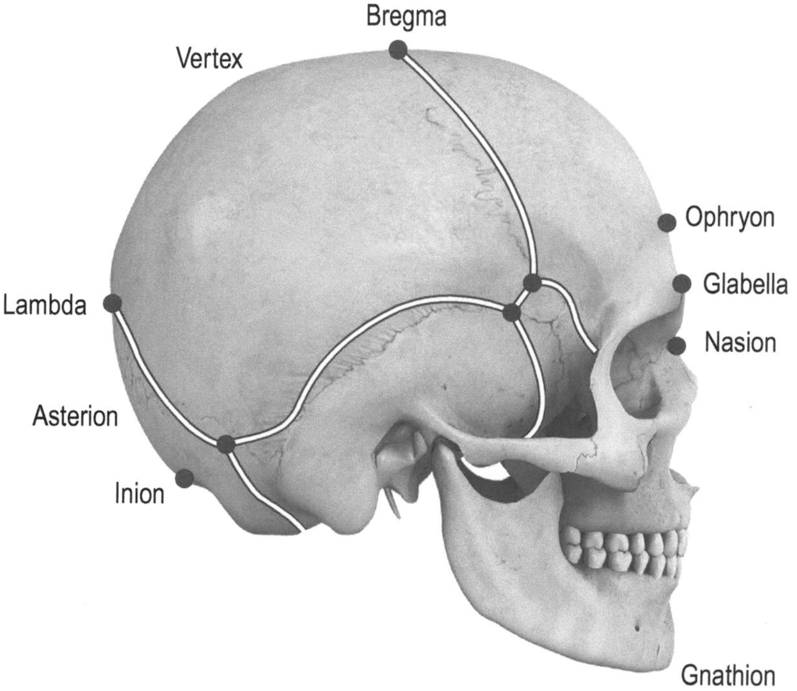

Osteometric points on the skull

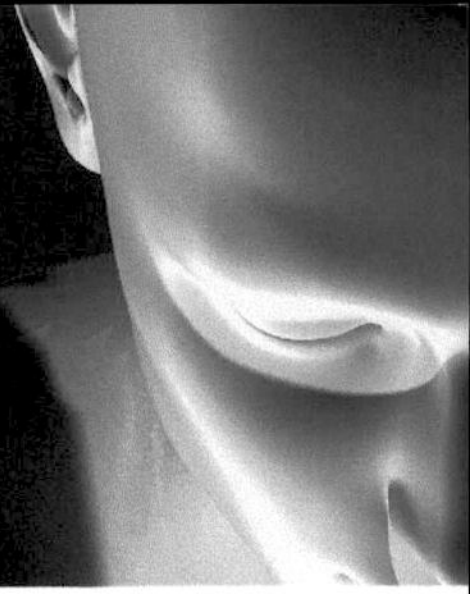

ABOUT THE AUTHOR

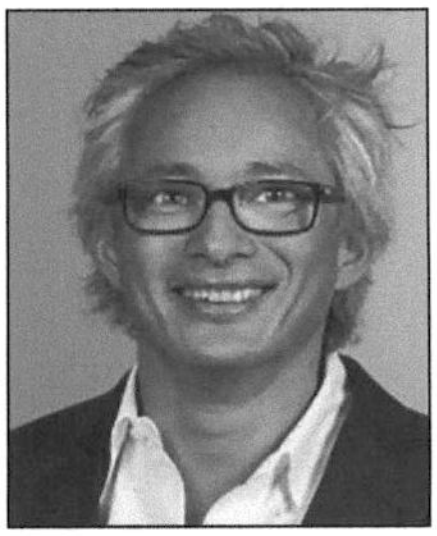

Torsten Liem BSc Ost, MSc Ost, MSc Ped Ost, D.O., DPO (DEU) founded the Osteopathie Schule Deutschland (OSD) and led it from 1999 to 2019. He is also recognized as an osteopath in the United Kingdom by the General Osteopathic Council. He founded and developed the first academic teaching programs in Germany for osteopathy, sports osteopathy, and pediatric osteopathy, the Institute of Integrative Morphology (2009) and the Institute of Psychosomatic Osteopathy (2023). He has also developed new approaches in osteopathic acupuncture and psychosomatic osteopathy. He has published numerous books, including *Foundations of Morphodynamics in Osteopathy*, and is author of the instructional DVD series *Rhythmic Balanced Interchange I–V.* He is co-editor of *Osteopathische Behandlung von Kindern*, *Differenzialdiagnosen in der Kinderosteopathie*, and *Kinder-Osteopathie: Sanfte Berührung in den ersten Lebensjahren.* He co-founded the journal *Osteopathische Medizin* (2000) and is a member of the editorial board of the *International Journal of Osteopathic Medicine.* He is also a member of numerous professional societies and a board member of the European and German Society for Pediatric Osteopathy as well as the Osteopathic Research Institute. He teaches different styles of yoga, meditation, and breathing therapy and has developed his own integrated teaching system, and also combines music therapy approaches with osteopathy. Besides his practice in Hamburg, he is currently conducting clinical research on the treatment of athletes and techniques of psychosomatic osteopathy while developing the osteopathic health blog: www.osteopathie-liem.de.

He has been an international teacher in the cranial field, morphodynamics, immunology, fascia, ENT, nutrition, osteopathic counseling, pediatric osteopathy, sport osteopathy, psychosomatic osteopathy, and many other areas of osteopathy for several decades. His book *The Osteopathic Self-Help Book* (2021) was an Amazon bestseller for five months.

1.1 General procedure 4
1.1.1 Balancing the autonomic nervous system 4
1.1.2 Intention 5
1.1.3 Focus 5
1.1.4 Resonance 5
1.1.5 Induction of the point of balanced membranous tension, fluid tension, or dynamic balanced tension 6
1.1.6 Fluid impulse 7
1.1.7 Further treatment modalities 7
1.1.8 Further hints for performing the techniques 8
1.1.9 Additional information 9

1.2 References 10

1

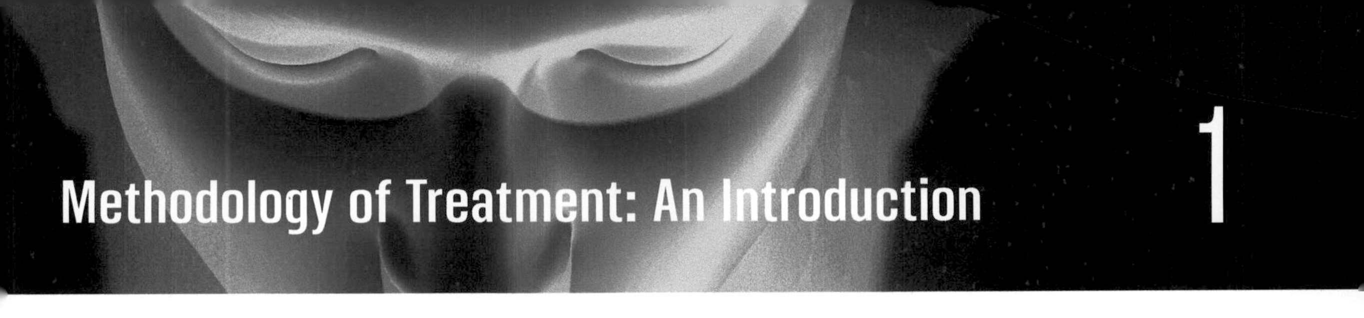

1 Methodology of Treatment: An Introduction

In this first volume of *Cranial Osteopathy* biophysical, neurobiological, and psychological interactions are discussed, as well as the interplay of developmental dynamics and further epigenetic influences on temporomandibular joint (TMJ) and mouth function, based on current studies.

- Developmental factors and the diagnosis and treatment of craniomandibular dysfunction (e.g., muscular, condylar, intraosseous, ligamentous and capsular, arterial, venous, and neural aspects) are described in detail. Self-help exercises for the patient are also presented.
- Treatment steps for specific disorders of the temporomandibular joint are examined, for example the consequences of trauma, osteoarthritis and degenerative processes, resistant occlusal stress, crossbite, progenic-type dysgnathia, backbite, open bite, deep bite, bruxism, dry lips.
- The use of occlusal splints in clinical practice is discussed.
- Developmental factors and the diagnosis and treatment of orofacial structures, the pharynx, and larynx are presented in detail. This includes, for example, techniques for the periodontium, in dental trauma, for the tongue, floor of the mouth, hyoid bone, thyroid cartilage, associated cranial nerves, arteries, veins, lymphatics, and tonsils, as well as specific indications such as inflammation. There are also exercise programs and self-help exercises.
- The location of each cranial bone is described as well as differential diagnoses and clinical presentations, including osseous, muscular, ligamentous, fascial, dural, neural, and vascular interactions.
- Comprehensive findings and techniques for each cranial bone are presented. This includes sutural techniques, intraosseous techniques, sphenobasilar synchondrosis (SBS), and dural and fluid techniques.

In order to address the stress on a patient's body we need to consider the factors affecting it from both the outside and from within; we must identify the interacting mechanisms and influences that work upon it, those that strengthen as well as those that are dysfunctional. From here we can move on to encourage the factors that promote strength and reduce the ones that create disease. As we do so, we should also enhance allostatic adaptation: the numerous adaptive and physiological changes that take place at the level of the tissues.

In order to achieve this, we need to support the body's inherent self-regulation system, and we can do this by addressing the system as a whole. To approach it in this way involves looking at the cybernetic control processes by which the body regulates itself. We do this through our palpatory approach and treatment, though we should bear in mind that this is just one part of clinical reasoning in osteopathy.

The roots of osteopathic treatment can be seen to lie in the fundamental principles and models of osteopathy. The dynamic, interoperating relationship between structure and function is one of the main principles of osteopathic thought and practice. The main focus here is on the individual; it is directed toward *one particular person*, seeking to perceive the specific contextual interactions, to place them in context, to differentiate and to integrate them into the treatment.

It is this understanding, within the osteopathic approach focusing on the promotion of health,[1] that forms the basis of the specific osteopathic clinical reasoning. Osteopathic treatment is based on understanding the way that various factors interact in a particular individual: (1) adaptive biomechanical and postural factors; (2) neurological control processes;

(3) respiratory and circulatory dynamics; (4) metabolic, energetic, and endocrine processes; and (5) biopsychosocial influences. Each of these five models is in turn based on the principles of anatomy, physiology, biochemistry, and psychology. Applying the models helps us arrive at a diagnostic and treatment approach and put it into practice.

When we examine the patient, we take these models into account. The clinical history is also essential, for osteopathy as elsewhere. It will include biomedical and biographical information (see e.g. History-taking, Volume 2, section 5.2.1), and should both focus on the problem and be solution-oriented.

We should not force world-views or inappropriate concepts on the patient. We should also avoid discussion or judgment or hasty interpretations, asking leading questions, giving instruction from on high, and either over- or underestimating the patient's resources. The following are, however, helpful:

- Listening empathetically, appreciatively, actively, and openly.
- Asking questions in a structured way.
- Framing our questions in a sympathetic way that will clarify and stimulate, and incorporate feedback.
- Repeating important statements and enquiring further.
- Taking account of the whole, without getting lost in the detail.
- Being aware of psychological projection.

Good history-taking provides:

- Clearly formulated treatment goals.
- Some chronological understanding of the associated conditions in the origin of the complaint.
- Biographical influences.
- Information on the resources available to the patient.
- Differential diagnosis and contraindications.
- The initial outline of a possible treatment plan.

It is important, even at this stage, to do everything we can to establish a high degree of patient compliance. Throughout the treatment session, we should pay attention to the patient's expression (gestures, facial expression, behavior, manner, etc.), whether or not the meaning or connection is evident.

The course of osteopathic treatment includes both the control processes that are centrally governed and peripheral interactions. It will be oriented along the lines of the fundamental principles and the five osteopathic models mentioned above. It will also involve exercise therapy and consideration of the patient's other life factors, habits, and environment. Psychoeducation can be used to improve compliance by helping the patient better understand the significance of lifestyle changes.

The osteopathic examination will determine the region to be treated (head, thoracic cage, vertebral column, pelvis, and/or limbs) and the possible order in which the steps in treatment should be taken.

The osteopathic diagnosis and treatment interact, involving qualitative subjective avenues of approach, for instance coherence, instability, and sensitivity,[5] together with objective findings. In all this, intuition is an important factor and develops over the course of the learning[6,9] that takes place during clinical experience.

The primary aim of treatment approaches in osteopathy is to improve the body's self-regulation, as a result of which the symptoms also improve. The algorithm that drives osteopathy is therefore geared to findings rather than symptoms. Nevertheless, this is not a matter of either/or, but of both/and. Consequently a treatment approach geared to findings and directed to the body as a whole can be combined with local treatment of regions displaying symptoms. This is just as true of functions of the jaw and mouth or orofacial structures as it is of other organs of the head discussed in this book.

The present book will therefore present the functional and structural interrelationships that are important for understanding and diagnosis, and will draw on them when dealing with treatment.

It presents theoretical patterns of dysfunction, diagnostic algorithms, local manual approaches for the tissues, bones, muscles, fasciae, blood vessels, nerves, etc. involved, as well as suggestions for therapeutic exercises and other helpful advice on treatment. The influence of supra-regional factors must not be forgotten; these are typically integrated into all osteopathic treatment, although this can only be hinted at in any written description.

A general procedure for carrying out the techniques described in this book is presented below.

1.1 General procedure

1.1.1 Balancing the autonomic nervous system

Balancing the autonomic nervous system reduces multiple activity, the adaptations arising from everyday demands, and the effects of sympathetic nervous stimulation. It supports the process of transition to a better balanced fundamental state. The reciprocal tensions in the body and aspects of body, mind, and soul interact with each other in a more coherent way. This then eases the way toward healing and the transformation of dysfunctional patterns.

Patient responsiveness to therapeutic impulses seems to be enhanced after balancing of the autonomic system; negative results are minimized and it becomes easier to sense when a particular treatment has reached its conclusion. In this state it also seems to be easier for the patient to perceive bodily sensations, emotions, and thought patterns.

A number of approaches can be used here, such as osteopathic heart-focused palpation, the neutral state, osteopathic "felt sense," or the butterfly hug.[10]

Osteopathic heart-focused palpation

1. Synchronizing perception Begin by helping patients to sense their own health, without making any judgment: physical (tensions, proprioceptive and interoceptive bodily sensations); vitality and energy level; and level of (autonomic) stimulation, emotions, and cognitive perceptions.
2. Palpation of the heart field Follow the dynamics of the heart field until equilibrium is reached.
3. Harmonization heart—abdomen—head Practitioner: place one hand about half an inch (1.5 cm) below the umbilicus and the other in the region of the heart, centrally on the sternum. Now ask the patient to imagine directing vitality upward from the lower abdomen to the heart region while breathing in, and directing love and empathy from the heart region to the lower abdomen while breathing out. Repeat for at least three breaths. Then follow the same essential procedure, but this time with one hand on the head region.
4. Heart palpation by the practitioner With one hand posterior and the other anterior, touch the heart region directly on the body and synchronize with the different qualities of the tissue. Rest your focus on the very innermost of the innermost in the heart (the eye of the whirlwind), locally on the heart, regionally on the environment of the heart, globally on the body as a whole, on the field around the body, to the horizon, expanding into the great yonder and beyond the horizon.
5. Heart palpation involving the patient During the heart palpation, ask the patient to direct their awareness to the heart region in the center of the chest. This will involve, for example, sensing the heart beating, or sensing the changes in sensation of the body as they direct their awareness to the heart and as you palpate the heart. Ask the patient to close their eyes, and to look with their closed eyes in the direction of their heart. The patient gives "permission" to the heart space to expand in all directions.
6. The end point is reached when the expansion and dynamics of the heart field and tissue tensions in the heart region enter a dynamic stillness, when a balance of tension is

established, locally, regionally, and globally, and when any emotional processes that may have arisen in the patient have arrived at a state of balance. The patient can then slowly, consciously, open their eyes. Meanwhile, maintain contact with the heart space.

7. Vertical balancing Finally the patient imagines inhaling from the crown of the head, breathing throughout the entire body, into the pelvis, and exhaling through the soles of the feet. Then the patient should inhale through the soles of the feet and pelvic region, and exhale through the crown of the head. Repeat for three cycles.

Osteopathic "felt sense"

By means of palpation, the osteopath identifies the regions with the greatest rhythmic flow, vitality, and sense of well-being. Let the patient's sense of how they feel confirm these. Accompany indirectly all the tissue, and fluid, and energy qualities. At the same time, the patient should focus concentration on interoceptive experiences relating to the regions palpated, together with visual, auditory, kinesthetic, olfactory, and taste sensations. The osteopath should observe whether these sensations enhance the patient's sense of well-being and reorganization of the patient's inner experience.

The butterfly hug

The patient places each hand on the opposite shoulder and taps each shoulder alternately with the hand that rests there. Repeat 20 times.

1.1.2 Intention

Clear intention focuses attention on the maneuver to be carried out and activates the energy needed to perform it.

1.1.3 Focus

Good focus demands sound anatomical knowledge of the structures to be examined and how they relate to each other. Without this, it becomes impossible to carry out the differentiated palpation that osteopathy involves: it requires the practitioner properly to locate the right level and identify the network of connections, and to recognize the qualities present, so that these can enter into palpatory focus. Try to create a detailed perception of the tissues you are to examine, recognizing their qualities and characteristics, and to harmonize that mental picture as accurately as possible with the living tissue.

1.1.4 Resonance

Resonance arises when the other factors are in place and the practitioner has attuned to the dynamics and qualities of the complex of interrelationships, in harmony and perceiving the necessary differentiation.[10]

When palpating, you need to distinguish which tissue you are in contact with. This involves either a conscious decision to contact those tissue levels, or allowing yourself to be led to the level where the dysfunction is located.

The following can help to achieve successful resonance:

- Letting the tissue come to you.
- Palpating the levels.
- Becoming one with the tissue that needs to be treated.
- Using compression, as with a tai-chi ball or when gently pressing a mango.
- Through perception and intensifying perception; a tissue dance.

Certain skills are essential here: empathy, active listening, and tuning in to the tissue. Adapt the force exerted by your hands to match the micromotions, tensions, elasticities, and vibrations of the complex of connections: bones, fasciae/membranes, fluids (viscera: cerebrospinal, etc.), and the electrodynamic field. A dialog is taking place, but it happens less through your hands and more through your entire body, as it imitates the micromotions and other phenomena that can be palpated. Your entire body—not just your hands—opens up to the dynamics you are palpating, enters into resonance with them, and copies them. Let your body dance with the dynamics of the connections you palpate, as you might dance in contact improvisation. Your clarity of perception is greatly enhanced; the complex of connections is clearer and resonance increases.

1.1.5 Induction of the point of balanced membranous tension, fluid tension, or dynamic balanced tension

The *PBMT* (point of balanced membranous tension) is the position in which the tension in the dural membrane and between the structures involved is in its optimum state of even distribution. The following techniques can be used to help achieve PBMT:

- Exaggeration technique.
- Direct technique.
- Opposite physiological motion.
- Disengagement of joint surfaces.
- Molding.

Where the restrictions are within the physiological range of motion, you should let yourself be led to the PBMT; when dealing with restrictions beyond the physiological, you should lead the structures concerned to the PBMT.

With increasing experience, practitioners usually find that less and less force is needed to induce the correction that is right for that patient's body. This is in accordance with Sutherland's method of procedure in his latter years of teaching. Sutherland placed special importance on the idea that it is not so much the direction by the therapist as the fluid fluctuations of the primary respiratory mechanism (PRM) that lead the structures to the PBMT. The practitioners' role is rather to allow themselves to be led by the fluctuations to the point of balanced tension (PBT).

We do not have to find the point of balance in the reciprocal tension membranes because the cerebrospinal fluid tide will do it for us. We merely initiate the movement and follow it as the fulcrum shifts. These membranes maintain a constant reciprocal tension for whatever pattern exists in the osseous elements of the cranial mechanism. If permitted by the proper manual application in the technic approach the tide will carry the mechanism to the balance point in that particular pattern. When the balance point is reached the cerebrospinal fluid has found its proper fulcrum and it is at this time that the correction takes place.[13:176]

Once the point of membranous balance has been achieved, the practitioner's task is to maintain the balance until a correction of the abnormal tension in the dural membrane has occurred and the tidal motion of the cerebrospinal fluid (CSF) has brought about a correction in the affected structures. This involves holding them in PBMT with the gentlest possible touch until the motion of the structures has ceased.[13:73]

At first, when the PBMT is established, your palpating hands usually sense a kind of growing unrest in the fluids. This comes to a point of rest as a *point of balanced fluid tension* (PBFT) is established. This is the moment when the correction occurs. The practitioner senses a softening of hardened structures and resolution of tissue resistance. There is a change in the fluctuations of the CSF, and a kind of new balance can be sensed in the tissue.

Finally, a slight increase in the patterns of rhythmic activity re-emerges. You can sense that the rhythmic activity patterns have become more symmetrical, freer, easier, and stronger, and that their amplitude has increased.

Sometimes, during the final stage of the correction, you may sense the fluctuations spontaneously coming to rest, rather as they do with a CV-4 technique, and other, slower rhythms may become evident.

Another, alternative approach might be to use *dynamic balanced tension* (DBT). To carry out DBT, you work during the inhalation phase of the inherent rhythm to gently reinforce any dysfunctional or asymmetrical, aberrant motions or tensions that may be present without altering the speed of these motions. During the exhalation phase, you passively follow the tissue tensions.

This process is repeated until, at the end of an inhalation phase, a clearly palpable disengagement occurs that is spontaneous and *not* induced by the practitioner. This disengagement is more marked than that which occurs at the end of each inhalation phase. It is usually accompanied by automatic shifting.

Forces not induced by the practitioner begin to take effect. During the following exhalation phase, these forces lead the affected tissue out of the dysfunction. What takes place, we might say, is a self-correction.

1.1.6 Fluid impulse

In addition, you can deliver a fluid impulse, as near as possible from a position diametrically opposite the structure to be treated. If you do not have a finger free to deliver it, you can deliver the fluid impulse using another part of your body or with the palm of one of your hands. Alternatively, the patient can be asked to assist the treatment by dorsally flexing the feet or by pulmonary breathing.

1.1.7 Further treatment modalities

According to the particular case, you might also choose to use a low thrust or recoil or other technique.

- To perform a *low thrust*, apply gentle pressure in the direction of the motion restriction in sutures, bones, muscles, fasciae, and other soft tissues. If you find motion restrictions in different directions, you can also deliver several low thrusts quickly one after another.
- To perform a *recoil*, bring the tissue into an initial state of tension during pulmonary inhalation. Then, as the patient breathes out again, you increase this. At the beginning of the next in-breath, you suddenly release the tension or pressure. The sudden change in pressure loosens old motion-related tensions, which goes on to make them accessible to further treatment.

> **FURTHER INFORMATION** An essential point to bear in mind is that osteopathic intervention should embrace both structural and functional, direct and indirect, general and specific, and maximal and minimal approaches. These do not contradict one another; rather, they represent the full spectrum of osteopathic thinking and practice. Osteopaths need to have every variation between these extremes at their command, like a virtuoso who knows every note of the piano. These approaches are often applied in combination. One aspect or another might predominate from one practitioner to another, from one patient to another, and indeed from one moment to another of the treatment, and considerations such as the state of the tissue. This means that there will to some extent be considerable differences in the way the techniques described are performed in practice. The reason for this is surely that the manner of performing a technique emerges from a direct dialog with the tissue, the forces at work, and the body as a whole. It is the tissue that tells us what it needs and what we should do. Establishing a point of balance, for example, may call for various techniques or combinations of techniques (see above).

There is often a tendency to adopt received procedures unquestioned—for example, using direct techniques when treating children. This is seldom based on proven research, but rather on values arising from the experience of individual osteopaths. They should therefore find their way into day-to-day practice as exactly what they are—the fruit of experience rather than fixed rules. For example, there are osteopaths who exert much more force on the cranium than is usually said to be appropriate. Some work almost exclusively with indirect techniques, even with small children. So, allow yourself to gather your own experience, do this in humility and empathy, respecting the uniqueness of the body and its tissues, but do not allow yourself to be limited by dogma. Test various models of working, and let your palpatory experience guide you.

The specific reaction of a tissue to traumatic force also provides indications as to the kind of therapeutic touch required.

Every technique will also vary according to its dynamic synchronization with inherent rhythms, whether it is partly or fully synchronized, or which other qualities and parameters you are observing. You should avoid dogmatically following unproven concepts such as the classification of frequencies with regard to rhythmic phenomena, or sphenobasilar synchondrosis (SBS) lesions; the risk is that you distance yourself from immediate experience.[11,12]

FURTHER INFORMATION There is an interesting example that illustrates this. A pilot study was carried out, which involved palpating tensions. Unexperienced lay participants achieved the best results and experienced osteopaths performed least well.[2]

All the techniques in this book can be carried out in dynamic synchronicity with micromotions and/or inherent rhythms (during the inhalation phase of the inherent rhythm or only during the exhalation phase) or independently of this. They can also be performed as direct or indirect techniques or a combination of both, or as structural or functional approaches, and in many other contexts.

The execution of techniques to treat dysfunctions may also differ significantly according to whether you are encountering motion barriers in your therapy, or are entirely allowing the activity of inherent homeodynamic forces, such as the "breath of life," to guide the therapy. Every structure can be treated without addressing a motion barrier. In these cases, the practitioner's attention is especially directed toward the naturally occurring disengagement during each inhalation phase. You can encourage the disengagement between the structures involved either by supporting it physically to a greater or lesser degree, or by an empathetic, mental granting of space, or by a pure focusing of attention on this process.

The retraction and "drawing closer" in the tissue can likewise be encouraged by providing physical support to whatever degree is necessary, or empathetic mental encounter with the forces at work in drawing closer, or pure focus of attention on the process occurring.

Another possibility for therapy is that, during a particular phase—usually the inhalation phase—you additionally support the expression of the forces involved in the dysfunction. These forces are usually expressed as chaotic or aberrant motions and tensions. In this case, you passively follow the exhalation phase. This unwinding and release of bound, fixed energy patterns can occur together with an integration and creation of a new order in the body.

The way in which a technique is performed is also influenced by the state of energy or of autonomic nervous excitation, emotional state, cognitive and belief patterns (e.g., regarding the concept of somatic dysfunction[8]), and other biographical matters that influence the person giving treatment; also, by both the practitioner's and the patient's consciousness of their own physical, mental, and spiritual experience.[3,4,6,7,9] Their perception of the forces and worlds at work within them, and of the dynamic interrelationship between inner and outer worlds, also plays a significant role.[4,5] With appropriate training we can achieve a greater awareness of these processes and interactions. This also enhances the capacity of the inner observer, the empathetic interaction with the patient, and self-reflective thought and action during the treatment. And practice can train us to develop a state of relaxed, non-invasive attention and empathy during palpation.

1.1.8 Further hints for performing the techniques

1. The dysfunctions of all the bones are named for the direction of greater mobility—the "direction of ease." For example, when there is motion restriction of the temporal bone in

internal rotation and greater ease of motion in external rotation, this is called an external rotation dysfunction.

2. "Inhalation phase" and "exhalation phase" are terms relating to the phases of inherent rhythms. (In the literature the alternative terms "inspiration phase" and "expiration phase" are also sometimes used.) The meaning is usually made clear in the text by adding "inherent rhythm," or "PRM (primary respiratory movement)." "Breathing in" or "inhalation" and "breathing out" or "exhalation" refer to pulmonary respiration; in most cases the fact that pulmonary respiration is meant is specifically added to make this clear.
3. The patient is assumed to be supine unless otherwise stated. However, most techniques can also be carried out with the patient in a different position.
4. Whenever possible, the practitioner's elbows should rest on the treatment table. This provides a fixed point. Both feet should rest on the floor so that, together with the sit (sitting) bones on the practitioner's stool, they create a fulcrum. Practitioners should sit upright, in no way supporting themselves on the patient—physically or psychologically. If it is necessary to stand to carry out the treatment the practitioner can also lean against the table as a support.
5. Whenever bilateral hand contact needs to be made, you should create a link by means of a fulcrum if at all possible (usually by placing the thumbs of your two hands in contact with each other).
6. Robert Fulford has pointed out in recent years that it can be important for treatment for the practitioner to touch the left side of the patient with the right hand and the right side of the patient with the left hand. This aspect of energy polarity has not been taken into account in the description of the techniques, but this might be done if required by having the practitioner stand and take up hand contact facing the patient.
7. Where the motion of the cranial bones is described on the basis of sutural, dural, muscular (and fluid) structures, this book uses the term "biomechanical" palpation. The term "developmental dynamic" is used to denote palpation where the motion of the cranial bones is described on the basis of embryological development. The description of the motion impulses is of course only roughly approximate to the reality. The above-mentioned explanation, too, is purely hypothetical. Most important for the practitioner's approach is to stand aside from theory and trust the experience of the palpation in as unprejudiced a way as possible.

FURTHER INFORMATION The term "motion," used here and in the text that follows to refer to the phenomena that are palpated, does not entirely cover what is meant. This "motion" can better be thought of as tension phenomena in the tissue.

1.1.9 Additional information

1. The palpation can be performed passively or actively as a test of mobility. These can be carried out in synchrony with inherent rhythms or independently of them. In active testing too, doing so makes it possible to avoid confronting motion barriers. Another possibility—when necessary—is to use motion barriers to help you put together your picture of additional information and resonance.
2. The bones of the viscerocranium, unlike those of the neurocranium, are not attached to each other by means of the dural membranes. This means that a PBMT cannot really be established there as it can for the neurocranium. Despite this, Sutherland does also

mention the PBT as a form of treatment for the bones of the viscerocranium. The explanation for this lies partly in Sutherland's own palpation experience and partly in the way the sutures themselves are constructed, with fibrous structures within the intrasutural joint. According to K. E. Graham D.O., "point of balanced fascial tension" would be a more comprehensive term, as every structure in the body is surrounded by fascia. Intraosseous dysfunctions are also treated according to the PBT concept. It is possible to induce a PBMT because the bone lies in a periosteal membrane, as well as a PBFT, because the bone itself consists of around 70% fluid, or a point of balanced electrodynamic tension (PBET).

3. The indications mentioned in this book should not be seen in categorical terms, as a different manner of establishing the findings has prime place in osteopathy. The guiding criteria are less based on the patient's symptoms; instead osteopathy looks to the findings from palpation and the interactions.
4. All the techniques presented in this textbook can—indeed should—be adapted in the process of dialog with the tissue.

1.2 References

1 Flatscher, M. and Liem, T. (2011) 'What is health? What is disease? Thoughts on a complex issue.' *J. Am. Osteopath. Assoc. 21*, 4, 27–30.

2 Hager, C. (2017) *Der Zusammenhang von osteopathischer Erfahrung und Spannungspalpation – eine experimentelle Pilotstudie*. OSD.

3 Liem, T. (2011) 'Osteopathy and (hatha) yoga.' *J. Bodyw. Mov. Ther. 15*, 1, 92–102.

4 Liem, T. (2011) 'Palpation des kraniosakralen Rhythmus.' *Osteopath. Med. 12*, 4, 12–17.

5 Liem, T. (2011) 'Wechselseitige Beziehungsdynamiken und subjektive Ansätze in der Osteopathie.' *Osteopath. Med. 12*, 2, 4–7.

6 Liem, T. (2014) 'Pitfalls and challenges involved in the process of perception and interpretation of palpatory findings.' *Int. J. Osteopath. Med. 17*, 4, 243–249.

7 Liem, T. (2014) 'Prozess der Wahrnehmung und Interpretation von Palpationsbefunden.' *Osteopath. Med. 15*, 4, 4–8.

8 Liem, T. (2016) 'Still's osteopathic lesion theory and evidence-based models supporting the emerged concept of somatic dysfunction.' *J. Am. Osteopath. Assoc. 116*, 10, 654–656.

9 Liem, T. (2017) 'Intuitive judgement in the context of osteopathic clinical reasoning.' *J. Am. Osteopath. Assoc. 117*, 586–594.

10 Liem, T. (2018) *Kraniosakrale Osteopathie. Ein praktisches Lehrbuch*, 7th Ed. Stuttgart: Thieme.

11 Liem, T. and Moser, M. (2016) 'Biologische Rhythmen und ihre Bedeutung für die Osteopathie.' *Osteopath. Med. 17*, 1, 22–26.

12 Liem, T., Hilbrecht, H. and Schmidt, T. (2012) 'Osteopathie und Wissenschaft.' *Osteopath. Med. 13*, 1, 4–10.

13 Magoun, H. I. (1951) *Osteopathy in the Cranial Field*. Kirksville, MO: Journal Printing Company.

2.1 Anatomy of the temporomandibular joint 12
2.1.1 Head of the mandible 13
2.1.2 Mandibular fossa and articular tubercle 14
2.1.3 The bone architecture of the masticatory system 15
2.1.4 The articular disk 16
2.1.5 The articular capsule 17
2.1.6 Ligaments 18
2.1.7 Muscles 21
2.1.8 Fasciae 26
2.1.9 Innervation of the temporomandibular joint 27
2.1.10 Mechanoreceptors 28
2.1.11 Blood and lymphatic vessels 28
2.1.12 Connections with other structures 29

2.2 Biomechanics of the mandible 30
2.2.1 Biomechanical demands on the temporomandibular joint 31
2.2.2 Opening and closing of the mouth 31
2.2.3 Protrusion and retrusion 34
2.2.4 Laterotrusion 35
2.2.5 Control of the act of chewing 36

2.3 The mandible as metamorphic reflection of the lower limb 37

2.4 Phylogenetic and ontogenetic influences on the development of the jaw 37
2.4.1 Phylogenesis 37
2.4.2 Embryology of the mandible and temporomandibular joint 37
2.4.3 Postnatal development of the cranium 41
2.4.4 The capsule, disk, and muscle complex 41
2.4.5 The influence of mandibular growth on disturbances of the TMJ, facial growth, and craniocervical balance 42

2.5 Craniomandibular dysfunction 42
2.5.1 Epidemiology 42
2.5.2 Comorbidities and relation to other systems of the body 43
2.5.3 Clinical features 43
2.5.4 The temporomandibular joint and body posture 45
2.5.5 Postural signs of craniomandibular dysfunction 55
2.5.6 Dynamic signs of craniomandibular dysfunction 58

2.6 Location, causes, and treatment of craniomandibular dysfunctions 63
2.6.1 Osseous, disk-related, and dental occlusion-related factors 66
2.6.2 Muscular dysfunctions 82
2.6.3 Dysfunction of the ligaments 89
2.6.4 Fascial dysfunctions 90
2.6.5 Dural dysfunctions 91
2.6.6 Disturbances of the nerves, sensitization mechanisms, and disturbances of pain processing 91
2.6.7 Central nervous system 94
2.6.8 Neurotransmitters/neuropeptides 95
2.6.9 Vascular disturbances 95
2.6.10 Disturbances of the salivary glands 96
2.6.11 Disturbances of the endocrine glands and immune system 96
2.6.12 Orofacial dyskinesias 97
2.6.13 Psyche; stress; sleep disturbances 97
2.6.14 Genetics 98

2.7 Diagnosis of craniomandibular dysfunction 98
2.7.1 The patient history 99
2.7.2 Inspection 101
2.7.3 Palpation 110

2.8 Treatment of craniomandibular dysfunctions 134
2.8.1 Treatment of the masticatory muscles 136
2.8.2 Treatment of the condyles 146
2.8.3 Intraosseous treatment 155
2.8.4 Treatment of the capsule and the ligaments of the lower jaw 156
2.8.5 Treating the arteries, veins, and nerves 158

2.9 Self-help techniques, exercise programs for CMD and other disturbances 161
2.9.1 Stretching and relaxation 162
2.9.2 Coordination exercises 164
2.9.3 Strengthening exercises 165
2.9.4 Chewing exercises 166

2.10 Treatment approaches for specific disturbances of the temporomandibular joint 167
2.10.1 Disturbances resulting from traumatic injury 167
2.10.2 Osteoarthritis and degenerative processes 167
2.10.3 Resistant occlusal stress 168
2.10.4 Types of transverse deviation: crossbite; scissorbite (non-occlusion) 168
2.10.5 Dysgnathias characterized by mandibular protrusion 169
2.10.6 Retrusive occlusion 169
2.10.7 Open bite 169
2.10.8 Extreme deep bite 170
2.10.9 Dry lips 170
2.10.10 Rhagades at corner of mouth 170
2.10.11 Bruxism 170
2.10.12 Treatment of children 173
2.10.13 Interdisciplinary cooperation in the production of occlusal splints and splint correction 174
2.10.14 Occlusal splints 175

2.11 References 178

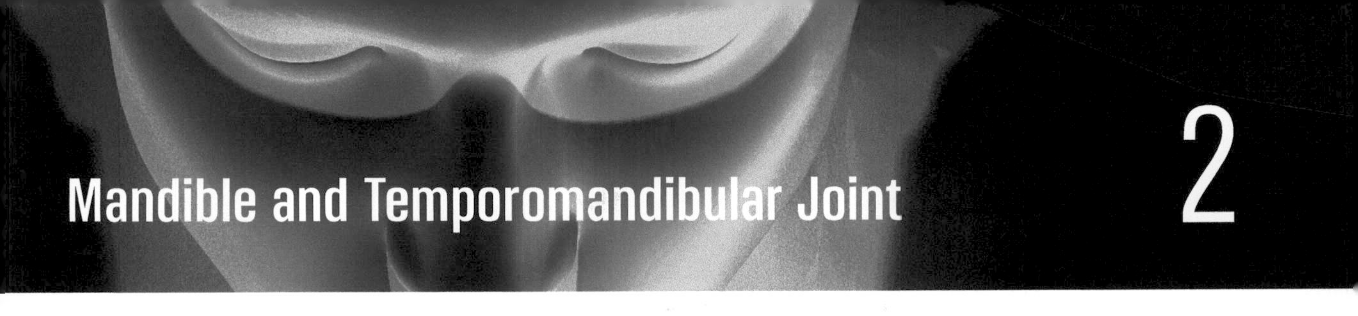

2 Mandible and Temporomandibular Joint

The temporomandibular joint (TMJ) is a component of the functions of the mouth; in view of this role it can only be understood in this context. Seen in primordial terms, the mouth is the place of life and the experiences that characterize it.[445] Extant from 541 million to 252 million years ago were a now extinct class of fish-like vertebrates, Placodermata. There is a direct line of development from the evolution of these creatures to animals with four limbs, and they were the first to develop a bony jaw. The head and trunk were also armored with bony plates.[275] At the time of the placoderms, the jaw was already significant for procreation, the ingestion of food, and communication. Today it is still associated with these functions.

Dysfunctions of the jaw can usually only be understood and treated by considering the way in which the act of living is expressed in the particular individual. This means that therapy emerges from an understanding of that person's development, habits, and everyday practice and experience of life, as well as their attitude to life. These aspects interact closely with the various functions taking place within them, so including, for example, their respiratory, locomotor, postural, and support systems, their gastrointestinal tract, circulatory, and hormone systems, the sensory nervous system, and psycho-mental and psychosomatic interrelationships.[445]

Dysfunctions of the temporomandibular (jaw) joint often have a long pathogenetic history; sometimes this may stretch back to the embryological stage or through to the time of birth (intrauterine displacement of position or spatial restriction).[445]

The TMJ, viewed as part of the body as a whole, has been a subject of attention from the beginning of osteopathy. To mention just a few examples, Still[429] and Sutherland[432] both mention techniques for the treatment of temporomandibular joint dysfunctions, while Magoun[284] and Fryette[140] describe possible causes and diagnostic and therapeutic methods for problems of the temporomandibular joint. In osteopathy—in contrast to the accepted treatments of traditional medicine—considerable importance is also assigned to the temporal bones in the development of temporomandibular dysfunctions.[101,284] Osteopaths Smith, Hruby, and Blood[41,182,418] all speak of a close association between dysfunctions of the temporomandibular joint and multiple disturbances affecting the whole body. A study by Vathrakokoilis et al.[450] provides an example; looking at osteopathic treatment of patients with chronic craniomandibular dysfunction (CMD), they found that there was an improvement in issues of pain and clicking of the jaw, general function of the jaw, and amplitude of mouth opening.

The estimated need of treatment for disturbances of the TMJ was found to have increased from 5% in 1983 to 8% in 2003.[224] One in six adults visiting a general dentist had experienced orofacial pain during the past year, the most prevalent types of pain being musculoligamentous and alveolar.[181] Clinical signs of temporomandibular joint disturbances were found in one in six children and adolescents.[90] Over 23% of children of preschool age were found to experience pain on chewing and to have joint sounds.[190]

2.1 Anatomy of the temporomandibular joint

The TMJ (Figure 2.1) plays a direct or indirect role in a number of functions, including chewing, swallowing and sucking, articulation of sounds, breathing, and facial expression. The joint is composed of the head of the mandible, which is cylindrical

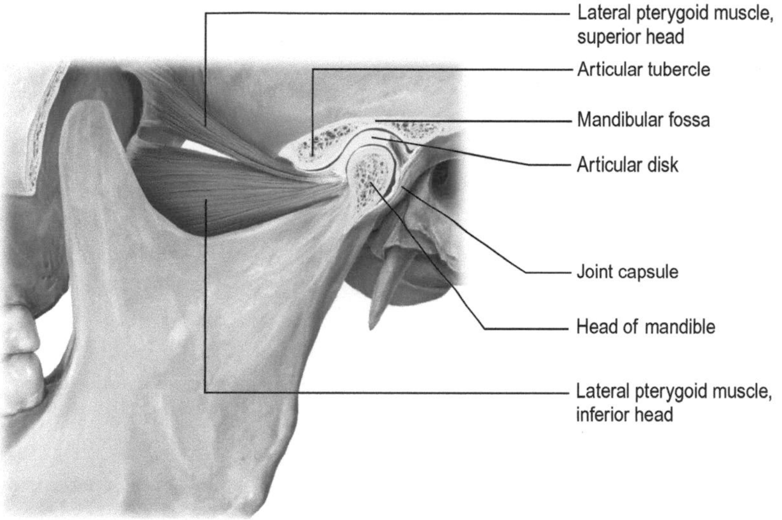

Figure 2.1
Temporomandibular joint. (Schünke, M., Schulte, E., Schumacher, U. (2015) *Prometheus LernAtlas der Anatomie. Kopf, Hals und Neuroanatomie.* Illustrations by M. Voll and K. Wesker, 4th ed. Stuttgart: Thieme)

in shape, and the mandibular fossa and articular tubercle of the temporal bone. Between these lies the articular disk, which divides the joint into an upper and a lower compartment, the meniscotemporal and meniscocondylar joint spaces.[265]

2.1.1 Head of the mandible

- The head of the mandible forms the cranial end of the condylar process (of the ramus of the mandible) (Figure 2.2). Its surface is convex, being cylindrical or ellipsoid in shape.[251:215] It protrudes medially. The cartilaginous layer is highly vascularized in newborns, a feature that decreases with age. There is a reduction in thickness of the cartilage at the articular head during the life of the individual.
- The anterior portion of the mandibular head is oriented anteriorly and superiorly. It is covered with fibrocartilage, and it articulates with the articular tubercle of the temporal bone. Between the two lies a disk.
- The transverse axis of the mandibular head runs from anterolateral to posteromedial, and obliquely downward. The extended axes normally intersect at the anterior border of the foramen magnum.[35:525]

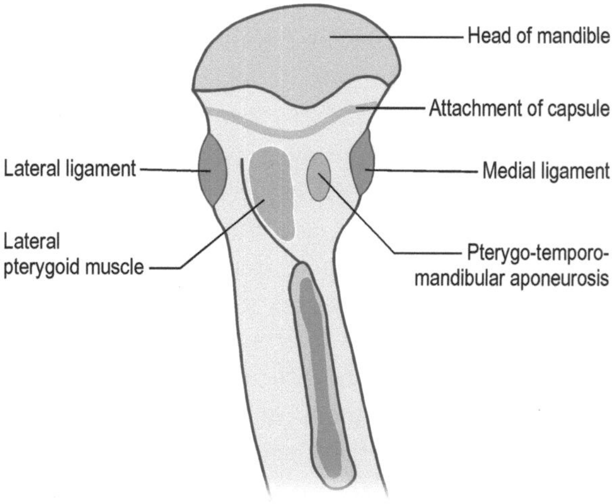

Figure 2.2
Right condylar process (anterior view)

- In its frontal and sagittal aspects the head of the mandible is convex. The two mandibular heads are seldom symmetrical. They are flat at birth, and only become hemispherical when the child begins to chew and the deciduous molars appear. The head of the mandible attains its final cylindrical form when the permanent dentition is complete.[390:368]

- The anterior surface of the mandibular head is the main articular surface. It is covered with fibrocartilage.
- The posterior, smooth portion of the mandibular head is oriented posterosuperiorly. Although it is enclosed in the articular capsule, it does not act as part of the joint. It is covered in taut connective tissue.
- The attachment of the articular capsule runs around the condylar process.
- Below the head, the bone is narrower and forms the neck of the mandible.
- Immediately below the head of the mandible, on the anterior surface of the condyle, is a small depression, the fovea, for the insertion of the lateral pterygoid muscle.

2.1.2 Mandibular fossa and articular tubercle

- The mandibular fossa (Figure 2.3) is situated on the inferior surface of the squamous part of the temporal bone. It is two to three times the size of the articular surface of the head of the mandible.
- Only the anterior portion of the mandibular fossa, belonging to the squamous part, forms part of the joint. The fossa runs from the articular tubercle dorsally to the petrosquamous fissure, and measures about 19 mm in the anteroposterior direction by about 25 mm wide. The posterior portion does not form part of the joint. It belongs to the tympanic part, and lies outside the articular capsule. It is covered in taut connective tissue. The chorda tympani emerges at the petrotympanic fissure.[35:526]
- The axis of the mandibular fossa, like that of the mandibular head, runs posteromedially. In its frontal and sagittal aspects the fossa is concave.
- Anteriorly the fossa gives way to the saddle-shaped articular tubercle, which has a slanting articular surface, oriented posteriorly and inferiorly.
- The anterior part of the fossa and the tubercle are covered in fibrocartilage. The fibers are mainly collagenous and run both obliquely and parallel, from the petrotympanic fissure and the superior anterior portion of the posterior zygomatic (postglenoid) tubercle to the articular tubercle. The intermediate zone is capable of proliferation and so of initiating repair processes throughout life.
- In sagittal section the fossa and the tubercle describe an S-shaped course (Figure 2.4).

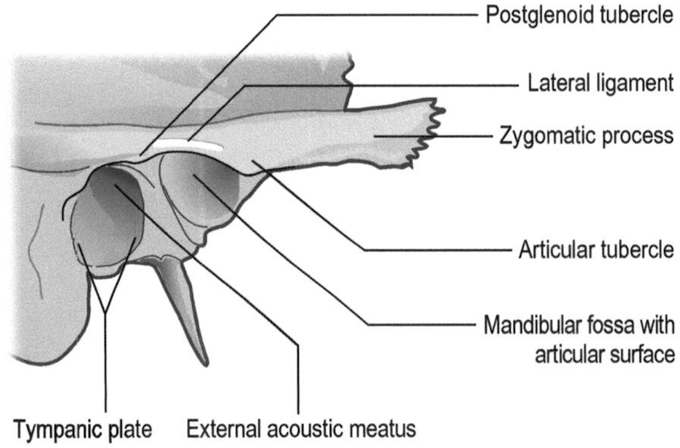

Figure 2.3
Mandibular fossa and articular tubercle of the temporal bone

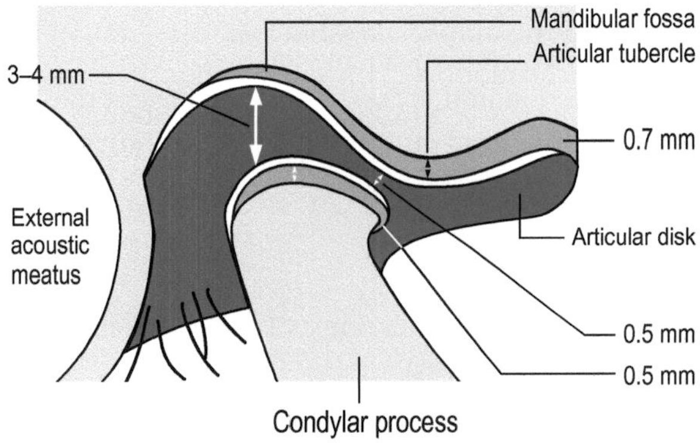

Figure 2.4
Temporomandibular joint, sagittal section

2.1.3 The bone architecture of the masticatory system

The structure of the cranium makes it highly resistant to the effects of force. A number of factors contribute to this resistance: the elasticity of the bone, the buttressed structure, the tensile restraint of the dural system, the absorption of vibration by the paranasal sinuses, and the way in which the viscerocranium articulates with the skull.[18,177,405]

The enormous forces generated by the muscles during mastication affect the middle and anterior cranial fossae in particular. The masticatory muscles exert a downward tension on the middle cranial fossa, while the pressure generated by chewing is transmitted upward by buttresses of the maxilla and mandible.

Maxilla In the case of the maxilla, the supportive elements are the buttress of the canine, the zygomaticomaxillary buttress, and the less robust pterygomaxillary buttress. The buttress of the canine transmits the forces from the alveoli of the canine teeth around the piriform aperture to the frontal process of the maxilla and medial orbital margin. The zygomaticomaxillary buttress distributes the forces from the alveoli of the molars to the zygomatic bone. From there, they are transmitted to the frontal bone via the frontal processes of the zygomatic bones, then onward to the inferior temporal line and forward to the lateral superior roof of the orbit. A second route leads from the zygomatic bone to the zygomatic arch and onward as far as the articular tubercle. The pterygomaxillary buttress, which is less robust, transmits the pressure from the rear molars to the middle of the cranial base.

Mandible In the mandible, the forces are transmitted to the basal arch, which comprises the base of the mandible, the central part of the ramus, and the condylar process. The bone fibers in the condylar process run in an oblique vertical direction from posterior cranial to anterior caudal. In addition to the basal arch, the mandible includes the apophysis for the insertion of the temporalis muscle, the masticatory muscle extending from the coronoid process to the body of the mandible, and the angular apophysis, on the angle of the jaw.

Temporal bone The course of the fibers in the temporal region of the joint is complex. In the horizontal plane the fibers are oriented along the course of the zygomatic arch. They divide at the roots of the zygomatic processes of the temporal bone. Transverse fibers continue into the infratemporal crest of the greater wings of the sphenoid, and combine with the pterygosphenoidal-frontal buttress. Other, longitudinally oriented fibers continue into the squamous part of the temporal bone. In the frontal plane, the fibers run vertically and link the laminae of the temporal bone.

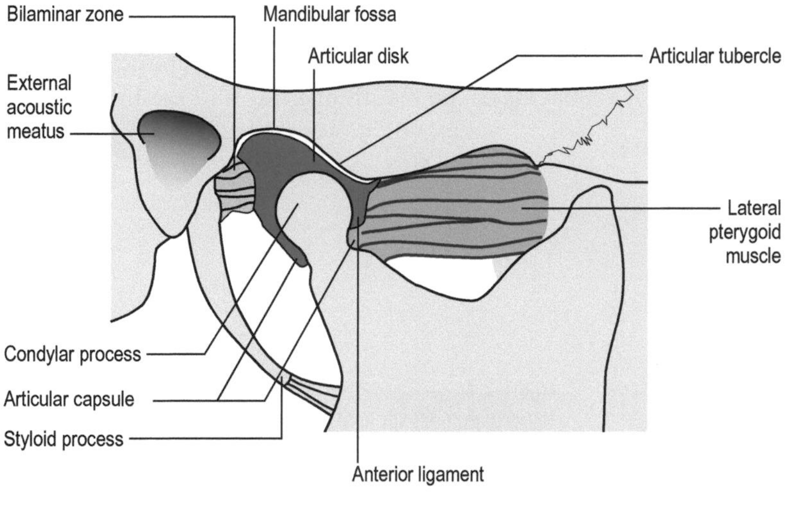

Figure 2.5
Lateral view of the right temporomandibular joint

2.1.4 The articular disk

The articular disk (Figures 2.4, 2.5) divides the TMJ into an upper and a lower compartment and forms the effective joint socket. The disk is biconcave and made of fibrocartilage. There are individual variations in shape, since the disk adapts to the adjacent components of the joint.[73,176,207,292] The central portion is shallow (1–2 mm). At birth, however, it is of even thickness throughout.[66,251:126,307,431] There are no pain receptors. The disk is more resistant than the cartilage in other joints; it consists of fibrous cartilage (collagen types I and II).

The disk consists of anterior, central (intermediate), and posterior parts or bands. The posterior part splits into two layers to create the bilaminar zone; however, there are differences in the structure of the bands. The peripheral parts are firmer than the central parts of the disk:[243]

- Ventral: taut connective tissue and cartilage.
- Middle: taut connective tissue.
- Dorsal, superior layer: loose connective tissue (collagen and many elastic fibers).
- Dorsal, inferior layer: taut, non-elastic connective tissue.

Adjacent structures of the disk

Ventral

- Anteriorly, medially, and laterally the disk is connected to the articular capsule.
- Anteriomedially the disk is in contact with the lateral pterygoid muscle (superior part), and anterolaterally with the temporalis and masseter muscles.
- The anterior part is thinner than other parts of the disk.

Dorsal

- Posterior to the disk is the bilaminar zone,[363] also referred to as the retroarticular or retrodiscal fat pad.[105]
- These retrodiscal structures consist of highly vascularized connective tissue.
- This zone can be subdivided into the superior and inferior layer and genu vasculosum.[168]
    - **Superior layer** This consists of elastic and collagenous fibers, fat, and blood vessels. It is attached to the postglenoid process, irregularly to the parotid fascia and typanosquamous, petrosquamous, and petrotympanic fissures, and to the osseous and cartilaginous acoustic meatus (discotemporal ligament). The superior layer and dorsal joint capsule (dorsocranially separate) attach in the fissures. (The variation most commonly found is a medial attachment to the joint.) In the lateral region of the joint, the superior layer usually attaches at the glenoid process, as the dorsal capsule fills the fissure.
    - **Inferior layer** This layer is composed of taut connective tissue. Posteriorly it is attached to the condyle, and stabilizes the disk on the condyle. Fibers of the superior and inferior layers radiate into the posterior part of the disk and link with transverse fibers of the posterior part and sagittal fibers of the intermediate part.
    - **Genu vasculosum** Between the superior and inferior layers is tissue rich in nerves and blood vessels.
- Posteriorly, the bilaminar (retrodiscal) zone gives way to loose, fat-rich connective tissue through which run blood vessels including a venous plexus (the retrodiscal pad).

Function of the bilaminar zone Both layers are involved in the production of synovial fluid. The superior layer is tautened on the abduction movements of the mouth opening and the inferior layer on the adduction movements of the mouth closing. This latter movement fixes the disk on the condyle. The retrodiscal (retroarticular) pad provides protection from pressure to the chorda tympani, which exits at the petrotympanic fissure. It also influences the movement of the TMJ.[390:370] Movements of the lower jaw also exert an effect via the condyle, leading to pumping motions in the bilaminar zone. This assists both joint metabolism and the capacity of the joint surfaces to glide. It may also serve as a receptor field.

Embryonic development The articular disk develops in the seventh week in utero.[424] During embryonic development it extends anteriorly to penetrate the tendons of the pterygoid muscle. Posteriorly, the superior lamina is attached in the region of the petrosquamous fissure, the medial lamina moves through the fissure to the malleus and the anterior ligament of the malleus in the middle ear, and the inferior lamina of the disk attaches to the condyle.

Function The disk serves the function of evening out the difference in size and shape between the head of the mandible and the joint cavity. It improves the distribution of pressure in the joint by enlarging the effective surface (and the three-dimensional course of the fibers), so reducing the forces on the TMJ from masticatory pressure.[212] It also serves as a movable joint cavity that changes its position with the movements of the condyle. The disk divides the joint compartment into an upper joint (gliding motion) and a lower joint (combined rotation and gliding motion). The taut discocondylar ligament maintains the disk in its location on the head of the mandible. This makes it highly important for the coordination between the disk and the condyle during movement of the jaw.

Biomechanics of the disk[250]

- Physiological closing of the mouth: the disk lies centrally in the mandibular fossa. During mouth closure, a physiological position exists between the condylar process and the joint surface of the temporal bone. The retrodiscal pad is folded and the discotemporal ligament relaxes. Increased load has the effect of making the disk tend to glide posteriorly. The lateral pterygoid muscle (superior belly) opposes this motion.
- Opening of the mouth: the discotemporal ligament is stretched, preventing further opening of the mouth.
- Middle stage of mouth opening: the disk glides anteriorly in absolute terms, but posteriorly in relation to the condyle.
- Maximum opening of the mouth: the disk glides posteriorly in relation to the condyle.

2.1.5 The articular capsule

The articular capsule (Figure 2.6) extends from the condyle to the disk and from the disk to the temporal bone, so that it is possible to distinguish an upper and a lower joint space. Only on the lateral side do true capsule fibers run directly from the condyle to the temporal bone. The joint capsule is fairly wide, looser above and somewhat tauter below the disk.[35:526,472] It can be seen as a peripheral, fibrous, and synovial continuation of the disk.[207]

The anterior attachment of the capsule allows plenty of room for motion to the articular head, especially in the anterior direction, and is usually able to prevent tearing of the capsule in the case of dislocation.[435,370]

Attachment to the temporal bone

- Circular.
- Anteriorly: to the tubercle. A layer of collagenous fibers runs medially. This layer can be described as a continuation of the disk or a thickening of the fascia of the lateral pterygoid muscle.
- Laterally the fibers of the disk and thickened fibers of the capsule connect with the lateral

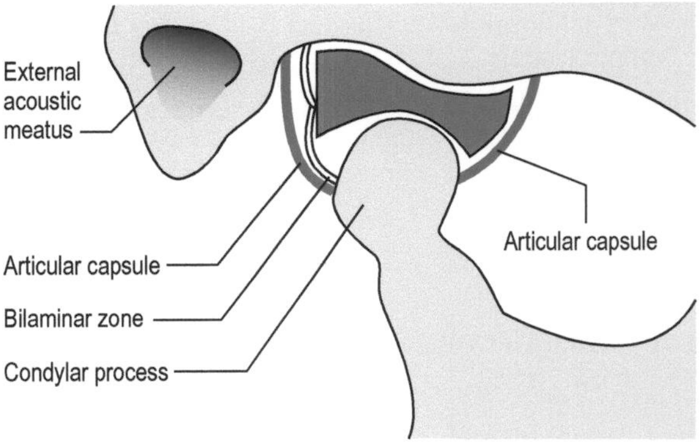

Figure 2.6
The capsule and disk of the temporomandibular joint

ligament of the temporomandibular joint and approach the masseter and temporalis muscles.[292]
- Medially and laterally: to the bone–cartilage boundary.
- Posteriorly: to the mandibular fossa and petrotympanic fissure.
- Some fibers of the capsule pass through the fissure to the malleus in the middle ear (called the meniscomalleolar ligament).[292]
- At the articular tubercle, the capsule thickens toward the inner part of the lateral ligament.[405]

Attachment to the mandible

- Anteriorly, medially, and laterally: to the bone–cartilage boundary.
- Posteriorly: to the transition between the head and the condyle. The posterior attachment of the joint capsule is approximately 5 mm deeper than anterior.
- Posteriorly there is transition of the capsule into the retrodiscal pad.[435]
- Fibers of the superior head of the lateral pterygoid muscle attach to the anterior side of the capsule.[435]

FURTHER INFORMATION There is no vascularization or innervation of the joint surfaces of the mandible and temporal bone, or of most of the disk. The **articular capsule** (auriculotemporal nerve; a small medial region is also innervated by branches of the facial nerve) and the **posterior bilaminar (retrodiscal) tissue**, in contrast, are highly vascularized and richly supplied with nerves, especially nociceptors; they are therefore extremely pain-sensitive. The posterior region (bilaminar zone) of the joint is more vascularized and innervated than the anterior; the lateral region, similarly, more than the medial region.
Stress, traumatic injury, and inflammation are registered in the capsule and bilaminar zone, and transmitted to the brain by afferent nerve signals. Mechanoreceptors in the capsule and bilaminar zone register tensile strain, which is regulated by reflex response via the effect on the muscles. The anterior attachment of the disk is also vascularized and innervated, but less so than the posterior attachment.[250,435] The outer borders of the disk, which do not bear any stresses, are innervated.
It is also clinically relevant to note that if the disk is ventrally displaced, this puts stress on the bilaminar zone. This can lead to formation of a pseudo-disk of firm connective tissue which is less well perfused. That, in turn, creates a greater risk of TMJ arthrosis.

2.1.6 Ligaments

See Figures 2.7 and 2.8.

- **Lateral ligament of the temporomandibular joint (lateral or temporomandibular ligament)[435]**
  - Origin: root of the zygomatic arch of the temporal bone.

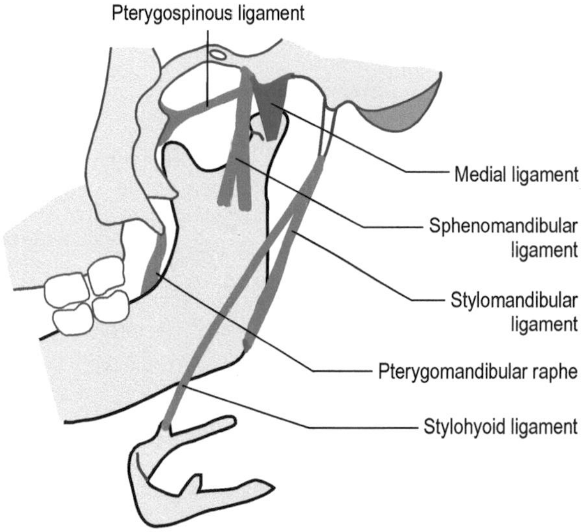

Figure 2.7
Ligaments of the temporomandibular joint

- Anterior part: surrounds the articular tubercle and runs from a point anterior to the tubercle on the zygomatic process of the temporal bone, in an obliquely posterior direction.
- Insertion: laterally and posteriorly on the neck of the mandible.
- Posterior part: runs behind the articular tubercle on the zygomatic process.
- Insertion: posteriorly and slightly inferiorly on the condyle, together with the middle and posterior part of the capsule. Posteriorly the ligament is firmly interlinked with the articular capsule.
- Function:
  * Strengthens the temporomandibular joint capsule.
  * Limits extreme protrusion and retrusion of the mandible.
  * Resists inferior movement of the mandible as the mouth begins to open.
  * Gives support during the transition from rotation to gliding movement and the reverse.
  * Stabilizes the mandibular head on the operative side during molar grinding movements.

- **Lateral collateral ligament**
  - The lateral collateral ligament can be distinguished from the lateral ligament of the temporomandibular joint.[321] This ligament is fairly thin and weak. The superior part is wider than the inferior part.
  - Origin: disk.
  - Insertion: condyle.
  - Function: pterygomandibular raphe; controls jaw movement.
- **Medial (collateral) ligament**
  - This ligament is significantly thicker than the lateral collateral ligament.
  - Origin: disk.
  - Insertion: medially on the condylar process.
  - Function: supports and limits condyle movement.
- **Stylomandibular ligament**
  - Origin: styloid process of the temporal bone.
  - Insertion: posterior border of the angle of the mandible; fascia of medial pterygoid muscle.
  - Function:
    * Limits protrusion, reinforces the parotid fascia and masseteric fascia.
    * Tensed on protrusion, mediotrusion.
- **Sphenomandibular ligament**
  - Thin, broad ligament, medial on capsule.
  - Origin: spine of the sphenoid.
  - Insertion: lingula of the mandible, mandibular foramen on the inner surface of the ramus.

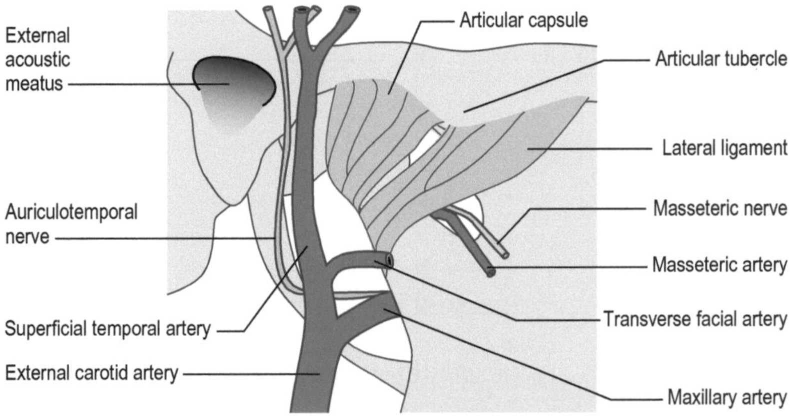

Figure 2.8
Lateral view of the right temporomandibular joint showing blood vessel and neural pathways

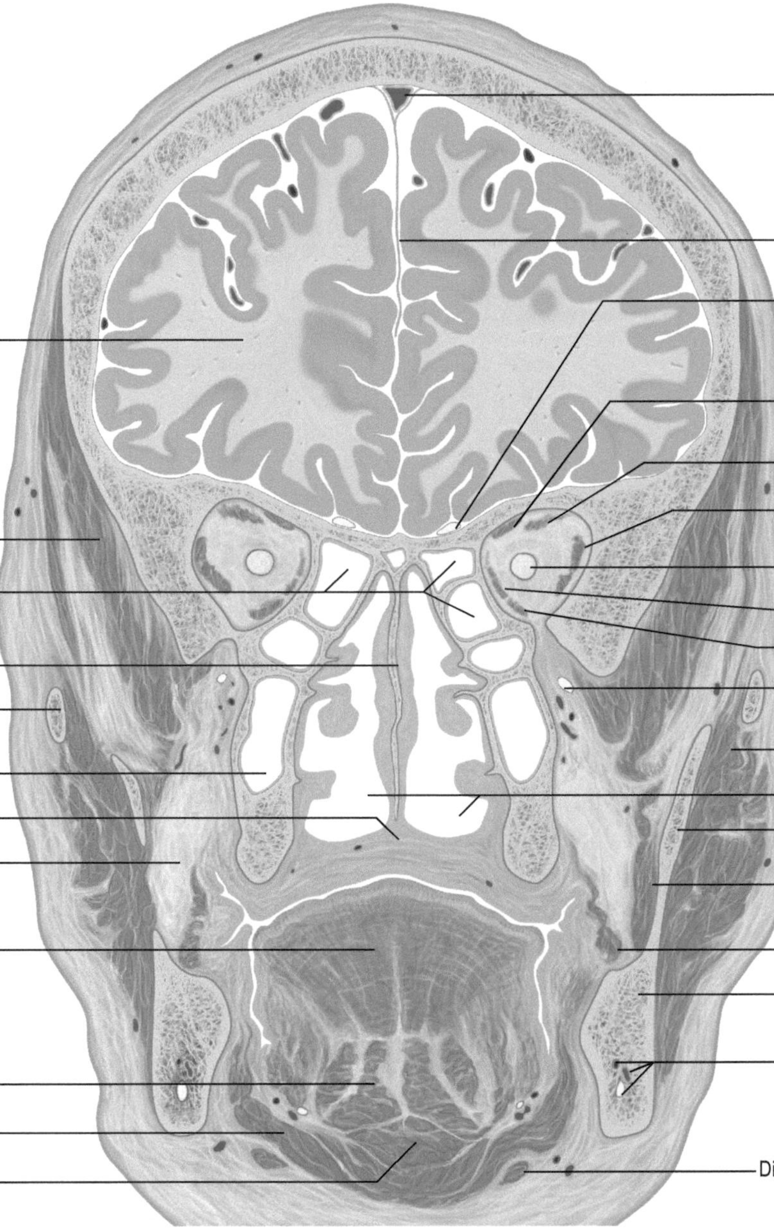

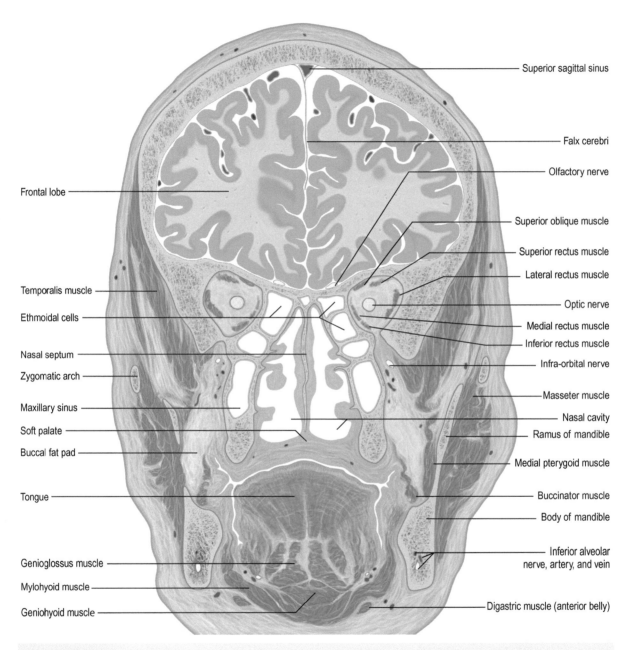

Figure 2.9
Frontal section at the level of the orbital pyramid, ventral view. [Schünke, M., Schulte, E., Schumacher, U. (2015) *Prometheus LernAtlas der Anatomie. Kopf, Hals und Neuroanatomie.* Illustrations by M. Voll and K. Wesker, 4th ed. Stuttgart: Thieme]

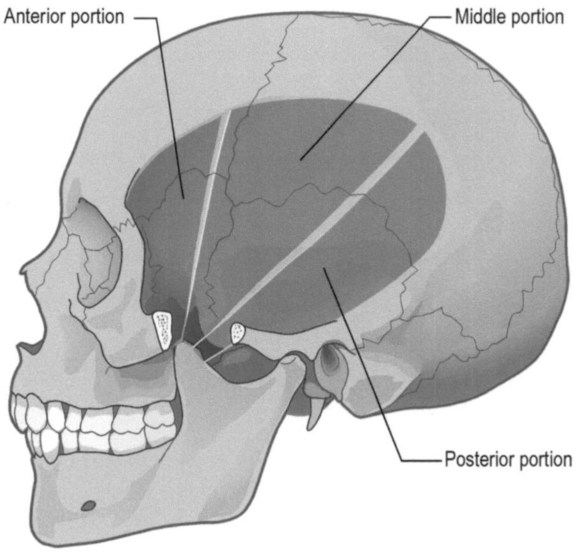

Figure 2.10
Temporalis muscle

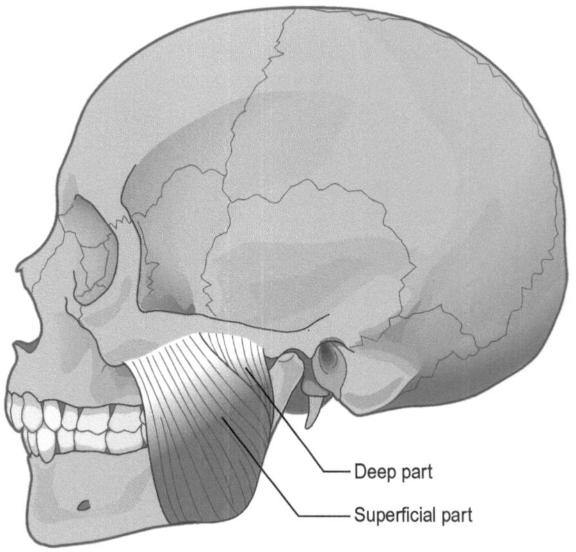

Figure 2.11
Masseter muscle

- Function:
  - Limits inferior movement and protrusion of the mandible.
  - Tensed on final stage of mouth opening, protrusion, mediotrusion.
- **Pterygomandibular raphe**
  - Origin: pterygoid hamulus of the sphenoid.
  - Insertion: inner surface of the body of the mandible, above the mylohyoid line.
  - Function: limits extreme movements of the mandible.
- **Tanaka ligament**[435]
  - Origin: medial ligament.
  - Insertion: wall of the middle fossa, immediately posterior to the attachment of the superior part of the lateral pterygoid muscle to the disk.
  - Course: medially and slightly anteriorly.
  - Function: provides medial reinforcement; holding function during the anterior and posterior movement of the disk.
- **Anterior ligament of the malleus**
  - Origin: anterior process of the malleus in the middle ear.
  - Insertion: petrotympanic fissure; a few fibers run to the spine of the sphenoid and onward with the sphenomandibular ligament to the ramus of the mandible. Continuity of connective tissue through to the tympanic membrane has been found to exist.[435]
- **Pintus ligament**
  - Occurrence not regular.
  - Origin: the malleus, in the middle ear.
  - Insertion: passes through the petrotympanic fissure to the head of the mandible.

2.1.7 Muscles

See Figure 2.9.

- **Temporalis** (Figure 2.10)
  - Innervation: mandibular nerve (CN V_3). Each of the three parts of the muscle has its own nerve branch.
  - Origin: temporal fossa (temporal, sphenoid, parietal, and frontal bones).
  - Fan-shaped origin:
    - Deep layer: inferior temporal line.
    - Superficial layer: temporal fascia.

    * Further origins: temporal fascia of the sphenoid and posteriorly on the zygomatic bone.
  - Insertion: coronoid process. Further fibrous attachments to the middle part of the anterior capsule (not directly to the disk).[292]
  - Course of fibers:
    * Anterior portion: vertically, from inferior to superior.
    * Middle portion: from anterior and inferior to posterior and superior.
    * Posterior portion: from anterior and inferior to posterior and superior or horizontally.
  - Function:
    * Elevation of the mandible. Active in posteriorly directed biting force (anterior and posterior portions).[212]
    * Adduction of the mandible.
    * Positioning of the mandible to ensure optimum bite using masseter and pterygoid muscles.
    * Tensing of capsule.[244] Posterior portion: retrusion.
    * Transverse tensing of the epicranial aponeurosis to brace/secure the zygomatic arch against flexing tension.
- **Masseter muscle, deep part** (Figure 2.11)
  - Innervation: mandibular nerve (CN V_3).
  - Origin: posterior third of the zygomatic arch.
  - Insertion: almost perpendicular at the masseteric tuberosity of the ramus of the mandible; lateral part of the anterior articular capsule (not directly to the disk).[292]
  - Course of fibers: vertical.
  - Function: elevation of the mandible, especially in the case of anteriorly directed biting force; laterotrusion; tensing of capsule.[244] Active in laterally directed biting force on the ipsilateral side.[212]
- **Masseter muscle, superficial part** (Figure 2.11)
  - Innervation: mandibular nerve (CN V_3).
  - Origin: anterior two-thirds of the zygomatic arch.
  - Insertion: obliquely at the angle of the mandible.
  - Course of fibers: from superior and anterior to posterior and inferior.
  - Function:
    * Elevation of the mandible and protrusion.
    * To prevent flexing of the zygomatic arch.
- **Medial pterygoid muscle** Covered by the deep fascia of the masseter muscle; forms a muscle sling together with the masseter muscle. The medial pterygoid forms part of the lateral pharyngeal wall (Figure 2.12). The pterygoid process serves as a fulcrum for the meeting point of the pterygoid fascia and buccopharyngeal fascia; also at the pterygomandibular raphe.
  - Innervation: mandibular nerve (CN V_3).
  - Origin: pterygoid fossa (inner surface of the lateral plate of the pterygoid process).
  - Insertion: inner aspect of the angle of the mandible (pterygoid tuberosity); may form raphe with the tendon of insertion of the masseter muscle.

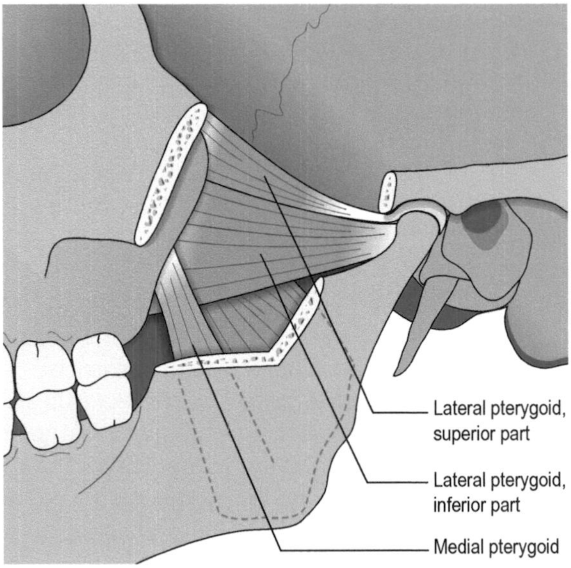

Figure 2.12
Medial and lateral pterygoid muscles

- Course of fibers: nearly vertical, obliquely to inferior and posterior and outward.
- Function:
  - Elevation of the mandible (together with masseter).
  - Protrusion when teeth occluded (opposing retrusion by temporalis muscle, posterior part).
  - Unilateral: medial movement of the mandible.[390:388]
  - Participates in swallowing.

NOTE Excessive medial movement leads to hypertrophy of the muscle.

- **Lateral pterygoid muscle, superior part** (Figure 2.12)
  - Innervation: mandibular nerve (CN V_3).
  - Origin: infratemporal surface and infratemporal crest of the sphenoid.
  - Insertion: upper border of pterygoid fovea, anterior and medial to the articular capsule; disk. (Attachment to the disk is a matter of some debate: is the attachment functionally effective, not functionally effective, or non-existent?)[292,172]
  - Course of fibers: slightly oblique, from inside, anterior and superior, running outward and posterior.
  - Function:
    - Elevation of the mandible (mouth closure).
    - Anterior movement of the disk and condyle and unilateral medial movement.
    - Stabilization of the capsule and disk at the terminal stage of mouth opening.
    - Positioning and stabilization of the condylar head and disk during mouth closure.[298]
    - Stabilization of the resting condyle on the operative side during molar grinding movement.
- **Lateral pterygoid muscle, inferior part** (Figure 2.12)
  - Innervation: mandibular nerve (CN V_3).
  - Origin: outer aspect of the lateral pterygoid plate.
  - Insertion: anterior of condyle in the pterygoid fovea.
  - Course of fibers: horizontally oriented, from inside, inferior, running outward and superior.
  - Function:
    - Protrusion with or without mouth opening.
    - Unilateral: molar grinding (medial movement).
    - Works in synergy with the suprahyoid muscles in movements of mouth opening.
    - Gives support in the translation of the condylar head caudad, anteriorly and contralaterally during the opening of the mouth.[298]
- **Sphenomandibular muscle**[172]
  - Innervation: mandibular nerve (CN V_3).
  - Origin: greater wing of the sphenoid.
  - Insertion: coronoid process or adjacent area.
  - Function: stabilization of the mandible if required.

Indirectly involved muscles

- **Suprahyoid muscles** (innervation in parentheses)
  - **Mylohyoid:** from the mylohyoid line of the mandible to the body of the hyoid bone and median raphe (CN V_3). The left and right portions of the mylohyoid form a mobile diaphragm in the floor of the mouth. When the mouth is closed, the fibers run in a superior, lateral, and slightly anterior direction from the hyoid to the raphe of the mandible. The course of the muscle fibers between their bony attachments is not straight, as is often stated, but curved. This is caused by the connection between the muscle and the geniohyoid above and the anterior belly of the digastric below.[109]

  - **Geniohyoid:** from the mental spine of the mandible to the body of the hyoid (CN XII, spinal nerve C1).
  - **Digastric:** from the mastoid notch of the temporal bone, via a tendinous loop at the hyoid, to the digastric fossa of the mandible (CN V_3, CN VII).
  - **Stylohyoid:** from the styloid process of the temporal bone to the lesser horn of the hyoid (CN VII).
  - **Hyoglossus:** from the body and greater horn of the hyoid to the sides of the tongue (CN XII).
  - **Chondroglossus:** from the lesser horn of the hyoid to the sides of the tongue (CN XII).
- **Infrahyoid muscles**
  - **Omohyoid:** from the upper border of the scapula to the body of the hyoid (spinal nerves C1–C3).
  - **Sternohyoid:** from the superior sternum and the sternoclavicular joint to the body of the hyoid (spinal nerves C1–C3).
  - **Thyrohyoid:** from the thyroid cartilage to the greater horn and body of the hyoid (spinal nerve C1 carried by CN XII).
  - **Sternothyroid:** from the sternum and first rib to the thyroid cartilage (spinal nerves C1–C3).
- **Muscles located behind the hyoid**
  - **Middle constrictor of pharynx:** from the greater and lesser horns of the hyoid bone (CN IX, CN X, cervical sympathetic trunk).
  - **Stylohyoid:** from the styloid process to the lesser horn (CN VII).
  - **Digastric** (posterior belly) (CN VII).
- **Muscles of the floor of the mouth**
  - **Mylohyoid, digastric, geniohyoid.** Function: opening of the mouth (rotation movement); provide foundation for movements of the tongue.
- **Muscles of the tongue**
  - **Genioglossus:** from the mental spine of the inner surface of the mandible into the tongue; fan-shaped (CN XII).
  - **Hyoglossus:** suprahyoid muscles (see above).
  - **Chondroglossus:** suprahyoid muscles (see above).
  - **Styloglossus:** from the styloid process into the sides of the tongue.
  - **Myloglossus (inconsistent):** posterior of the mylohyoid line to the base of the tongue.
  - **Palatoglossus:** from the palatine aponeurosis into the sides of the tongue.
  - **Superior and inferior longitudinal muscles, transverse muscle of the tongue, vertical muscle of the tongue.**
- **Muscles of facial expression (facial, skin, or mimetic muscles)** as related to function of mouth (CN VII)
  - **Buccinator:** from the pterygomandibular raphe and upper and lower jaw to the corner of the mouth and orbicularis oris. Function: assists moving food within the mouth, and sucking and blowing.
  - **Depressor anguli oris:** from the mandible to the corner of the mouth.
  - **Depressor labii inferioris:** from the mandible; platysma, to the lower lip.
  - **Levator labii superioris alaeque nasi:** from the orbit to the upper lip.
  - **Levator labii superioris:** from the infraorbital foramen to the upper lip.
  - **Levator anguli oris:** from the canine fossa to the corner of the mouth.
  - **Mentalis:** from the inferior root of the incisor to the lower lip and skin of the chin.
  - **Risorius:** from the parotid fascia to the corner of the mouth.
  - **Zygomaticus major and minor:** from the zygomatic arch to the corner of the mouth.
- **Other muscles**
  - **The facial muscles** (Figure 2.13)—facial expression; muscle system of the lips and cheeks (CN VII), e.g., buccinator: from the

pterygomandibular raphe and the maxilla and mandible to the angle of the mouth, and orbicularis oris muscle (assists movement of food in the mouth; also sucking and blowing).

- Pharyngeal muscles (swallowing) (CN IX, CN X).
- Muscles of the palate and pharynx: levatores/tensores veli palatini and the superior, middle, and inferior constrictor muscles—muscles of the soft palate, palatoglossal and palatopharyngeal arches (CN V, CN IX, CN X).
- Muscles of the larynx (articulation/formation of sounds) (CN X).
- Nuchal muscles: indirect opening of the jaw, by drawing the head/nape of neck backward (cervical spinal nerves).
- Sternocleidomastoid: indirect opening of the jaw by extension of the head on bilateral contraction[390:382] (CN XI, cervical plexus).

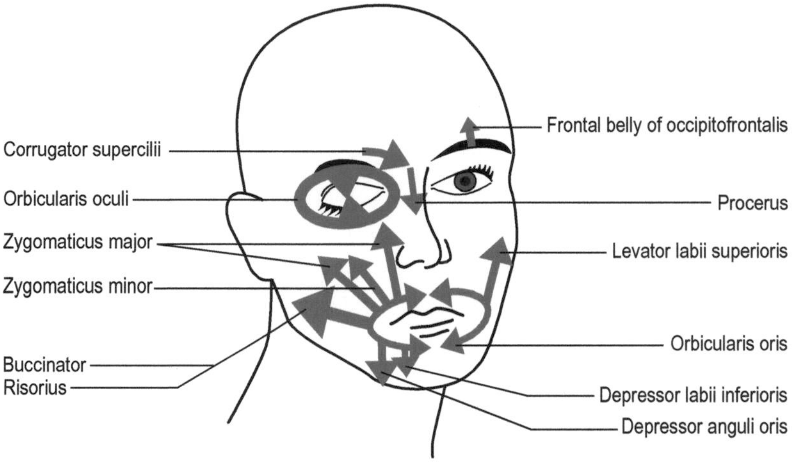

Figure 2.13
Function of the facial muscles

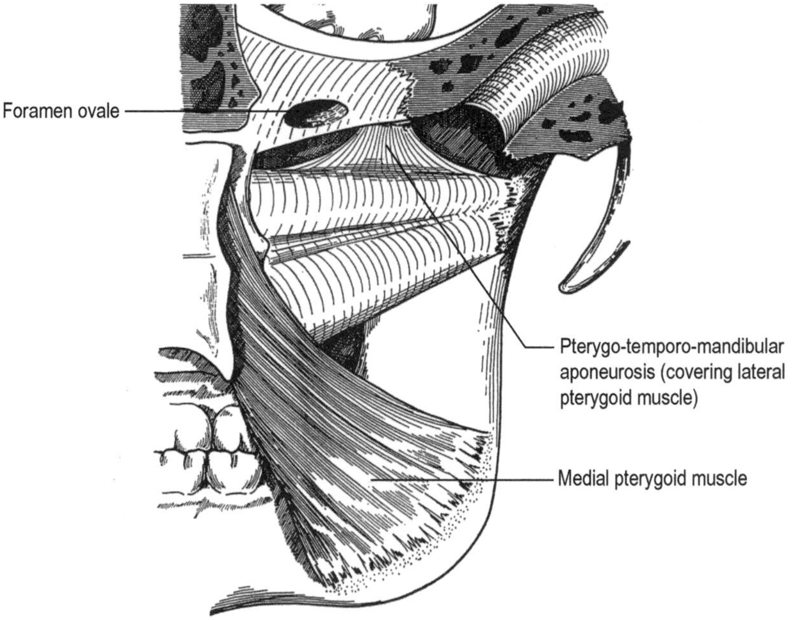

Figure 2.14
Interpterygoid region, pterygo-temporo-mandibular aponeurosis. (Perlemuter, L., Waligora, J. (1980) *Cahiers d'anatomie 1. Système nerveux central*, 4th ed. Paris: Masson)

2.1.8 Fasciae

- **Temporal fascia** of the deep fascia of the cranium
  - Fibrous layer covering the temporal muscle.
  - Cranially, partly at the superior temporal line. and caudally, (outer layer) runs as the superficial layer and (inner layer) runs as the deep layer, with attachment to the zygomatic arch.
  - The zygomatico-orbital artery (branch of the superficial temporal artery) and zygomatico-temporal branch (CN V_2) run through the fat pad that lies between these layers.
  - Superior to the zygomatic arch is the deep temporal fat pad, which extends caudally. This serves as a layer that allows the temporal muscle to glide smoothly and also to protect the masticatory space.
  - The temporoparietal fat pad lies in between the superficial and deep layers of the temporoparietal fascia.
  - The fascia extends cranially into the epicranial fascia and caudally into the paratideomasseteric fascia.[41]
- **Paratideomasseteric fascia** of the deep facial fascia: see Volume 2, section 4.2.2.
- **Pterygoid fascia** of the deep facial fascia: see Volume 2, section 4.2.2.
- **Pterygomandibular raphe**
  - This ligamentous band runs between the pterygoid hamulus of the sphenoid and the mandible.
  - Medially it also runs across the TMJ. A portion of the constrictor muscles of the pharynx arise on its posterior aspect; the buccinator arises on its anterior aspect.
- **Pterygo-temporo-mandibular aponeurosis** (Figure 2.14)
  - Dorsally, this is attached at the ventral border of the neck of the condylar process of the mandible, and ventrally at the lateral plate of the pterygoid process.
  - The superior border is reinforced by Hyrtl's ligament (pterygoalar ligament).
  - The inferior border is free, running out onto the medial aspect of the lateral pterygoid muscle.

There are also functional links with the falx cerebri, falx cerebelli, and tentorium cerebelli, and the nuchal muscles. The intracranial structures may transmit the balance of forces between the weight of the viscerocranium and the compensating tone of the nuchal muscles. One effect of this may be to influence the function of the temporomandibular joint and the occlusion patterns of the upper and lower jaw (Figure 2.15).

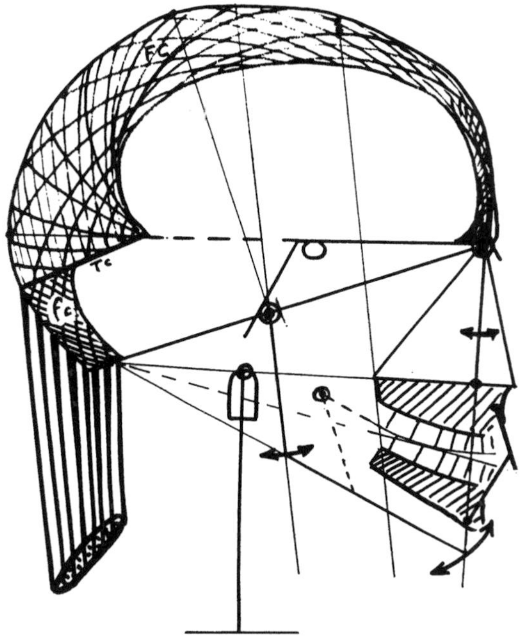

Figure 2.15
Diagrammatic representation of the balance between the neurocranium and viscerocranium and the cervical spine. The weight of the viscerocranium is compensated via the tone of the nuchal muscles. The effect of these extends into the interior of the cranium via the falx cerebri and cerebelli and tentorium cerebelli. (From: Delaire, J. (1978) 'L'analyse architecturale et structurale cranio-faciale.' *Rev. Stomatol. 79*, 1–33)

2.1.9 Innervation of the temporomandibular joint

- **Auriculotemporal nerve** (branch of the mandibular nerve, CN V_3): the articular branches of the auriculotemporal nerve run from outside, inward, and from posterior to enter the articular capsule[33] (Figures 2.16, 2.17).
- **Masseteric nerve and deep temporal nerve** (both branches of the mandibular nerve, CN V_3): their articular branches run from anterior to enter the articular capsule.
- **Facial nerve (CN VII):** a twig of this nerve sometimes enters the joint from outside.
- Autonomic innervation via the **otic ganglion:** preganglionic parasympathetic fibers begin in the lesser petrosal nerve (CN IX), are reoriented in the otic ganglion, and pass into the articular capsule from medially. These are concerned with the production of synovial fluid. Sympathetic innervation is supplied from the carotid plexus without reorientation in the otic ganglion.
- The lateral ligament of the TMJ and surrounding fatty tissue are also richly innervated.
- **Additional nerves** of the mandible
  - ◆ Buccal nerve (from CN V_3) (entirely sensory branch).

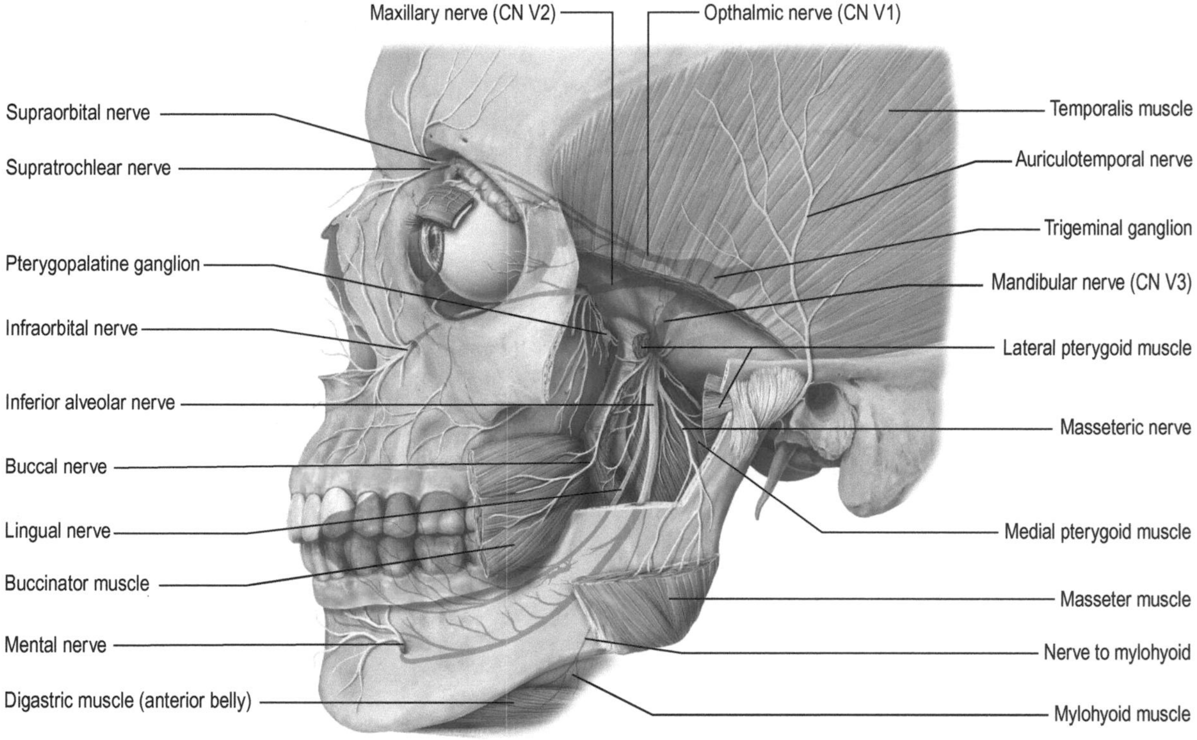

Figure 2.16
Innervation of the masticatory muscles. (Schünke, M., Schulte, E., Schumacher, U. (2015) *Prometheus LernAtlas der Anatomie. Kopf, Hals und Neuroanatomie*. Illustrations by M. Voll and K. Wesker, 4th ed. Stuttgart: Thieme)

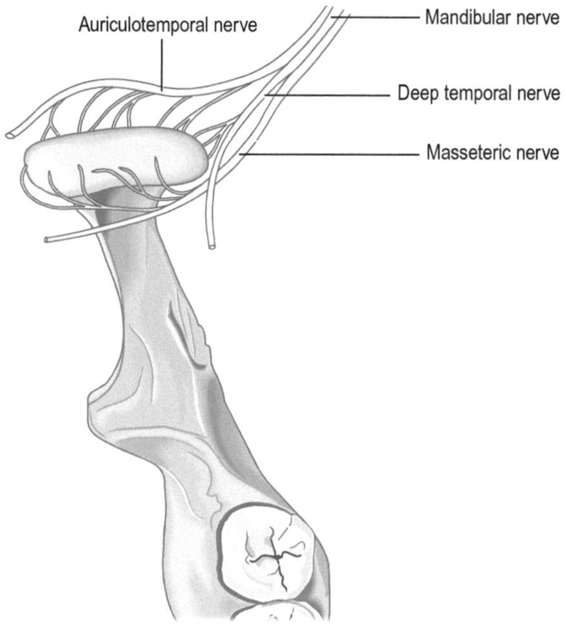

Figure 2.17
Innervation of the temporomandibular joint

- Nerve to the medial pterygoid muscle (from CN V_3).
- Inferior alveolar nerve (from CN V_3): in the mandibular canal.
- Mental nerve (branch of inferior alveolar nerve) (from CN V_3): at the mental foramen.
- Nerve to mylohyoid (branch of inferior alveolar nerve): in the mylohyoid groove.
- Masseteric nerve (from CN V_3): at the mandibular notch.
- Otic ganglion and submandibular ganglion supply innervation to the salivary glands.

2.1.10 Mechanoreceptors

Four different types of mechanoreceptor are found in proximity to the joint:[25,44,57,165,218,219,220,488]

- Ruffini corpuscles (endings): information relating to present position of the joint and its movement (direction, speed, amplitude of condylar movement).
- Lamellated (pacinian) corpuscles: dynamic receptors in the articular capsule register acceleration of TMJ movements.
- Golgi tendon organs: isolated receptors in the lateral articular capsule reinforcement; in response to maximum forces they bring about reflex relaxation of the masticatory muscles. The condyles can then glide freely sideways.
- Numerous free nerve endings: depolarization occurs in sudden pronounced translation movements in the TMJ.

The proprioceptive impulses produced by these structures (TMJ, together with the complex comprising the capsule, disk, and muscles, the anterior ligament of the malleus, and the sphenomandibular ligament), which derive from the first branchial arch, are mainly transmitted to the nucleus of the trigeminal nerve (Volume 2, section 7.5).

This connection means that any disturbance of the masticatory system may also affect the proprioceptive system of the entire first branchial arch.

Of the three following muscles, the lateral pterygoid, masseter, and temporalis, it is the temporalis that possesses the greatest number of neuromuscular spindles. 1A and 1B fibers continue to the posterior horn of the spinal cord. These react to stretching of the muscles and to the speed of stretch.

2.1.11 Blood and lymphatic vessels

See Figures 2.18 and 2.19 (also Figure 2.8 and Volume 2, Figure 3.18):

- The **maxillary artery** (branch of the external carotid artery) has branches to the mandible and masticatory muscles.
- The **inferior alveolar artery** (branch of the maxillary artery): in the mandibular canal.

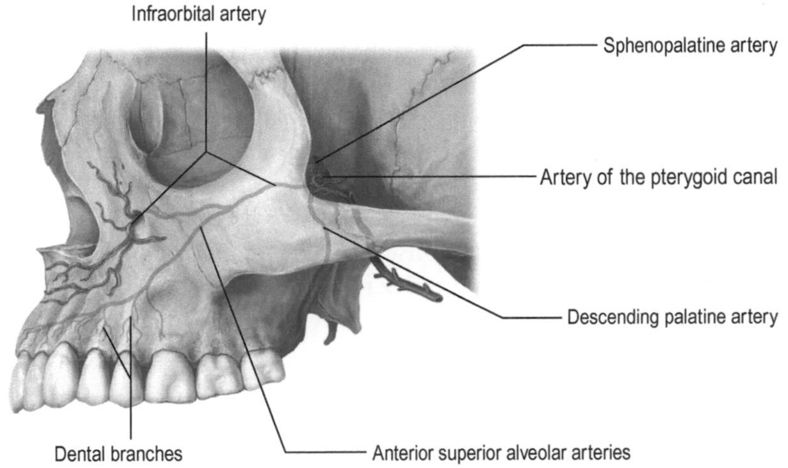

Figure 2.18
Infraorbital artery, left. (Schünke, M., Schulte, E., Schumacher, U. (2015) *Prometheus LernAtlas der Anatomie. Kopf, Hals und Neuroanatomie*. Illustrations by M. Voll and K. Wesler, 4th ed. Stuttgart: Thieme)

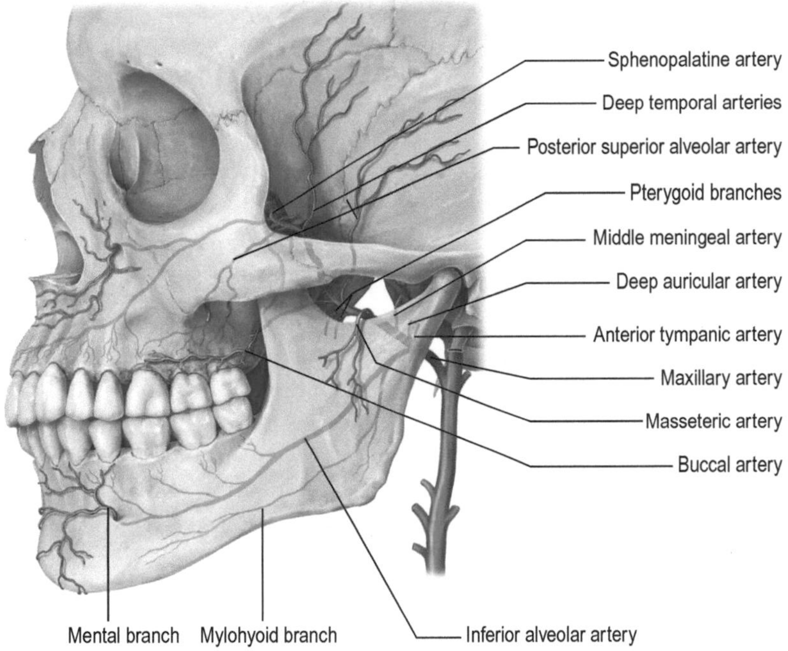

Figure 2.19
Maxillary artery and its branches, from left. (Schünke, M., Schulte, E., Schumacher, U. (2015) *Prometheus LernAtlas der Anatomie. Kopf, Hals und Neuroanatomie*. Illustrations by M. Voll and K. Wesler, 4th ed. Stuttgart: Thieme)

- The **mental branch of the inferior alveolar artery**: at the mental foramen.
- **Mylohyoid branch** (branch of the inferior alveolar artery): in the mylohyoid groove.
- The **masseteric artery** (branch of the maxillary artery): at the mandibular notch.
- The **superficial temporal artery** (branch of the facial artery): structures supplied include the TMJ.

Lymphatic outflow

- The retropharyngeal, sub- and preauricular, and submandibular lymph nodes.
- The occipital lymph nodes.
- Also: the cervical lymph nodes.

2.1.12 Connections with other structures

- **Parotid gland** (Figure 2.20) at and behind the ramus of the mandible.

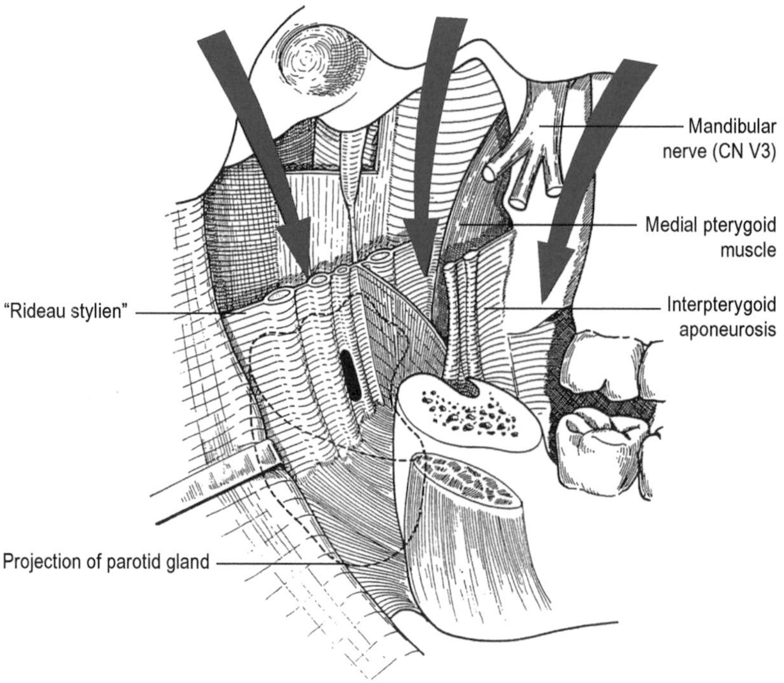

Figure 2.20
The interpterygoid region. Location and connections of the parotid gland. (Perlemuter, L., Waligora, J. (1980) *Cahiers d'anatomie 1. Système nerveux central*, 4th ed. Paris: Masson)

2.2 Biomechanics of the mandible

The articular surfaces of the TMJ are highly incongruent, and the articular capsule is very lax. As a result the joint has considerable mobility, with a large range of motion.[230,341] Joint movement options include opening and closing, protrusion/retrusion, and laterotrusion/mediotrusion.[34,154,158,301] The temporomandibular joints enable movement around three axes.[391,416] Rohen[370] and others have described the temporomandibular joint as a turning and sliding joint. There is no fixed centralized position of the condyles in the mandibular fossa.[410]

Movements of the jaw are always a combination of movements, making it impossible to define static axes of jaw movement. On the contrary, according to Koolstra and van Eijden,[229] the patterns of muscle contraction determine the helical axis of motion (immediate rotational/shifting axis) for the open–close movement.[34,142,229] This means that not only does the muscle function of the TMJ depend on the immediate helical axis of motion, but conversely the helical axis depends on the muscle function.[230]

Opening of the jaw, for example, begins with movement around an axis of rotation about 1 cm posterior and inferior to the condyle. At the end of mouth opening, the axis of rotation lies below the coronoid process, approximately at the transition from the ramus to the body of the mandible. Many of the movements of the human TMJ are not symmetrical. An example of this is lateral movement of the TMJ. Here, the contralateral condyle moves anteriorly, to the articular tubercle, while the ipsilateral condyle remains in the mandibular fossa and moves only slightly toward the ipsilateral side.[34,158,278]

Koolstra and van Eijden developed a biomechanical model of the human masticatory system which does not limit its movements to fixed, immutable axes. Their model combines effects of the joint surfaces, muscle forces, dynamic properties of the muscles, and the mass of the structures moved. However, the primary factor for the movements of the TMJ is the direction of movement of the involved muscles.[227,228,229,230]

All movements of the mandible involve both the superior and the inferior joint compartment. In the superior joint compartment, mainly sagittal gliding movements take place, and in the inferior compartment, mainly rotation movements.

NOTE Certain main movements can be distinguished:

- Opening and closing of the mouth (abduction and adduction).
- Forward and backward movement (protrusion and retrusion) of the mandible.
- Sideways movement (laterotrusion).

In the rest position there is no contact between the teeth. The mandibular head is located at the posterior slope of the articular tubercle. The posterior part of the disk fills the fossa.[35:527]

2.2.1 Biomechanical demands on the temporomandibular joint

The act of chewing imposes loads on the TMJ.[57,122,126,175,226,413,442] This fact explains overloading of the joint, as in parafunctional activities.[297,322,323,340] However, loading of the TMJ is highly variable from one individual, and habit, to another,[48,54,189] since the mandible operates like a balance beam together with the adjacent muscles of the TMJ[23,56,58,138,155] and the muscles of the floor of the mouth and other hyoid muscles, and numerous other regulatory mechanisms, and so is integrated into a supraordinate regulatory system. The smooth functioning of all the components in the regulatory equation, which are being constantly adjusted to current requirements by processes of feedback and adaptation, is fundamental to normal TMJ function.

Various muscle forces can be activated to produce a particular masticatory pressure. The physiological contact forces can vary between zero and 50% of total masticatory force. With a contact force of 0% and when the condyle is supported on the articular tubercle while biting onto a solid piece of food, almost no load is imposed on the joint.[238,318,319] The positioning of the condyle on the articular tubercle is in turn dependent on the angle of opening of the TMJ.

Simulation of static load with jaw closed indicates that the transmission of stress and tension primarily affects the intermediate zone of the disk (especially the lateral parts). Even relatively minor joint loading is stated to produce distinct deformations, and relatively large differences in the direction of the loads on the joint was found to have little influence on the distribution of the deformations.[27]

The smooth functioning of the virtual neuromuscular axis that governs the masticatory apparatus is fundamental to normal TMJ function. Without it, overloading of the system and damage to the temporomandibular joint occur.[318]

2.2.2 Opening and closing of the mouth

NOTE Combined rotation and gliding movements are involved in the opening and closing of the mouth.[390:372]

When the mouth is opened, the first movement is a rotation of the condylar process (inferior discomandibular joint). This produces an opening of about 12° (Figure 2.21).[10:52] The next stage is a protrusion movement. The condylar process and disk are drawn anteriorly, under the articular tubercle (superior discomandibular joint). The lateral pterygoid muscle, aided by the digastric muscle, produces protrusion of the disk and condylar process. Closing of the mouth involves retrusion and posterior rotation of the condylar process. Mouth closure is controlled by the lateral pterygoid muscle (superior part) (Figure 2.22).[10:52]

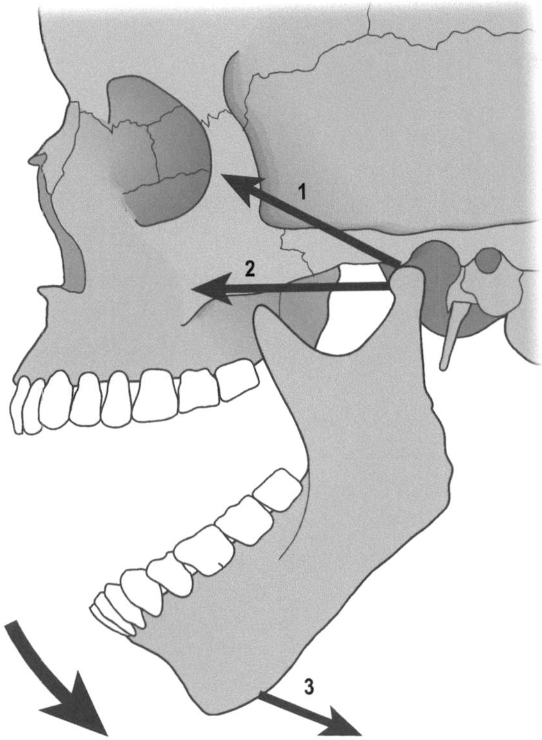

Figure 2.21
Opening of the mouth according to Amigues. **1** Superior part of the lateral pterygoid muscle relaxes. **2** Inferior part of the lateral pterygoid muscle contracts. **3** Digastric muscle (anterior belly) contracts

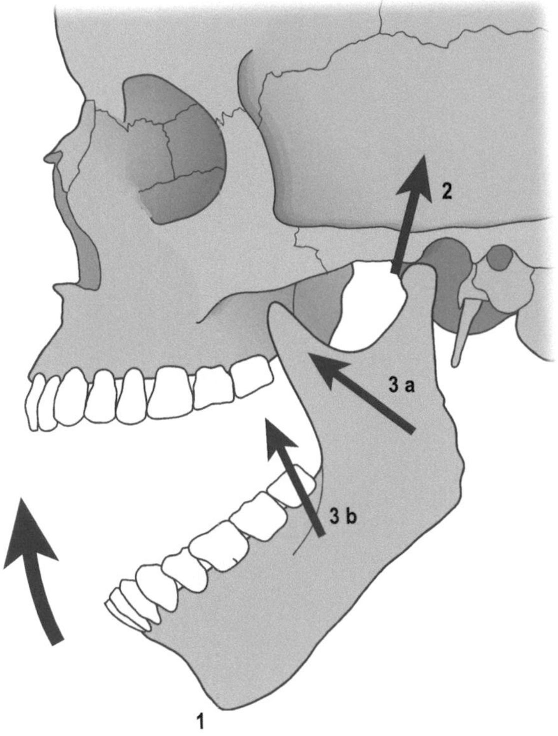

Figure 2.22
Closure of the mouth according to Amigues. **1** Suprahyoid muscles relax. **2** Temporalis muscle contracts. **3a** Medial pterygoid muscle contracts. **3b** Masseter muscle contracts

A more detailed analysis of mouth opening and closing is given below. The structures involved are shown in Figure 2.23.

Mouth opening

- **Initiation of mouth opening**
  - The superior part of the lateral pterygoid muscle relaxes.
  - Forward rotation of the condylar process.
  - Posterior translation of the disk relative to the gliding movement of the condyle.
  - The digastric muscle (in particular the anterior belly) contracts to initiate mouth opening, assisted by the mylohyoid and geniohyoid muscles. The hyoid bone acts as a fixed point, stabilized by the infrahyoid muscles.
- **Middle stage of mouth opening**
  - The condylar process rotates forward and glides anteriorly and inferiorly.
  - Forward translation of the disk (along the oblique course created by the articular tubercle of the temporal bone and condyle). The distance traveled is less than that of the condyle, resulting in posterior movement relative to the condyle.[35:527]
  - Contraction of the lateral pterygoid (inferior part) and digastric muscles, assisted by the mylohyoid and geniohyoid muscles, enable the middle stage of mouth opening.[390:402]

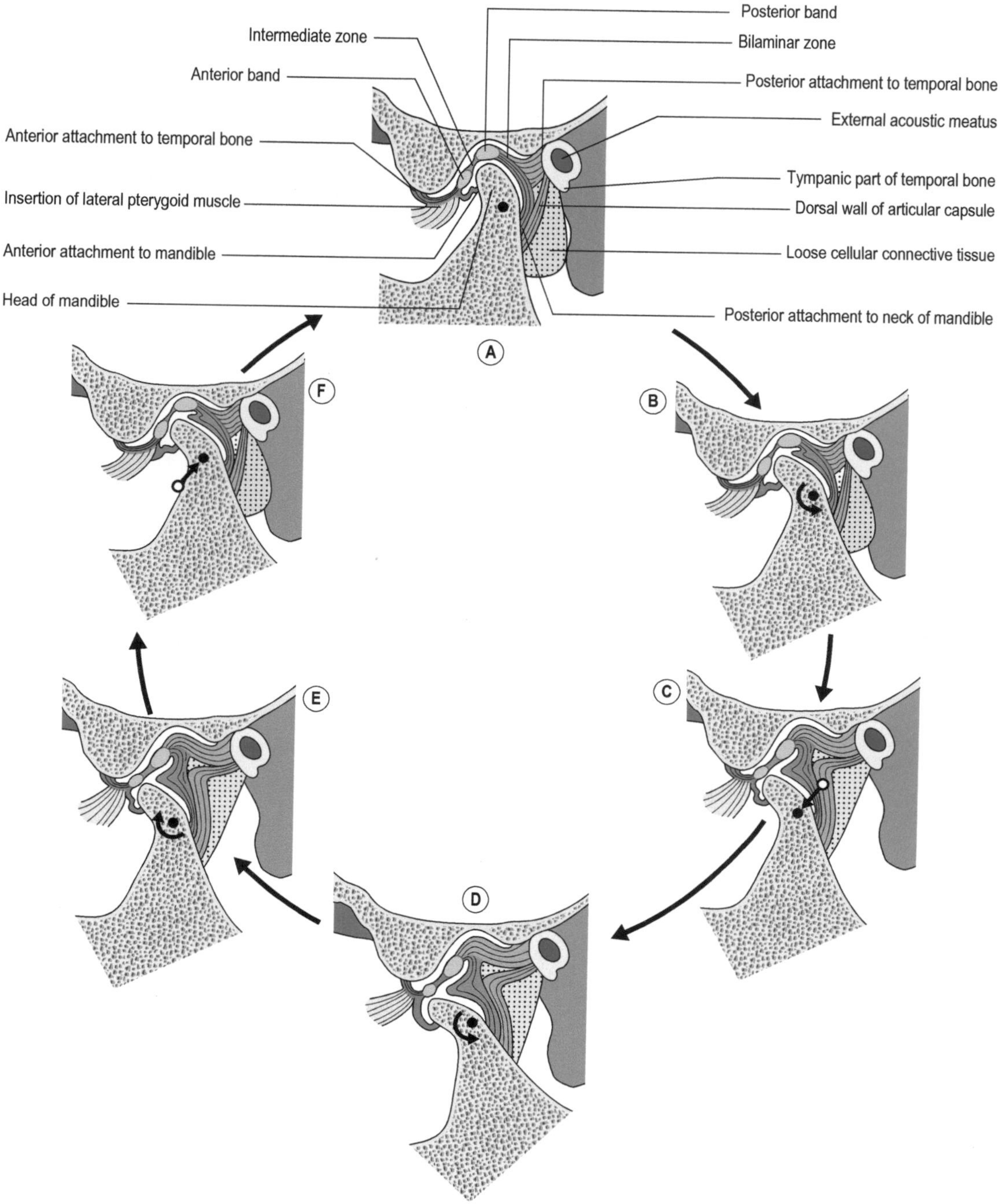

Figure 2.23
Diagrammatic illustration of the effects in the temporomandibular joint of opening and closing of the mouth, according to Rees. **A–D** Opening of mouth. **D–F** Closing of mouth

- **Maximum opening of the mouth**
  - Forward rotation of the condylar process; this transmutes into a gliding movement.
  - Posterior translation of the disk relative to the gliding movement of the condyle.
  - Contraction of the digastric muscle (assisted by the mylohyoid and geniohyoid muscles) produces the final stage in mouth opening.
  - Opening of the mouth is limited by the lateral ligament of the temporomandibular joint, the retrodiscal connective tissue (discotemporal ligament), and the temporalis muscle (posterior fibers).

If tensing of the masseter and temporalis muscles restricts the opening of the mouth, a change in the fixed point leads to flexion of the head and cervical spine.

Mouth closing

- **Initiation of mouth closure**
  - The condylar process rotates backward.
  - Anterior translation of the disk in absolute terms.
  - Anterior translation of the disk relative to the gliding movement of the condyle.
  - Relaxation of the suprahyoid muscles begins closure of the mouth.
  - Maximum tension of the discotemporal ligament.
- **Middle stage of mouth closure**
  - The condylar process rotates backward and glides posteriorly and superiorly.
  - Posterior translation of the disk. The distance traveled is less than that of the condyle, resulting in anterior movement relative to the condyle.
  - Contraction of the temporalis muscle enables the mouth-closing movement.
  - The discotemporal ligament increasingly relaxes.
- **Final position**
  - Closing rotation of the condylar process.
  - Relative anterior translation of the disk.
  - The final position is produced by contraction of the temporalis and masseter muscles, lateral pterygoid (superior part), and medial pterygoid.
  - The movement is limited by the lateral ligament of the TMJ and discocondylar ligament.
  - The vascular retrodiscal pad empties.

NOTE The disk glides more slowly than the condyle when the mouth is opened or closed, so as to maintain the balance of form and function.[237]

2.2.3 Protrusion and retrusion

The movement involved in protrusion of the mandible is relatively slight. An anterior and inferior gliding movement of the condylar processes occurs (in the superior discomandibular joint). The angle of inclination is between 5° and 55°. A slight turning around a transverse axis also occurs in the TMJ, so that the lower incisors can slide downward on reaching the upper incisors. The lower incisors are raised again once they have passed the upper front teeth (Figure 2.24). Retrusion is the reverse of the protrusion process.[10:54]

Protrusion

- Anterior translation of the condylar process, together with slight rotation.
- The disk glides anteriorly. The distance traveled is less than that of the condyle, resulting in posterior movement relative to the condyle.
- Protrusion is enabled mainly by contraction of the lateral pterygoid muscle (inferior part), assisted by the medial pterygoid and masseter muscles and the anterior fibers of the temporalis muscle.
- Protrusion is limited by the discocondylar, sphenomandibular, and stylomandibular ligaments.

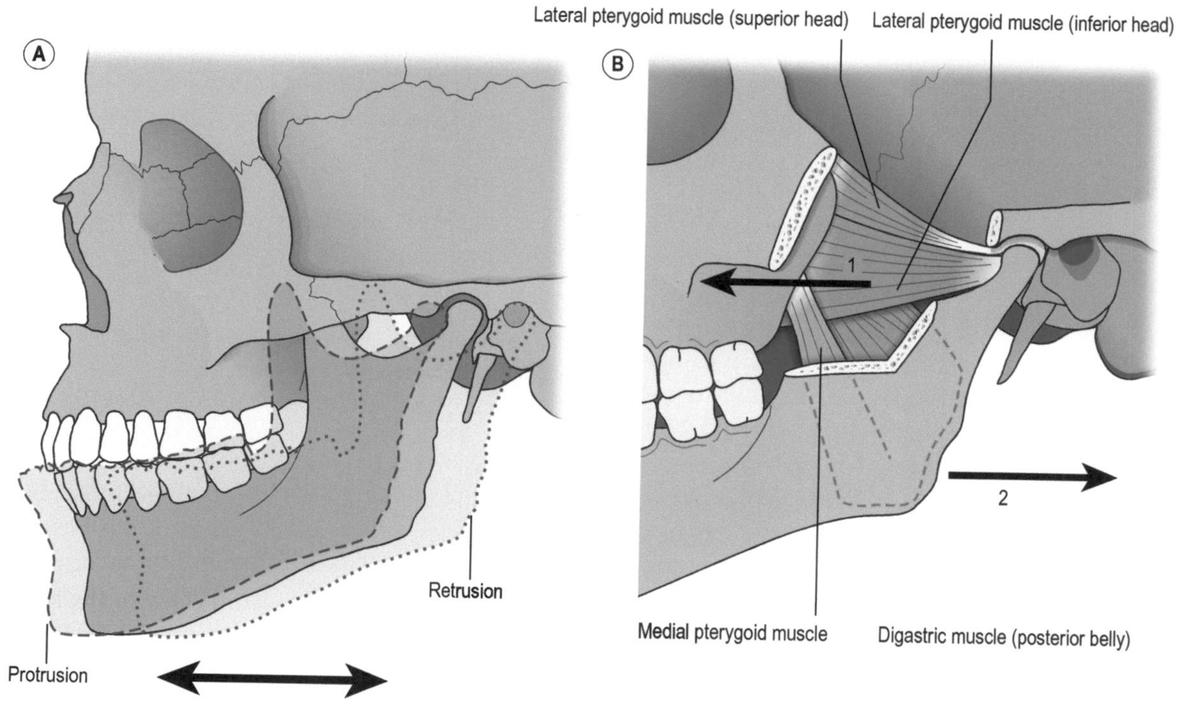

Figure 2.24
A Protrusion and **B** retrusion, according to Amigues

Retrusion

- Posterior translation of the condylar process occurs, together with slight rotation.
- The disk glides posteriorly. The distance traveled is less than that of the condyle, resulting in anterior movement relative to the condyle.
- Retrusion is enabled mainly by contraction of the lateral pterygoid muscle (superior part) and medial pterygoid and masseter muscles (deep part), assisted by the posterior fibers of the temporalis muscle and the posterior belly of the digastric muscle.
- Retrusion is limited by the discocondylar ligament and lateral ligament of the TMJ.
- The vascular retrodiscal pad empties.

2.2.4 Laterotrusion

See Figure 2.25.

- **On the side of the laterotrusion**[10:52]
  - The condylar process turns in the joint cavity, rotating around a vertical axis through the neck of the mandible.
  - The condylar process moves slightly laterally and posteriorly or anteriorly; also superiorly or inferiorly as required.
  - Lateral rotation of the disk. Relative to the movement of the condyle the disk moves in a medial and anterior direction.
  - Contraction of the lateral pterygoid muscle (superior part), the posterior fibers of the temporalis muscle, masseter, and digastric.
  - Laterotrusion is limited on the side of laterotrusion by the lateral ligament and discocondylar ligament.
- **On the side of the mediotrusion**
  - The condylar process moves in an anterior, inferior, and slightly medial direction.

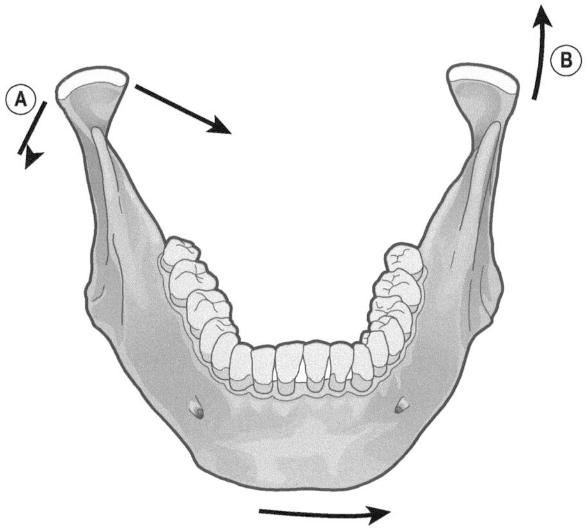

Figure 2.25
Laterotrusion according to Amigues.
A Side of mediotrusion: condylar process moves anteroinferiorly and slightly medially. Contraction of lateral pterygoid (inferior part), medial pterygoid, masseter, and anterior part of the temporalis.
B Side of laterotrusion: condylar process moves laterally and posteriorly. Contraction of lateral pterygoid (superior part), posterior part of temporalis, masseter, and digastric muscles

- There is anterior and medial translation of the disk in absolute terms, but in relation to the movement of the condyle its movement is posterior and lateral.
- Contraction of the lateral pterygoid muscle (inferior part), the medial pterygoid and masseter muscles and the anterior fibers of the temporalis.
- Laterotrusion is limited on the side of mediotrusion by the sphenomandibular and stylomandibular ligaments.

2.2.5 Control of the act of chewing

A biological system of feedback control governs the operation of the TMJ and integrates its many functions (chewing, swallowing, sucking, speaking, facial expression, etc.).[57] The biomechanical parameters governed by this control system are not limited to the joint itself, but have to include all neighboring structures (muscles of mastication, tongue, hyoid and facial muscles, the teeth and periodontium, and the mucous membranes of the cheeks and mouth); all of these must be registered and processed.

The extrapyramidal system is mainly responsible for neural control, which means that chewing and swallowing do not take place under voluntary control, although conscious control can be achieved via the cerebral cortex.

Afferent information is conveyed by means of mechanoreceptors, chemoreceptors, and thermoreceptors. Mechanoreceptors are present in muscles, in the articular capsule, in the mucosa of the mouth, and in the periodontium. Thermoreceptors are located in the mucosa of the mouth and dentinal canals, and chemoreceptors in the taste buds.

The afferent information is transmitted to the cranial nerve centers and so to the CNS by the trigeminal (CN V), facial (CN VII), glossopharyngeal (CN IX), and vagus (CN X) nerves. On reaching the CNS this information is passed to the thalamus in the diencephalon or to the masticatory center (probably in the pons). In the thalamus impulses are directed as appropriate to the extrapyramidal system, basal ganglia, or cerebral cortex on the basis of the afferent information from the sensory organs.

From the basal ganglia, the efferent stimuli pass via the red nucleus to the origins of cranial nerves V, VII, IX, X, and XII and spinal nuclei of the first three cervical nerves, which regulate and control the act of chewing and swallowing.

The process of mastication can be governed consciously in the cerebral cortex. The information passes from the primary somatosensory cortex to the primary motor cortex. From there the stimulus can be transmitted by way of the corticospinal tract to the origins of the cranial nerves already mentioned, and of the cervical nerves, and on to the structures involved in mastication.

2.3 The mandible as metamorphic reflection of the lower limb

The two evident design principles in the function of the lower limbs[371] are the use of arches as a means of support to the upright body, and of angled levers for locomotion. Rohen sees these functions of the lower limbs as having their metamorphic equivalents in the dynamics of the mandible. In the case of the lower limbs, it is only for dynamic reasons that both sides are required to work functionally together (in this the legs and arms differ). In the case of the mandible, this cooperation is complete in that both halves fuse to form a single bone during embryonic development.

The architecture of the mandible, the arch, with its alveolar and coronoid (muscle) processes, is metaphorically equivalent to the supporting and load-bearing arch structures of the lower limbs.

These mandibular structures are, however, mainly responsible for the work of mastication. Rohen sees this work as the beginning of the digestive process, expressing the "dissolution of an object in space" in contrast to the function of the lower limbs, which is characterized more by the act of "integration into three-dimensional space."

The principle of the angled lever, too, which is important for locomotion, can be seen in the mandible on account of its unmistakable angled shape and the condylar process that connects it to the TMJ. Here the relationships are reversed, according to Rohen, in that the human TMJ is largely relieved of mechanical stress during chewing by the extended length of the angled lever. This gives us a relatively freely movable temporomandibular joint, combined with a kind of physiological dislocation on wide opening of the mouth, while further movement combinations of the joint are made possible by the disk.

The remarkable angled construction of the mandible therefore releases it from three-dimensional space, quite unlike the lower limbs. The movable joint of the human jaw, relieved as it is of stress, in combination with the development of an arched palate, continuous row of teeth, mobile tongue, and lowered position of the larynx, also provides the basis for the development of language. These dynamics can be seen as a kind of anti-movement, in which the development of language serves as a new framing of the powers with which we shape physical space.

2.4 Phylogenetic and ontogenetic influences on the development of the jaw

2.4.1 Phylogenesis

The development toward upright gait produced certain structural changes in the body, including the development of the clavicle, the use of the upper limbs in place of the jaw for defense and for grasping objects, and the development of the mouth and laryngeal region to become a highly specialized organ of speech.

For Delattre and Fenart, the most important change in the skull in the development of human beings was the posterior rotation of the occiput.[96] This completely alters the intracranial volume and leads to further changes, for example those to the masticatory apparatus:

- The extension of the pterygoid processes.
- The increase in height of the maxillae and rami of the mandible, combined with a lowering of the hard palate and horizontal body of the mandible.
- The reinforcement of the nasal spine of the maxilla and the mandibular symphysis, with a retreat of the alveolar parts (superior and inferior) relative to the maxilla and mandible.
- The outward and downward rotation of the external petrous (mastoid) part.[96]
- The gliding hinge movement of the TMJ is only found in humans.

2.4.2 Embryology of the mandible and temporomandibular joint

The temporomandibular joint in human beings is a recent development in their history.[57] In this they are unlike primitive vertebrates, in which the posterior and anterior parts of the first branchial arch connect in the primary jaw (differentiating to form the malleus–incus joint). In humans, however, the mandible connects with the temporal bone.[425,265]

The mandible develops from mesenchymal tissue, around Meckel's cartilage (cartilage of the first branchial arch), by membranous ossification. The maxilla, zygomatic bone, and squamous part of the temporal bone develop by membranous ossification from the mesenchymal maxillary process of the first branchial arch. Movements of the jaw can be detected in the embryo at two months in utero.[112]

The masticatory muscles develop from the somitomeric mesoderm of the mandibular process of the first pharyngeal arch. These are the mylohyoid, digastric (anterior belly), tensor veli palatini, and tensor tympani. The muscles of facial expression (mimetic muscles), digastric (posterior belly), stylohyoid, and stapedius develop from the second pharyngeal arch. The stylopharyngeus develops from the third pharyngeal arch. The muscles of the soft palate (except the tensor palatini), those of the pharynx (except the stylopharyngeus), the cricothyroid, and cricopharyngeus develop from the fourth pharyngeal arch. The infrahyoid (and suboccipital) muscles develop from the cranial somites.

Until the seventh week the face is confined between the growing brain and the bulge of the early heart, leading to the broad embryonic face with its widely spaced eyes and nose and crooked mouth opening. When the embryonic heart and viscera migrate progressively downward with the diaphragm, and the brain ascends as it continues to grow, there is at last room for the face to elongate (Figure 2.26).

Regions of growth

The development of the craniofacial structures can be traced back to three functional mechanisms:[202:15]

- Increase in size: by appositional growth at periosteal (outer) and endosteal (inner) surfaces.
- Bone remodeling: on the one hand by processes that add to the external cortical bone, and on the other, by processes that remove tissue from the inner cortical bone.
- Repositioning of bones: brought about by divergent movement of neighboring bones, caused by their increase in size, in the region of sutures, synchondroses, and condyles. In this category we can distinguish primary repositioning (together with growth of the bone itself) and secondary repositioning (taking effect from a distance, due to expansive forces from non-neighboring bones and soft tissue).

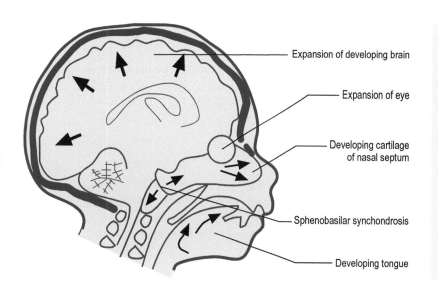

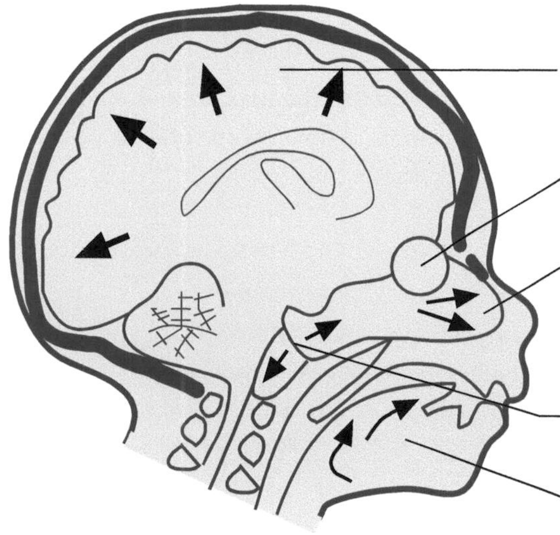

Figure 2.26
Influences on the growth of the skull: effect on the growth of the maxillary complex of the downward and anteriorly directed force associated with growth of the nasal septum

The control of bone growth lies in the soft tissue, which operates as a functional matrix. Certain growth centers are particularly active regions of growth: the sutures, maxillary tuberosities, alveolar processes, and synchondroses.[202:17ff.] Particular attention should be paid to these regions when treating children. Growth of the maxillae is dependent on the growth of the maxillary sutures, and these can only actively contribute to this as growth centers until the fourth year of life. Their closure is functionally dependent. The synchondroses play a significant role, as they are primary growth centers for the jaw. The sphenobasilar synchondrosis (SBS) is the most important of these, and remains active for longest.

Growth movements and factors affecting the growth of the lower third of the face

- Growth of the ramus posteriorly and superiorly (Figure 2.27). *Explanation*: bone formation in the condyles of the mandible.
- Overall downward and anterior repositioning of the mandible. *Explanation*: growth of the ramus in a posterior and superior direction in relation to the cranial base.
- Posterior separation of the two halves of the body of the mandible (Figure 2.28). *Explanation*: posterior growth of the condylar heads.

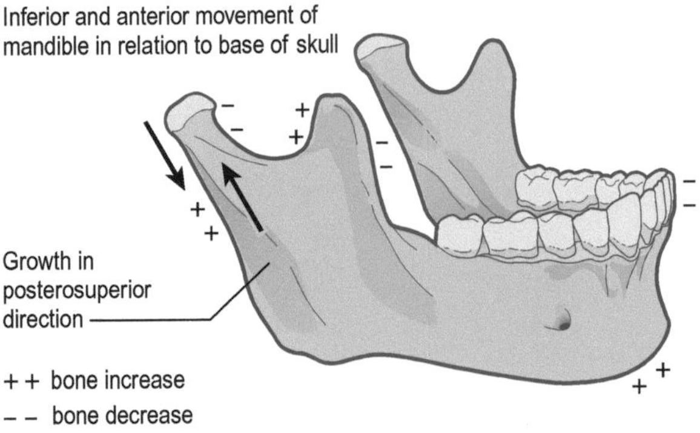

Figure 2.27
Growth movement of the mandible

Further factors involved in the growth of the mandible

- The mandibular nerve is the first structure to form in the mandibular region. It probably induces the formation of the bulge of the early mandible from a membranous thickening of the ectomesenchyme (mesectoderm). In the sixth week an ossification center for each half of the mandible is formed (near the bifurcation of the inferior alveolar nerve and artery). Ossification proceeds along the alveolar nerve and its branches, and the cartilage of the branchial arch almost completely disappears (Figure 2.29).
- The transformation of woven bone into lamellated bone takes place at an earlier stage in the mandible than in other bones in response to the fetus's early swallowing and sucking activity (fifth month in utero).

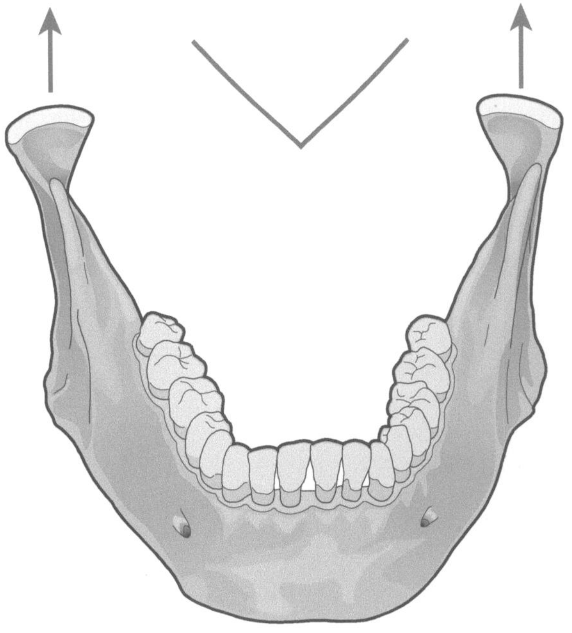

Figure 2.28
Lateral expansion of the ramus of the mandible.
[Liem, T., Schleupen, A., Altmeyer, P., Zweedijk, R. (ed.) (2012) *Osteopathische Behandlung von Kindern*, 2nd ed. Stuttgart: Haug]

- In the 12th week in utero, secondary cartilage appears, independently of the pharyngeal arch cartilage, as precursors to part of the condylar process, for the head of the mandible and the mental protuberance. The secondary cartilage of the condyle is replaced by bone, but the upper part remains as articular cartilage and as a growth center. This growth center is of particular importance for the further shaping of the mandible.
- The activity of the lateral pterygoid muscle regulates the development of the condylar process.[347]
- The activity of the temporalis muscle influences the development of the coronoid process.
- The activity of the masseter and pterygoid muscles influences the development of the angle and ramus of the mandible.
- The primordial teeth form the basis for the development of the alveolar part.

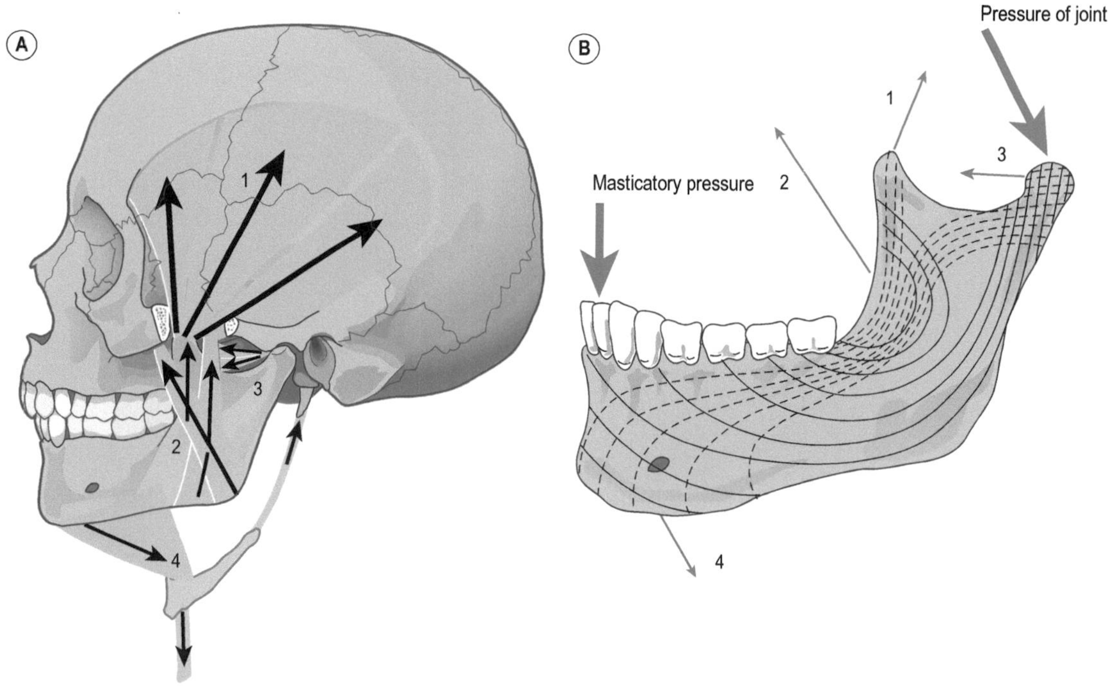

Figure 2.29
Effects of forces on mandibular growth and course of trajectories. Dotted lines: trajectories of pull. Solid lines: pressure trajectories.
A Effects of forces on mandibular growth. **1** Superior and posterior pull of temporalis. **2** Superiorly and anteriorly directed force of masseter and medial pterygoid. **3** Inferior and anterior pull of the lateral pterygoid in interaction with the temporalis (posterior part). **4** Directions of force of the suprahyoid and infrahyoid muscles.
B Effect of forces on course of trajectories. **1** Superior and posterior pull of temporalis. **2** Superior and anterior direction of force of the masseter and medial pterygoid muscles. **3** Inferior and anterior pull of the lateral pterygoid in interaction with the temporalis (posterior part). **4** Directions of force of the suprahyoid and infrahyoid muscles. Dotted lines: trajectories of pull. Solid lines: pressure trajectories. (Liem, T., Schleupen, A., Altmeye, P., Zweedijk, R. (ed.) (2012) *Osteopathische Behandlung von Kindern*, 2nd ed. Stuttgart: Haug)

- Vertical movement of the teeth.
- The growth and movement of the tongue also affect the development of the maxillae.

Cartilaginous growth of the mandibular head

The type of growth undergone by this cartilage is unlike normal cartilaginous growth by interstitial cartilage cell division. Cartilage cells are present which divide very little but do produce important ground substance and fibers. The secondary cartilage develops from the mesenchyme, as does the secondary mandible. Like the mandible, it is covered with a layer of connective tissue. Cartilage cells differentiate from this connective tissue layer, subsequently leaving the layer and forming the cartilage of the mandibular head. In a sense this process corresponds to the growth of bone that occurs on the surface, the periosteum (appositional bone growth), rather than by interstitial cell division. Consequently the head of the mandible reacts like any cartilage and yet also has properties of bone.

Growth of the temporal joint components

The ossification center of the squamous part (with the zygomatic process) appears in the neurocranium when the embryo is 30 mm long. Membranous ossification begins when it reaches a length of 35 mm. The zygomatic process of the temporal bone appears and extends anteriorly. The mandibular fossa is formed medially.

Synchronicity of ossification

When an embryo reaches a length of 28 mm (vertex–coccyx) the ossification centers of the zygomatic bone, squamous part, and ramus of the mandible appear, along with the masseter muscle.[86,112,294,328]

The tooth-bearing parts of the bone, the alveolar process of the maxilla and alveolar part of the mandible, begin membranous ossification at the same stage of embryonic growth (around the 40th day in utero). The premaxilla appears around the 45th day.

The ossification centers of what will become the greater wing, pterygoid process of the sphenoid, condylar process, and pyramidal process of the palatine bone appear when the embryo reaches 40 mm, along with the temporalis and the medial and lateral pterygoid muscles.

Although the origin and ossification of the condylar process and the temporal joint surface differ, ossification of both begins around the same time and same place. This synchronous ossification also reflects the functional destiny and design of these structures.[86]

2.4.3 Postnatal development of the cranium

Around the fifth to sixth year (girls slightly earlier than boys) the "sixth year" molar appears. (This is the first molar of the second dentition to erupt behind the deciduous molars.) It is at this time that growth dominance transfers from the neurocranium to the viscerocranium. The neurocranium ceases to grow in the eighth year. The viscerocranium grows, shifting inferiorly by translation of the upper and lower jaw.

2.4.4 The capsule, disk, and muscle complex

In the course of ontogenesis the tissue of the first branchial arch—which is to become the capsule, disk, and muscle complex—develops between the ossification centers of the mandible and the temporal bone. The unity of tissue is apparent not only during the embryonic stage, but also during childhood and adulthood.[83,84,85,94]

Phylogenetically, the masticatory muscles form anteriorly on the blastema. Fibers of the lateral pterygoid, temporalis, and masseter muscles attach to capsule and disk.

In the newborn the masticatory apparatus is sufficiently mature to enable sucking. In the adult the complex of capsule, disk, and muscle has adapted to the mechanical demands of the form of nutrition.

Histologically the disk corresponds to the surface of the TMJ. The connective tissue fibers of the capsule run parallel and in continuity with the fibers of the disk, and with the tissue covering the articular surfaces.

NOTE An understanding of the functional, structural, and dynamic unity of the capsule, disk, and muscle complex and the bony parts of the TMJ is of key importance when treating disturbances of the masticatory system.

2.4.5 The influence of mandibular growth on disturbances of the TMJ, facial growth, and craniocervical balance

As described above, the growth of the mandible plays an important role in the development of the face. Both genetic and epigenetic factors govern the growth of the mandibular head. Biomechanical factors play a large role.

Dibbets showed that in objectively established symptoms of a craniomandibular dysfunction (CMD) (this volume, section 2.5), no morphological changes or disorders of growth of the jaw are found. However, subjective symptoms of CMD are often associated with changes in the shape of the jaw: with a blunter shape for the angle of the mandible or a deeper location of the TMJ.[100:104ff.]

The head of the mandible normally grows quickly, but if this is retarded, compensation immediately takes place in the form of heightened appositional bone growth activity, which is normally slower. Dibbets demonstrated that this process is not sufficient to compensate completely, resulting in disorders.[100] The mandible is no longer able to perform its functions of support for the adjacent tissues at the right time. These include support to the teeth, the functional relationship of the upper and lower teeth, as a relay point for the masticatory and hyoid muscles, holding open the digestive and respiratory tracts. The consequence is that the adjacent parts adapt more than normally to the mandible, leading to altered growth of the middle part of the face, altered craniocervical balance (muscular and in terms of growth), and the emergence of CMD.

Displacement of the respiratory tract alters the growth of the face, and produces an elongated profile, open mouth, and retruding mandible.[100:104ff.,268] To this is added an anteverted posture of the head and neck and extension of the head, so as to ease breathing.[388:77ff.]

A prominent chin leads to backward tilting of the head (the process is the reverse of the retruding chin). It has been shown that the backwardly tilted head position was associated with altered growth of the head and mandible.[422]

2.5 Craniomandibular dysfunction

Craniomandibular dysfunction (CMD) is a multifactorial disease.[312] It is ultimately the sum of causative factors and their interaction that leads to the emergence of symptoms. CMD as an overall concept comprises various different elements: the TMJ, the masticatory muscles, and associated tissues (such as ligaments and connective tissue structures), which can cause pain, restricted movement, or joint sounds on movement of the TMJ.

Antczak-Boukoms's[12] review of the literature between 1980 and 1992 finds more than 4000 instances of temporomandibular disorder. There is no agreed single definition of this concept in the literature.

2.5.1 Epidemiology

The following is a summary of an overview by Fernández-de-las-Peñas and Svensson[123] of the epidemiology of myofascial CMD.

The occurrence of a craniomandibular syndrome is common and widespread.[64,80,199,260,280] Its prevalence in the western population is between 3% and over 40%,[64,260] with an incidence rate of 2–4%.[260] Women between the ages of 20 and 45 years are particularly affected.[386]

The reported figures for prevalence in the studies show a wide variance, which may be due to any of a number of causes: different study methods, variation in the criteria used (indicating symptoms, number and type of symptoms), genetic variation in different countries, differences of dental health/hygiene, different dietary habits, age, and other social factors.[64,327]

Myofascial CMD pain appears to be the most common diagnosis, at 42%, in patients with orofacial pain (single or repeated diagnosis). Disk dislocation with reduction follows, at 32.1%, followed by arthralgia (30.5%).[354]

A meta-analysis looking at orofacial pain produced an overall prevalence for myofascial CMD pain of 45.3% and, for disk dislocation, of 41.1%.[286] Syndromes related to whiplash injury[293] and gastroesophageal reflux[152] predispose to developing myofascial CMD. Comorbidities with myofascial CMD are common. This is one of the reasons for the lack of agreement over prognosis.

2.5.2 Comorbidities and relation to other systems of the body

Following a narrative review by Landzberg et al.,[248] a connection was demonstrated between temporomandibular disorder (TMD) and **whiplash injury**.

Instances of TMD where **sleep bruxism** is assumed are frequent: Yeler[480] found 52% of mild cases, 33% moderate, and 11% pronounced. Unilateral chewing appears to be a factor for the development of sleep bruxism and TMD.[480] If bruxism occurs both during sleep and during the day, this increases the risk of temporomandibular pain. Account should also be taken of concomitant factors.[36]

Symptoms of TMD occur more frequently in patients who suffer from **migraine**, episodic **tension headache**, or chronic daily **headache**.[157] Up-to-date studies have confirmed this. TMD symptoms are associated with migraine.[132] A combination of TMD and headache occurs in patients with severe TMD due to central pain processing, and in 29.3% of cases.[456] There is a higher prevalence of systemic disease and nonspecific physical symptoms in patients with painful TMD and migraine.[81]

Patients with **irritable bowel syndrome** show a three-fold increased risk of developing TMD compared with healthy study participants.[143]

Amongst TMD patients there is an increased prevalence of **pain** in other regions of the body, especially the knee joint, but also the shoulder, hip, wrist, and elbow.[43]

Patients with **tinnitus** report pain in the cervical spine more frequently than those without tinnitus.[46] In contrast to the results of earlier individual studies, there appears to be no strong evidence for any association between TMD and tinnitus.[46] Different positions of the joint relative to the cervical spine did produce a reduction in loudness of the tinnitus. Somatosensory associations are thought to play a central role in patients with tinnitus whose hearing is not greatly reduced and whose previous history of TMD or problems at the nape of the neck is positive.[360]

Existing cervical spine symptoms are often accompanied by TMD. Treatment of the TMD brought improved range of motion and reduced pain in the cervical region.[459] The craniomandibular system was also found to influence body balance.[160] Intervertebral disk disorders in the lumbar region are thought to affect the movement of the mandible (maximum mouth opening and speed of movement).[423]

2.5.3 Clinical features

In 1934, Costen described a set of symptoms which he linked with malfunction of the TMJ. Costen's syndrome, as it is known, involves otological symptoms such as loss of hearing, dizziness, tinnitus, otalgia (usually due to altered pressure equalization between the internal and middle ear), restriction of the jaw, preauricular pain, burning sensation of the tongue, and globus sensation.[82]

In 1968, Schwarz grouped together the involvement of all the structures of the masticatory system together with psychological factors in the development of increased muscular tension; he termed this concept temporomandibular joint pain dysfunction syndrome.[395]

Hülse[184] describes the situation where disturbances of the afferent nerves from the temporomandibular joint and associated muscles can affect the regulation of body balance and can therefore be associated with a number of symptoms (Volume 2, section 6.2).

Laskin introduced the concept of myofascial pain dysfunction syndrome, which he used to denote unilateral TMJ symptoms with painless palpation of the TMJ and after excluding radiological changes.[252]

The present book combines the definition of TMJ dysfunction given by Solberg (1982) and De Boever and van Steenberghe (1988) and the definition of CMD given by Dibbets.[100:99,475:341] This definition provides no information on the affected structures (myogenic, arthrogenous, occlusal, neurogenous, ligamentous, etc.) and the underlying causes (this volume, Chapter 3).

CMD is not an isolated condition. In simple terms it can be said to be due to a disturbance of the temporomandibular joint, the masticatory muscles, and/or occlusion and associated neighboring structures (also more distant structures such as the lower limbs). In the majority of cases of CMD, the cause involves myogenic disturbances.

Diagnostic criteria laid down by the International Headache Society state that at least one of the following criteria must apply in order to demonstrate that head pain is due to disorders of the TMJ:[192]

- The pain is precipitated by jaw movements and/or chewing of hard or tough food.
- Reduced range of, or irregular, jaw opening.
- Noise from one or both TMJ during jaw movements.
- Tenderness of the joint capsule(s) of one or both TMJs.

Possible **clinical signs** of myofascial CMD are deviations or deflection during mouth opening and closing,[353] tenderness to pressure, or pain on palpation of the muscle structures, especially the masticatory muscles,[125] and restriction/limitation of mouth opening, parafunctions, and clenching the teeth, the last of these often associated with arthralgia.[353]

FURTHER INFORMATION Muscle pain is often concentrated in the region of the masseter (in females, in the lateral part of the muscle and in the eye region), spreading to the temporalis.[8,125] Pain in the masticatory muscles can potentially also be traced to mechanisms causing sensitization and the presence of trigger points.[125]

The main symptoms of oromandibular dysfunctions are clenching the teeth, bruxism, and irregular opening and closing movements of the jaw.[198]

Tip for practitioners

Craniomandibular dysfunction (CMD) is said to exist if one or more of the following symptoms are present:

- Subjective symptoms (reported by the patient): **pain and sensitivity** in the region of the masticatory muscles and TMJ at rest, on chewing, and on biting; **clicking, crepitation,** and **restriction of movement** (or deviation) of the TMJ.
- Objective signs (observed by the examiner): **palpation of clicking and crepitation** and observation of **movement restriction** ("blockages")[39] and **abnormal movement patterns** of the TMJ.
- Abnormal shape and position of the mandibular head on a radiograph performed for the purpose.

From the pathophysiological point of view, many factors may be simultaneously at work. Parafunctions, neuromuscular, central, and peripheral neural sensitization, myofascial and skeletal influences, the form and position of the condyle, occlusion, and psychological factors or stress are important **etiological factors** of CMD. Other factors to consider are sutures, dural folds, venolymphatic, arterial, and ascending and descending chains ("continuities"). (See this volume, sections 2.5.4 and 2.6; and Figure 2.65.)

2.5.4 The temporomandibular joint and body posture

There is a close interrelationship between body posture and the function and structure of the temporomandibular joint, and myofascial tone of the masticatory and hyoid muscles (see also Figure 2.49).[145:96] The effect of body posture on the masticatory system in the course of human development, with the development of upright posture and of the cerebrum, has already been described.

It is important to take comprehensive account of body posture—looking at the entirety of the body—when treating oromandibular dysfunctions, since ascending chains can directly affect occlusion. This includes dysfunctions of the lower limbs, e.g., of the sacroiliac joint, hip, and foot; footwear can also play a part.

Posture of the head

The most common faulty posture found is anterior translation of the head. This can be either the result or the cause of various disturbances.

Translation of the head is accompanied by a decrease in lordosis at the middle cervical spine and increased kyphosis of the upper thoracic spine (this volume, section 2.5.4).

CMD is linked with anterior shifting of the head, which considerably increases the load on the cervical and lumbar spine (Figure 2.40). The resulting force of compression can lead to the compression of nerves.[61, cited in 334]

Chain of dysfunction Shortening of the cervical extensors → excessive stretching and weakness, as well as deficits of motor control, of the cervical flexors. This is especially the case in chronic or mechanically caused neck pain,[115,408] especially involving the longus colli and infrahyoid muscles → displacement of the hyoid.

Littlejohn model

Littlejohn described a gravity line linking the symphysis of the mandible with the pubic symphysis (Figure 2.30).[463] He also identified functional triangles in the body that establish an interrelationship between the TMJ and other body structures (Figure 2.31). The polygon of forces is made up of several lines of force:

- **Descending anteroposterior gravity line**
  - **Course:** from the anterior border of the foramen magnum through the body of T11 and T12 and the articulations of L4/L5 to the tip of the coccyx.
  - **Function:** unites the spine into a single functional joint system, centered on T11 and T12.
- **Ascending posteroanterior gravity lines**
  - **Course:** beginning bilaterally at the hip joint, as a result of the pressure of the head of the femur in its articulation with the acetabulum. These lines run anterior to L3 and anterior to T4 to end at the posterior border of the foramen magnum.
  - **Function:** reinforces support for the organs of the pelvis and abdomen; directs the forces at the atlanto-occipital joint to T2 and the second rib. The double line removes stress from L3 by directing tensions toward the head of the femur.

Polygon of forces These lines of force cross to form two triangles, balanced one above the other. L3 acts as the center of gravity, while T4 is the crossing point of all the functional lines and the balance point between the upper and lower triangle. These vertebrae play a special role in the static balance of the body.

Function The triangles support the vertebral column and organs. The upper triangle contains the joint structures with links to the foramen magnum,

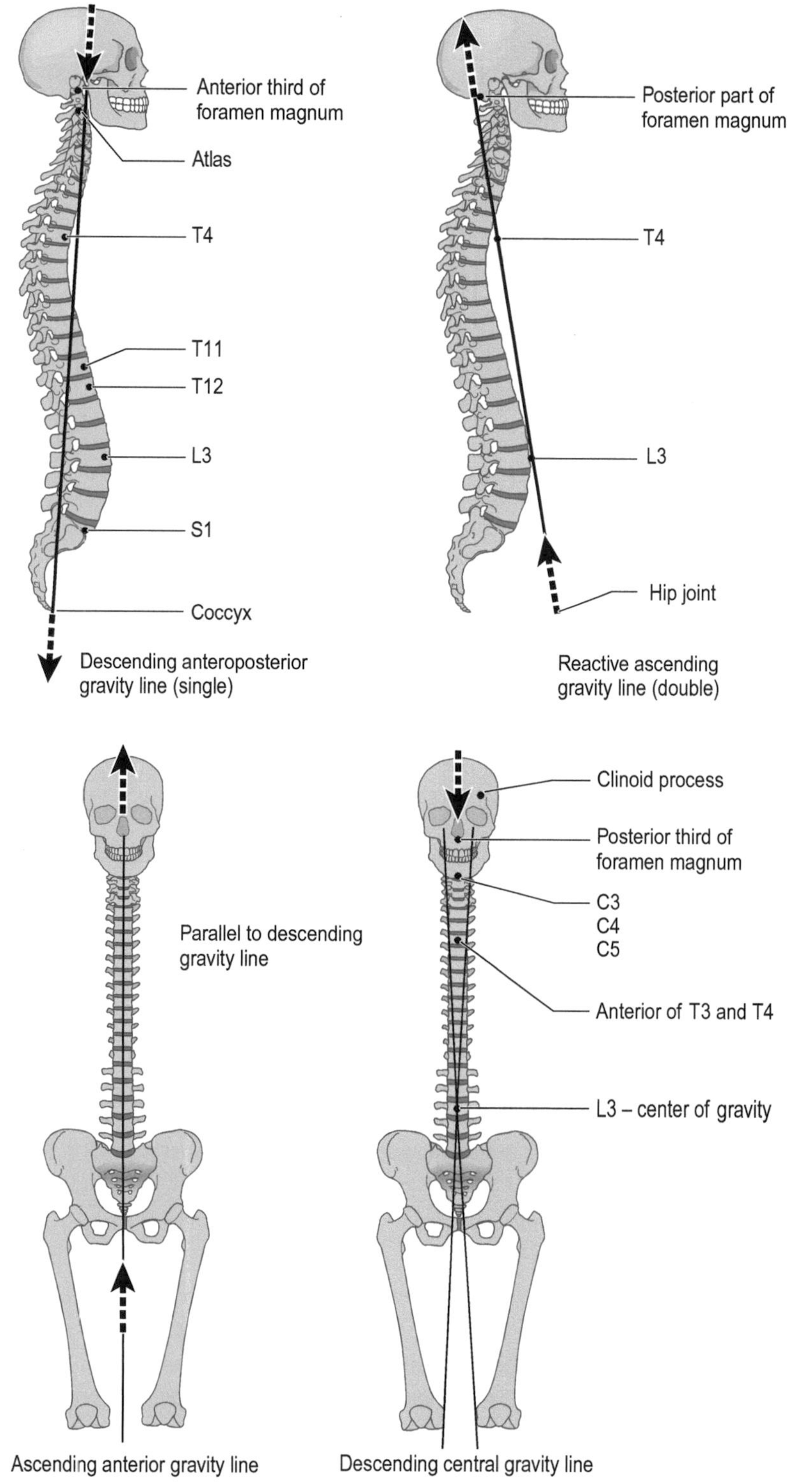
Anterior third of foramen magnum
Atlas
T4
T11
T12
L3
S1
Coccyx
Descending anteroposterior gravity line (single)
Posterior part of foramen magnum
T4
L3
Hip joint
Reactive ascending gravity line (double)
Parallel to descending gravity line
Ascending anterior gravity line
Clinoid process
Posterior third of foramen magnum
C3
C4
C5
Anterior of T3 and T4
L3 – center of gravity
Descending central gravity line

Figure 2.30
Gravity lines

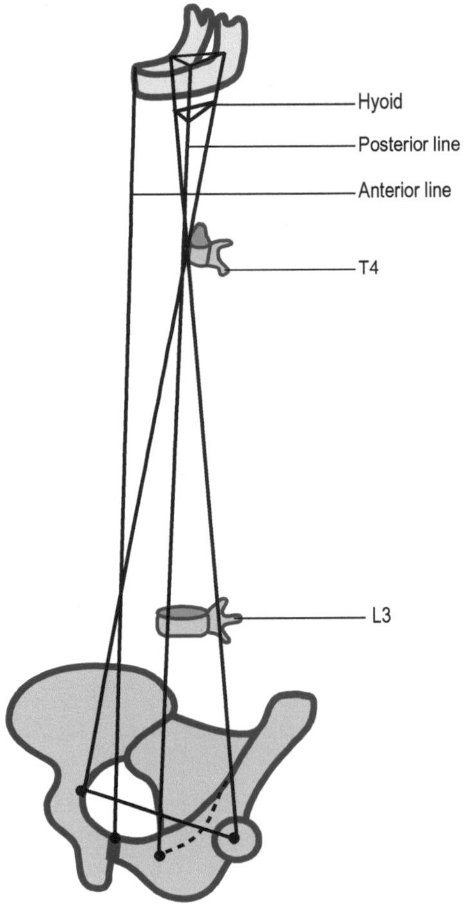

Figure 2.31
Polygon of forces acting on the spine, according to Littlejohn

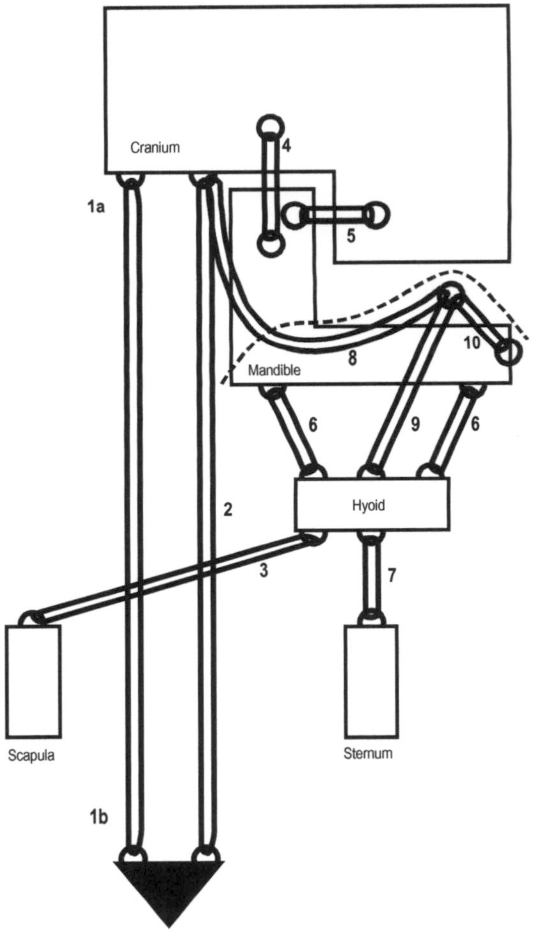

Figure 2.32
Samoian model, modified. **1a** Nuchal muscles. **1b** Muscles of the back. **2** Prevertebral muscles. **3** Omohyoid. **4** Temporalis, masseter, and medial pterygoid. **5** Lateral pterygoid. **6** Suprahyoid muscles. **7** Infrahyoid muscles. **8** Muscles of the tongue (styloglossus) that move tongue posteriorly and superiorly. **9** Hyoglossus and chondroglossus: lower and retract tongue. **10** Genioglossus

providing a base for the skull, which is balanced on T4. Effects of rotation of the skull are felt down as far as T4. Any imbalance in the hyoid and its muscles affects the function of the upper triangle. The lower triangle helps maintain abdominal function by transmitting the rhythmic activity of the thorax. Normal posture of the pelvis (base of triangle) is necessary for support of abdominal tension.

- **Ascending anterior gravity line**
  - **Course:** parallel to the descending gravity line.
  - **Function:** links the symphysis of the mandible with the symphysis pubis.
- **Descending central gravity lines**
  - **Course:** from the vertex, passing posterior to the clinoid processes, posterior third of the foramen magnum, transverse processes

of C3–C6, anterior to T3 and T4, past the lower border of the third rib, body of L1–L4, and inside of the knee, to the feet.

- **Function:** L3 is the center of gravity of the body.

Samoian model, modified

Robert Samoian produced a model to demonstrate the integration of the TMJ in vertical body posture (Figure 2.32).

Additional models and theories

- Functional links also exist with the falx cerebri, falx cerebelli, and tentorium cerebelli, the nuchal muscles, and vertebral column[21:28] (see also Figure 2.33). Delaire[95] states that the intracranial structures serve to transmit the balance of forces between the weight of the viscerocranium and the compensating tone of the nuchal muscles, although this hypothesis is the subject of controversy.[127] The function of the temporomandibular joint and the bite configurations of the upper and lower jaw are dependent on this balance (Figure 2.33; see also Figure 2.15). Incorrect posture should be redressed in order to ensure long-term success of treatment.[231]
- Crooked pelvic posture and unequal leg length affect occlusion to an electromyographically measurable degree.[430]
- Bahnemann[21:28] sees the overwhelming majority of cases of dysgnathia as being due to a spinal syndrome, which can be considered to be a "gnatho-vertebral syndrome."
- Dysfunctions of the cervical spine can exert an effect on the TMJ via the cervical fasciae or the hyoid.
- Mouth breathing usually produces extension of the head according to Lawrence and Razook,[257] to ensure the best airway in the

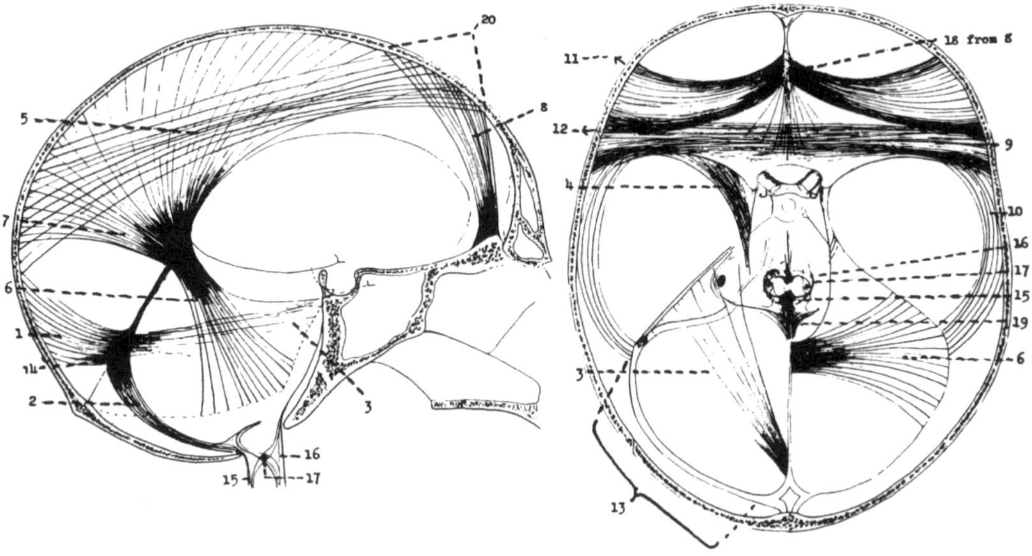

Figure 2.33
Stress fibers of the dura mater. **Horizontal: 1** Falx cerebri inferior. **2** Falx cerebelli. **3** Tentorium cerebelli. **4** Sphenoidal. **5** Falx cerebri superior. **Vertical: 6** Tentorium cerebelli. **7** Falx cerebri posterior. **8** Falx cerebri anterior. **9** Transverse. **Circular: 10** Squamosal. **11** Roof of skull anterior. **12** Roof of skull medial. **13** Roof of skull posterior. **14** Cranial fossa posterior. **15–17** Spinal. (Arbuckle, B. (1994) *The Selected Writings of Beryl E. Arbuckle DO, FACOP.* Indianapolis: American Academy of Osteopathy)

mouth area. The shortening of the nuchal muscles and resulting extension of the head causes accommodative protrusion of the head to maintain the horizontal line of sight. Hypertonicity of the nuchal muscles results. The combination of the forward inclination of the head, neck, and pectoral girdle also leads to backward and downward displacement of the mandible, through the tension of the hyoid muscles. This leads to compression of the condylar process into the joint cavity of the TMJ, and increased tonicity of the masticatory muscles.

- Sidebending with contralateral rotation of the head causes the mandible to shift contralaterally to the direction of sidebending, as in congenital torticollis.[402:377–378]
- Dysfunction of the pectoral girdle can affect the TMJ via the omohyoid muscle to the hyoid bone and via the suprahyoid muscles. Further possible effects of pectoral girdle dysfunctions are to the temporal bone via the sternocleidomastoid muscle and so to the TMJ.[419]

FURTHER INFORMATION According to Schöttl and Broich, the following associations can be found between functional units, on the basis of studies by Haberfellner, Bahnemann, Rocabado, and Treuenfels:[388:95,59]

- Retrusive occlusion (prognathism) and anteflexion of the head (70% of cases according to Rocabado).
- Temporomandibular joint and occipito-atlanto-axial joints: crossbite and raised shoulder.
- Open bite (side) and crooked pelvic posture.
- Head and neck posture and speech.
- Mouth breathing/open bite and lymphatic reaction and digestive tract disturbances.
- Motor function of the tongue and skeletal muscles/total body posture.
- Ear, pupillary, and occlusal planes and spine.
- Temporomandibular joint and hyoid.

The relationship between the functional triangles and the temporomandibular joint

Posterior functional triangles

- **Posterior-superior triangle:** the trapezius (descending part) and the more deeply

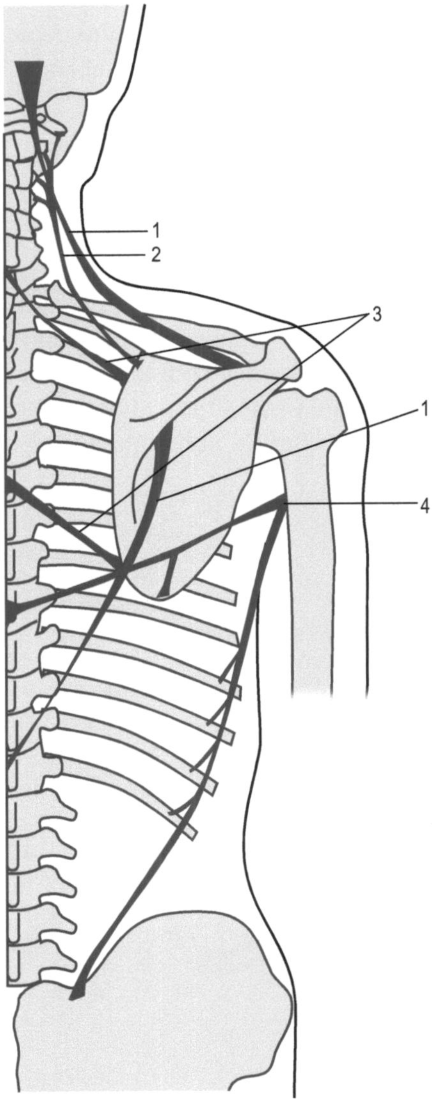

Figure 2.34
Muscles of the posterior functional triangles. **1** Trapezius. **2** Levator scapulae. **3** Rhomboid major and minor. **4** Latissimus dorsi

located cervical muscles link the occiput with the scapula (Figure 2.34).

- **Posterior-inferior triangle:** the trapezius (ascending part) and the deeper-lying pectoral muscles continue to the lumbosacral transition and coccyx. Lateral support is given by the latissimus dorsi (Figure 2.34).

Anterior functional triangles

- **Superior inframandibular triangle:** the digastric (anterior belly), mylohyoid, and geniohyoid muscles link the mandible with the hyoid. The superior inframandibular triangle also incorporates the muscles of the tongue (Figure 2.35).
- **Inferior inframandibular triangle:** the sternocleidomastoid, thyrohyoid, sternohyoid, and sternothyroid muscles link the hyoid and the thyroid cartilage with the sternoclavicular and sternocostal joints (Figure 2.35).
- **Lateral triangle**
    - The digastric muscle links the mastoid with the hyoid and the mandible.
    - The sternocleidomastoid links the occiput and the mastoid with the sternum and clavicle.
    - The stylohyoid muscle links the temporal bone with the hyoid.
    - Further muscles of the neck[265] (Figure 2.36).

Myers describes the TMJ as part of the deep front line,[316] whose function is the balancing of the head and neck on the body, the stabilization of the thorax, support of the lumbar spine, stabilization of the leg segments, and raising the medial arch of the foot.

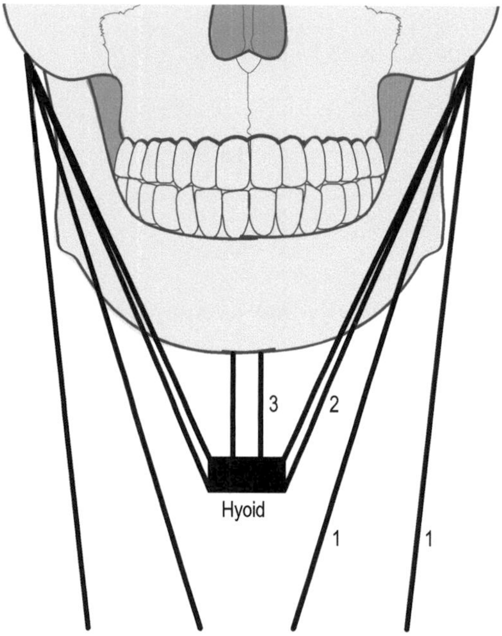

Figure 2.35
Anterior functional triangles. **1** Sternocleidomastoid. **2** Stylohyoid. **3** Digastric

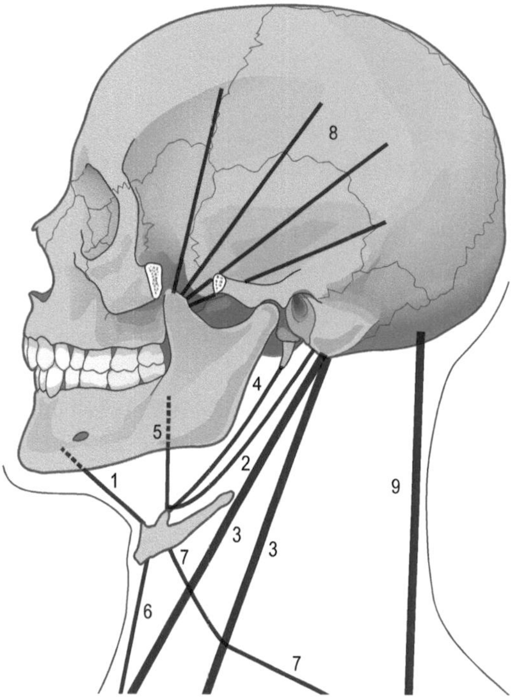

Figure 2.36
Lateral functional triangle. **1** Digastric (anterior belly). **2** Digastric (posterior belly). **3** Sternocleidomastoid. **4** Stylohyoid. **5** Suprahyoid muscles. **6** Infrahyoid muscles. **7** Omohyoid. **8** Temporalis. **9** Muscles of the back

Course of the deep front line in the superior region: cranium → masticatory muscles → mandible → suprahyoid muscles → hyoid → infrahyoid muscles → pretracheal layer of cervical fascia → posterior border of subcostal cartilage, xiphoid process → anterior diaphragm, lumbar part with crura of diaphragm → body of the lumbar vertebrae.

Postural patterns, according to Hall and Wernham

Studying body posture, Hall developed a concept that summarized his findings and presented a scheme of postural patterns. These he subdivided into a ventral and a dorsal postural type. The patterns can be negatively influenced by posture. Seeing lines of gravitational force that had become shifted forward or back, Hall's treatment approach sought to bring these back into better balance.[464,465]

Normal gravity line

The **gravity line** runs from the dens of the axis via the sacral promontory, through the middle of the hip and knee to the calcaneocuboid joint. The gravity line is derived from the combination of forces holding the body upright. The cranium is aligned with the center of the pelvis and the pectoral girdle is aligned with the pelvic girdle (Figure 2.37).

The **central gravity line** runs through the tragus, ventral to the mastoid process, through the promontory, through the greater trochanter, through the middle of the knee joint, and ventral to the lateral malleolus. The starting point for measurement is the tragus.

The **Frankfurt plane** (or auriculo-orbital plane: line between the cranial point of the external acoustic meatus and orbitale) is horizontal.

The **anterior line** runs from the tip of the mental protuberance to the pubic symphysis. It runs parallel to the gravity line and perpendicular to the pubic line, and is the result of thoracic and abdominal tensions. Thoracic and abdominal pressure is normal.

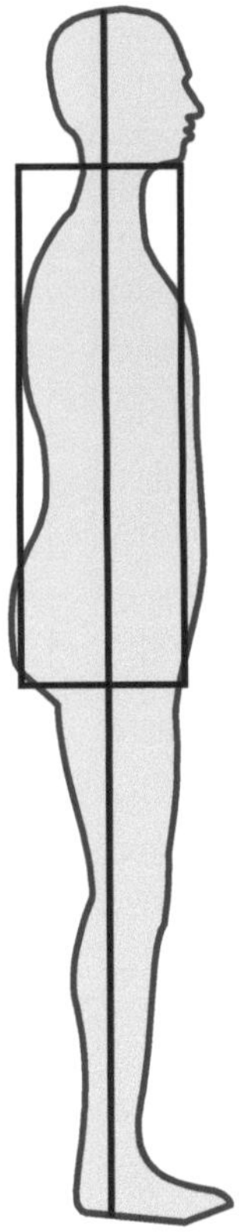

Figure 2.37
Postural pattern according to Hall and Wernham: normal gravity line

Ventral pattern

- Central gravity line: as compared to the normal central gravity line, the greater trochanter and middle of the knee joint lie in a more posterior position. The upper body lies further forward (Figure 2.38).
- Frankfurt plane: runs obliquely in a ventral and cranial direction.
- Anterior line: runs in a caudal and dorsal direction.
- Posterior line: runs in a caudal and dorsal direction.

This postural pattern is linked with a tendency to crural hernia; inguinal hernia; visceral ptosis; bladder irritation.

Dorsal pattern

- Central gravity line: as compared to the normal central gravity line, the greater trochanter, the middle of the knee joint, and the lateral malleolus lie in a more anterior position. The upper body lies more posterior (Figure 2.39).
- Frankfurt plane: runs obliquely in a ventral and caudal direction.
- Anterior line: runs in a caudal and ventral direction.
- Posterior line: runs in a caudal and ventral direction.

This postural pattern is linked with a general enfeebled appearance; tendency to constipation, hemorrhoids, and rectal prolapse (Table 2.1).

Effects of craniomandibular dysfunction on body statics

Craniomandibular dysfunction (CMD) can of course affect body posture and statics, in its turn (Figures 2.41 and 2.42). For example, anterior shifting of the head can be a postural adaptation, secondary to disturbances causing pain on swallowing.[334] The effect of shifting the head forward by 2.5 cm almost doubles the load imposed on the vertebral column. Thus, if the weight of the head is 5.5 kg, the load is increased by about 4.5 kg. Shifting the head forward by 7.5 cm, the weight increase is doubled: a load of 13.5 kg (Figure 2.40).

There is a close connection between the occipitocervical transition zone and the tonicity of the muscles of the neck, and the position and function

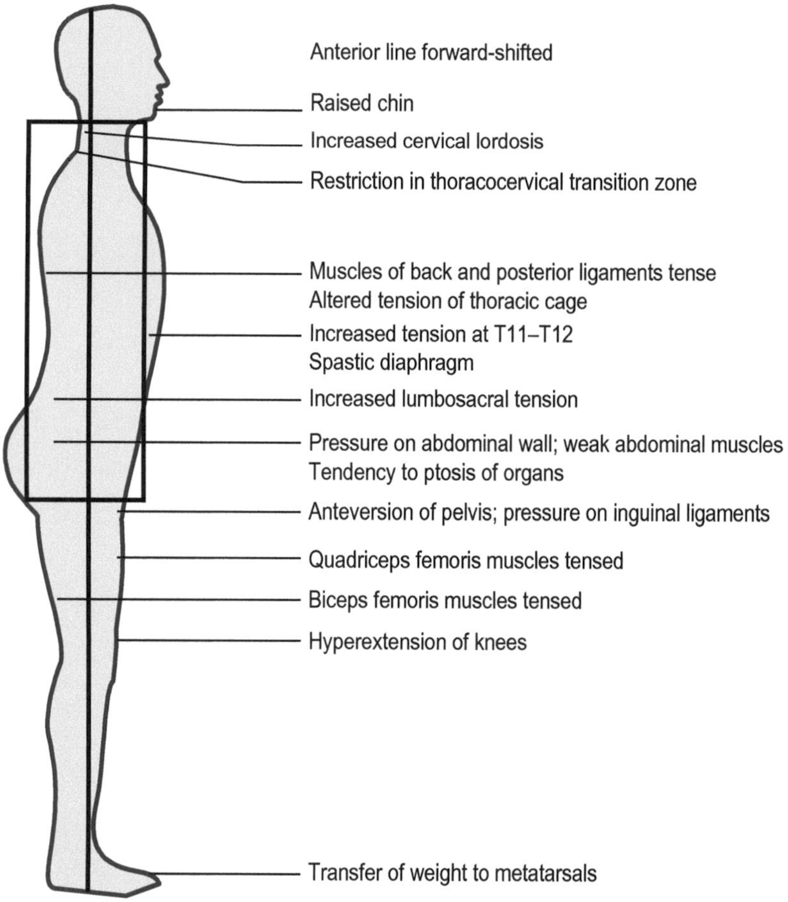

Figure 2.38
Ventral pattern

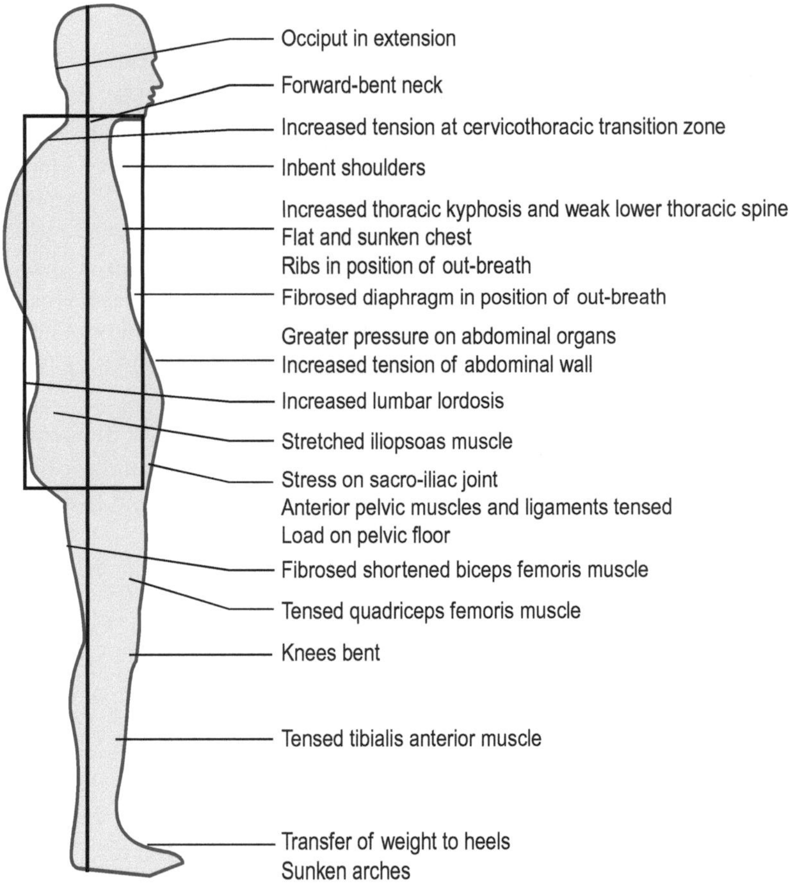

Figure 2.39
Dorsal pattern

Table 2.1 Posture types according to Hall, Wernham, and Littlejohn (Fossum 2002)

Posture type	Ventral (anterior type)	Dorsal (posterior type)
Joint problems	• Increased cervical lordosis* • Restriction in cervicothoracic transition zone • Increased tension of posterior muscles of the back and ligaments • Restriction and increased tension at T11 and T12 (T10–L1) • Increased lumbar lordosis: load on lumbosacral transition zone	• Occiput in extension (and compression) • Reduced lordosis of cervical spine: stress in cervicothoracic transition zone • Increased thoracic kyphosis and weakened lower thoracic spine • Compression of sternocostal joints • Increased lumbar lordosis or flatter lumbar spine**

Continued

Table 2.1 Posture types according to Hall, Wernham, and Littlejohn (Fossum 2002) *Continued*

Posture type	Ventral (anterior type)	Dorsal (posterior type)
	• Pelvis tips forward; sacrum more horizontal • Hyperextension of knee, IR thigh, genu valgum, IR lower leg, valgus position of foot • Weight mainly displaced forward, onto ball of foot • Tendency to shortening of posteromedial chains: calves, ischiocrural and gluteal muscles, thoracolumbar fascia	• Pelvis tips backward; sacrum more vertical • Load on iliosacral joints • Tendency to bend knee, ER thigh, genu varum, ER lower leg, varus position of foot • Weight mainly displaced posteriorly, onto heels
Respiratory-circulatory	• Tensions in diaphragm (often inhalatory) • Weak overstretched abdominal muscles	• Tensions in diaphragm (often in exhalation) • Disturbed pressure relationships between abdominal and thoracic cavities • Increased tension of abdominal wall
Visceral	• Tendency to ptosis of organs • Reduced tension of parietal peritoneum • Tendency to hernias and irritation in the lesser pelvis	• Increased pressure on abdominal and pelvic organs • Tendency to circulatory disorders • Tendency to respiratory problems • Tendency to obstipation

IR, internal rotation; ER, external rotation.

* Supine patients whose chin is lying cranially displaced. In the anterior type, cervical lordosis usually increases over the course of the person's life.

** A flattened lumbar spine can be accompanied by increased tendency to shift body weight backward (as seen in individuals who are pregnant).

of the temporomandibular joint. The head is involuntarily held in the position that ensures the best occlusion of the teeth. Bahnemann[21:28] was almost always able to demonstrate changes in spinal posture in cases of malpositioning of the jaw. It is very important in this connection that not only the masticatory muscles in the wider sense, but also the specialized muscles of mastication, can be used to stabilize the head[388:106] (see also this volume, section 2.6.1 on dysfunction of the cervical spine).

In cases of prognathism (projection of the mandible), or of extreme open bite, what is termed inferior position of the atlas is found with a frequency of 30%. The suggested cause is the frequent inflammation of the nasopharyngeal region found with this dysfunction of the jaw, because of the proximity to the atlas.[444:119f.] This corresponds to the extension position of the occiput (occipital condyles located anteriorly on the atlas). In this position the posterior arch of the atlas is approximated to the occiput.

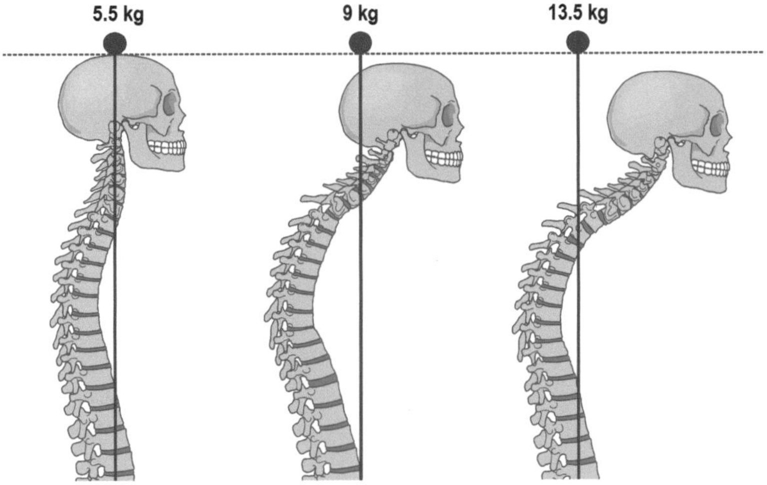

Figure 2.40
Increase in load on vertebral column from weight of head when anteriorly shifted

Sequelae

- Ligament strain between the anterior arch of the atlas and the dens axis, which is common, can impinge on the space of the cerebrospinal fluid in the subarachnoid space, at the level of the second cervical vertebra.[444:119f.]
- The vertebral arteries (supplying the cerebellum and brainstem), the meninges of the brain and spinal cord, spinal cord, medulla oblongata and adjacent cranial nerve nuclei, the hypoglossal nerve (CN XII), superior cervical ganglion, and vagus nerve (CN X) can be compromised.

Clinical presentation Disturbances to speech and swallowing, or to movement of the tongue, dizziness, headache, autonomic symptoms.[59:34]

Effect of mandibular position on the cervicothoracic transition zone

See Figure 2.41.

- Class I Abnormal position of teeth with neutral occlusion.
- Class II Maxillary prognathism (retrusive/distal occlusion).
- Class II/1 With proclined upper front teeth ("buck teeth").
- Class II/2 With deep overbite of upper front teeth.
- Class III Mandibular prognathism (progenism) (protrusive/mesial occlusion).

2.5.5 Postural signs of craniomandibular dysfunction

Signs that may indicate involvement of the jaw include a positive Dorrance test or deviation/deflection of mouth opening.

Methodology of postural testing

- General findings.
- Test using two scales.
- Barre's vertical alignment test.

General findings

- Differently raised eyebrows.
- Crooked posture of the head.
- Unilaterally raised clavicle.
- Lateral deviation of tip of chin.
- Facial asymmetries.
- In the case of ipsilateral CMD: sidebending in the atlanto-occipital joint and secondary compensation of the atlantoaxial joint.

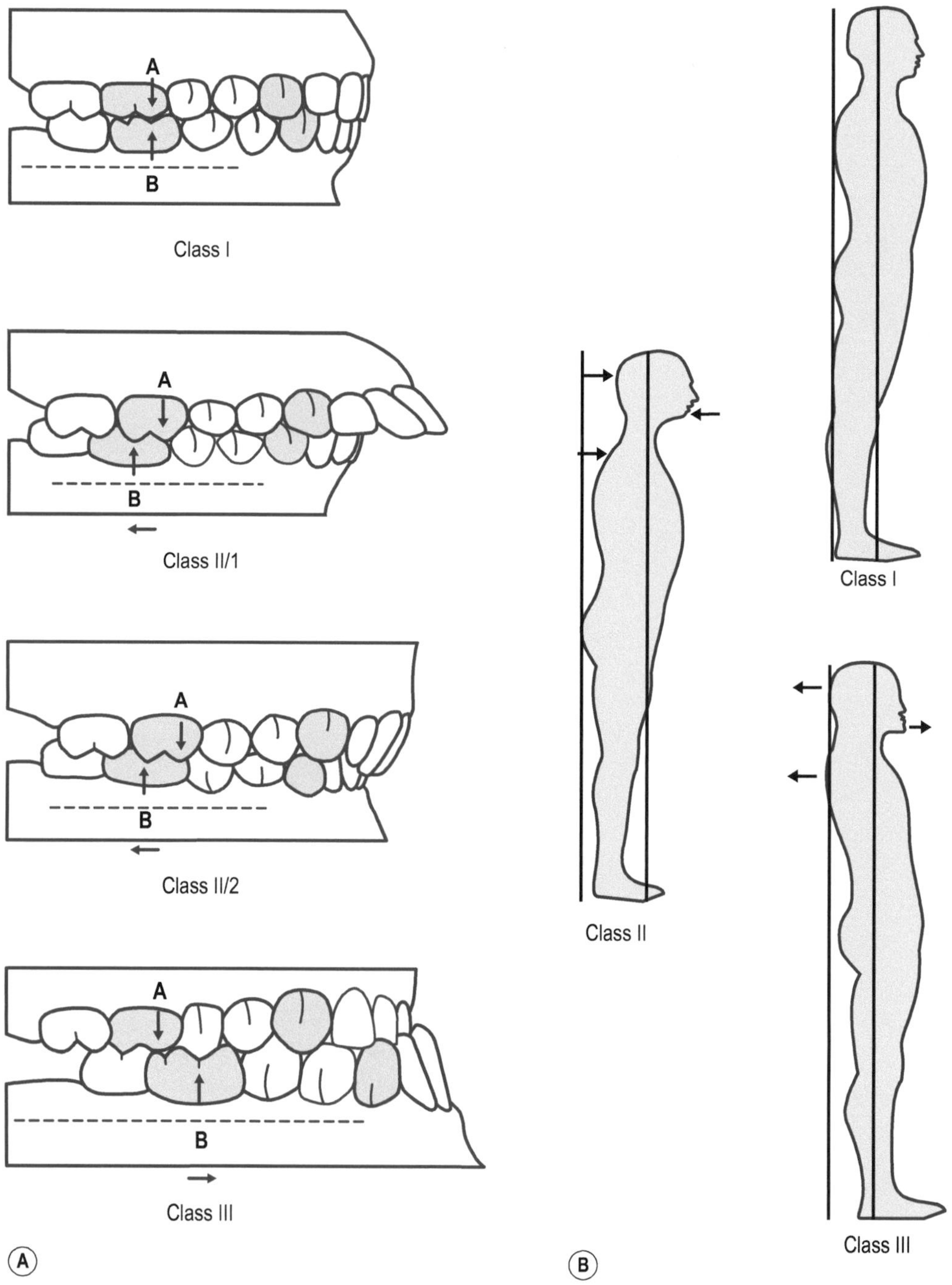

Figure 2.41
Effect of mandibular position on the cervicothoracic transition zone

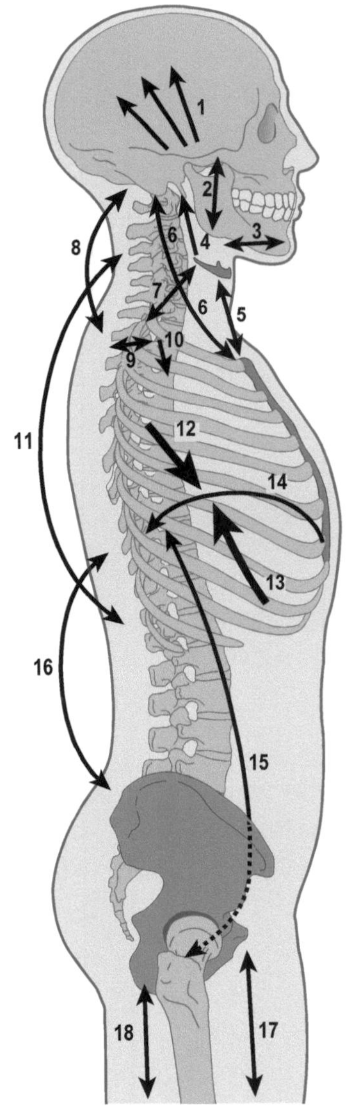

Figure 2.42
Myofascial interaction between TMJ and body.
1 Temporalis. **2** Masseter. **3** Suprahyoid muscles. **4** Stylohyoid; digastric (posterior belly). **5** Infrahyoid muscles. **6** Sternocleidomastoid. **7** Omohyoid. **8** Cervical muscles (posterior and anterior). **9** Infraspinatus/supraspinatus. **10** Biceps brachii. **11** Thoracic back muscles. **12** Serratus anterior. **13** External oblique. **14** Diaphragm. **15** Iliopsoas. **16** Lumbar back muscles. **17** Adductors. **18** Biceps femoris

- In the case of maxillary prognathism (retrusive/distal occlusion): gravity line anteriorly displaced, especially at the head, cervicothoracic transition zone, and shoulders; hyperlordosis of the cervical spine and lumbar spine.[21:28]
- In the case of mandibular prognathism (progenism/protrusive occlusion): gravity line posteriorly displaced, especially at the head, cervicothoracic transition zone, and shoulder; cervical and lumbar spine extended.[21:28]
- Restriction of the hyoid.
- Cephalad and medial movement of the scapula.
- In the case of ipsilateral CMD dysfunction: development of latent scoliosis.[234]
- In the case of ipsilateral CMD dysfunction: imbalance of the pelvic girdle.[234]
- In the case of crossbite: asymmetry of the face and scoliosis.[21:28]
- In the case of open bite: atlas–axis dysfunction.[21:28]

Test using two scales

For this test of balance, the patient stands with a foot on each of two separate scales and tries to distribute body weight equally between both. According to Lewit, a difference of more than 4 kg between the two sides, with dizziness, indicates vertebral column involvement and proprioceptive disturbance.[262]

Differential diagnosis to explore the effect of the TMJ involves placing a cotton wool roll between the molars on each side, so that the inserted roll creates separation, disengagement, and anterior shifting of the joint. If repeat testing using the two scales produces an improved result, this is a possible indication that the TMJ is involved as a descending dysfunction.

Barre's vertical alignment test

This test is quick and simple to perform.

Method

- The patient stands with heels touching, and forefeet apart.
- The gaze should be unfocused so as to exclude any influence from the eyes and increase the demand on the proprioceptive system; the patient can perform the test with eyes closed.
- To determine the measurement, sketch in a plumbline running upward from below, with its starting point between the heel bones.
- Measurement looks at three reference points: the intergluteal cleft, spinous process of C7, and vertex.

Assessment of findings Negative: all reference points lie on the plumbline. The patient should be able to maintain this for at least 4 s.

The following dysfunctions may be found (Figure 2.43):

1. **Ascending dysfunction** (pelvis deviates to one side):
   - Short leg, lumbar pain, dysfunction of the foot, knee, hip, or pelvis (sacroiliac joint).[169]
   - The ascending chain can briefly be inhibited if the patient stands on a neck cushion.
2. **Descending dysfunction** (head/neck deviate to one side):
   - Cervical pain, upper cervical dysfunction, dysfunction of the clavicle, shoulder, first rib, mandible; also old craniocervical trauma, disturbance of eyes or vision.
3. **Dysfunction ascending and descending** (head/neck deviate to one side; pelvis to the opposite side).
4. **Compensatory state:**
   - In this state any therapeutic intervention brings with it a risk of decompensation.
5. **Unilateral hypertonicity** (head, upper body, and pelvis deviate to the same side):
   - Occurs in central or vestibular disturbance, possibly also severe toxic stress, disturbance of organs, or autonomic dystonia.
   - Examination of the autonomic nervous system is required to exclude autonomic dystonia.

2.5.6 Dynamic signs of craniomandibular dysfunction

Mobility or motion restriction of body structures is far more important to the osteopath in diagnosis and treatment than static positional findings

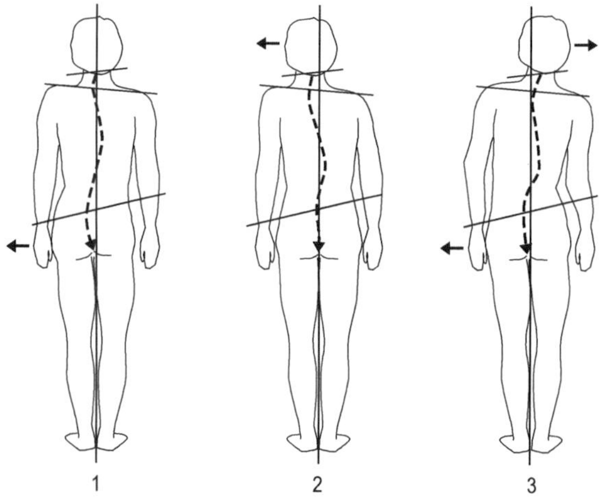

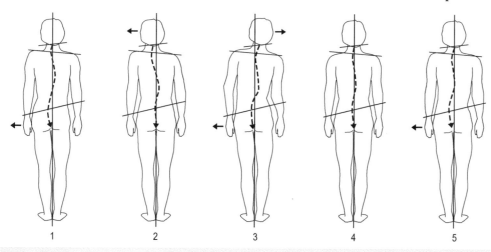

Figure 2.43
Barre's vertical alignment test

relating to individual body structures, or to the posture of the body. It is therefore essential to the success of osteopathic treatment to carry out dynamic local and global motion tests in addition to positionally based diagnosis.

Methodology of the dynamic test

- Fascial organization.
- Differential diagnosis
  - Testing mouth opening, standing, and sitting.
  - Scapula test (paper test).
- Meersseman test.
- Fukuda test.
- Test of the functional triangles: passive/active.
- Deep front/medial line: fascial testing passive/active.
- Flexion test sitting.
- Test of oculomotricity.

> **NOTE**
> 1. Rotation restriction of the head on the side of the raised scapula.
> 2. The atlas and axis are usually rotated toward the side of the lowered scapula.
> 3. Lateral redistribution of weight leads to instability of the lower limb on the side of the lowered scapula.

Fascial organization according to Zink

Zink described the interaction between fascial patterns and postural organization. He ascribes particular importance to the transition zones—the craniocervical (atlanto-occipital/O-A joint), cervicothoracic, thoracolumbar, and lumbosacral regions—for diagnosis and therapy.

The ideal fascial organization would be a body without fascial motion restrictions, in which rotation in both directions is equally possible in all the above regions (Figure 2.46). The ideal is not found in practice; fascial organization in fact reflects not only traumatic injury, but asymmetry of gait, disturbances of organs, and a host of other factors in life.

Compensatory fascial organization Compensatory fascial organization is the most common situation in healthy individuals (Figure 2.44). The direction of fascial mobility varies from one region to another. The fascial organization most frequently found (80% of cases) is expressed in greater ease of rotation in left craniocervical, right cervicothoracic, left thoracolumbar, and right lumbosacral (L/R/L/R) rotation. The compensatory pattern of fascial organization arranged R/L/R/L is less frequently found.

Decompensatory fascial organization This is characterized by the situation in which the direction of fascial mobility does not change from one region to the next (Figure 2.45). This may arise, for example, as the result of traumatic injury.

Diagnostic procedure

Test the regions described with the patient standing, sitting, and lying down. Locate the areas of compensatory fascial organization and identify the levels that deviate from this type of organization.

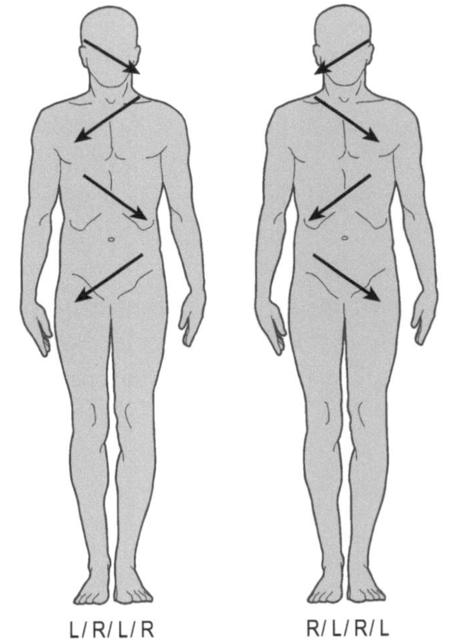

Figure 2.44
Compensatory fascial organization

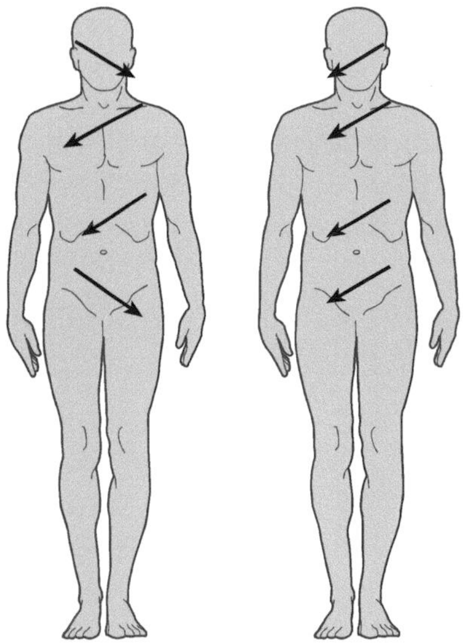

Figure 2.45
Decompensatory fascial organization

The success of treatment is usually accompanied by the re-establishment of compensatory fascial organization.

Diagnosis, standing/sitting/lying down If the parameters remain unchanged when the patient has sat/lain down, a descending dysfunction is more likely. Improvement in the parameters indicates that an ascending dysfunction is probable.

Diagnosis, paper test Place a piece of paper between the teeth on the side of the raised scapula. An improvement in the parameters means that a dysfunction of the masticatory apparatus can be assumed as the origin of symptoms.

Meersseman test (differential diagnosis of ascending or descending dysfunction)

Patient standing

- Posterior: compare the height of the superior iliac crests, shoulders, and ears.
- Lateral: set against a body plumbline; holding this laterally to the body, observe the position of the shoulder, greater trochanter, and lateral malleolus.

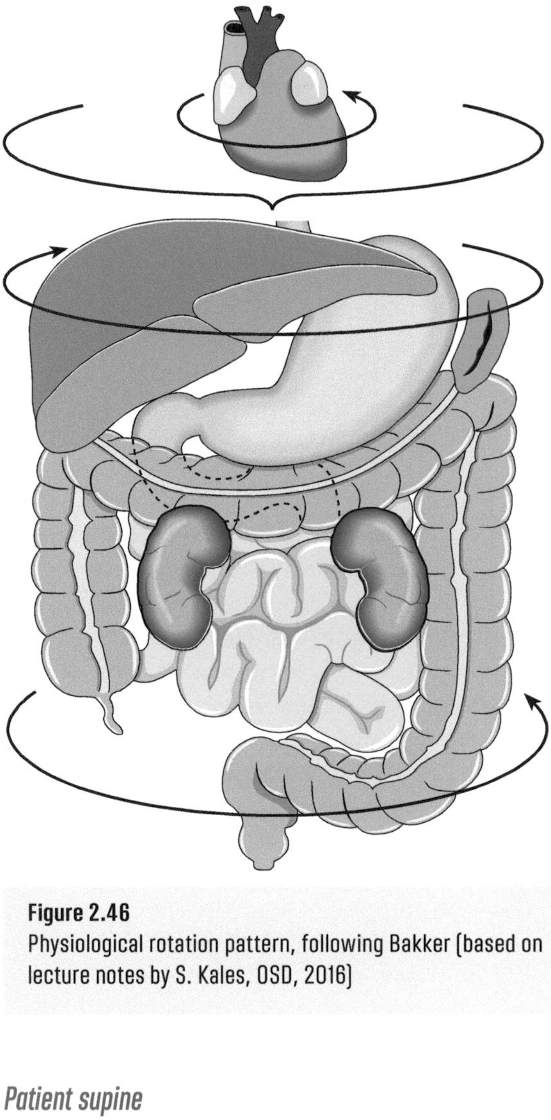

Figure 2.46
Physiological rotation pattern, following Bakker (based on lecture notes by S. Kales, OSD, 2016)

Patient supine

- Examine leg length and the position of the medial malleoli.
- Compare the abduction and internal rotation of the legs.
- Compare the active bending of the hip with legs extended.
- Compare the turning of the head.

Establishment of contact between the teeth of the upper and lower jaw

- With the patient supine, insert a separator of maximum thickness 3 mm between the teeth of the patient's upper and lower jaw, extending over the whole row of teeth (to prevent posterior displacement of the mandible) immediately posterior to the incisors.

- Ask the patient to take a few steps while biting gently together and swallowing the saliva.

Then repeat the test

- Evident improvement of the parameters: descending dysfunction (cranium; TMJ).
- No change: ascending dysfunction.
- Partial improvement only: further general osteopathic examination is needed.

Fukuda test

This test shows whether the functional mechanics or dysfunction of the TMJ is affecting the statics or dynamics of body posture, particularly if the following symptoms are present: bruxism, pain in the joint or masticatory muscles, trigger points in the head or nape of neck, sounds such as clicking or crepitation, headache, neck pain or back pain, tinnitus, or following dental procedures or during orthodontic treatment.

Stage 1 The patient stands, eyes closed and mouth closed (but without contact of the teeth), in a room with minimal sound disturbance (ideally a dark, soundproof room). Ask the patient to step quickly from one leg to the other about 40 times, arms outstretched and raising the knees as high as possible with each step.

The practitioner stands facing the patient. Look for any rotation to one side. Rotation up to 30% is physiological; if the angle is greater, this is pathological. If the finding is pathological, continue to stage 2.

Stage 2 The procedure is the same as for stage 1, but this time you should use a cotton wool roll to separate the joint on the side of the pain or dysfunction so as to disengage and shift it anteriorly. If rotation improves, the Fukuda test is positive. If not, this is a negative result and the TMJ dysfunction is not primary.

Summary Rotation of the body is mainly performed by the psoas. The connectivity that operates is mainly contralateral, so that a dysfunction in the right TMJ is associated with relative shortening in the left psoas. Ipsilateral connectivity may also be found, but this is rare.

Test of the functional triangles: passive/active

Passive test

Patient: Standing, eyes closed.

Practitioner: Behind the patient, standing well centralized on both legs.

Hand position: Place one hand on the vertex and the other on the upper cervical spine.

Method: With your cranial hand and your entire body reaction, sense whether your hand is drawn in an anterior, posterior, or lateral direction toward the neck region.

Active test:

Testing the anterior triangles: the patient extends the neck, mouth closed. *Normal:* the surface of the forehead should exhibit an angle of about 80°. Reduced extension indicates dysfunctional tension of the anterior triangles.

Testing the posterior triangles: the patient stands, back against a wall, and lets the head sink gently forward. *Normal:* the distance between chin and sternum should be no more than 3 finger-widths. If the distance is greater, this indicates dysfunctional tension in the posterior triangles.

Testing the lateral triangles: the patient stands, back against a wall, and gently lets the head sink to the side. *Normal:* the distance between ear and shoulder should be no more than 4 finger-widths. If the distance is greater, this indicates dysfunctional tension in the contralateral lateral triangles. If the difference is symmetrical, the prognosis is more positive than if it is asymmetrical.

If the test is positive

1. Repeat the test, this time with a 3–5 mm insert between the molars of both sides. An improved result is a possible indication that the TMJ is involved as a descending dysfunctional factor.
2. Testing mouth opening: if mouth opening improves relative to initial testing, this is a possible indication of an ascending dysfunction stemming from the region of the neck triangles.

Deep front/medial line: fascial testing passive/active

Passive test

Patient: Standing, eyes closed.

Practitioner: Behind the patient, standing well centralized on both legs.

Hand position: Place one hand on the vertex and the other on the region of the sacrum, or, if you intend to test the lower limbs as well, this hand is not in contact.

Method: With your cranial hand and your entire body reaction, sense whether your hand is drawn in an anterior direction toward particular regions of the deep front line or, as appropriate, medial line.

Active test:

The patient lies prone, palms of the hands on the treatment table underneath the shoulders; then, by stretching the elbows, lifts up into extension.
Normal: the distance between the anterior superior iliac spine and the table should not be more than 3 finger-widths.
If the distance is greater, this is an indication of dysfunctional tension of the deep front/medial line. Here, beside the rectus abdominis, you should also consider possible visceral dysfunctions, giving particular attention to the esophagus, for example, and also the stomach, small and large intestines, bladder, or uterus.

If the test is positive

Proceed as for the testing of the functional triangles (see above).
Also test hip extension for the iliopsoas, knee flexion, and plantar flexion of the foot using the appropriate method corresponding to the one described.

NOTE The chains that should particularly be tested in relation to the TMJ are the spiral lines, since, in the author's experience, positive findings in ascending or descending chains are often encountered in the spiral lines in CMD. A description of this testing would exceed the scope of this book.

Flexion test sitting, to test descending dysfunctional chains

Patient: The patient should sit on a chair, feet in contact with the ground.

Practitioner: Take up a position behind the patient.

Hand position: Position your thumbs inferiorly to the posterior inferior iliac spine.

Method:

1. The patient leans forward. As they do so, palpate both iliac spines. The result is positive if the iliac spine on one side moves forward.
2. If the result is positive, carry out a follow-up test, this time with inhibition of the TMJ (e.g., by placing an insert between the molars on both sides, or a 3–5 mm insert on the side of the positive test). If the test is now negative, the TMJ may be involved.

Test of oculomotricity

Patient: The patient should stand and stretch out both arms. The patient's mouth should be closed, but without closing the teeth together.

Method: Ask the patient to look slowly alternately to left and right, without moving the head but keeping it centered. During the glance to the right, tonicity on the opposite side should increase, i.e., the tonicity of the left extensors and in the posterior side of the limbs on the left.

If contralateral tonicity does not increase, the test is positive. That can happen if the postural function relating to the eye muscles is overstressed.

(See Table 2.2.)

2.6 Location, causes, and treatment of craniomandibular dysfunctions

Causes The etiology of CMD rests in particular on osseous, articular, occlusal and dentally related, muscular, ligamentous, fascial, and neurogenic disturbances. Venolymphatic, arterial, and psychological influences should also be considered.

The development of CMD is usually multifactorial, and these factors interact (Figure 2.47). For example, disbalances, compensation within the structures of the TMJ, or dysfunctions of the jaw may in time lead to structural TMJ changes (e.g., due to altered muscular activity). Pain states of the joint may also induce reactions (neurological, muscular) that can give rise to a vicious circle or give rise to psychological changes.

Table 2.2 Differentiation of ascending and descending dysfunctions associated with the temporomandibular joint

	Functional restriction and/or pain in masticatory apparatus	Positional or dynamic signs in TMJ	Tissue and motion changes of parietal/ visceral structures	After treatment of identified dysfunction
Ascending dysfunction	Yes	No	Yes	Improvement of TMJ signs
Ascending dysfunction with CMD	Yes	No	Yes	Dynamic and positional TMJ signs → TMJ therapy
Descending CMD	Yes, in parietal system, e.g., pain in cervical spine	Yes		Improvement of parietal system signs
Descending CMD with dysfunction of the parietal/ visceral system	Yes, in parietal system	Yes		Partial or no improvement of parietal signs and posture → therapy for parietal and visceral dysfunction

TMJ, temporomandibular joint; CMD, craniomandibular dysfunction.

Parietal system: skeleto-musculofascial system of the body. Visceral system: internal organs and associated structures.

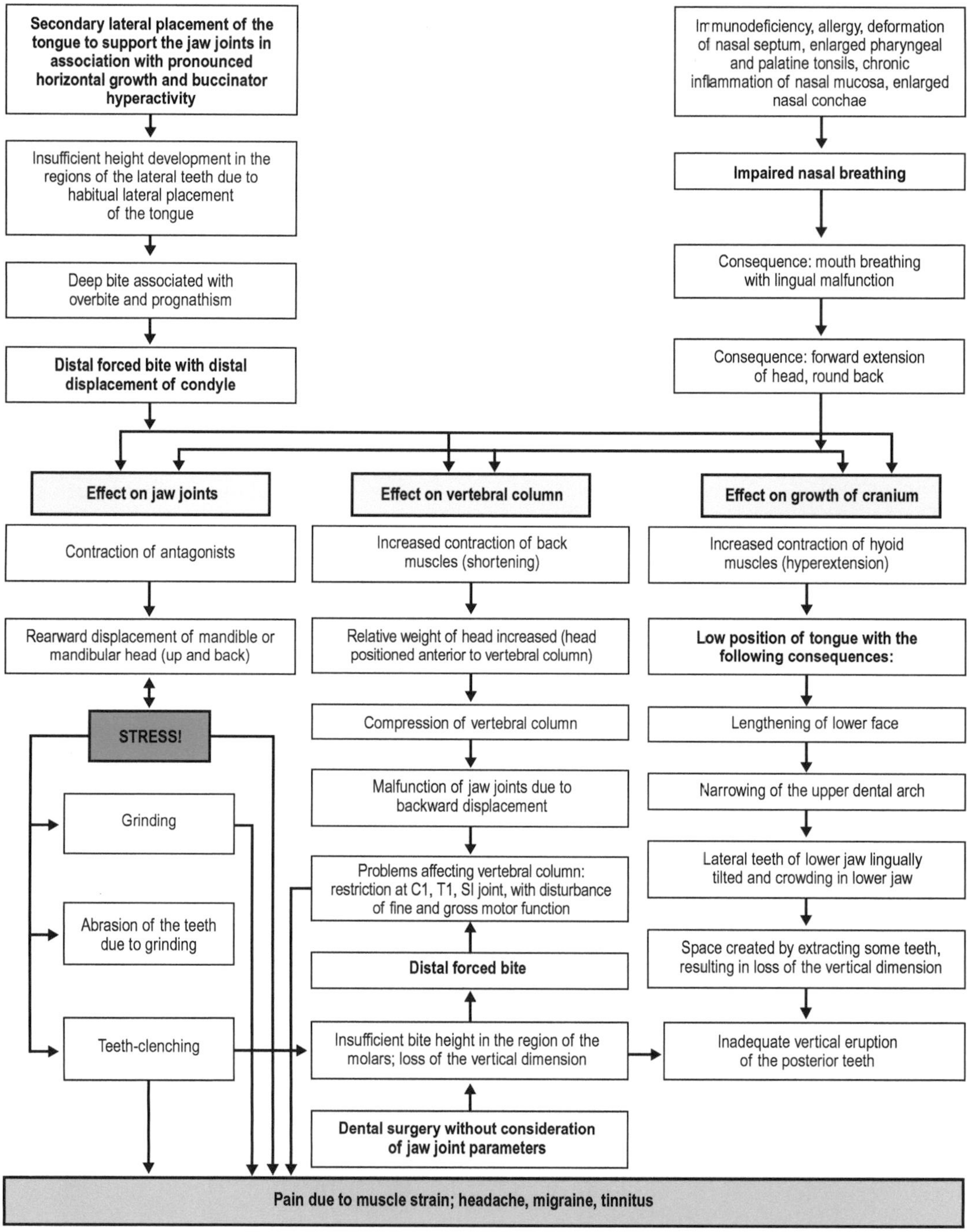

Figure 2.47
Causes of jaw joint-cervical spine dysfunction (Garry, Yerkes, and Bowbeer, modified by Wolz from references 47 and 145)

Primary CMD

- Congenital: the treatment of choice is usually orthodontic surgery.
- Traumatic:
  - **Perinatal trauma**, affecting the whole cranium; however, intraembryonic or postnatal causes are also possible; these may involve dysfunctions of the TMJ or intraosseous dysfunctions (the mandible originally consisted of two parts).
  - **Falling or blows to the face**, with the possible consequence of one TMJ moving in an anterolateral direction and the other posteriomedially. Other sequelae could be muscular disbalances and damage to the capsule or disk.
  - **Tooth extractions**, or other forceful interventions on the lower jaw.[78]
  - **Extreme mouth-opening movements**, e.g., during dental surgery, intubation, etc.
  - Blows to, or falling onto, the **pelvis** may also trigger restrictions of the lower jaw.

This may lead both to intra-articular and to intraosseous dysfunctions.

Secondary CMD

- Orofacial dyskinesia, especially mouth breathing and infantile patterns of swallowing, affect craniofacial development. Sequelae may include crowding of teeth and lack of space for the third molars.
- Disturbance of **nasal breathing** or of the **diaphragm**: allergies, asthma, and chronic infections of the upper respiratory tract should be considered. Consequences are mouth breathing, impairment of swallowing, an alteration of lip position, possibly an alteration of tongue position, a lower jaw that is drawn down slightly, vertebral column in an extension position, and, sometimes, altered growth of the lower and middle thirds of the face[21:28] (Volume 2, section 2.3.5).
- Nutritional defects can be significant causes, e.g., **elevated sugar consumption**,[144] **vitamin and mineral deficiencies**: C, D, E, F, calcium, magnesium, phosphorus.[388:30–35]
- Dysfunctions of the **bones of the cranium** and the cranial sutures, in particular of the temporal bone and occipital bone; this results in restriction of the TMJ and changes its position.
- Generalized hypermobility may occur in some circumstances.[467,167]
- Abnormal tensions in the **masticatory muscles, hyoid muscles** and ligaments of the TMJ.
- Poor **chewing and swallowing habits**, or a dysfunction of the **tongue**, especially the anterior position of the tongue: this may lead to dental misalignment and malocclusion.
- Disturbances of the **teeth**: malocclusions (premature contact, etc.), orthodontic appliances,[398] dental prostheses, etc.
- **Bottle-fed babies** who have not been breastfed: breast-feeding is an important stimulus to the growth of the mandible, which is as yet relatively underdeveloped, and it encourages closure of the mouth; it also stimulates the development of all organs involved in sucking, insalivation, chewing, and swallowing.[22] Dysfunction of the **upper cervical spine** and of the atlanto-occipital joint: the cervical spine has a major influence on the TMJ, for example hypertonicity of the muscles of the cervical spine can lead to hypertonicity of the masticatory muscles.
- Dysfunction of the pectoral girdle (scapula, clavicle, first rib, e.g., via the omohyoid muscle, etc.).
- **Static dysfunctions**: poor posture, poor working position, scolioses and dysfunctions of the pelvis, sacrum, and lower limbs (e.g., a difference in leg length[402:377f.]) may lead to CMD via myofascial links.
- **Visceral dysfunctions**, via their fascial connection with the cranium, via the influence on the statics of the human body or on the meridian system.

- **Disposition of the tissues:** hyperlaxity of the capsular/ligamentous apparatus, laxity of the connective tissue (opinions vary[188,75]).
- Faulty tension of the intracranial **dural membrane**.
- **Psychological-emotional factors:** stress, bullying, or emotional harm may lead directly or indirectly to increased muscle tonicity (e.g., in association with nocturnal clenching or gnashing of the teeth, nail-biting).
- Psychosocial factors.
- **Neurological disturbances**, e.g., overactivity of the trigeminal ganglion, or reticular formation.
- Endocrine disturbances.
- Physical strain or exhaustion.
- **Foci/disturbance fields:** scars, dental foci, septic tonsils, and diseases of the stomach and small intestine can have a remotely acting influence on the TMJ.[388]
- Genetic factors.
- Degenerative and inflammatory **rheumatic** disorders: osteoarthritis (the commonest rheumatic development), rheumatoid arthritis, psoriatic arthropathy, primary Still disease, soft-tissue rheumatism, Bechterew disease (spondylitis deformans).
- **Other causes:** infectious osteitis, osteopathies (toxic, endocrine, cancerous), endocrine disturbances, and allergies.[388:30–35]
- See also this volume, section 2.5.2.

Factors that can disturb the relative position of upper and lower jaw (following Morales and Brondo, modified)

- Hypotonicity of cervical muscles, visual disturbances → abnormal head position, backward tilting of head → anterior shifting of mandible.
- Laxity of TMJ ligaments → hypotonicity of temporalis and masseter muscles → dropping of mandible.
- Smallness of the nasal sinuses, polyps, tonsillar hypertrophy → narrowing of the upper airways, mouth breathing → extension and forward inclination of the head → dropping and anterior displacement of the mandible.
- Smallness of the oral cavity, large and/or thick tongue → prolapse of the tongue, tongue presses against the lower lip → anterior displacement of the mandible.
- Birth trauma, falling, blows, tooth extractions → dysfunction of the SBS (lateroflexion-rotation, vertical strain).
- Difference in leg length, pelvic obliquity → transmission via the muscle chains to the TMJ.

Sequelae Atypical deglutition and disturbances of articulation, CMD.

The presentation of etiological dysfunctional patterns is conjectural.

2.6.1 Osseous, disk-related, and dental occlusion-related factors

Clinical presentation Pain, TMJ restrictions, joint sounds.

Teeth; disturbances of occlusion

See also this volume, Chapter 15.

Some key terms explained

- **Gnathology:** science of the function of the masticatory organ (or stomatognathic system) as a functional entity; comprising the TMJ, teeth, and associated framework of neuromuscular relations.
- **Occlusion** (closure of dentition): any contact between the teeth of the upper and lower jaw.
- **Static occlusion:** dental contact/meeting of teeth without movement of the lower jaw.
- **Maximum intercuspation:** static occlusion with maximum multipoint contact between the teeth of the upper and lower jaw.
- **Dynamic occlusion:** dental contact with movement of the lower jaw (mediotrusion, laterotrusion, protrusion, etc.).
- **Habitual occlusion:** static occlusion usually adopted.

- **Centric occlusion:** maximum intercuspation with centric position of condyles: position of both condyles not shifted to the side when condyle–disk relation is normal—the ideal position for achieving lifelong, trouble-free occlusion.
- **Centric condyle position:** designation of an idealized position of both condyles of the temporomandibular joints in the mandibular fossae.

FURTHER INFORMATION Definitions and nomenclature are the subject of some discussion, with no clear agreement. There have been changes of opinion regarding condyle position: from posterior (distal contact) through cranial to ventrocranial. Current practice, for example, in order to determine myocentricity when the muscles are in a state of chronic excessive tension, is to relax the muscles using TENS before deciding what is optimum occlusion. Using manual methods, this can be done using myofascial release techniques (this volume, section 2.8.1).

- **Incisal guidance:** movement of the anterior teeth of the lower jaw relative to those of the upper jaw (during protrusion movement).
- **Canine guidance:** dynamic occlusion between canines of the upper and lower jaw. In lateral chewing movements (laterotrusion), a gap is created between upper and lower molars. Canine guidance in laterotrusion represents a gliding tooth contact route for the opposing teeth and guides the lower jaw while the lateral teeth are not in contact. In *good canine guidance*, there should only be *guiding contact* between the *canines* of the upper and lower jaw.
- **Malocclusion:** complex, functionally determined disturbances in the dental, mandibular, and temporomandibular joint system.
- **Non-occlusion; infraocclusion:** lack of contact between opposing teeth; i.e., teeth or groups do not meet vertically.
- **Premature contact:** contact occurring too soon in static or dynamic occlusion.
- **Centric premature contact:** premature contact of the teeth in the central condyle position, the effect of which leads the condyle into an eccentric position when assuming habitual occlusion.
- **Mesial occlusion:** Angle's Class III occlusion; underbite; anterior occlusion.
- **Disto-occlusion:** Angle's Class II occlusion; retrusive, posterior, or distal occlusion: retrognathic occlusion.
- **Forms of transverse occlusal deviation:** crossbite; scissorbite (non-occlusion).
- **Deep bite:** lower incisors and canines bite deep (i.e., high) into palate of upper jaw, whether or not they pierce the gum.
- **Cover-bite; extreme deep overbite:** incisors of upper jaw overlap (in vertical dimension) the lower incisors, usually with retrusion. Cover-bite is always deep bite, and generally only a vertical overbite, not a horizontal one.
- **Overbite (informal usage):** this relates to the cutting edge of the incisors, which are separated either in the horizontal plane or in terms of height. Informally it can describe the horizontal relationship of the front teeth, where the upper incisors are in front of the lower incisors (**overjet**), as when sucking a thumb, or a vertical overlap (**overbite**).
- **Horizontal overbite:** often associated with disto-occlusion (Angle's Class II occlusion); sometimes with Class I, when the incisors are inclined (upper incisors forward, lower ones backward, in which case anterior open bite or deep bite).
- **Underbite:** anterior teeth of the lower jaw set forward relative to those of the upper jaw, in the horizontal or vertical plane (Angle's Class III occlusion).

- **Open bite:** the opposite of deep bite; the teeth do not make contact, either anteriorly or laterally, even when biting together, making it impossible either to bite something off with the front teeth or to chew at the side of the mouth. Placing the tongue between the teeth can be either a cause or a consequence.
- **Edge-to-edge bite:** neither posterior (disto-) nor anterior (mesial) occlusion, but occlusion in which the edges of the teeth meet exactly, not moving past each other.
- **Overbite:** not a misalignment, but a description of the relative vertical position of the anterior teeth.
- **Overjet:** a horizontal (sagittal/anteroposterior) separation; not a misalignment, but a description of the relative horizontal position of the anterior teeth.

Causes of malocclusion and disturbances of occlusion

Secondary to disturbances of the TMJ or muscles,[62] following dental extractions, maxillofacial surgery, traumatic injury, biting on something hard, as a result of CMD, poorly fitting dental prostheses and dental fillings,[204] genetic factors, dietary factors, and birth trauma.[357]

Afferent neural connections, e.g., in the periodontium, may cause these etiologies to produce peripheral sensitization of the trigeminal nerve; also central sensitization and/or postural adaptation of the head and neck (see also this volume, section 2.6.6). With advancing age, tooth loss and displacement, wearing down of articular cartilage, and disk defects can make disturbances of occlusion more likely.

Laughlin mentions that, if certain conditions exist, some dental surgery and orthodontic operations are capable of inducing cranial dysfunctions.[253] These include, e.g., rigid dental bridges, especially ones which span the front teeth, solid metal or non-metal dental prostheses or partial prostheses, amalgam fillings, and rigid dental braces and dental crowns. In addition, dysfunctions of body statics, mental and physical stresses, etc.

- Causes of a bite that is too low are abrasion of the teeth, defects in dental fillings, or dental prostheses that are too low.
- Causes of a bite that is too high are "high" dental fillings, "high" prostheses (full or partial), crowns, or bridges.

Disturbances of occlusion were traditionally held to lead to muscular dysfunctions or spasms, resulting in CMD.[187,261] This implied that patients who had had dental treatment would more often suffer from CMD than patients with intact teeth.[204] However, a review published in 2016 cast some doubt on the existence of a causal connection between disturbances of occlusion and muscular dysfunctions. The authors come to the conclusion that occlusal changes are usually secondary to disturbances of the joints and muscles.[62]

There is a positive correlation between the extent of TMJ dysfunctions as well as of occlusal disturbances, and parafunctional habits; a correlation also exists between occlusal disturbances and parafunctional habits.[381] It was found that occlusion of the upper and lower teeth more seldom occurs simultaneously, and even more seldom symmetrically, in TMJ patients than in healthy individuals.[72]

To give a simple analogy, we can compare the functional unit of the upper and lower jaw and temporomandibular joints in simplified terms with a door, door frame, and hinges: over time, a door that can only be closed with the application of force inevitably damages the components.[97]

A correlation exists between a muscle imbalance of the anterior part of the temporalis muscle and TMJ symptoms. In association with maximum voluntary bite, the anterior part of the temporalis has a more significant effect on tooth contact than the masseter.[72] However, as already discussed, occlusal relationships alone cannot be seen as responsible for the occurrence of TMJ dysfunctions.[92]

Crossbite appears to cause neither symptoms nor disease in the TMJ. This means that crossbite

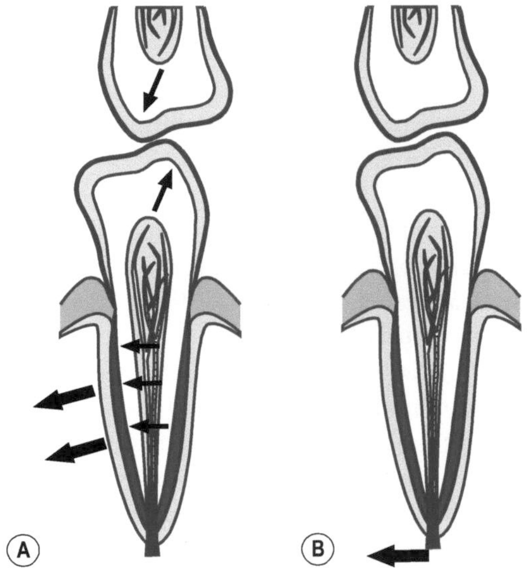

Figure 2.48
Effect of premature contact on the TMJ. Compensatory contraction of the muscles of the jaw.
A Premature contact: information is conducted via nerve endings in the periodontal ligament. Masticatory muscles contract.
B In some circumstances, this contraction counterbalances the premature contact. This can cause a displacement of the mandible

should, if possible, not be corrected unless there is pain. Nor is there any evidence that an overbite influences non-arthritic disturbances of the TMJ in any way, whereas a clear association exists between a skeletal, anterior open bite and osteoarthritic changes of the TMJ.[399]

A combination with other factors (such as emotional states, stress, dysfunction of the cervical spine, joint disease, cold or damp, metabolic disturbance, and hormonal factors) can produce additional contraction of the masticatory muscles, and ultimately triggering or exacerbating symptoms. The consequences are bruxism (grinding or gnashing of the teeth without a functional purpose), pain, tendinomyopathies, further compensation, and degenerative processes (joint diseases) (Figure 2.48).

Possible, theoretical, mechanisms of myofascial dysfunction

- Joint and muscle disturbances → disturbance of occlusion.
- Disturbance of occlusion ↔ contraction of the neck muscles → dysfunction of the cervical or thoracic spine.
- Disturbance of occlusion ↔ contraction of the cervical flexors and suprahyoid muscles → reduction of lordosis of the cervical spine, displacement of the hyoid in a posterosuperior direction, lowering and posterior displacement of the tongue → the consequence may be to encourage bruxism, especially if conditions are favorable due to simultaneous contraction of the retrohyoid muscles and posterior part of the temporalis muscle → the infrahyoid muscles follow the suprahyoid muscles and, via their influence on the scapula and thorax, can impair breathing.
- Change in position of mandible → disturbance of occlusion → impairs body posture and musculoskeletal system → pelvic obliquity; difference in leg length.

Laughlin's dysfunction mechanism[253] Excessively narrow maxilla and mandible → extraction of the bicuspids to create more space → posterior displacement of the anterior teeth and premaxilla by orthodontic measures → possible compression of cranial sutures, flattening of the facial profile and lateral compression of the facial structures[47,134,147,113,477] → possible compression of the sphenobasilar synchondrosis → posterior displacement of the mandible due to posterior displacement of the maxillary complex → TMJ syndrome with displacement of the disk, and cervical and sacral imbalance.[147,197]

Premature contact and reduced contact of teeth

Any premature contact of the teeth is communicated to the central nervous system via the nerve endings (mechanical stimuli, pain) in the periodontal ligament. In response to this, the jaw muscles contract. Abrasion of the impeding tooth surface or the exertion of force on the tooth are two ways of trying to correct the premature contact (Figures 2.48 and 2.49); alternatively, the chewing surfaces involved are avoided by hypertonicity of the muscles. These reactions usually achieve little or no success. Contraction of these muscles causes a displacement of the mandible (laterotrusion, protrusion). This can affect the TMJ, temporal bone, and C0/C1/C2, and can activate descending dysfunctional chains (continuities).

An occlusal obstruction 0.1 mm in height fixed on a healthy tooth produced a significant rise in epinephrine (adrenaline), norepinephrine (noradrenaline), and hydrocorticosteroid levels and pain in the masticatory muscles, clicking of the TMJ, and extended periods of apnea during sleep. After one week, the body appeared to have adapted to the change, and levels returned to normal.[223]

FURTHER INFORMATION Premature contact → mechanical irritation/pain stimulates nerve endings in periodontal ligament → branches of trigeminal nerve → contraction of jaw muscles → bruxism or clenching of teeth → displacement of mandible → dysfunction of TMJ, temporal bone, C0/C1/C2, and activation of descending dysfunctional chains.

- **Premature contact in the anterior region** There should be no contact of the incisors on maximum occlusion. This can be checked by placing your finger on the anterior surface of the front teeth and asking the patient to close their bite. You will be able to sense whether contact occurs.
  - Causes: deep bite due to greater length of upper anterior teeth, crowns on upper anterior teeth, crowding at front of upper jaw with rotation and inclination of individual teeth, greater length of lower anterior teeth, or slight palatal displacement of upper lateral anterior teeth.[427:253,264]
  - Sequelae: posterior displacement of the condyles with anterior displacement of the disk and compression of the retroarticular region.
  - The farther posterior the premature bite is located, the greater the stress or compression of the contralateral TMJ. At the same time, the ipsilateral TMJ is subjected to less pressure and greater strain.
- **Premature contact of distal molar** Premature contact of the distal cusps (superior) produces compression of the condyle in the dorsocranial, cranial, and slightly ventral direction.
  - Sequelae: premature contact of mesial cusps (anterior) produces displacement of the condyle in a ventrocranial and ventromedial direction and to compression of the disk (Figure 2.48).
- **Reduced support of molars** Reduced posterior tooth contact, e.g., due to dental extraction or treatment, leads to increased activity of the temporalis, masseter, medial, and lateral pterygoid muscles (superior head) and increased compression of the TMJ.[91]
  - Sequelae: reduced tooth contact in the molar region can lead to a greater effect of force at the TMJ and possibly to an increase in tension in the dural system and cervical spine.

FURTHER INFORMATION There is some discussion as to how far occlusal factors do indeed affect bruxism.[150,399:96,447] Correlations between bruxism as a central nervous phenomenon and CMD, as well as headaches—independently of occlusal factors—are being considered.[151,183,314,452]
Dysfunctions of central nervous regulation → bruxism or gnashing of teeth → CMD, headaches.

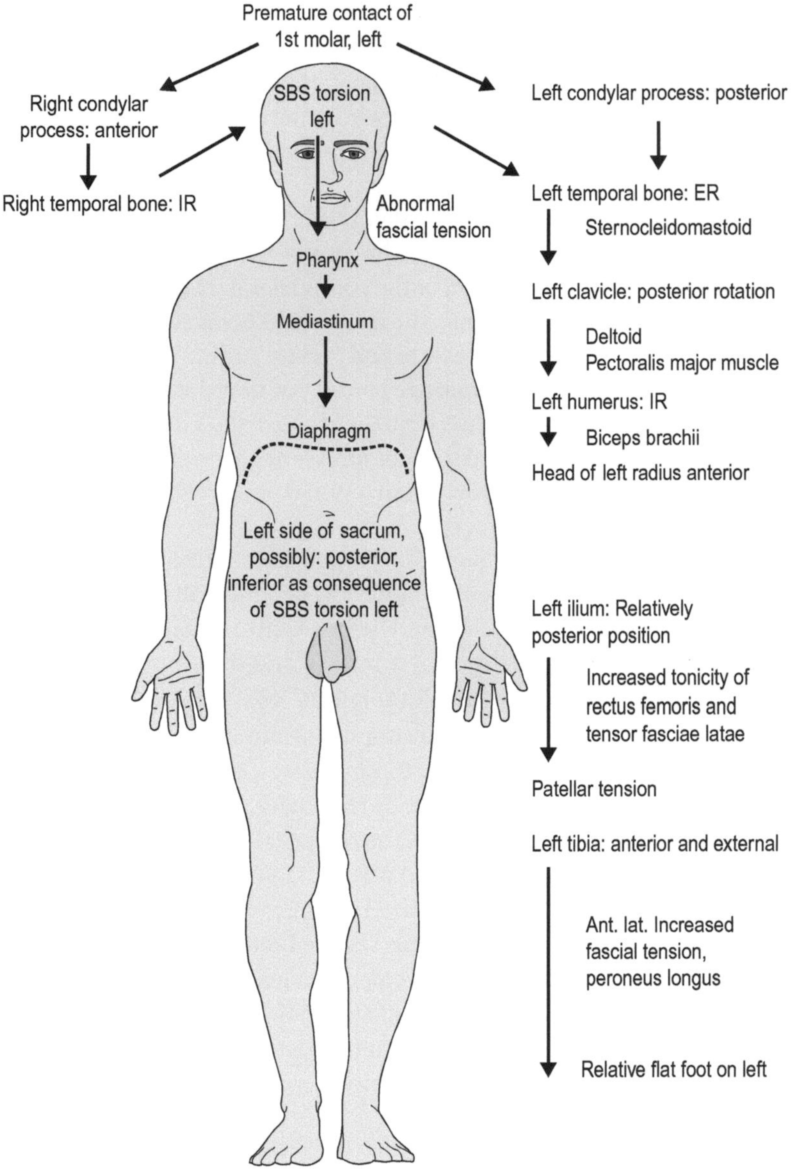

Figure 2.49
Myofascial adaptation in the example of premature contact of the first molar on the left

Occlusal disturbances due to malposition of teeth between upper and lower jaw

Main causes: genetic (cleft lip/jaw/palate; crooked molars), hormonal (mandibular prognathism, acromegaly), orofacial dyskinesias (damaging habits, e.g., mouth breathing, dysfunctional patterns of swallowing and tongue movements, thumb-sucking: this volume, section 2.10), dental extraction without prosthesis, infectious diseases, and chronic vitamin deficiency.

Sequelae: altered vectors of force during mastication, aesthetic changes affecting the individual emotionally/psychologically, etc.

Classification

The sagittal position of the jaws is classified according to Angle's classes of occlusion. The occlusal relationship assesses the occlusion of the first molar of the lower jaw with that of the upper jaw:

- **Neutro-occlusion Class I** Neutral bite or normal occlusion, with ideal occlusion in which the mandible is in the normal position relative to the maxilla, present from the end of the first year of life. (Neutral bite should not change for the rest of an individual's lifetime.)
- **Angle's Class II/1** The anterior cusp of the upper first molar lies anterior to the anterior cusp of the lower first molar. The upper incisors protrude noticeably.
- **Angle's Class II/2** The relationship between the first molars is as described for II/1, but the upper incisors are markedly inclined in the palatal direction.
- **Angle's Class III** The anterior cusp of the upper first molar is dorsal to the second cusp of the lower first molar. The lower anterior teeth may be anterior to the upper incisors.

Angle's classification is a purely descriptive one and looks at the two-dimensional picture, however, and only in static occlusion, whereas disturbances of occlusion occur in a three-dimensional context; static occlusion is insufficient for diagnostic examination and treatment. The static view also disregards functional disturbances and other criteria relevant to treatment.

In cases of CMD, the position of the condyles should also be considered together with occlusion.

Van Caille's model of the six-legged table[5,110,300,308,350,396,485,486]

Given the variety and complexity of occlusion, and of the concepts and diagnosis of occlusion, we need to turn to the use of models. Although models are not the same as reality, they do allow us to create a simplified picture of complex realities. Using a particular model enables us to answer certain questions relevant to treatment, and can help us understand complex processes. Here, Dr. Sebald's model of the six-legged table (Figure 2.50) is helpful. It shows a way to evaluate the craniomandibular system in its totality and complexity so that we can develop a therapeutic strategy:

- First pair of legs: represents anterior/canine tooth guidance, or the occlusion between the anterior teeth of the upper and lower jaw.
- Second pair of legs: represents molar occlusion.
- Third pair of legs: represents the jaw joint, including the whole TMJ complex that makes up the joint itself; that is, the anatomical structures such as bone, cartilage, synovial membrane, disk, capsule, ligaments, muscles, fasciae, and receptors, along with the control system that governs its highly complex function.

The more balanced the stomatognathic system in the way it operates in its active function, the more protective of the joint the associated occlusion will be. When this does not happen, it can lead to degenerative changes in the intra-articular structures (e.g., disk, cartilage, bilaminar zone) and extra-articular structures (e.g., apparatus of the capsule, muscle, fasciae). If we place our six-legged table on the patio, we know what is going to happen: the table will easily tend to wobble. The solution for

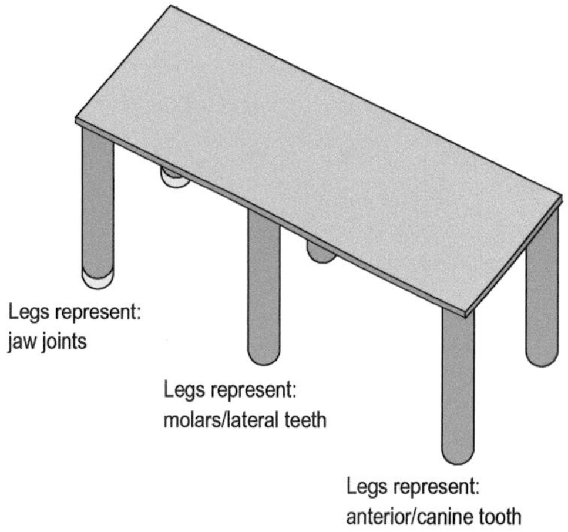

Figure 2.50
Model of the six-legged table

our garden table is to put a beer mat under the leg. What can we do for the craniomandibular system?

The ideal would be for all the legs to be the same length, so that the table rests stably on them. The third pair of legs, the "jaw joints," could compensate for slight differences. The joint is certainly capable of neutralizing minor discrepancies to enable the best possible occlusion. In reality, problems could happen in any of the three pairs of legs. The third pair, the TMJ joints, might be impaired because of degenerative changes, for example, or because chronic hypertonicity of the masticatory muscles massively limits the capacity to adapt. The other two pairs could give rise to problems, maybe because they are too "long" or too "short." Possible consequences might be that the system "wobbles" if the TMJ joints cannot compensate for the degree of imbalance, or the table surface becomes distorted due to the force of the masticatory muscles as we chew.

Practical application of this thought model
The TMJ joints are very often neglected as the structures that need to be treated. When patients open their mouths, the teeth are easy to assess while the joints are hidden. Consequently, occlusion (or the teeth) will often be treated, perhaps with the aim of neutralizing the forces exerting a retrusive effect on the joints. Such treatment tries to create greater room to allow adaptation, which can indeed be helpful. Treatment of the joint itself, however, remains unaddressed.

1. The two TMJ joints are, as it were, the table legs that can allow the table to adapt so that it "wobbles" less or not at all. Factors that can hinder this include degenerative changes in the joint or disk, dysfunction of the disk (subluxation or dislocation), and muscular imbalances or hypertonicity.
2. The first two pairs of legs determine occlusion. It is often possible to adapt to small divergencies or irregularities, but the capacity to adapt is limited. This is so, for example, when there is no lateral support on one side. If the six-legged table has two legs missing on the same side, it needs support, and treatment has to use a splint.
3. If the table has legs of very different length, and the TMJ joints are not able to compensate, strong forces may cause the table to "buckle" or cause the table surface to become distorted. These intraosseous changes and tensions can be treated via the individual bones of the viscerocranium, mainly the maxilla and mandible, the trajectories of pressure and tension relating to them, and the supportive pillars built into the viscerocranium. The loss of intraosseous elasticity or intraosseous tensions can be treated using gentle compression, divergence, and listening techniques (this volume, section 2.8).

The mandible

Powerful blows to the mandible, or falling and hitting the lower jaw, may lead to fractures or subluxation. Less powerful blows or less serious falls usually cause an asymmetric displacement of the lower jaw, resulting in one side moving anterior and the other posterior. The consequence—expressed in terms of traditional cranial osteopathy—is one temporal bone in internal rotation (IR) (on the side with the anteriorly displaced condyle) and one temporal bone in external rotation (ER) (on the side with the posteriorly displaced condyle), with disturbance of the tentorium cerebelli. Other sequelae may be intraosseous dysfunction of the mandible, and disturbances of the intracranial membranes, SBS, hyoid bone, and sacrum. But many other causes may also lead to dysfunctions of the TMJ.

Secondary dysfunctions at the mandible may be caused by **ascending chains of myofascial dysfunction** or **occlusal disturbances**:

- Ascending myofascial/neural chains relating to the lower limb,[330] vertebral column, or viscera → dysfunctions of the cervical fasciae, suboccipital muscles, and/or hyoid

muscles → dysfunction of the cranium → dysfunction of the mandible and TMJ.
- Occlusal disturbances → dysfunction of the mandible and TMJ.
- Temporomandibular disturbance → changes to the equalization of pressure between internal ear and middle ear → otological symptoms[108] and headaches.[428]

Inflammatory or degenerative processes in the TMJ lead, via pain receptors and mechanoreceptors, to an alteration of muscular contraction, which causes a change in the position of the TMJ as a way of avoiding pain. Inflammation of the TMJ has been associated with irritable bowel syndrome.[143] Intraosseous dysfunctions of the mandible can also be involved in producing pain.

The condylar process

Chronic contraction of certain masticatory muscles, establishment of a posteriorly displaced position of the condyle, or traumatic injury can cause the condyles to become locked in a certain position. This phenomenon may be unilateral or bilateral.

Restriction of the condyle in the anterior position (Figure 2.51)

- Causes This dysfunction arises when the mouth is opened too wide, whether in tooth extractions or as a result of a fall or a blow on the tip of the chin, with spasm of the lateral pterygoid muscle.
- Sequelae
  - Temporal bone in internal rotation.
  - Posteriorization of the hyoid, e.g., via the digastric muscle and stylohyoid muscle.
  - Dysfunction of the fourth thoracic vertebra;[265] symptom: possible disturbances of cardiac rhythm.
  - Secondary contraction of the sternocleidomastoid.
- Clinical/hypothetical pathology: venous stasis of the cranial vessels, or vagal problems and functional disturbance of the thyroid.

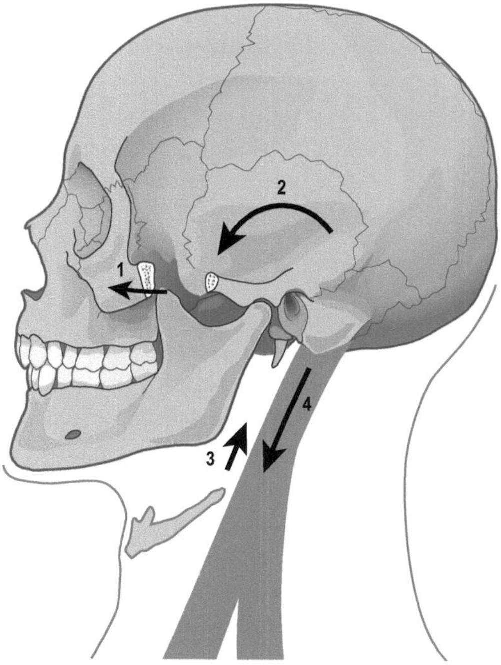

Figure 2.51
Restriction of condyle in anterior position. **1** Condyle in anterior position. **2** Temporal bone in internal rotation. **3** Posteriorization of hyoid bone. **4** Contraction of sternocleidomastoid

Restriction of the condyle in a posterior position (Figure 2.52)

- Causes This dysfunction usually arises in association with traumatic injury or a dysfunction of the atlanto-occipital joint, and is sustained by spasm of the posterior fibers of the temporalis muscle. For the role of the lateral pterygoid muscle, see this volume, sections 2.1.7 and 2.6.2. A posterior position of the condyle may also come about with advancing age, if a reduction in vertical tooth height has occurred due to wear of the teeth, or if in the past, abrasion may have been carried out as a therapeutic measure because this was seen as the way to achieve the best centric relation. The posterior displacement of the condyle is associated with anterior displacement of the disk during mouth-closure movement in the intercuspal position (see also The disk, this volume, 2.6.1). For Weinberg, posterior displacement of the condyle is an important factor in TMJ pain syndrome.[118 (Cf.29,31,40,119,120,121,163,211,351,358,366,394,404,407,440,457)]

- Possible sequelae
  - Temporal bone in external rotation.
  - Discal dysfunction with the possibility of compromising the bilaminar zone: dislocation or clicking. The clicking usually precedes locking of the jaw joint.
  - Reciprocal clicking during mouth-opening is the result of unlocking the TMJ. Reciprocal clicking during the closure movement is due to a displacement of the disk and condyle.

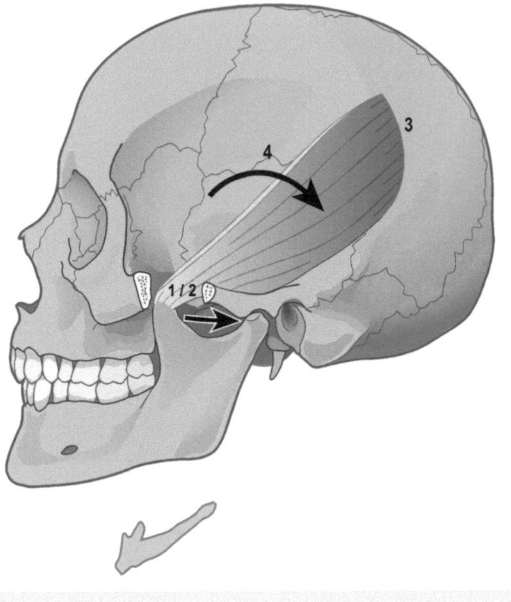

Figure 2.52
Restriction of condyle in posterior position. **1** Condyle in posterior position. **2** Contraction of lateral pterygoid muscle. **3** Contraction of temporalis muscle (posterior portion). **4** Temporal bone in external rotation

  - In cases of chronic reciprocal clicking and locking, the disk remains dislocated anterior during the normal extent of movement of the mandible (see The disk, this volume, 2.6.1).[118]
  - Dysfunctional strain of the petrosphenoidal ligament with disturbances of the sixth cranial nerve.
  - The pterygoid process of the sphenoid is shifted posterior (and in a lateral, inferior direction).
  - Disturbance of the hamulus in the middle ear, e.g., via the anterior ligament of the malleus: auditory disturbances.
  - Dysfunction of the carotid sympathetic plexus.
  - Dysphagia.
  - Descending myofascial chain.

Restriction of the condyle in a lateral position (Figure 2.53)

- Causes This dysfunction usually arises in association with traumatic injury.
- Possible sequelae
  - Asymmetric motion of the temporal bones.
  - Compression of the squamous suture.
  - Torsion of the tentorium cerebelli.
  - Asymmetric opening and closure of the jaw.
  - Limited opening of the jaw.
  - Lateralization of the hyoid to the side of the laterally displaced condyle.

Possible sequelae of TMJ dysfunction

- Increased tonicity of the orbicularis oris and buccinator.
- Increased tonicity of the constrictor muscles of the pharynx may occur via the pterygoid process of the sphenoid.
- Dysfunction of the basilar part of the occipital bone can lead to a dysfunction of the cervical spine.

Factors that may cause TMJ pain Joint effusion, fractures, disturbances of occlusion (premature contact due to high or reduced dental fillings, crowns, bridges, or loss of dental hard tissue),

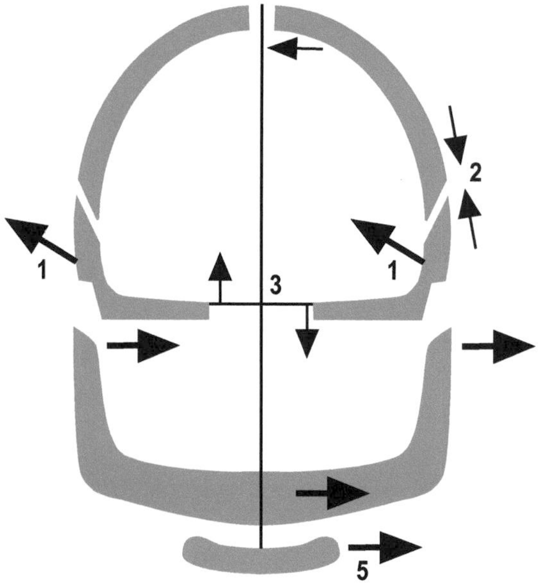

Figure 2.53
Restriction of condyle in a lateral position. **1** Asymmetric motion of the temporal bones. **2** Compression of the parietotemporal suture. **3** Torsion of tentorium cerebelli. **4** Lateralization of mandible and asymmetric opening and closure of jaw. **5** Lateralization of hyoid to the side of the laterally displaced condyle

anterior displacement of the disk, excessive posterior compression of bilaminar structures.

Factors that may cause temporomandibular osteoarthritis Many factors can lead to this, including malpositioning of the joint (especially posterior displacement of the condyle), tooth extraction, especially of molars (leading to distortion of stress on TMJ), poorly adjusted dental fillings or replacement, caries, periodontal inflammation, traumatic injury, inflammation, (age-related) abnormal stress, bruxism, local tumors, or rheumatic conditions (osteoarthritis or arthritis).

The temporal bone

Osteopathy ascribes great importance to the temporal bones in the development of craniomandibular dysfunctions (CMD).[284:162f.,424] All disturbances of the temporal bones, or restrictions in their adaptation, are capable of impairing the TMJ. Primary or secondary impairment of the temporal bone can arise due to ascending chains.

The most common dysfunction, according to traditional cranial models, is IR of both temporal bones (associated with perinatal trauma). In IR, displacement of the mandibular fossae in an anterolateral direction occurs, resulting in anterior displacement of the mandible. In ER of both temporal bones, the mandible is displaced posteriorly. Secondary dysfunctions of the mandible are usually only manifested once the child begins to chew.

Mechanism of neuromuscular dysfunction

- Dysfunction of temporal bone and sphenoid leads, via the facial nerve (CN VII), to abnormal tension of the digastric muscle (posterior belly), resulting in CMD.
- Dysfunction of the temporal bone and sphenoid leads, via the trigeminal ganglion and mandibular nerve (CN V_3), to abnormal tension of the temporal muscle, masseter muscle, pterygoid muscle, and digastric muscle (anterior belly), resulting in CMD.

Synchondroses of the cranial base The significant factor here is the developmental dynamic influence of the cranial base on the growth of the middle and lower face. This takes place in an anteroinferior direction. As well as the SBS, the sphenoethmoid and sphenofrontal synchondroses also have a significant influence here.

According to traditional cranial osteopathic models, the occipital bone influences the temporal bone, which in turn influences the mandible. For example: occipital bone in extension draws the temporal bones into internal rotation; this causes anterior displacement of the mandible (Figure 2.54).

Traditional cranial osteopathic models tell us that the sphenoid influences the anterior bones of the face (including the maxilla), but not the mandible.

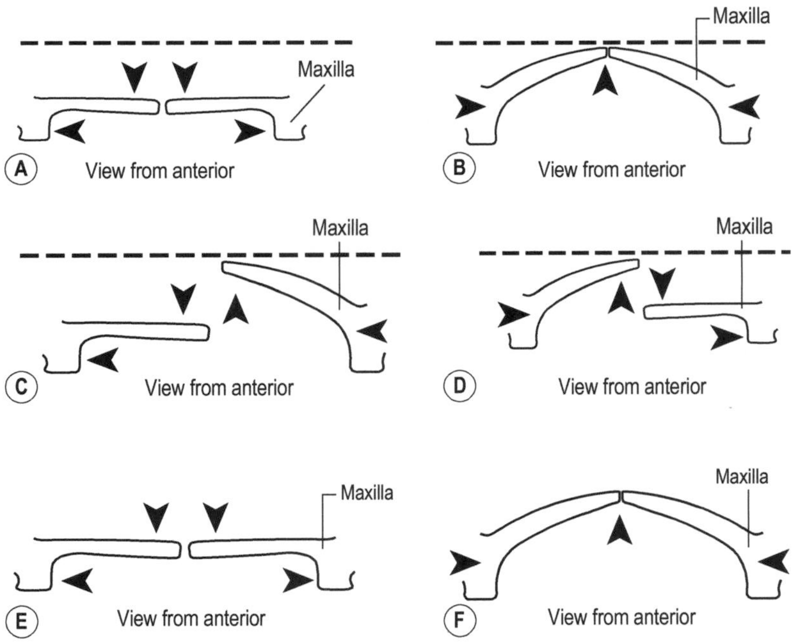

Figure 2.54
Influence of the sphenobasilar synchondrosis on occlusion.
A Flexion of the SBS.
B Extension of the SBS.
C Torsion right of the SBS.
D Sidebending/rotation right of the SBS.
E Superior vertical strain of the SBS.
F Inferior vertical strain of the SBS

Mechanism of neuromuscular dysfunction

- Via the accessory nerve (CN IX) and the cervical plexus, dysfunction of the occipital bone causes abnormal tension of the sternocleidomastoid muscle, which may lead to a restriction of the temporal bone with consequent CMD.
- Via motor nuclei of cranial nerve V_3, dysfunction of the occipital bone is believed to produce abnormal tension of the temporalis, masseter, lateral and medial pterygoid muscles, and digastric muscle (anterior belly), with consequent CMD.
- Via the mandibular nerve (CN V_3), torsion of the SBS with compression of the foramen ovale causes spasm of the masticatory muscles with consequent CMD.

Mechanism of myofascial dysfunction

- Torsion of the SBS leads, via the pterygoid process, to abnormal tension or hypertonicity of the lateral pterygoid muscle, as a result of which the condylar process is restricted anterior.
- TMJ dysfunctions also affect the contralateral sphenoid and occipital bones
  - Via the pterygoid process of the sphenoid, increased tonicity of the pharyngeal constrictor muscles can arise.
  - Dysfunction of the basilar part of the occipital bone can lead to dysfunction of the cervical spine.

The disk

The effects of stress and of the transmission of tension are produced primarily in the intermediate zone of the disk (especially in its lateral parts). Even relatively minor loading of the joint can induce distinct deformation.[27]

During a forceps delivery, the disk may be damaged by the pressure of the forceps on the preauricular region.[145:96] As a rule, however, the damaged tissues of the baby quickly regenerate.

Extreme mouth-opening movements, or holding the mouth fully open for long periods (e.g., during dental treatment, etc.), can lead to overextension of the bilaminar structures. Traumatic injuries caused, e.g., by falling or by blows may lead to excessive posterior compression of the bilaminar (retrodiscal) structures, resulting in inflammation, pain, and swelling which in some circumstances may cause anterior displacement of the disk. Another consideration is that, with age, the disk becomes thinner.

As a result of malocclusion, tooth extractions, muscle imbalances (e.g., hypertonicity of the posterior part of the temporalis muscle), and dysfunctions of the musculoskeletal system, etc., sustained asymmetric forces (extension or compression) may affect the related disk (monolateral or bilateral), leading to increased discal wear and problems with the bilaminar (retrodiscal) structures. Another cause quoted as leading to anterior dislocation of a disk is orthodontically induced retrusion of the mandible, resulting in histological and macroscopic changes in the disk and its attachments, e.g., flattening of the posterior discal region.[193] Anterior displacement of the disk may be induced by excessive contraction of the superior part of the lateral pterygoid muscle.[243,466] However, the associated posterior displacement of the condyle can also be caused by the temporalis muscle (see restriction of the condyle in the posterior position, above).[174]

For anterior displacement of the disk to occur, there must previously have been strain due to dorsocranial displacements of the condyle. In the long term, anterior displacement of the disk damages the bilaminar zone. That can often lead to hyalinization of the retrodiscal tissue, and so to diminished vascularization of the temporomandibular joint, which in turn predisposes to arthritic changes.

Changes in the position of the menisci are frequently encountered, but are usually symptomless.[466] Retrodiscal disturbances may exist with or without alteration of the disk–condyle relationship. However, investigations have confirmed that anterior displacement of the disk in static occlusion represents the most common intra-articular symptomatic disturbance of the TMJ.[29,31,40,119,120,121,163,211,313,342,351,358,366,394,404,407,420,440,457,461] While an anterior dislocation of the disk does not necessarily coexist with CMD, it is frequently associated with a convex disk shape and perforation of the posterior disk attachment, as well as with an increased susceptibility to the development of CMD.[4,65,277,421]

It has been demonstrated that lateral and medial disk displacements, in contrast to the rare posterior displacements, are found more frequently than had been assumed in the past.[29,31,40,119,120,121,163,211,351,358,366,394,404,407,437,440,457] An anteromedial position of the disk is more common than the anterolateral position.

Clinical presentation/hypothetical pathology Joint sounds (clicking, crepitation), subluxation, motion restriction, and pain may occur (severe restriction and pain occur particularly in association with discal dislocation).[241] In the anteromedial position of the disk, there is usually (80%) a retral position of the condyle. Also, the head of the condyle is shifted laterally somewhat and therefore appears to be more prominent.[240] In the anterolateral disk position, the head of the condyle is displaced medially and is less prominent. This is associated with severe trismus (locked jaw).[474]

Where the condition is chronic, we find osteoarthitis (crepitation; grating), or—due to persisting dysfunctional stresses—disk perforation with additional deviation (see this volume, section 2.7.2 on divergencies in the midline of the incisors on mouth opening and closing).

Secondary abnormal contractions of the masseter and temporalis muscles arise as an arthrokinetic protective reflex associated with an abnormal disk position.[194]

Analysis of temporomandibular joint clicking

Jaw clicking can be traced to joint-related CMD, e.g., changes in the articular surfaces of the TMJ, hypermobility of the condyle, hypermobility of the disk, disk displacement with or without repositioning, and via the lateral ligament (Table 2.5):

- Normal movement of the jaw joint (Figure 2.55).
- Clicking begins immediately on opening the mouth (**initial clicking**): the bilaminar

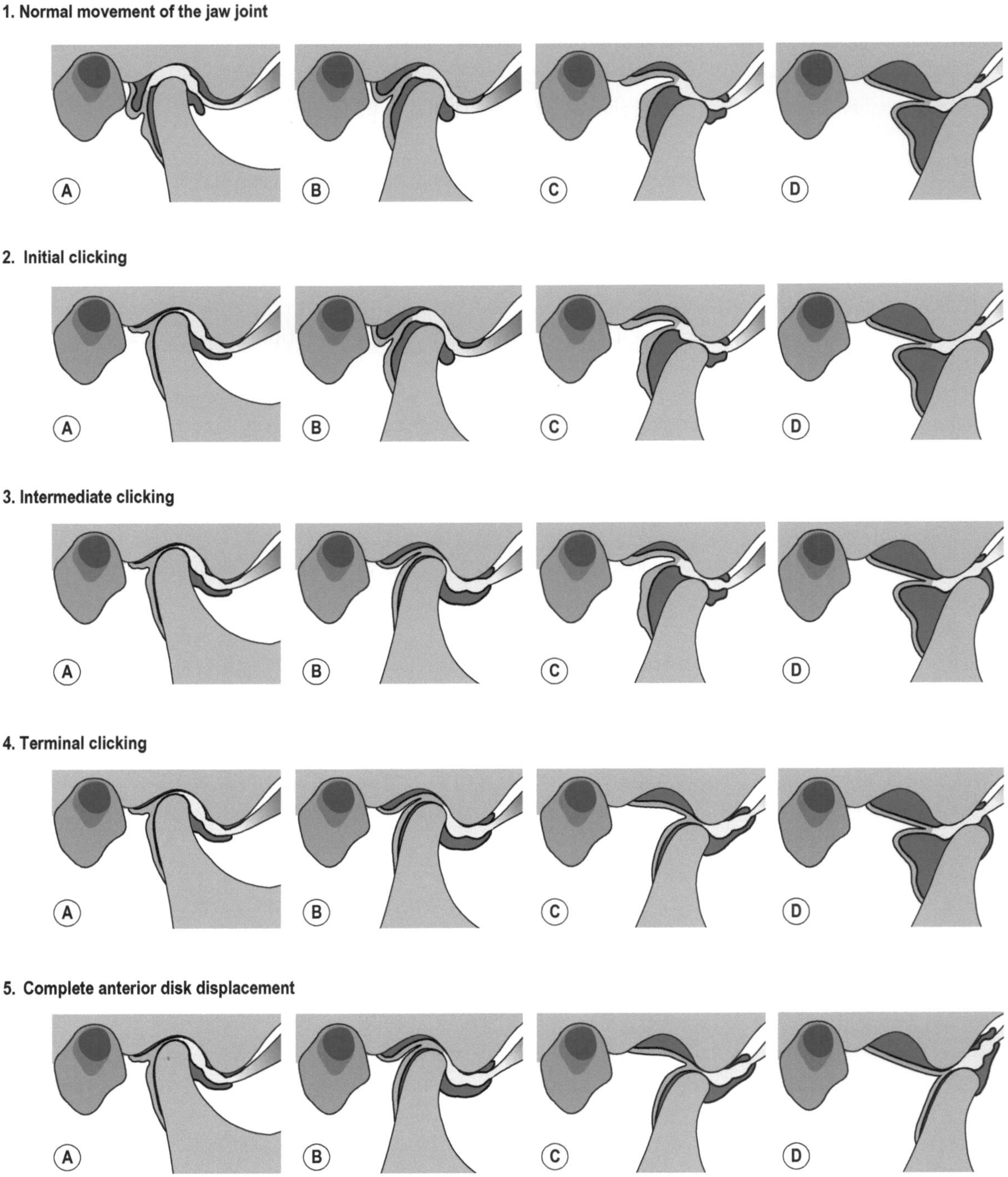

Figure 2.55
Analysis of jaw joint clicking. **1** Normal movement of the jaw joint. **2** Initial clicking. **3** Intermediate clicking. **4** Terminal clicking. **5** Complete anterior disk displacement

(retrodiscal) tissue has been displaced immediately in front of the condyle. The sound is due to the condyle shifting into position into the disk.

- Clicking during mouth opening (**intermediate clicking**): the bilaminar (retrodiscal) tissue has moved a greater distance in front of the condyle. The condyle must therefore travel further to locate in the disk.
- Clicking during the end of mouth opening (**terminal clicking**): the disk has moved further forward beneath the articular tubercle of the temporal bone. The condyle regains contact with the disk only at the end of mouth opening. The sound is indicative of damage to the disk.
- Complete anterior disk displacement: the disk is positioned in front of the articular tubercle of the temporal bone. The condyle is no longer able to locate in the disk. At this stage, there is normally no longer any clicking noise. This stage can progress to a true arthrosis.

Hyoid bone

The hyoid may be dysfunctional owing to temporomandibular joint disturbances (disturbances of swallowing or vocalization, etc.) and transmit CMD via myofascial chains (Figure 2.56). However, it may also participate in the development of CMD.[265]

Maxilla

Cause Traumatic injury (a fall or a blow). The fact that the maxilla is displaced posterior can lead to ER of the zygomatic bone and compression of the maxilla–palatine–pterygoid process complex. The consequence is an ipsilateral displacement of the condyle anterior.

Clinical presentation Clicking sounds, reduced mouth opening, pain on chewing.

Intraosseous dysfunctions of the maxilla may also be involved where there is pain.

Further cranial structures

In the treatment of children, from the developmental dynamic point of view special attention should be paid to dysfunctional tensions in sutures, maxillary tuberosities, alveolar processes, and synchondroses, which are regions of growth.

The most important mechanical stimulus in distortions of the cranium (apart from traumatic injury) comes from the cranial muscles, especially the masticatory muscles.[141] In this respect it is possible for myogenic CMD to lead to dysfunctional influences on the cranium.

The cranium as a whole should be taken into consideration in connection with CMD, as should further cranial bones in addition to those mentioned above, especially the palatine, zygomatic,

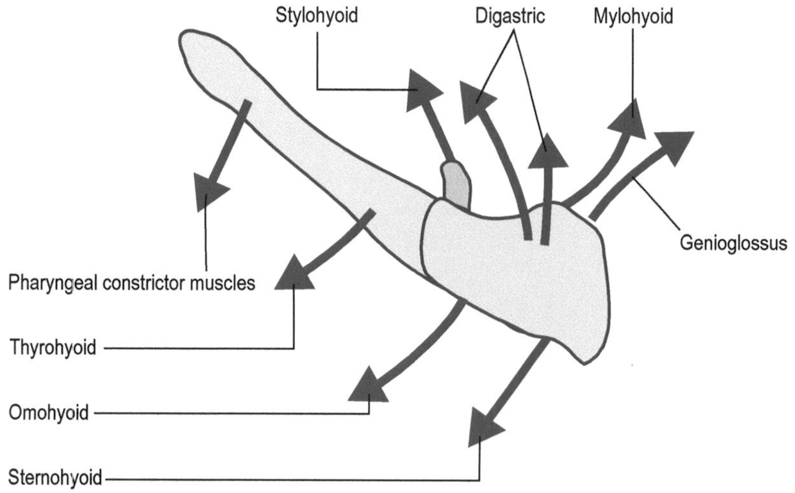

Figure 2.56
Effects of muscles on the hyoid bone

sphenoid, occipital, ethmoid, and frontal bones and vomer.

The cranial base and vomer, for example, are important from the developmental dynamic perspective, and exert an anteroinferior growth impulse. Malocclusion could potentially compress the vomer. From the point of view of osteopathy, in the chains of lesion relating to CMD, all the sutures of the bones mentioned can be affected or can play a role. In CMD and disturbed functioning of the mouth/jaw, the following are particularly important: transverse palatine suture, median palatine suture, sphenopalatine suture, palatomaxillary suture, frontozygomatic suture, vomeromaxillary suture, and incisive suture.

Points of passage for any nerve tracts or blood vessels involved should be considered (for example, in the case of the sphenoid, the foramen rotundum, the point of passage for the maxillary nerve and foramen ovale for the mandibular nerve) (see also this volume, Chapter 3).

Clinical presentation For example, disturbances or pain of the masticatory muscles, toothache, and sensitive or viscerosensitive disturbances of the anterior three quarters of the tongue and adjacent gingiva, soft palate, and cheek.

Bruxism and CMD can potentially bring about changes or localized increases in the effects of force on intraosseous or intrasutural structures in the regions of the mandible, nasomaxillary buttress, zygomatic buttress, and pterygomaxillary buttress (see also this volume, section 2.1.3). Conversely, it is conceivable that reduced elasticity in the bone could negatively affect resorption and the distribution of mechanical stresses caused by masticatory pressure.

Points of passage

- **The carotid canal in the petrous part of the temporal bone**
  - CMD and bruxism can lead to intraosseous dysfunctions of the temporal bone, and as a result possibly also affect the carotid plexus and internal carotid artery in the carotid canal.
  - Clinical/hypothetical pathology: disturbances of the oral and nasal cavities, lacrimal gland (the sympathetic system has an inhibitory effect on secretion), and the ear.
- **Foramen rotundum**
  - Can in some circumstances be affected in CMD.
  - Clinical/hypothetical pathology: atypical facial pain in the maxillary region, nose, and upper lip.
- **Foramen ovale**
  - Can in some circumstances be affected in CMD.
  - Clinical/hypothetical pathology: atypical facial pain in the lower third of the face.
- **Foramen spinosum**
  - Can in some circumstances be affected in CMD and increased tension of the lateral pterygoid muscle.
  - Clinical/hypothetical pathology: headache.
- **Jugular foramen**
  - Causes: in association with the occipital bone; primarily traumatic, e.g., tooth extraction with mouth very wide open.
  - Clinical/hypothetical pathology: disturbance of the jugular foramen and foramen lacerum, and the nerves and vessels passing through these, e.g.:
    - CN XI: pain at nape of neck; torticollis.
    - CN IX: disturbances in the sense of taste, dry mouth (parasympathetic fibers serving the parotid gland), disturbed swallowing (sensory fibers to the pharynx).
    - CN X: cardiac, digestive, and respiratory dysfunctions, disturbances of speech and swallowing.
- **Incisive foramen**
  - Causes: early traumatic influences or use of dental braces.
  - Clinical/hypothetical pathology: impairment of the nasopalatine nerve (CN V_2) with pain affecting the maxillary front

teeth, in the region of the mucosa at the anterior palate and the nasal septum.

- **Mental foramen**
  - Clinical/hypothetical pathology: impairment of the mental nerve (branch of the inferior alveolar nerve from CN V_3) or the mental artery and vein with pain affecting the teeth of the lower jaw.

Other points of passage can also be affected indirectly in cases of CMD.

Cervical spine

Mechanism of neuromuscular dysfunction

- Dysfunction of the upper cervical spine leads, via the cervical spinal nerves C1 to C3, to an abnormal tension of the infrahyoid muscles. These restrict the hyoid bone and affect the suprahyoid muscles, resulting in CMD (see below).
- Dysfunction of the upper cervical spine leads, via the accessory nerve (CN IX) and cervical plexus, to abnormal tension of the sternocleidomastoid with restriction of the temporal bone, resulting in CMD.
- Mutual reinforcement of dysfunctions of the neck muscles and TMJ via the trigeminal nucleus.

Mechanism of myofascial dysfunction

- Dysfunction of the upper cervical spine leads to CMD via the suprahyoid muscles, or the superficial layer, pretracheal layer, or deep layer of cervical fascia.
- A dysfunction of the upper cervical spine may also give rise to stimulation of the auriculotemporal nerve, with consequent pain in the TMJ, and earache.
- Hyperlordosis of the cervical spine can give rise to distocclusion.[21:28]
- A hyperextended/kyphotic cervical spine may lead to prognathic occlusion.[21:28]
- Scoliosis may cause ipsilateral CMD and crossbite.
- Atlas–axis dysfunction can give rise to an open bite.

Pectoral girdle

There is a close functional relationship between the pectoral girdle (shoulder girdle) and the function of mouth and jaw.

Mechanism of myofascial dysfunction

- Dysfunction of the scapula leads, via the omohyoid muscle, to restriction of the hyoid bone and, via the suprahyoid muscles, to CMD.
- Via the sternocleidomastoid and through the continuity of the infrahyoid muscles with the digastric muscle (posterior belly) and stylohyoid muscle, dysfunction of the clavicle and sternum causes restriction of the temporal bone, resulting in CMD.
- Drawn-back shoulders can bring about protrusion.

2.6.2 Muscular dysfunctions

A number of investigations have concluded that most temporomandibular joint pain[29,30] and occlusal disturbances[62] are of muscular origin. It is also possible that muscle imbalances give rise to pain and ultimately to masticatory disturbances[30] or inflammatory and degenerative changes in the joints.[393] However, there is no consensus as to whether muscle hyperactivity is of local (occlusal, articular) or central causation (stress; psychoemotional factors).[481] Myogenic CMD can also be assumed to exert an influence on skull distortions and sutures (this volume, section 2.6.1). Apart from this, muscle continuities are a significant factor in the formation of the osseous structures. Account should be taken of asymmetries.

There are significant associations between sensitivity to palpation of the masticatory muscles (including the sternocleidomastoid and suboccipital muscles) and headache.[38] This need not necessarily mean that the association between these is one of cause and effect. In both, it is possible that the underlying factor may be a disturbance in pain processing, with a reduction of the pain perception or tolerance threshold.[447]

The **masseter, lateral pterygoid, and temporalis muscles** are the muscles of mastication most commonly involved in CMD.

Causes of muscular hypertonicity

- Malocclusion, bruxism.
- Dysfunction of the cervical spine, as well as of the rest of the vertebral column and the limbs.
- Faulty posture (this volume, section 2.5.4).
- Stress and psychological factors (gnashing of the teeth and grinding of the teeth).
- Traumatic injury: fall or blow to the mandible or head; also, supporting one's head with the hand or arm under the lower jaw, or in consequence of tooth extraction or wear; this can result in acute or persistent muscle spasm.
- Poorly adjusted dental prostheses.
- CMD.
- Degenerative and inflammatory diseases of the TMJ (pain leads to further muscular contraction).
- Neurovascular: associated with dysfunction of the sphenopetrosal synchondrosis or foramen ovale. This leads to compression or edema affecting the mandibular nerve (CN V_3) either directly or via circulatory stasis.
- Hormonal influences: menopause, puberty, thyroid dysfunctions.
- Metabolic influences.
- Other influences: cold, damp, and climate.
- Shaper[402:377f.] states that shortness of one leg is the commonest single cause of spasm of the masticatory muscles.

Clinical presentation Pain; motion restrictions.

- **Temporalis muscle** (Figure 2.57)
  - Causes: psychoemotional factors, dental malposition, premature tooth contact, immobilization of the jaw, bruxism, gnashing of the teeth, cold, or traumatic injury, secondarily in association with dysfunction of the upper trapezius and of the sternocleidomastoid.[443:240]
  - Sequelae: in hypertonicity, the muscle may compress the squamous suture and then the disk and articular surface of the temporomandibular joint. A further possibility is that contraction of the temporalis muscle in bruxism can increase the transverse tension of the epicranial aponeurosis. This in turn leads to an increase in pressure on the calvaria (roof of skull): bruxism → contraction of temporalis muscle → increase in transverse tension of epicranial aponeurosis → increased pressure on roof of skull.
  - **Clinical presentation/hypothetical pathology:** pain in the maxillary sinus and in the molars of the upper jaw; pain in the temporal region; hypersensitivity and pain in the upper teeth:[120,121]
    - * Anterior part: parietal headache (compression of the sphenoparietal and coronal sutures); malocclusion;[72] grinding, central teeth-clenching; limited mouth opening. Muscle spasm draws the

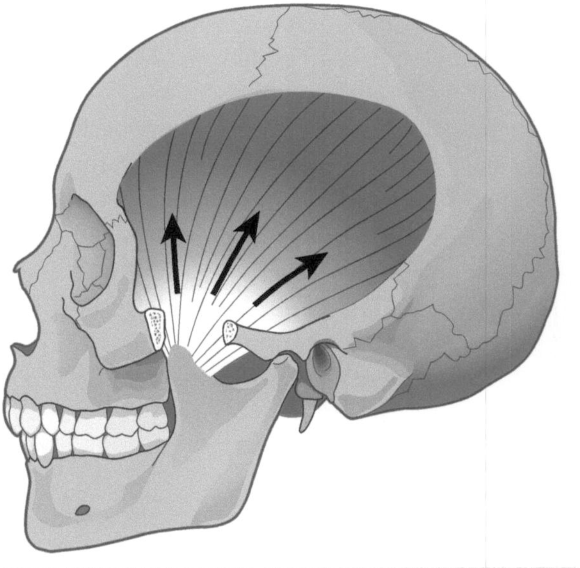

Figure 2.57
Hypertonicity of the temporalis muscle

mandible cephalad; possible compression in the TMJ, with discal dysfunction; possibly jaw clicking; disturbance affecting the bilaminar zone; temporal bone in anterior rotation.
    * Medial part: headache focused on the temporal bone. Muscle spasm draws the mandible cephalad (with the anterior part). Pain radiating into the larynx.
    * Posterior part: headache focused on the temporal bone or occipital bone (compression of the occipitomastoid suture); disturbance of venous drainage of the cranial vessels; muscle spasm draws the mandible posterior; limited mouth opening. Temporal bone in external rotation (as the condyle is positioned posterior), while the parietal bone is in internal rotation; pain radiating into the larynx.
- **Masseter muscle** (Figure 2.58)
  - Causes:

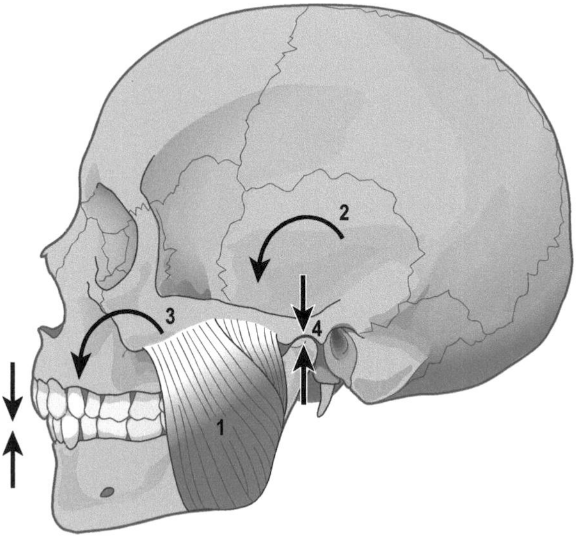

Figure 2.58
Hypertonicity of the masseter muscle. **1** Hypertonicity of the masseter muscle. **2** Temporal bone in anterior rotation. **3** Zygomatic bone in external rotation. **4** Compression of the TMJ

    * Chronic muscle strain (bruxism, excessive gum-chewing, pacifier/soother/dummy-sucking).[24]
    * Sudden strong contraction (cracking nuts), disturbances of occlusion, premature contact, mouth breathing, emotional trauma, CMD, overextended opening of the mouth during dental surgery, traumatic injury, secondarily in association with trigger points of the sternocleidomastoid.[443:223f.]
    * Pain in the TMJ is very often associated with increased muscle activity (sometimes with simultaneous contraction of the neck muscles).[389]
    * Interaction with the contralateral gluteus medius (Rossaint and Thie).[388:63]
  - Clinical presentation/hypothetical pathology:
    * Increased tension in the masseter muscle,[389] grinding of the teeth (protrusive bruxism), pain in the upper jaw and lower molars, and in the mid-facial region (maxillary nerve [CN V_2]) and maxillary sinus, and retro-ocular pain.[235]
    * Limited mouth opening.
    * In cases of unilateral hypertonicity, the mandible may deviate to the ipsilateral side.
    * Compression of the TMJ.
    * Deep part: unilateral tinnitus, frontal headache. Radiation into the TMJ and deep into the ear.
    * Superficial part: radiation into the eyebrow region, maxilla, mandible, and upper and lower molars.
- **Lateral pterygoid muscle** (Figure 2.59)
  - Causes: premature contact, bruxism, excessive gum-chewing, secondary to dysfunction of the sternocleidomastoid and nuchal muscles;[443:264] interaction with the adductor muscles (according to

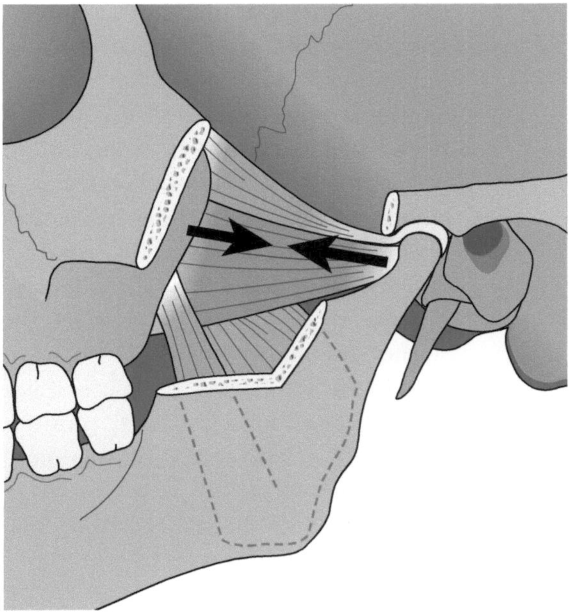

Figure 2.59
Hypertonicity of the lateral pterygoid muscle

Rossaint and Thie).[388:63] The lingual nerve may run through the belly of the muscle and therefore sometimes be compressed.[195]

- Clinical presentation/hypothetical pathology: grinding and clenching of the teeth, pain in the TMJ, maxilla, floor of the mouth, and earache; protrusion of the lower jaw, with slightly reduced mouth opening; reduced medial motion of the lower jaw; malocclusion:
  - **Inferior part:** mouth opening very slightly reduced, reduced laterotrusion to the contralateral side. On opening the mouth, the midline between the incisors deviates laterally. Muscle hypertonicity anteriorizes the condyle, resulting in premature contact of the contralateral front teeth and malocclusion of the ipsilateral back teeth. As a result, full bite closure usually triggers pain on the ipsilateral side. The more strongly the teeth are pressed together, the greater the pain. Possible dysfunction of the pterygopalatine ganglion. Dysfunction of the anterior ligament of the malleus.
  - **Superior part and pterygoid fascia**: muscle hypertonicity may displace the disk anterior, resulting in joint clicking. Although the masseteric fascia and temporalis fascia are connected with the articular disk, [387] these connections appear to be too weak to affect the movement of disk. Rather, their muscle spindles register the position of the disk and TMJ and transmit this information via afferent fibers to the brain.

- **Medial pterygoid muscle** (Figures 2.60 and 2.61)
  - Causes: malocclusion, bruxism, excessive gum-chewing and post-childhood thumb-sucking, emotional stress and anxiety, rarely muscle spasm in the pterygomandibular fossa; secondarily in association with dysfunction of the lateral pterygoid muscle or contralateral medial pterygoid muscle,[443:252] interaction with the contralateral adductor muscles/psoas (Rossaint and Thie).[388:63]
  - Clinical presentation/hypothetical pathology:
    - Similarly to masseter muscle, pain in the TMJ and floor of the mouth.
    - Mouth opening as a rule reduced and painful.
    - Dysphagia.
    - Radiation into the posterior region of the mouth, the pharynx, the region inferior and posterior to the TMJ, and deep into the ear.
    - Deviation of the midline of the incisors. (A displacement of the mandible to the contralateral or ipsilateral side, or to neither side, has been described.[30])

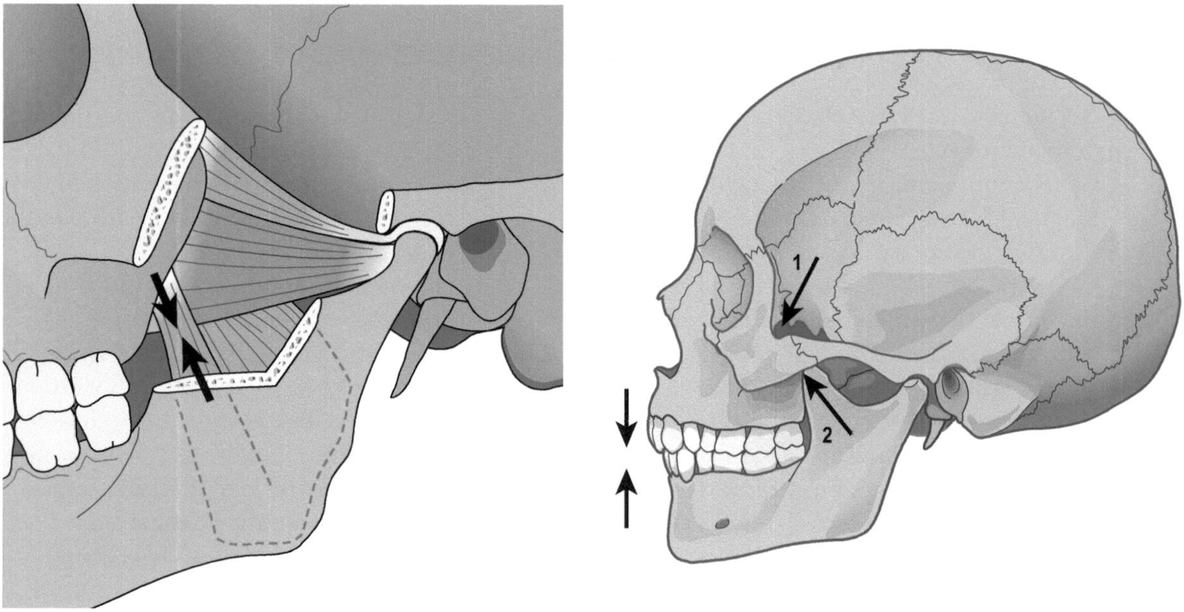

Figure 2.60 and Figure 2.61
Hypertonicity of the medial pterygoid muscle. **1** Muscle spasm restricts the pterygoid process of the sphenoid posterior and therefore the greater wing in flexion position. **2** Muscle spasm restricts the condyle anterior and cranially

    * Muscle spasm moves the condyle in an anterior and cranial direction, and the pterygoid process of the sphenoid in a posterior direction.
    * Possible dysfunction of the pterygopalatine ganglion.
    * Disturbances of the process of swallowing.
- **Sphenomandibular muscle**
  - Causes: muscle spasm, with compression of the maxillary nerve against the posterior wall of the maxillary sinus.[172]
  - Clinical presentation: retro-orbital pain, possible involvement in the causation of cluster headache.
- **Mentalis muscle**
  - Causes: incomplete mouth closure due to lip incompetence (a too-short upper lip), especially in mouth breathing.
  - Clinical presentation: amplifies or encourages Angle's Class II occlusion. Visible signs of the strong tension are the formation of a marked labial fold below the lower lip and a dimple in the middle of the chin. When the lips are clenched, the overpronounced role of the mentalis muscle causes inversion of the upper incisors.
- **Orbicularis oris muscle**
  - Causes: mouth breathing; oral dyskinesia.
  - Clinical presentation: dental malposition, etc.
- **Buccinator muscle**
  - Causes: mouth breathing; oral dyskinesia.
  - Clinical presentation: dental malposition; CMD symptoms, etc.
- **Other facial muscles in the region of the mouth**
  - Causes: dyskinesias, etc.

- Clinical presentation: trigeminal neuralgia; atypical facial pain (Volume 2, section 4.3.3); pain in the region of the upper canines (levator labii superioris alaeque nasi muscle).

• **Mylohyoid muscle**
  - Causes: functional disturbances of the tongue,[145:94] dysphagia, tightness of the throat or globus sensation, sore throat, TMJ symptoms. Glossoptosis (pressure of the root of the tongue against the cervical spine, resulting in mouth breathing).

• **Digastric muscle**
  - Causes: bruxism (tenderness, unilateral: anteroposterior bruxism; bilateral: lateral bruxism), mouth breathing, secondary to dysfunction of the masseter muscle,[443:273,276] elongated stylohyoid process. (Posterior belly.)
  - Clinical presentation/hypothetical pathology: grinding of the teeth, pain and functional disturbances of the mouth floor, tongue, and pharynx, pain in the lower incisors (anterior belly); difficulty swallowing, TMJ symptoms, possibly pseudo-pain in the sternocleidomastoid (posterior belly). Hypertonicity of the muscle can restrict the hyoid bone in a cranial position, cause difficulty in closing the mouth, and cause external rotation of the temporal bone.
  - Hypertonicity of the posterior belly draws the mandible towards the ipsilateral side. This does not usually become manifest, however, as other muscles compensate for the effect (e.g., contralateral temporalis muscle, posterior part, and masseter muscle, deep part).

• **Geniohyoid muscle**
  - Clinical presentation: TMJ symptoms, similar symptoms to digastric muscle (see above).

• **Stylohyoid muscle**
  - Causes: bruxism (tenderness, unilateral: anteroposterior bruxism; bilateral: lateral bruxism), elongated stylohyoid process.
  - Clinical presentation/hypothetical pathology: pain/discomfort on swallowing, pain in upper region of neck, dizziness:
    * Associated with muscle spasm: cranial motion of the hyoid bone and difficulties closing the mouth. Radiation of the pain into the tongue, floor of the mouth, pharynx, and larynx.
    * Hypertonic suprahyoid muscles may draw the mandible posterior. During the growth phase, this leads to reduced sagittal growth by comparison with the maxilla, resulting in distocclusion and withdrawal of the tongue from the palate due to the loss of its counterpart.
    * Hypertonic suprahyoid musculature may also compress the articular surfaces and disk of the TMJ, as well as the vessel-conducting retrodiscal pad, by moving the articular processes of the mandible into the posterior part of the TMJ groove. The infrahyoid muscles and middle constrictor of the pharynx must then produce a counterforce in order to hold the hyoid bone in position in response to contraction of the suprahyoid muscles. This reactive tension can in turn produce symptoms in the infrahyoid muscles. A reactive chronic hypertonicity of the middle constrictor of the pharynx can, via its connections with the neck, lead to strain in this region.
    * The suprahyoid muscles are often affected together as a functional unit.
    * The suprahyoid muscles also interact with the opposite psoas muscle (Rossaint and Thie).[388:63]

• **Superior pharyngeal constrictor**
  - Clinical presentation/hypothetical pathology:
    * Pain and functional disturbance of the floor of the mouth and the pharynx.

    * In association with hypertonicity: via the pharyngeal raphe, dysfunctions of flexion and extension of the SBS.
- **Genioglossus muscle**
  - Clinical presentation/hypothetical pathology: functional disturbance of the tongue.
- **Sternohyoid, thyrohyoid, omohyoid muscles**[265] (Figure 2.62)
  - Clinical presentation/hypothetical pathology. In muscle spasm: cephalad movement of hyoid bone and difficulties closing the mouth; possibly thyroid disturbances.
- **Tongue** (see this volume, section 3.1)
  - Clinical presentation: dysphagia.
- **Sternocleidomastoid** (Figure 2.63)
  - Causes: postural imbalance due to a difference in leg length and pectoral girdle dysfunction, disturbances of breathing (asthma), dyskinesia, a sequela from CSF puncture, chronic sinusitis, dental abscess, herpes simplex in the mouth region.[443:207]
  - Clinical presentation/hypothetical pathology:
    * Soreness of the neck (patient lies in bed, usually on the side of the dysfunction).
    * Tension headache, sweating of the forehead on the ipsilateral side, conjunctival redness, lacrimation, rhinitis, blurred vision.
    * Sternal part: pain at the temple, cheek, and orbit.
    * Clavicular part: frontal headache, disturbance of balance, postural dizziness, sea-sickness or travel sickness, possibly with nausea.

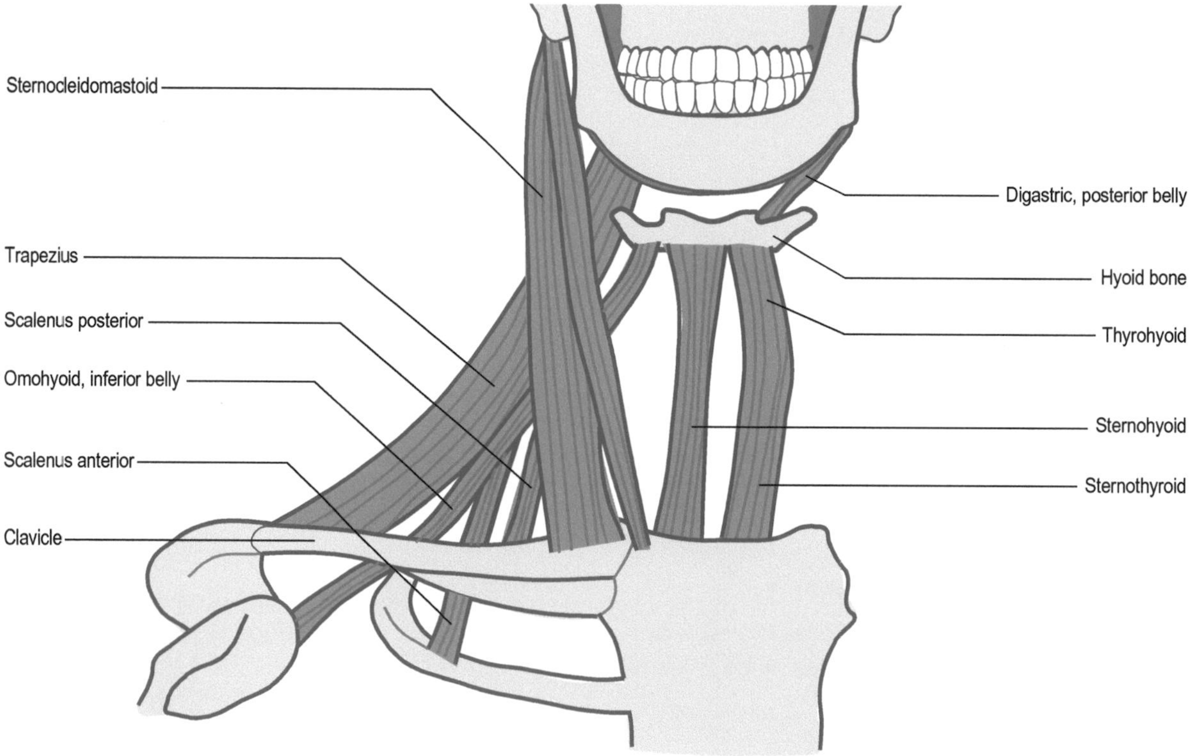

Figure 2.62
Hyoid muscles

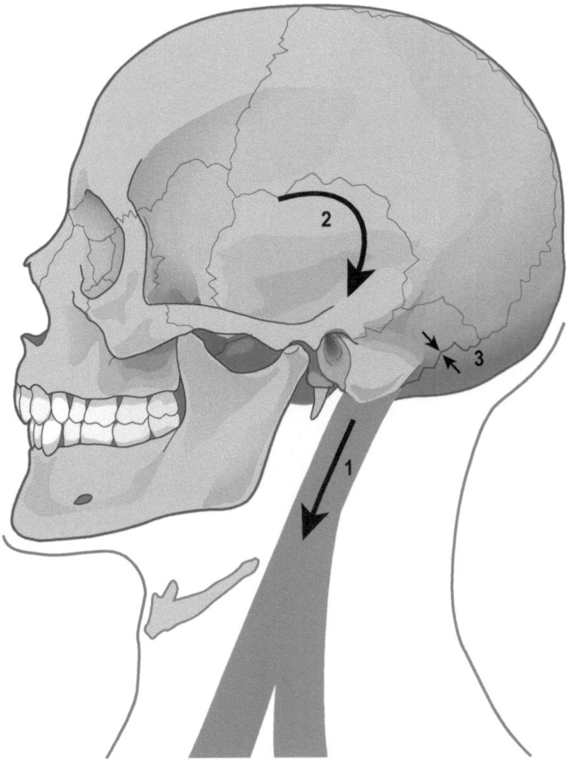

Figure 2.63
Hypertonicity of the sternocleidomastoid. **1** Contraction of the sternocleidomastoid muscle. **2** Internal rotation of the temporal bone. **3** Compression of the occipitomastoid suture

  - * Associated with hypertonicity: internal rotation of the temporal bone with secondary TMJ disturbance and compression of the occipitomastoid suture.

2.6.3 Dysfunction of the ligaments

Clinical presentation: pain, motion restrictions (possibly joint sounds, associated with dysfunctions of the articular capsule).

- **Stylomandibular ligament**
  - ◆ Causes: dysfunctions due to prolonged mouth opening, dental extractions, associated with anterolateral displacement of the disk. The ligament can also calcify or the styloid process can be elongated (Eagle syndrome, stylohyoid syndrome).
  - ◆ Clinical presentation: neuralgic pain, dysphonia, earache, eustachian tube dysfunction with pressure affecting the ear, dysphagia, and carotodynia;[249] also possibly sensitivity to pain at the styloid process. In Eagle syndrome, vague neck pain, cervical dysphagia, and chronic orofacial pain; rarely vertigo and syncope.[19]

> **CAUTION** In Eagle syndrome, turning the head can cause compression or even dissection of the internal carotid artery. This can potentially lead to transitory ischemic attack (TIA) or stroke.[179]

- **Sphenomandibular ligament**
  - ◆ Causes: dysfunctions due to prolonged mouth opening, dental extractions, or treatment in the posterior molar region: immobilization of the head, and having the mouth open wide, result in restriction of the temporal bones in internal rotation:
    - * Extraction of a tooth in the lower jaw creates a pull on the sphenomandibular ligament on the contralateral side. Since the ligament is attached to the sphenoid posterior to the transverse flexion/extension axis, the traction on the ligament causes a cranial movement of the greater wing on this side (= opposite side to the dental extraction).
    - * Extraction of a molar from the lower jaw: cranial motion of the greater wing on the contralateral side (torsion).
    - * Extraction of a molar from the upper jaw: cranial motion of the greater wing on the same side (torsion). This results in stretching of the petrosphenoidal ligament on the side of the cranial greater wing.

- Clinical presentation/hypothetical pathology: restriction of protrusion and mouth opening, narrowing of the mandibular foramen with stimulation of the inferior alveolar nerve (pain in the lower jaw, around the teeth), facial pain (CN V, trigeminal ganglion), visual disturbances (CN VI), disturbances of blood outflow in this region, eustachian tube dysfunction with pressure affecting the ear, tinnitus.
- **Articular capsule and lateral ligament**
  - Causes: traumatic injury from fall or blow, excessive strain and subluxation of the TMJ, premature contact, grinding, gnashing or clenching the teeth, lateral capsulitis, diseases (e.g., polyarthritis).
  - Clinical presentation/hypothetical pathology: on account of the good nerve supply, particularly of the articular capsule and lateral ligament, but also of the other structures, inflammation (mostly anterior and lateral), strain, and subluxation of the temporomandibular joint can cause severe pain. This massive sensory input is transmitted to the trigeminal ganglion, which consequently acts as a kind of facilitated segment and contributes to maintaining the CMD.
  - Atrophy (mostly of the posterior part of the capsule) leads to slowly increasing limitation of jaw opening.
  - If the bilaminar zone is affected, pain and/or joint effusion can develop.
  - If the condyle is posteriorly displaced: clicking sounds or restricted mouth opening.

FURTHER INFORMATION A "facilitated segment" describes a spinal cord segment that has become more easily excited due to certain factors, so that a much smaller stimulus is sufficient to evoke a reaction at this segment. This results in tissue changes and symptoms in regions of the body innervated by this segment.

- **Anterior ligament of the malleus and Pintus ligament**
  - Clinical presentation: hearing difficulties, tinnitus.
- **Sphenopetrosal ligament:** at the sphenopetrosal synchondrosis.

2.6.4 Fascial dysfunctions

All fascial structures are capable of transmitting tensions caused by CMD or, conversely, of conducting dysfunctions from other regions of the body to the TMJ (see also section 2.5). There is a close functional connection between the fasciae of the head and neck and they are clinically significant in CMD and TMJ pain as well as pain on chewing and swallowing, tension headache, pain affecting the nape and shoulders, tinnitus, dizziness, visual disturbances, sinusitis, pharyngitis, and laryngitis. The most important connections are explained below (see also reference [265]).

- **Carotid sheath:** increased tension can sometimes affect the internal jugular vein, internal carotid artery, or vagus nerve.
- The **superficial (investing) layer of cervical fascia** arises ventrally at the hyoid, at the mandible, acromion, and spine of the scapula, clavicle, and anterior border of the manubrium of the sternum. It attaches to the dorsal side of the clavicles, sternum, and hyoid. Interacting tensions can occur between these parts and are involved in, for example, dysphagia and globus sensation, possibly also in association with the thyropericardial lamina.
- Increased tension of the **pretracheal layer** of the cervical fascia can be involved in dysphagia, and may possibly—e.g., via the thyropericardial lamina—impair cardiac function. In addition, here there is also indirect contact with the diaphragm. There is also contact with the thyroid gland via the continuity with the thyroid fascia.
- The visceral compartment, trachea, and esophagus are surrounded by a visceral fascia in

continuity with the **buccopharyngeal fascia** (Volume 2, section 4.2.2).

The buccopharyngeal fascia covers the buccinator muscle and continues posteriorly into the **pterygomandibular raphe** and fascia of the constrictor muscles of the pharynx; caudally it is connected with the parietal pleura and cervical pleura (pleural cupula). These fasciae are of importance in connection with tensions of the pharynx and oral cavity, dysphagia, and possibly neck pain.

- The **deep (prevertebral) layer** of the cervical fascia lies behind the visceral compartment (esophagus, trachea, thyroid), which is in turn secured to the diaphragm. This fascia is involved in interactions between the upper cervical region, craniocervical transition, and disturbances of occlusion.
- **Pterygoid fascia** of the deep fascia of the face: see lateral pterygoid muscle (section 2.6.2).
- **Parotideomasseteric fascia** of the deep fascia of the face: when there is increased tension, this could continue via fibrous septa to the parotid gland, and can potentially impair the function of the gland.
- **Temporalis fascia** of the deep fascia of the neurocranium: if there is dysfunction, this can impair the ability of the temporalis muscle to glide. Tensions of the temporalis, masseteric, and paratideomasseteric fasciae and of the superficial (investing) layer of cervical fascia also affect each other.
- Attachments of the **pterygotemporomandibular aponeurosis** create a route by which tensions of the TMJ could exert an effect at the cranial base.
- The **interpterygoid aponeurosis** may be involved where there is pain in the temporomandibular joint, clicking sounds, and potentially also where there is discoordination or deviation of the lower jaw. (See also medial and lateral pterygoid muscles, section 2.6.2.)
- **Epicranial aponeurosis:** chronic tension of the temporalis muscle can increase transverse tension in the epicranial aponeurosis; this in turn increases pressure on the roof of the skull. The epicranial aponeurosis links the muscles of the head (frontalis and occipitalis bellies of the occipitofrontalis muscle, and the auricularis superior to the ear, and, indirectly, the orbicularis to the eye). Attention should be paid to impairment from interactions where there is increased suboccipital muscle tension and tension of the temporalis muscle; also where there is headache, dizziness, or visual disturbances.
- The shoulder and jaw influence each other via the **clavipectoral fascia**.

2.6.5 Dural dysfunctions

Because dural innervation is provided via the trigeminal nerve (CN V), CMD may also result in headache. Dural dysfunctions and CMD may lead to facilitation of the **trigeminal ganglion**.

Evidence has been produced that the tentorium cerebelli plays a role in disk dislocation; in post-mortem investigations, a correlation has been reported between disk dislocation, the degree of ossification of the petrotympanic fissure, and fibrosis of the tentorium cerebelli.[245]

2.6.6 Disturbances of the nerves, sensitization mechanisms, and disturbances of pain processing

Dysfunction of the joints, sutures, dura mater, and fasciae may directly impair the neural structures and facilitate motor innervation in such a way as to give rise to CMD. However, such disturbances may also be caused indirectly by venous stasis, e.g., in the cavernous sinus, or by stimulation of the periarterial sympathetic nerves. This leads, either directly or indirectly, to edema or compression of the nerve. The consequence could be a change in pH at the nerve, and altered stimulus conduction.

In association with dysfunction: due to the many nerve connections at the TMJ, the lateral ligament and the surrounding adipose tissue, dysfunctions, or inflammation of the jaw joint may be associated with severe pain.

Mechanisms of sensitization and disturbance of pain processing

There are clear empirical indications that peripheral and central sensitization mechanisms play a role in myofascial CMD.

Peripheral sensitization Peripheral sensitization arises when the activation threshold of primary afferent nociceptors (A-delta and C fibers) becomes lower.[470] This is characterized by increased spontaneous activity, a reduced response threshold and greater response readiness of peripheral nociceptors to noxious stimuli, or stimulation of their receptive fields (which may be enlarged). This means that the expression of muscle pain mainly occurs through a mechanism where there is peripheral sensitization of nociceptors. Hyperalgesia in more deeply located tissue of the injured area can be traced to this mechanism.[164] Muscle injuries and nociceptive nerve endings are the means by which inflammation mediators are released.[186] Peripheral sensitization in myofascial CMD indicates dysregulation in the trigeminal system[483] due to a raised trigeminal nociceptive input (see below).

Central sensitization If the increase in activated sensitized nociceptors leads to structural and functional modifications in the course of the pain pathway of neurons in higher centers, dorsal root ganglia, and in the posterior horn, this gives rise to central sensitization.[401] This is seen in a higher response to pain stimulation, brought about by a strengthening of the signals coming to the CNS. The result is increased stimulation (sensitization) and/or reduced inhibition of pain (descending facilitation). Central sensitization of regions farther away from the TMJ which were previously pain-free arises via extra-trigeminal hypersensitivity. The high rate of comorbidities between clearly different pain syndromes (e.g., fibromyalgia) could also be traceable to sensitization mechanisms.[478] It is therefore assumed that widespread pain, CMD, and fibromyalgia syndrome could be grouped together as "central sensitivity syndromes."[484] Central sensitization mechanisms could also be an explanation for the fact that fibromyalgia, CMD, and craniocervical dysfunctions are closely linked.[276]

There is clear evidence that peripheral and central sensitization are both involved in the pathophysiology of myofascial CMD.[377] For example, patients with myogenic CMD show not only trigeminal (peripheral) sensitivity, but also extra-trigeminal hypersensitivity to various stimuli[124,377,433] and persistent pain in several regions of the body.[448]

CMD patients exhibit either peripheral sensitization (non-sensitive patients, who essentially respond well to manual approaches) or central sensitization (sensitive patients);[348] the prognosis for manual approaches in these patients is less favorable.[201] A disturbance of pain processing, with a lowering of the pain perception or pain tolerance threshold, may possibly also be a factor underlying the interaction between increased sensitivity to palpation of the masticatory muscles (including the sternocleidomastoid and suboccipital muscles) and the development of headache.[447]

Pain sensitization also leads to changes in the mid-brain (section 2.6.7).

Neuropathic pain as related to axon and nerve root: see Volume 2, section 4.4.8.

Trigeminal nerve; trigeminal ganglion

The majority of cases of sensitization appear to be concentrated in patients with myogenic CMD in the trigeminal region[124,285,433] and can be considered to be peripheral sensitization (see above).

Pain in the TMJ and dental structures may spread throughout the entire region innervated by the trigeminal nerve. For example, nociceptive information may be conducted via the trigeminal nerve (CN V) to the trigeminal nucleus, which extends to the height of the second or third segment of the cervical spinal cord, and may even reach the upper thorax via intermediate neurons. It is also the case that the nerve receptors in the mouth region are much more sensitive than in other regions of the body. The trigeminal nucleus in the mid-brain simultaneously receives afferent proprioceptive information from the periodontal ligaments and from the muscle spindles. The stimuli may be mutually reinforcing in this trigeminal nucleus. The ganglion too may facilitate and give rise to a vicious circle (Volume 2, section 7.5).

The effects of various stimuli such as pressure or thermal stimuli experienced by myogenic CMD patients are possibly due to trigeminal hypersensitivity to pain;[116,304,376,454] there is some discussion and no clear agreement regarding the results for thermal pain sensitivity.[166]

Repeated mechanical stimulation of the region of the masseter muscle causes pain to mount and extends the duration of the pain.[378]

One-sided chewing, e.g., as a result of extracting the last molar, can possibly lead to an increase of pressure in the trigeminal ganglion (and in the temporomandibular joint); however, impairment of the ganglion due to nociceptive stimuli from the one-sided chewing is more likely.

In close proximity to the trigeminal ganglion, the trigeminal nerve may be impaired by high pressure within the internal carotid artery or by venous congestion at the level of the cavernous sinus.

In addition, the branches of the trigeminal nerve could be impaired by dysfunctions of the temporal bones and sphenoid, by abnormal dural tensions and venous congestion of the sinus, as well as by disturbances of outflow in the cranium.

Pathologies Tumors, infections, and metabolic diseases such as diabetes mellitus.

Mechanism of neuromuscular dysfunction Dysfunction of the temporal bone and sphenoid leads, via the trigeminal ganglion and mandibular nerve (CN V_3), to abnormal tensions of the temporalis, masseter, and pterygoid muscles and digastric muscle (anterior belly), resulting in CMD.

Additional nerves

- **The mandibular nerve (CN V_3) and its branches: masseteric nerve, the deep temporal nerves, and the lateral pterygoid, lingual, and inferior alveolar nerves**
  - Causes:
    - The causes include hypertonicity of the lateral pterygoid muscle, dysfunction at the foramen ovale (sphenopetrosal synchondrosis), abnormal dural tensions, dysfunction of the pterygospinous ligament, and CMD.
    - The lingual nerve may course through the belly of the lateral pterygoid muscle, and so be compressed in some circumstances.[195]
    - The inferior alveolar nerve may become compressed within the mandibular canal.[471,412]
    - Accelerated demyelination of the mandibular nerve (generation of abnormal impulses).
  - Mechanism of neuromuscular dysfunction: via motor nuclei of the mandibular nerve (CN V_3), dysfunction of the occipital bone leads to abnormal tension of the temporalis, masseter, and pterygoid muscles and digastric muscle (anterior belly), with consequent CMD.
  - Clinical presentation/hypothetical pathology: pain in the TMJ and pain referral, abnormal tension in the muscles of mastication (sequelae: CMD, malocclusion), pain in the teeth of the lower jaw, disturbances of salivation, sensory disturbances and pain in the skin of the lower facial region, headache (innervation of the dura of the middle cranial fossa).
- **Auriculotemporal nerve (CN V_3)**
  - This nerve runs between the neck of the mandible and the sphenomandibular ligament, winds around the neck of the mandible in a lateral direction, and courses upward beneath the parotid between the TMJ and the external acoustic meatus.

    - Clinical presentation: pain in the side of the face and temporal regions, and earache.
- **Maxillary nerve (CN V_2)**
    - The maxillary nerve passes through the foramen rotundum into the pterygopalatine fossa; there it subdivides further into the infraorbital nerve, zygomatic nerve, and ganglionic branches.
    - Causes: congestion at the cavernous sinus, dysfunction at the foramen rotundum and pterygopalatine suture, spasm of the sphenomandibular muscle with compression of the maxillary nerve against the posterior wall of the maxillary sinus.[172]
    - Clinical presentation: disturbances of lacrimation, disturbances of secretion into the nasal and paranasal sinuses, toothache in the upper jaw, disturbances of sensitivity and pain in the skin of the mid-facial region, mucosa, and teeth of the upper jaw, retro-orbital pain.
- **Infraorbital nerve (CN V_2)**
    - Through the inferior orbital fissure into the infraorbital canal, and on through the infraorbital foramen into the soft tissue of the face.
    - Clinical presentation: disturbances of sensitivity and pain in the skin of the mid-facial region, mucosa, and teeth of the upper jaw.
- **Superior alveolar nerves (CN V_2)**
    - In the alveolar canals on the back of the infratemporal surface. These branches which supply the teeth and gums of the upper jaw branch off from the infraorbital nerve in the pterygopalatine fossa.
    - Clinical presentation: toothache and painful gums.
- **Greater palatine nerve**
    - Clinical presentation: disturbances of sensitivity and pain in the mucosa of the hard palate.
    - Sympathetic fibers: from the deep petrosal nerve, via the pterygopalatine ganglion, ganglionic branches, maxillary nerve, and zygomatic nerve to the lacrimal nerve (lacrimal gland).
    - Clinical presentation: disturbance of the lacrimal gland.
- **Chorda tympani (CN VII)**
    - Causes: dysfunction of the temporal bone, CMD, in association with its course from the petrotympanic fissure, infratemporal fossa, and under the lateral pterygoid muscle.
    - Clinical presentation: disturbance of taste (anterior two thirds of the tongue) and of salivation (submandibular ganglion) affecting the submandibular and sublingual glands.
- **Zygomatic nerve**
    - Clinical presentation: disturbances of sensitivity and pain in the skin in the region around the temporal and zygomatic bones.
- **Otic ganglion**
    - Clinical presentation: disturbance of secretion of the parotid salivary glands, and pain referral.

2.6.7 Central nervous system

In myogenic CMD patients, extensive changes of brain morphology were found in regions associated with pain.[149,267,483] Patients with chronic pain often show a diminution of gray matter; the brain areas so affected vary according to the causal pain. There is overlap in some areas, reduction being found, for example, in the cingulate cortex, thalamus, insula, basal ganglia, dorsolateral prefrontal cortex, and brainstem.[296] These are regions that can also be localized when there is CMD pain.

Information from the brainstem is conducted via spinothalamic fibers to the mediodorsal nucleus of the thalamus and on into the anterior cingulate gyrus, where the experience of pain influences the regulation of motivation. The lateral spinothalamic fibers transmit the information to the ventrodorsal nucleus of the thalamus and on to the insula. Functional MRI showed that pain modulation goes back to a network extending from the periaqueductal gray, hypothalamus, and parabrachial nucleus to regions of the brainstem (C8).[208] Neuropathic pain leads to changes in the cortex and also in the thalamus and brainstem, in the raphe nucleus, locus caeruleus, and cuneiform nucleus. Experiences of anxiety also change the pain processing in caudal neural structures down as far as the spinal cord.[60] Areas of the periaqueductal gray and rostral ventral medulla are involved in descending pain modulation pathways.[324]

The fact that most imaging studies of chronic pain revealed significant correlations between changes in the gray matter of the brain and the duration or intensity of the pain invite the assumption that these changes in the brain may be not the cause but the result of pain.[13,438]

Trigeminal sensory nuclei, thalamus, and primary sensory cortex In myogenic CMD pain, dysregulation in the trigeminal system occurs, together with a reduced volume of gray matter in several regions of the trigeminothalamocortical pathways including the trigeminal sensory nuclei of the brainstem[483] and of the thalamus and primary sensory cortex.[267,483] There is assumed to be a somatotopic or structural reorganization in the thalamus and primary sensory cortex.

Limbic system (e.g., cingulate gyrus, anterior insula) In myogenic CMD pain, dysregulation and potential somatotopic or structural reorganization have also been reported in the limbic system. There is an increased volume of gray matter in some limbic regions, e.g., the cingulate gyrus and left anterior insula.[483] This last correlates with a local rise in the amount of glutamine.[148] These changes were also drawn upon as an explanation for the appearance of psychological symptoms and interactions in myofascial CMD.

The pain intensity of myogenic CMD appears to be associated with an increase in gray matter in the rostral anterior and posterior cingulate gyrus.[483] However, in the left anterior and right posterior cingulate gyrus and right anterior insular cortex, a reduction in gray matter was recorded.[149]

Basal ganglia An increased volume of gray matter was recorded in the posterior putamen and globus pallidus.[483]

Frontal gyrus and temporal gyrus A reduction in the volume of gray matter appears in the left inferior frontal gyrus and superior temporal gyrus in patients with myogenic CMD pain.[149]

2.6.8 Neurotransmitters/neuropeptides

The neuropeptides involved in myofascial CMD pain are glutamate, serotonin, bradykinin, substance P, prostaglandin, calcitonin gene-related peptide (CGRP), leukotrienes, and cytokines.[111] In myofascial CMD, glutamate is found in higher concentration in the masseter muscle[67] and appears to play a significant role in the emergence of pain, for example by activation of peripheral N-methyl-D-aspartate receptors (NMDA receptors).[68] A rise in serotonin in myofascial CMD pain could also be related to the emergence of pain and thresholds of tenderness to pressure.[111]

Myositis of the masseter muscle induced in an animal study led to increased capsaicin receptor activity in the trigeminal ganglion; these receptors belong to the superfamily of transient receptor potential (TRP) channels and are important for viscerosensitivity. This was expressed in the form of bilateral allodynia.[167] A capsaicin injection, by activating these receptors in muscles, produced sensations of pain and sensitization.[15]

2.6.9 Vascular disturbances

Although the arteries are not as susceptible to dysfunction as the veins on account of their stronger walls, they nevertheless also merit consideration.

- **Superficial temporal artery** This vessel is important for the TMJ.
- **Infraorbital artery and vein** Clinical presentation/hypothetical pathology: functional disturbance of the front teeth, bones, and gums of the maxilla.
- **Anterior superior alveolar arteries** Clinical presentation/hypothetical pathology: functional disturbance of the front teeth.

- **Posterior superior alveolar artery** Clinical presentation/hypothetical pathology: functional disturbance of the maxillary sinus, upper molars, bones, and gums of the maxilla.
- **Descending palatine artery** in the greater palatine canal Clinical presentation/hypothetical pathology: functional disturbance of the pharyngeal mucosa and gingivae of the front teeth and soft palate.
- **Additional arteries**
  - Inferior alveolar artery (branch of the maxillary artery): in the mandibular canal.
  - Mental artery (branch of the inferior alveolar artery): on the mental foramen.
  - Mylohyoid branch (branch of the inferior alveolar artery): in the mylohyoid groove.
  - Masseteric artery (branch of the maxillary artery): at the mandibular notch.

Venous structures can be affected by CMD (including disturbances of the disk), bruxism, dental extractions, prolonged mouth opening, and numerous myofascial and articular dysfunctions of the neck and craniocervical and cervicothoracic transitions:

- **Internal jugular vein** Clinical presentation/hypothetical pathology: impairment of venous return can lead, inter alia, to headache due to congestion or pressure.
- **Pterygoid venous plexus** Clinical presentation/hypothetical pathology: congestion in the facial region.
- **External jugular vein** Clinical presentation/hypothetical pathology: congestion in the facial region.
- **Occipital vein** Clinical presentation/hypothetical pathology: secondary tensions in the nape region in CMD can also impair venous outflow in the region of the occipital vein, with signs of congestion at the back of the head.
- **Submandibular vein** Clinical presentation/hypothetical pathology: congestion in the lateral facial region.
- **Superior and inferior labial vein** Clinical presentation/hypothetical pathology: congestion in the region of the lips.
- **Retromandibular vein; maxillary vein** Clinical presentation/hypothetical pathology: congestion in the region of the cheeks.

FURTHER INFORMATION According to Wittlinger,[476] the body has somewhat over 600 lymph nodes, more than 160 of which are located in the neck region. The outflow of lymph from the masticatory organ is reduced, in particular by elevated myofascial tensions in the neck region and cervicothoracic transition, and by the masticatory muscles.

2.6.10 Disturbances of the salivary glands

Those affected are the parotid gland, sublingual gland, and submandibular gland.

2.6.11 Disturbances of the endocrine glands and immune system

According to Kopp,[232] interrelationships between the immune system, sensory and sympathetic nerves of the peripheral nervous system, and local cells play a major role in the modulation of pain and inflammation.

Altered basal and stress-induced activity of the HPA (hypothalamus–pituitary–adrenal) axis may possibly lie at the root of myofascial CMD. This assumption is supported by Fernández-de-las-Peñas and Svensson in a detailed analysis of the literature,[123] summarized below. So, for example, patients with myofascial CMD show a heightened cortisol response to psychological stress[200] and higher levels of plasma cortisol and epinephrine (adrenaline).[233,482] Controversial findings show connections between higher salivary cortisol levels and more strongly pronounced anxiety in patients with myofascial CMD pain.[196,317] Normal pain management appears insufficient to treat impairments of the HPA axis in patients with CMD pain.[103]

Estrogens appear to play a role in myofascial CMD.[87] The lowering of the estrogen level raises the threshold of TMJ nociception.[131] Testosterone plays a protective role in TMJ pain.[130]

Impairment of the thyroid and parathyroid glands, e.g., via the thyrohyoid muscle, is speculative.

2.6.12 Orofacial dyskinesias

See sections 2.10 and 3.2 in this volume.

2.6.13 Psyche; stress; sleep disturbances

From the biopsychosocial point of view, myofascial CMD is a complex disease.[409] There is a connection between myofascial CMD and psychosocial factors, and similarly with disorders due to anxiety, depression, stress, mood, and somatization.[53,129,153,162,213,361] Psychological disorders such as depression can lead to the development of symptoms in the region of the teeth and jaw.

> **NOTE** If mental illness is suspected, the patient should be referred to a specialist for further investigation. TMJ treatment is contraindicated in such cases.[162]

Expressions such as "to grit one's teeth," "to get one's teeth into something," and "to show one's teeth," as well as the fact that primates use baring of the teeth to threaten an opponent, are all indications that the biting apparatus is also used as a form of expression to defuse aggressive confrontations, and as a kind of release valve for excessive emotional tension.[161]

Huter sees the mandible as an expression of impulsiveness, power, stamina, dignity, pride, and stability[3,259] (Figure 2.64). The limbic system in particular appears to play a key role in muscle hypertonicity caused by stress and psychological factors. Elevated muscle tone has been induced, for example, by stimulating the reticular formation, thalamus, hypothalamus, and amygdaloid body.

Chronic stress and psychological–emotional overload lead to muscle hypertonicity, which can in turn trigger bruxism, with the possible consequence of tendinomyopathies and joint disease.

In patients with orofacial pain, **anxiety** and **depression** can also potentially lead to increased muscle tenderness and hypersensitivity in terms of tenderness to pressure.[311] There is a close connection between pain and anxiety as well as pain and depression.[281,282] In turn, pain and depression impair pain tolerance.[32,137,217,451]

Constant stimulation of the nociceptive system at the peripheral and central levels leads to changes in the processing of stimuli, and thus to altered pain perception.[6,344,389] (section 2.6.7). Chronic pain will also impair other brain functions.

Around half of patients with CMD show **reduced sleep efficiency**, which is connected with psychological stress and a worsening of pain symptoms or reduced inhibition of pain.[107,367] In myofascial CMD patients, sleep disturbances could be directly involved in central sensitization and reinforcement

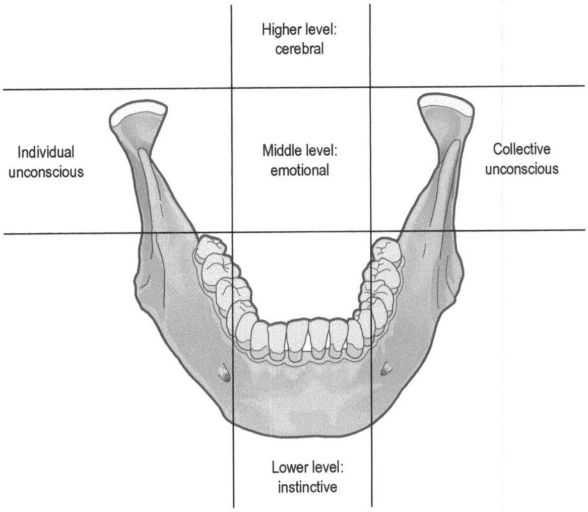

Figure 2.64
Symbolism of the mandible according to Lejoyeux, modified

of pain. Thus, CMD patients and patients with diagnosed primary insomnia demonstrate generalized hyperalgesia.[415]

Possible clinical presentation Psychological symptoms, hypertonicity of the masseter, pain in the TMJ, spasmophilic signs, grinding surfaces on teeth.

2.6.14 Genetics

The genetic factors that can influence the TMJ are complex.[417] Pain in CMD appears to be connected with various genetic variations mainly related to disturbances of catecholamine, serotonin, opioid, and cytokine metabolism.[98,99,332]

The gene sequence most often investigated in connection with pain is a polymorphism of the COMT gene that codes for the enzyme catechol-O-methyltransferase (COMT). COMT directs the catabolism of dopamine in the orbitofrontal cortex. This polymorphism affects around 25–40% of the population. It is assumed that one of the three resulting genotypes, the valin/valin genotype, is predisposed to pain and that the variability of the COMT gene may play an important role in the development of hyperalgesia.[489]

2.7 Diagnosis of craniomandibular dysfunction

Since CMD is a multifactorial disorder, accurate diagnosis is difficult.[312] No joint, especially not the TMJ, can be regarded as an individual joint in isolation; rather it must be understood in the context of the structure and function of the body as a whole.

Further, we need to take account of the fact that the emergence of CMD derives from multifactorial events. In order to achieve successful therapy that is not simply directed at the symptoms, we should study the whole body, and must recognize and understand the links and interactions between the body's structures and functions. The practitioner must try to judge the significance and weighting of the various causal factors with reference to the TMJ problem in order to be able to decide on a suitable course of treatment and carry it out.

Examination of the temporomandibular joint always comprises history-taking with the aid of standardized questionnaires (Figure 2.65), visual assessment, palpatory diagnosis, auscultation, and X-ray examination. Other diagnostic methods are: MRI[214] (nuclear magnetic resonance imaging), CT (computed tomography), arthrography, psychometric testing, bioelectronic testing, liquid-crystal thermography, EMG, etc. A reliable diagnosis of the observed signs is only possible with a combination of various diagnostic parameters. A study by Maghsudi also confirms this.[280]

Investigation of Krogh-Poulsen's "small functional analysis" as a screening test for CMD[236,352] produced no valid results with respect to sensitivity and specificity. When a summary of findings in combination was used, however, high sensitivity was found where there was more than one positive finding, but specificity was only moderate. From this, Maghsudi concluded that a combination consisting at least of motion restriction of the mandible, pain on palpation of the masticatory muscles, and screening of noises should be used.[280] In addition he recommends completing investigation by considering occlusal noises, traumatic eccentricity, and symmetry of mouth opening.[280]

The **diagnostic criteria** most commonly applied are the Research Diagnostic Criteria for Temporomandibular Disorders (RDC/TMD),[123] formulated by Dworkin and LeResche in 1992[106] and subsequently replaced by the validated diagnostic criteria for TMD (RC TMD).[331,382] In the RDC/TMD, the main diagnostic criteria under Axis I were myofascial pain, disk displacements, and joint pain, osteoarthritis, and osteoarthrosis.[106] In clinical settings, the classification of the American Academy of Orofacial Pain (AAOP) is usually used.[123]

When diagnosing CMD pain in adults in **osteopathy**, the influences differentiated are in particular those of posture (ascending and descending chains), of occlusion, and of the temporomandibular joint.

Interdisciplinary cooperation is especially important when dealing with disturbances of the mouth and jaw, both in diagnosis and treatment. The range includes dentistry, orthodontics, ear, nose, and throat medicine, osteopathy, physiotherapy, and others. For example, when treating CMD patients by osteopathic means, treatment using dental braces is often indicated.

2.7.1 The patient history

General

- The age of the patient. (The preconditions for occlusal disturbances usually increase with advancing age.) Start of the symptoms, identification of possible causes of the symptoms, or what may have triggered them.
- Family history.

> **FURTHER INFORMATION** Occlusal disturbances can emerge early in life, after the arrival of the second dentition. However, CMD symptoms often only first appear following an accident, dental or orthodontic procedure, cranial deformation, etc.

Symptoms of myofascial CMD[123]

- Spontaneous pain in the TMJ
  - Mainly concentrated in the regions of the masseter and of the temporalis muscle.
  - Joint clicking (more common in joint disorders).
- Other associated symptoms such as parafunctional habits (one-sided chewing, grinding, gnashing, or clenching the teeth, or clamping the tongue) can be involved in the etiology of CMD.[480] However, these are not always present.

Disturbances of the articular structures of the jaw

(articular surfaces, articular capsules, articular ligaments; retrodiscal pad)

- Pain in the TMJ or retrodiscal zone, associated with trismus, pain on opening the mouth or when biting into solid food, specific pattern of pain.
- Restriction of the TMJ: motion restriction after waking up is an indication of nocturnal teeth-grinding, or similar; if the mouth can be opened further after clicking of the jaw joint, this is evidence of a disk problem.
- Joint sounds (although no joint sounds occur in association with disturbances of the retrodiscal pad): clicking of the jaw is associated with CMD from an articular cause, e.g., dislocation of the disk
  - Clicking while opening or closing the mouth is indicative of a disk problem; rarely of alterations of the joint surfaces.
  - Loud clicking audible to those standing nearby, usually gives rise to social difficulties, but rarely to pain.
  - Quiet clicking perceptible only to the patient by bone conduction, very often arises in conjunction with pain and functional disturbance of the TMJ.
  - Crepitation is an indication of changes in the joint (breakdown of the articular cartilage). It is seldom pathological and seldom associated with further symptoms. In individual cases it can occur when there is perforation of the disk and/or of the retrodiscal tissue.
- Malocclusions.
- Bruxism (grinding, gnashing, or clenching the teeth).
- Disturbances of the temporomandibular joint muscles: pain in the muscles of mastication and restriction of the TMJ. In particular, radiating pain in the lateral pterygoid, masseter (deep part), sternocleidomastoid, or medial pterygoid muscles may induce pain in the TMJ.
- Triggering factors: for example, orthodontic and/or dental surgery (e.g., extraction of molars, bridges, etc.), alterations of bite, stress, accidents, falls or blows, whiplash, or surgery to the cervical spine or head region, face, back, pelvis, and lower limbs.[461]

Symptoms in other regions

CMD can favor the development of symptoms in other regions, or interact with them, or they can predispose to CMD:

- Cervical spine,[459] thoracic spine, and shoulder region: e.g., as radiating pain in the head, back of the neck, shoulder, and lower lumbar spine;[133,134] in the case of occlusal disturbances or possible central sensitization; cervical spine and tinnitus.[46]
- Disk injuries in the lumbar spine can impair mandibular function.[422]
- Whiplash injuries favor the development of CMD.[173,221,245]
- Physical exhaustion, depressive mood, possibly also an indication of central sensitization.
- Increase in the prevalence of pain in other regions of the body, especially the knee joint; also the shoulder, hip, wrist, and elbow;[42] simultaneous pain in other regions of the body and non-musculoskeletal pain may be an indication of central sensitization.
- Static-dynamic changes in the vertebral column.[133]
- Headache,[134,147,456] e.g., from gnashing or clenching the teeth; atypical facial pain; trigeminal neuralgia. Occipital headaches are the common symptom most frequently met with (at 94%) in cases of temporomandibular pain.[11]
- Symptoms of TMD can arise in migraine,[131] episodically occurring tension headache, or chronic daily headache.[155]
- There is increased prevalence of systemic disorders and unspecific physical symptoms in painful TMD and migraine.[79]
- Symptoms in the mouth and neck region: disturbances of swallowing and sucking.
- Organ of hearing and balance: otalgia, tinnitus.[43,358] Tinnitus and hearing impairment can accompany CMD;[133] also pressure in the ear or dizziness, e.g., in retromandibular compression; effect of CMD on balance.[157]
- Nasopharynx: disturbance of breathing, polyps, adenoid vegetations, sinusitis.
- Pharynx: speech disturbances and dysphagia, globus/pressure/foreign body sensations, neck pain, scratching the neck (e.g., in hypertonic tension of the hyoid muscles).
- Disturbances of the immune system.[55]
- Autonomic nervous system: autonomic symptoms, autonomic dystonia, and mood swings, which may be accompanied by bruxism, clenching the teeth, biting the fingernails, or chewing a pencil top.
- More rarely, e.g., eyes: eye ache (e.g., due to activation of trigger points of the masticatory muscles; gnashing or clenching the teeth), twitching/flickering of the eyes, blurred vision due to disturbances of drainage of the cavernous sinus, dry or burning eyes due to dysfunction of the ophthalmic nerve.
- Heart: disturbances of cardiac rhythm, racing heart rate, sensation of pressure in the heart region (may be an indication of central sensitization, possibly in compression syndromes in the TMJ).
- Gastrointestinal system: connection between gastroesophageal reflux and bruxism, which may be associated with depression, anxiety, and reduced quality of sleep,[141] irritable bowel syndrome,[260] upper or lower abdominal pain (potentially a sign of central sensitization, and possibly associated in cases of bruxism).
- Rheumatic disorders.
- Paresthesia, motor dysfunctions; important differential diagnoses for TMJ pain.
- Habits (parafunctions) such as grinding, gnashing, or clenching the teeth, crushing or biting the tongue, thumb-sucking, biting the cheek or lips, and chewing pencils or the fingernails can lead to such effects as oversensitivity of the dental neck or damage to the teeth (wearing down, cracking, splintering, or loosening of the teeth or breakage of tooth edges); more rarely to periodontal disorders and pain

in the TMJ, muscles of the neck and shoulders, headaches, sinusitis, tinnitus, pressure in the ear, otalgia, dizziness, and eye ache.
- Sleep disturbances, morning tiredness (potentially a sign of central sensitization); bruxism during sleep and by day increases the risk of temporomandibular pain.[34]
- Obstructive sleep apnea: associated with an increased prevalence of temporomandibular disturbances[89] and converse.[414] Symptoms of both appear to be related.[373,468] Indications of obstructive sleep apnea are a dry mouth on waking, morning headache, and nocturia.
- Psychological stress and psychological disorders such as anxiety and depression: anxiety can, for example, be predictive of CMD myogenic pain.[213]
- Various authors point out that TMJ patients often exhibit other somatic symptoms alongside their TMJ symptoms.[245,389]

> **NOTE** Differentiation between peripheral and central sensitization is important for treatment. More complex clinical reasoning is required for patients with central sensitization than for those with peripheral sensitization.[326] (See also section 2.6.6)

Patients can complete a questionnaire on their state of health, pain, and pain location (Figure 2.65) at home, in advance of the consultation, or in the waiting room, and bring it to the first consultation.

Diagnosis of pain by means of visual analog scale (VAS)

The intensity of pain in each of the affected region(s) is assessed according to the VAS scale; scores range from 1 to 10, representing the following degrees of pain:

1: No pain
2–3: Pain that becomes evident at rest or when doing nothing
4–6: Pain that cannot be masked by normal activities
7–9: Severe pain
9–10: Extreme pain

The following **pain modalities** are noted:
- Location of pain.
- Frequency: constant; several times a day/week; timing of pain, attacks.
- Onset of pain: is there a trigger or possible connection to events?
- Effect: to what extent does the pain affect everyday activities?
- Pain made worse by.../improved by...?
- Quality of the pain: burning, stabbing, dragging, racking, boring, radiating.
- Has the pain changed in the course of the illness?

> **Tip for practitioners**
>
> **Summary of possible TMJ symptoms**
> Pain at and around the TMJ and in the TMJ muscles, motion restriction of the TMJ, joint sounds, prominent condyle, pain in the head and face, nape of the neck and shoulders, paresthesias in the facial and mouth region, aural symptoms, dizziness, presence of triggering factors, other somatic symptoms.
>
> **The following disorders must be excluded in the differential diagnosis**
> Tension headache, migraine, temporal arteritis, spondylarthrosis or Bechterew disease of the cervical spine, sinusitis, otitis media, trigeminal neuralgia, tumors, the rheumatic disorders (acute arthritis, chronic rheumatism, primary rheumatoid arthritis, gout, psoriasis), infection (infectious otitis), true psychological illnesses.

2.7.2 Inspection

- Visual assessment of the face, oral cavity, teeth, tongue, lips, facial and masticatory muscles, etc.
- Includes, for example, evidence indicating non-specific hyperactivity: generalized hyperkinesia in the facial region, wear of

Date ______________________ Patient's main concern ______________________
Patient ______________________
Date of birth ______________________

Age ______________________ Previous osteopathic, dental, orthodontic treatment ______________________
Referred by ______________________
Case report form by ______________________

Localization of pain ______________________
Pain in ______________________
Headache ______________________

Tooth alignment	Jaw shape – Upper jaw	Jaw shape – Lower jaw	Occlusion	Facial development
☐ Straight teeth ☐ Crowding in upper jaw ☐ Crowding in lower jaw; midline correct ☐ Deviation of midline	☐ Normal ☐ Narrow ☐ Flat	☐ Normal ☐ Narrow ☐ Flat	☐ Normal ☐ Deep bite ☐ Overjet ☐ Open bite ☐ Crossbite ○ frontal ○ lateral left ○ lateral right	☐ Good facial development ☐ Deficiency in middle face ☐ Mandibular retrognathia ☐ Vertical growth
Note	Note		Note	Note

Breathing and posture	Tongue	Swallowing	Lips and cheeks
☐ Light nasal breathing ☐ Heavy nasal breathing ☐ Mouth breathing ○ by day ○ at night ○ Snoring ○ Tooth-grinding ○ Enlarged tonsils ○ Sleepy by day ☐ Good posture ☐ Poor posture ○ Head held forward ○ Shoulders forward	☐ Correct rest position ☐ Faulty rest position ○ displaced ○ interdental ○ addental Attachment of frenulum of tongue ☐ Sufficient room for movement ☐ Inadequate room for movement	☐ Correct pattern of swallowing ☐ Faulty pattern of swallowing ○ Compressing tongue ○ Mentalis muscle activity ○ Cheek activity	☐ Correct lip closure ☐ Faulty lip closure ○ No lip closure at rest ○ Muscle tension at rest with lips closed ○ Lack of muscle strength
Note	Note	Note	Note

Habits	TMD	L	R	Treatment notes
☐ No history	☐ Temporalis muscle			
☐ Thumb or finger-sucking	☐ Masseter muscle			
	☐ Lateral pterygoid muscle			
☐ Pacifier/dummy	☐ Sternocleidomastoid			
	☐ Trapezius			
☐ Bottle	☐ Posterior muscles of the neck			
☐ Headache	☐ TMD pain			
☐ Other ______	☐ TMD clicking			
Duration of treatment	TMD consultation Y/N			Proposed cost

Figure 2.65
Case report form

chewing surfaces, indentations in soft tissues, fingernails, nail beds, pencil-chewing.

External visual assessment

This can provide indications as to the presence of CMD, facial development, breathing and posture, and function of lips and cheeks, and enables conclusions to be drawn as to the function and position of the tongue and pattern of swallowing.

CMD

- The three most important clinical signs of myogenic CMD are[123]
  - Restriction of mouth opening.
  - Deviation or deflection during movements of the mouth.
  - Tenderness to palpation of the joint or masticatory muscles.
- In the case of crossbite (differential diagnosis is necessary in relation to cranial dysfunctions), facial asymmetry may be evident.
- Visible hypertrophy of the masseter muscle (due to gnashing or clenching the teeth; excessive gum-chewing).

Facial development

- Underdevelopment of the middle face (look at size of upper and lower jaw).
- Retrognathia of lower jaw.
- Vertical growth.
- Asymmetries of lower jaw.

Breathing

- Light or heavy nasal breathing.
- Mouth open or closed (daytime; at night).
- Is there formation of a crease under the lower lip? Or of a dimple under the crease? This is a sign of overactivity of the mentalis muscle (shortened upper lip in the case of mouth breathing).
- Rhagades (fissures or fine scars) at the angle of the mouth: may accompany incompetent lip closure or reduced mouth closure.
- Snoring, bruxism, size of tonsils, daytime tiredness.
- Dark rings round eyes (possibly a sign of poor sleep due to mouth breathing).

Posture

- Posture of body: shoulders inclined forward or asymmetry in shoulder region; see also Barre's vertical alignment test (section 2.5.5).
- Posture of head: inclined forward or to the side (asymmetry of ears). See also section 2.5.4.

Function of lips and cheeks

- Lips: hypotonic or atonic.
- Lip closure competent (lips touch effortlessly, without muscle contraction) or is effort required to maintain mouth closed?
- Lip closure incompetent (lip—usually the upper lip—anatomically too short).
- Lip closure potentially incompetent (lip contact hindered, usually by protrusion of upper incisors).
- Lips rolled up.
- Sucking of lips (lower lip held behind the upper incisors, causing these to be forward displaced).
- Pressing of lips (inversion of upper incisors due to strong mentalis muscle).
- Dry lips: possibly a sign of mouth breathing; incompetent mouth closure (upper lip too short; section 2.6.2).
- "Hamster" cheeks; one side or bilateral? Indicates tension of buccinator muscle (leads to a narrow upper jaw and the risk of crossbite).

Visual assessment of position of chin tip

Deviation to the side of the CMD, or to the side on which the temporal bone is in internal rotation (Figure 2.66).

Visual assessment of position of midline between the incisors

Ask the patient to open the lips, teeth resting above each other. Compare the midline between the

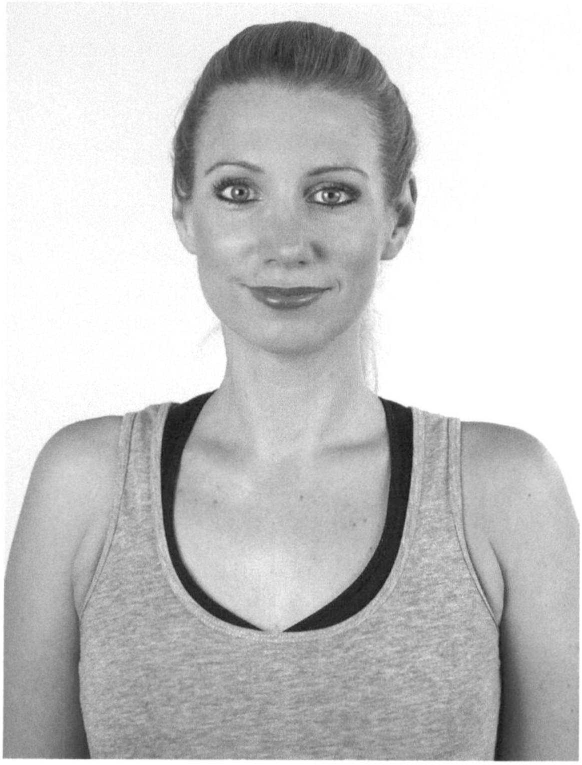

Figure 2.66
Visual assessment of position of chin tip

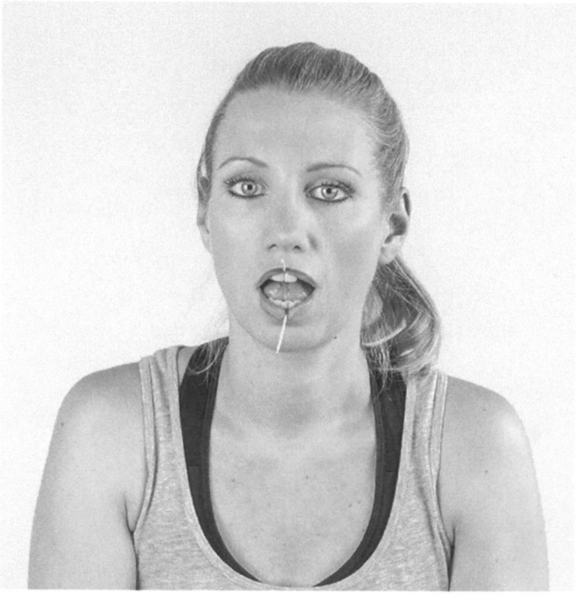

Figure 2.67
Visual assessment of position of midline between the incisors

upper incisors with the midline between the lower incisors (Figure 2.67).

The test is positive if the two midlines do not coincide. The midline of the lower incisors is displaced toward the dysfunctional TMJ side. If no asymmetric movement is observed when the mouth is opened, the deviation may be caused by a maxillary dysfunction.

> **NOTE** In this test, it is necessary to exclude divergent positioning of the teeth.

Cotton wool roll test

Ask the patient to bite down on two thin cotton wool rolls. A change in the position of the lower jaw is another sign of CMD.

Differential diagnosis: when examining for a dysfunction which could have arisen secondary to CMD, you can test for this first in occlusion (with tooth contact) and then with a cotton wool roll between the patient's front teeth. If the dysfunction is then improved, this is an initial indication of CMD.

Visual assessment in the oral cavity

Shape of jaw

- Shape of upper jaw: normal, narrow, flat.
- Shape of lower jaw: normal, narrow, flat.

Occlusion

- Normal.
- Deep bite.

- Overjet.
- Open bite.
- Crossbite: frontal, lateral.

Teeth

- Straight teeth.
- Crowding in upper or lower jaw.
- Midline normal or deviation.
- Wear faceting on surfaces: frequently on canine and front teeth where there is parafunction such as bruxism; less frequently in loss of height of molars; leading to abrasion (loss of dental hard tissue), which may result in lowering of the bite (→ damage to temporomandibular joint; formation of rhagades).
- Cracks in enamel: a good way to show vertical, hairline cracks in the enamel is by using a torch (flashlight); caused by pressure (bruxism) or temperature changes.
- Bruxism: signs of clenching or grinding the teeth.
- Teeth worn down and indentations in soft tissue.
- Tooth-grinding: distinct wear faceting of the teeth and wear of chewing surfaces.
- Low premolars, with canine "drop-off."
- Teeth-clenching: no wear faceting, and little wear of chewing surfaces.
- Visible hypertrophy of the masseter muscle.
- Possibly biting or sucking the cheeks.
- Possibly cracks in tooth enamel.
- Possibly key-in-the-lock phenomenon, in which teeth are worn in such a way that they catch on each other when the person bites together. This results in a uniformity of movement and stress in the craniomandibular system.

Tongue

- Indentations from clenching the teeth or clamping the tongue (also occurring more easily as a result of gaps from tooth loss); possibly dysfunctional patterns of swallowing (→ occlusal disturbances), macroglossia.
- Normal rest position.
- Displaced, interdental, addental.
- Frenulum of tongue: normal or inadequate room for movement.
- Deviation on protruding the tongue: local muscle imbalances or neural disturbances (CN XII).

Cheek Biting or sucking the cheek creates linear impressions in the mucosa of the cheeks seen at the level of the bite (bruxism, poorly fitting dentures, tooth fillings that are too high or low; psychological stress).

Hypomobility and hypermobility

General test for initial assessment

The three-finger metacarpal-joint test according to Dorrance

Ask the patient to open the mouth sufficiently wide to accommodate the metacarpal joints of the index finger, middle finger, and ring finger between the upper and lower incisors (Figure 2.68). The test is positive when this is not achieved, and indicates a CMD of articular or myogenic origin.

Mouth opening and laterotrusion should be performed first actively, then passively, and then isometrically.

Assess (measure or sense):

1. The amplitude and symmetry of mouth opening/closing and laterotrusion.
2. Any sounds created on doing so.
3. Pain (location; at which point during action does pain occur; does pain recur, etc.).
4. End feel on passive testing (see also Table 2.4).

Test of mouth opening and closing

Use a ruler to establish the distance between the lower edge of the upper teeth and the upper edge of the lower teeth in each case.

- **Mouth opening and closing, active** Ask the patient to open the mouth.
- **Mouth opening and closing, passive** Using a scissors hold (thumb on the upper teeth, index finger on the lower teeth), open the mouth passively.

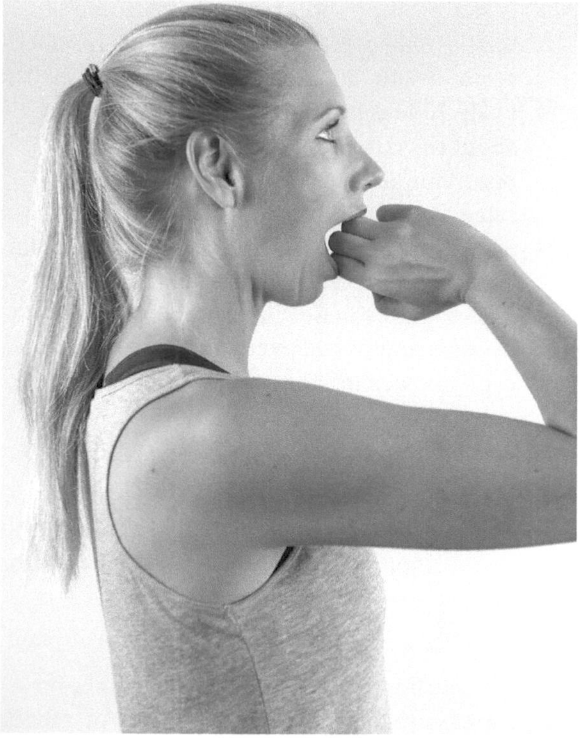

Figure 2.68
The three-finger metacarpal-joint test according to Dorrance

- **Normal range of mouth opening** >40 mm (passive opening 1–4 mm more than by active movement).

Cardonnet and Clauzade's interpretation of reduced mouth opening (and laterotrusion)[63]

- A slight reduction in mouth opening usually does not require treatment, unless there are other symptoms and positive test results.
- Reduced mouth opening (up to 35 mm) indicates muscular and discal/arthrogenous dysfunction.
- A distinct limitation of mouth opening (35–21 mm) indicates a relatively acute dislocation.
- A severe limitation of mouth opening (<21 mm) is usually present if there is ankylosis or acute muscle spasm (often with underlying dislocation).
- The ratio of the amplitude of mouth opening to the minimum possible laterotrusion should be 4:1. A deviation of more than 2 mm is a clear sign of disk displacement.

Test of isometric mouth opening

- Note pain and force.
- If pain occurs, is the cause arthrogenous or myogenic? To differentiate further, the mouth should be opened a little further and, from this position, apply isometric counterforce.
- If the test produces no pain: this indicates arthrogenous disturbance.
- If the test causes pain: this indicates myogenic disturbance.

Further tests and findings

- **Joint sounds** Joint sounds during mouth opening and closing may indicate a hypermobile joint, disk disturbance, disturbance of the lateral ligament, or path of joint movement. Clicking at the end of mouth opening and beginning of mouth closing are indications of a hypermobile joint (Table 2.11).
- **Interpretation of enlarged mouth opening** This can occur in the case of a hypermobile joint or over-rotation, retrodiscal ligamentous strain, and subluxation.
- **Testing laterotrusion** This too can be done actively, passively, and isometrically. First, a vertical line is applied to the upper and lower front incisors, marking the middle. The normal range of laterotrusion is around 10 mm.
- **Pain** Pain indicates disturbances in the region of the capsule, ligaments, and masticatory muscles. Pain on the side of laterotrusion indicates an arthrogenous disturbance (brought about by slight compression of the joint). Pain on the opposite side indicates myogenic disturbances (pain due to strain/stretching).
- **Active laterotrusion** Ask the patient to move the jaw to one side and then the other.

Measure the difference in distance traveled in each case.

- **Passive laterotrusion** Ask the patient to move the jaw to one side. Then, with your thumb and index finger on the patient's chin (holding the patient's head in place laterally with your other hand), move the jaw passively further into laterotrusion. Note the distance, end feel, and any pain.
- **Isometric laterotrusion** Ask the patient to move the jaw to one side. Here, apply counter-pressure with your thumb and index finger on the patient's chin (holding the patient's head in place laterally with your other hand). Compare pain and force as between the two sides.

Overbite

- Measuring (vertical) overbite With the patient's mouth closed in the habitual way, draw a line on the lower teeth at the point where the upper teeth end. The patient now opens the mouth. Measure the distance between the line and the upper edge of the lower incisors. The normal range is 2–3 mm.
- Measuring overjet With the patient's mouth closed in the habitual way, measure the distance from the edge of the upper incisors to the lower incisors. Here, too, the normal range is 2–3 mm.

Establish whether there is deep overbite (cover-bite) or edge-to-edge bite.

Watt's test

Ask the patient to close the teeth together quickly several times.[388:10–14]

Interpretation

- Sharp, clear sound (teeth come together at high speed): high-quality occlusion or high-quality regulating function (proprioceptive integration).
- Soft sound (teeth come together at low speed): poor-quality occlusion or poor-quality regulating function (proprioceptive integration).
- A sharp sound indicates only that, when the teeth come together, the same, large number of points (40–50) always meet simultaneously. It does not necessarily say anything about the condition of the occlusion, as a poor-condition occlusion can be compensated for by a high regulation function.
- We know that, in the case of a soft sound, the occlusal points do not come together evenly. This suggests malocclusion, an impairment of centering or overexertion of the proprioceptive mechanisms.

Deviation of the incisor midline during the opening and closure movement according to Sebald and Kopp

The following observes the procedure according to Sebald and Kopp.[397:45–48] Figure 2.69 illustrates discoordination, deviation, and deflection.

Discoordination

Deviations from the midline occur during the opening and closure movement. At the end of mouth opening, the lower jaw is once again in the midline position. Frequently encountered.

Interpretation Myogenic dysfunction/CMD. The greater the deviation, the greater the dysfunction of the muscle component of the masticatory system.

Prognosis Very good. A greater or lesser degree of incapacity during active movements and isometric contractions may indicate discoordination.[246]

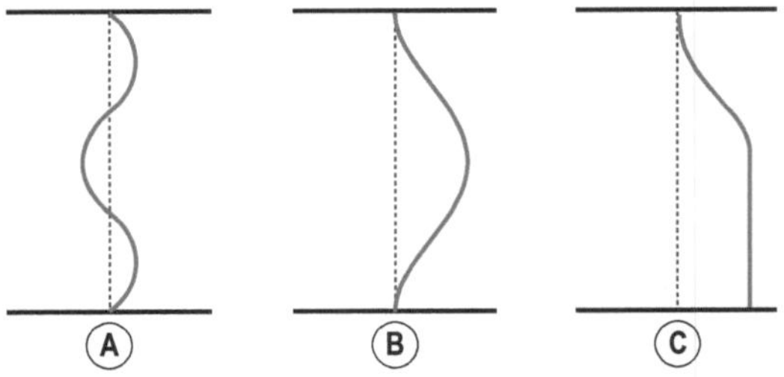

Figure 2.69
A Discoordination. **B** Deviation. **C** Deflection

Active movement Inability to perform isolated protrusion, mouth opening from maximum protrusion, closure in maximum protrusion, or sideways movement of the mandible (lateral pterygoid muscle). The degree of incapacity is evaluated as follows:

- Much activity in the auxiliary muscles without movement of the mandible.
- Much activity in the auxiliary muscles with movement of the mandible, but jerky, abrupt, atactic, etc.
- Little activity in the auxiliary muscles and relatively free mandibular movement.
- Little activity in the auxiliary muscles and smooth, free movement of the mandible.

Isometric contraction of the lateral pterygoid muscle (Figure 2.69) Evaluate the capacity for muscular response. The best result is when the mandible remains in a stable position in response to the application of variable pressure by the practitioner. A dysfunction is indicated if the mandible is not capable of maintaining its position in response to variable pressure.

> **NOTE** Discoordination never occurs without muscle hypertonicity or hyperactivity. On the other hand, hypertonicity and hyperactivity can occur without discoordination.

Deviation

During the opening and closure movement, a unilateral distinct deviation from the midline occurs. At the end of mouth opening, the mandible is once again in the midline position. Frequent.

Interpretation Usually myogenic dysfunction/CMD; here the deviation may be ipsilateral or contralateral to the side of the dysfunction. Less often there may be a disturbance of the joint surfaces (e.g., cartilaginous obstruction in the joint surfaces, intermediate clicking); in this case the deviation is to the side of the TMJ disturbance.

Prognosis Moderate.

Deflection

During the opening movement, a unilateral distinct deviation from the midline occurs. At the end of mouth opening, the mandible has deviated most distinctly from the midline.

Interpretation Discopathy/arthrogenous CMD, ankylosis (e.g., terminal clicking), deviation to the side of the TMJ disturbance.

Prognosis

- Acute discopathy: very good.
- Chronic discopathy: uncertain.

Ankylosis: indication for surgery If, on mouth opening, the midline of the incisors deviates, a test can be performed to establish whether the lateral pterygoid muscle is responsible for this deviation. (This muscle is very often involved in CMD.) Ask the patient to move the tongue to the posterior part of the roof of the palate. If mouth opening is now more symmetrical, the cause is very likely to be the lateral pterygoid. If mouth opening remains asymmetrical, the cause lies elsewhere.

> **NOTE** This position of the tongue prevents translation of the condyle over the articular tubercle.

Photographic analysis

Planes of reference form part of all temporomandibular work. These are usually established by means of X-rays; also by digital volumetric and CT imaging of the head. A simpler method that can be used in osteopathy to gain an impression of the planes of reference is to analyze this by means of photographs.

En face photograph

Method: If possible, the patient's heels, buttocks, and back (at shoulder blade level) should be touching the measuring staff (Figures 2.70 and 2.71). The head should rest free.

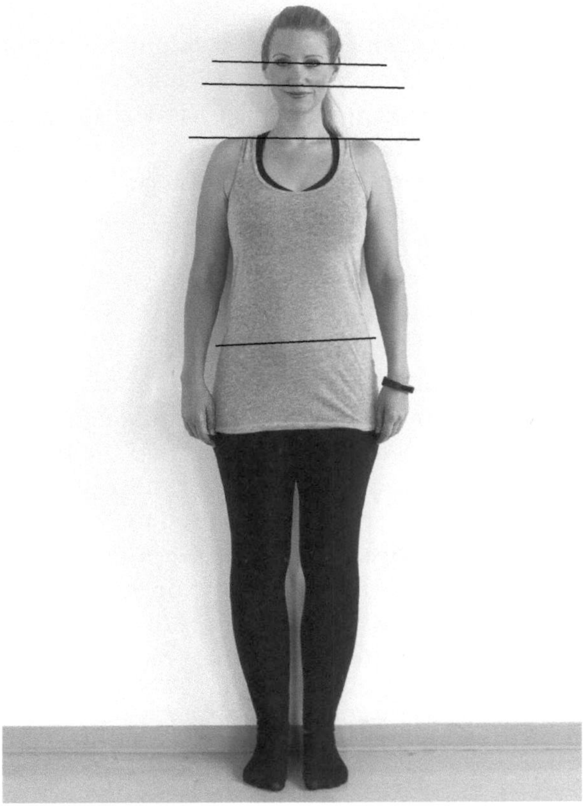

Figure 2.70 En face photograph, whole body

Draw the following lines:
- A horizontal line through both pupils.
- A horizontal line through the left and right corners of the mouth.
- A horizontal line under the front teeth.
- Starting from the bipupillar line, a vertical line in the region of the nasion.
- Assess the symmetry and even distribution of the thirds of the face.

In the en face photograph of the whole body, a line can also be drawn between the root of the two ears, the shoulders, and the iliac crests.

Symmetry:
- Normal: nasion, subnasion, and gnathion all lie on this line.
- Positive finding: any divergencies from the midline, especially of the lower jaw.

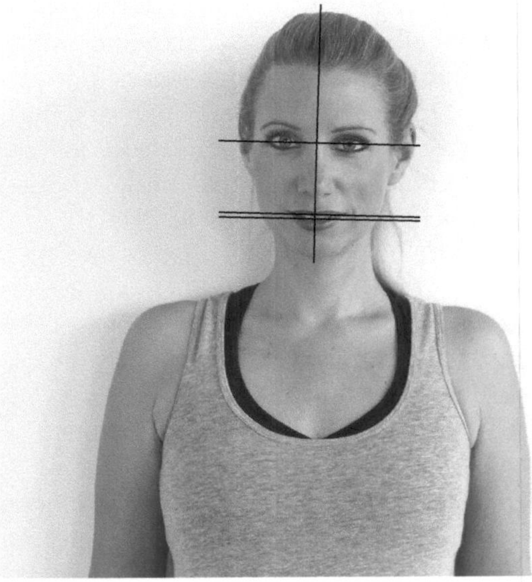

Figure 2.71 En face photograph

Causes: unilateral hypertonicity of the muscles, unilateral capsule restriction, TMJ dysfunction, differences in occlusal height, disk displacement or repositioning, genetically caused.

Distribution of thirds of face:
- Upper third of face: from hairline to nasion.
- Middle third of face: nasion to subnasion.
- Lower third of face: subnasion to gnathion.
- Assessment: an enlarged or reduced third of the face.

Profile photograph

Method: An ideal method for the profile photograph is to provide a mirror and ask the patient to look into their own eyes. This ensures that the head is held steadily in line. The lower edge of the orbits and tragion (ear opening) should lie on the same horizontal line (Figure 2.72).

Draw the following lines:
- Frankfurt plane: from the superior margin of the bony auditory meatus to the infraorbital ridge (plane of reference for the cranium).

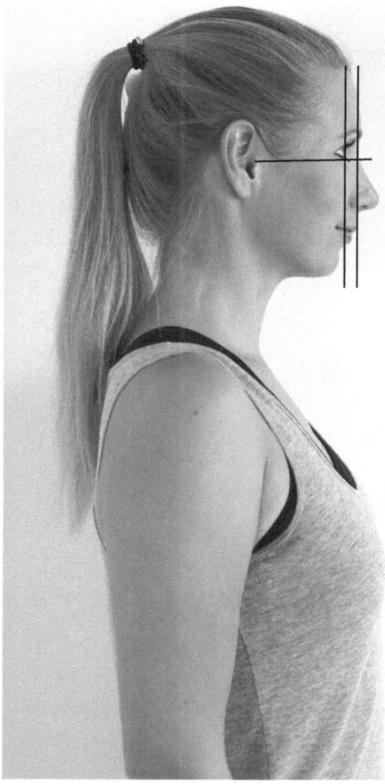

Figure 2.72 Profile photograph

- A vertical line at right angles to the Frankfurt horizontal, from the orbit.
- Another vertical line at right angles to the Frankfurt plane, running through the nasion.
- **Normal:** the tip of the chin should lie midway between the vertical line from the nasion and subnasion and the vertical line from the orbit.

Further lines:

- **Plane from tragus–corner of eye:** running from the tragus to the outer corner of the eye.
- **Camper plane:** notional plane running through the tragus of both sides, from the tip of the anterior nasal spine. It runs parallel to the occlusal plane and forms an angle of 15–20° to the Frankfurt plane.
- **Curve of Spee:** curve linking the cutting edges and cusps of the upper teeth and tangent to the head of the mandible. The midpoint of the notional circle lies at the front of the orbit, but this cannot be established by photographic analysis.
- **Occlusal plane**
  - Touches the incisal edges of the middle lower incisors.
  - Tips of the distobuccal cusps of the second lower molars.
  - Usually at the level of the line of lip closure.
- **Simon's orbital plane:** plane through the orbitale, perpendicular to the Frankfurt plane (establishment of sagittal divergencies).

2.7.3 Palpation

Test of the position of the TMJ

Hand position: Place your index or middle fingers on the temporomandibular joints or each side, and note the position of the condyles (Figure 2.73).

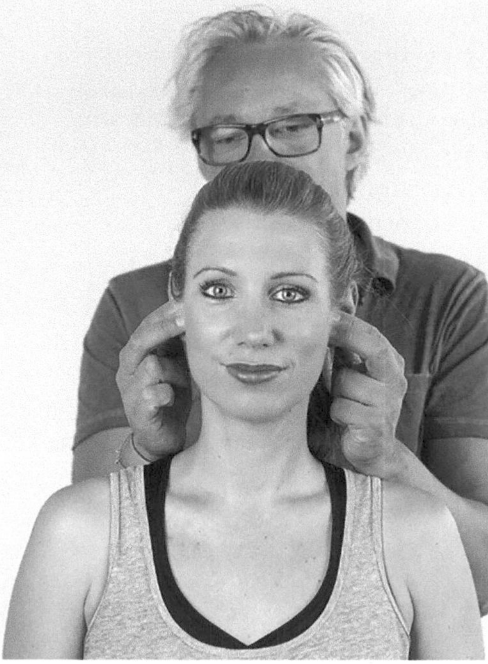

Figure 2.73 Testing the position and movement of the temporomandibular joints

Differential diagnosis of tenderness of the TMJ

Palpation or application of pressure is always bilateral (Table 2.3). The pressure should be applied not only statically, but also during mouth opening and mouth closure. If pressure induces pain, the test is positive.

The reflex arm length test as a method for testing stress from occlusion and depression of the jaw according to van Caille

The reflex arm length test is a method used in kinesiology.[37,258,403] Investigations performed in kinesiology observe the changes in patterns of motor

Table 2.3 Differential diagnosis of tenderness of the TMJ

Palpation	Finger position	If tenderness is present
From the side	Middle finger 1.5 cm anterior to the margin of the tragus	Minor arthrogenous disturbance, disturbance of the lateral ligament, discal ligaments, or lateral displacement of the mandible
From a posterolateral direction	Mouth slightly opened; middle finger posterior to the condyle (at several points)	Disturbance of the bilaminar zone, posterior capsular inflammation, acute luxation with pull on the bilaminar zone, tendinopathy of lateral pterygoid
From posterolateral on mouth opening and closing	As described	Disturbance of the bilaminar zone, path of condyle, disk displacement with or without repositioning
From a dorsal direction	Little finger in external acoustic meatus, pressure applied in an anterior direction	Severe arthrogenous disturbance, posterior inflammation of capsule,* posterior inflammation of the disk
From a dorsal direction on mouth opening	As described	Disk displacement without repositioning, sometimes with reduced mouth opening
From a dorsal direction with mouth opening	Little finger in external acoustic meatus, pressure applied in an anterior direction	Retrodiscal disturbance, muscular disturbance
From a dorsal direction with movement of mouth closing	Little finger in external acoustic meatus, pressure applied in an anterior direction	Capsulitis, subluxation

* Often with joint clicking.

movement as responses to a stimulus, or "challenge." These are understood to stimulate sensory receptors and to be experienced by the body either as stressors or as a neutral stimulus. The reflex arm length test aims to differentiate between these perceptions of the stimulus by the body. The test is therefore not designed to test the actual arm length or the muscles.

Although this is not an evidence-based test method, the effect can be explained as follows: the reflex arm length test provides information relating to unconscious regulation via the Golgi apparatus. A stress factor that is activated by the challenge changes the result of the test, which is assessed as positive when a reaction to the challenge is detected; i.e., if the arm length changes.

Method in the context of TMJ evaluation This test is not looking for faults of occlusion or jaw depression. Many people exhibit imbalances (e.g., minor faults of occlusion) that impose no stress on the body. The reflex arm length test aims to investigate whether the occlusion or depression of the jaw does constitute a stress factor for the body.

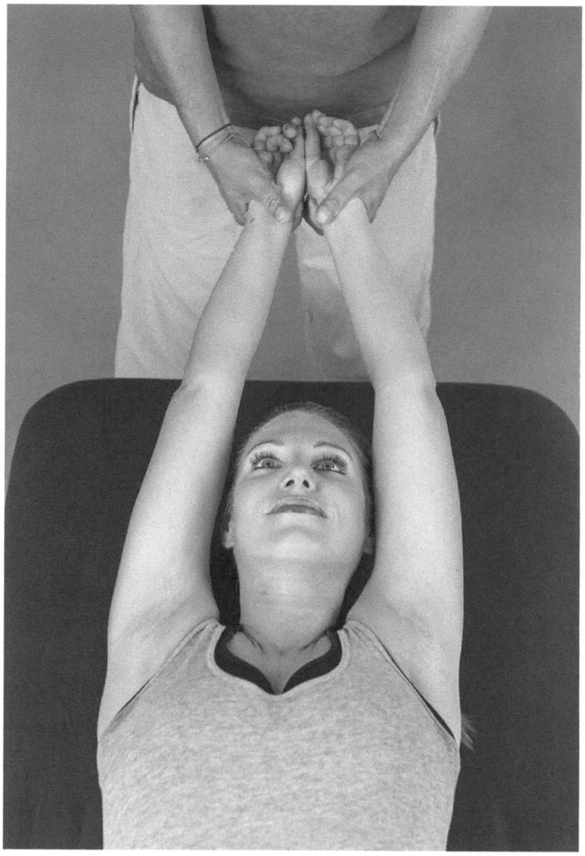

Figure 2.74
Reflex arm length test: determining the baseline

Practitioner: At the head of the patient.

Patient: Supine.

1. Determining the baseline

- Ask the patient to extend the arms and reach back (outward and upward) above the head.
- Take hold of the patient's two wrists and exert gentle longitudinal traction on the arms (Figure 2.74).
- To establish arm length, place the patient's two thumbs side by side.
- In carrying out the test, you are looking to see whether a difference in arm length occurs.
- There are two possible results
  - No difference in arm length is found.
  - The test shows unequal arm length.
- The result is the baseline value.
- In subsequent testing, the test is assessed as positive if the arm length changes relative to the baseline in reaction to the challenge. If there is no change, the test is negative.

2. Testing occlusal stress

- To present the challenge, ask the patient to clamp the teeth together a few times, and then to clench the teeth or bite down hard. This activates the muscles responsible for mouth closing and produces occlusion.
- While the patient is clamping the teeth, test arm length (as described above) (Figure 2.75).

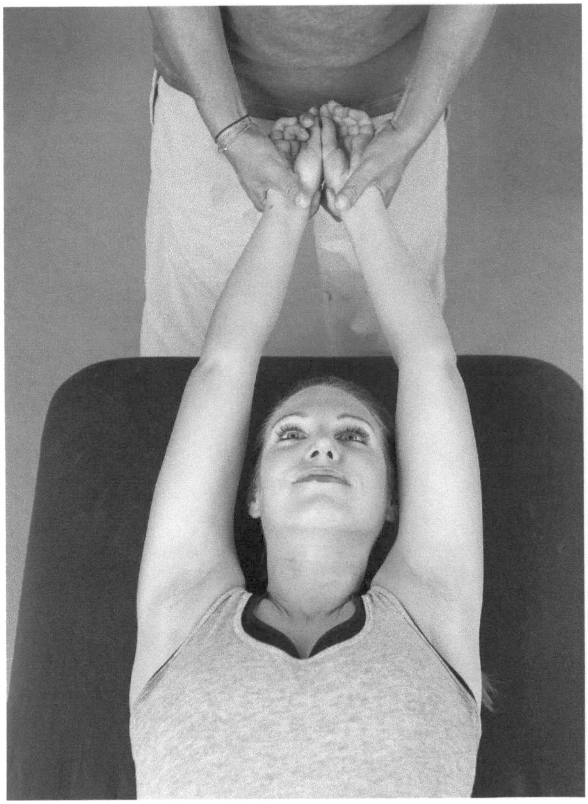

Figure 2.75
Reflex arm length test: testing occlusal stress

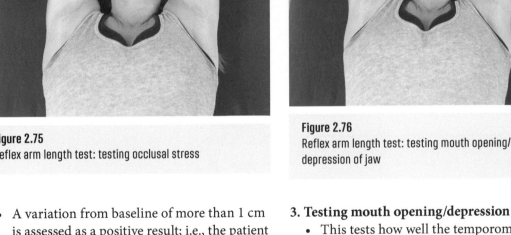

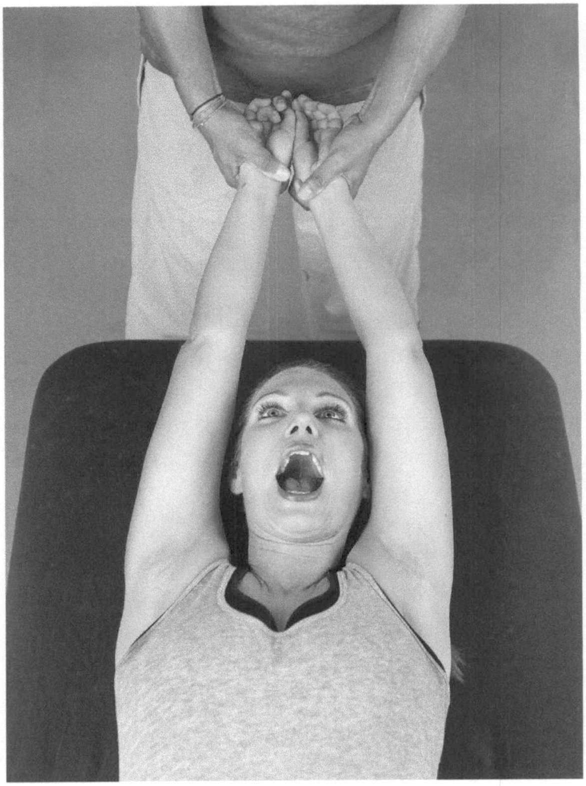

Figure 2.76
Reflex arm length test: testing mouth opening/ depression of jaw

- A variation from baseline of more than 1 cm is assessed as a positive result; i.e., the patient experiences occlusion as a stress factor.
- Conclusion: every occlusion (chewing, swallowing, gnashing, clenching, or grinding the teeth) creates a stressor, which produces negative somatogenic afferent nerve impulses. These stressful afferent impulses lead to adaptations or even decompensation, which take place in a craniocaudal direction. It cannot be predicted when and in which region the decompensation and symptoms caused by these repeated negative afferent impulses will appear. In our experience it is often the head and neck that are affected.

3. Testing mouth opening/depression of jaw

- This tests how well the temporomandibular joint is regulated in its movement during the phase of mouth opening; i.e., in the symmetrical release of the masticatory muscles and symmetrical activation of the muscles responsible for mouth opening. These abilities are necessary for smooth, functionally symmetrical TMJ movements.
- To present the challenge, ask the patient to open the mouth as wide as possible and to keep it open. This activates the muscles responsible for mouth opening.
- While the patient is keeping the mouth wide open, test arm length (Figure 2.76).

- A variation from baseline of at least 1 cm is assessed as a positive result; i.e., the patient experiences mouth opening as a stress factor.
- Conclusion: if the phase of mouth opening produces stress, this can usually be interpreted as a consequence of ascending negative afferent impulses from the periphery.

4. Combining the reflex arm length test with location of treatment

- This is carried out to determine the side of the stressor and to allow the test result to appear more clearly.
- To do this, palpate the structure to be tested. Touching the skin in the jaw region is done to activate the brain region for the temporomandibular joint.
- The rest of the testing is performed as before. As an example, for the test of occlusion, the patient clamps the teeth together and then bites down hard. Briefly touch the left TMJ (for example) or rub the skin in the region of the joint and then carry out the arm length test.
- Possible results from the test: occlusion stress at one or both temporomandibular joints; also in combination with jaw depression stress at one or both TMJs.

Palpating patterns of intraosseous tension

Practitioner: At the head of the patient.

Hand position:

- Place the flat of each hand bilaterally on the mandible and so as to cover the TMJ.
- Your index fingers should meet at the gnathion (the inferiormost median point of the chin) and span the chin.
- Your other fingers should lie alongside with your little fingers on the angles of the lower jaw.

Method: Evaluate intraosseous tensions of the mandible.

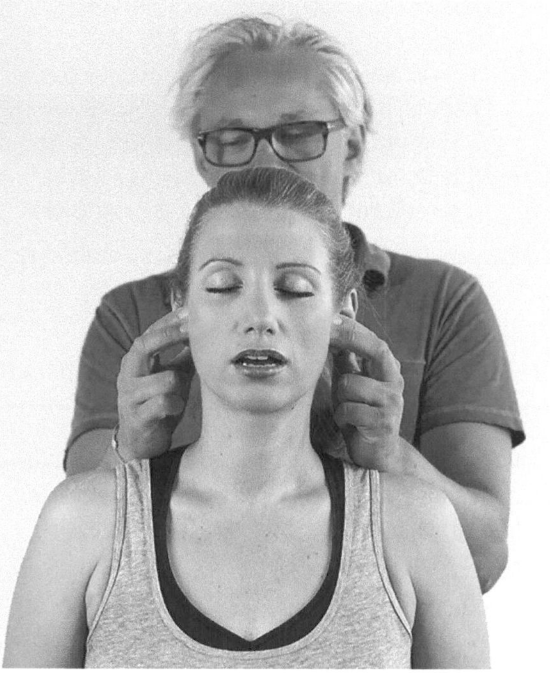

Figure 2.77 Mouth-opening palpation test

Testing the motion of the TMJ

Restricted mobility of the mandible does not in itself provide any relevant information for a specific diagnosis, as it can be traced to a number of causes.[123] Mobility tests can only be integrated into the investigation in combination with other tests.

Patient: Seated.

Practitioner: Take up a position behind the patient.

Hand position: Place your middle fingers in the ears, or your index and middle fingers immediately in front of the ears on the temporomandibular joints.

Method:

- Ask the patient to open and close the mouth slowly (Figure 2.77).
- Assess the rolling and gliding motion in the temporomandibular joints. Normally the

condyle should glide in a caudal and ventral direction.
- Any asymmetry or uneven movement or pain, or any palpable or audible noise (grinding or clicking, etc.), is an indication of CMD.
- Other movements of the mouth may also be palpated (protrusion, retrusion, laterotrusion).

Testing the passive motion of the TMJ

If mouth opening is limited, the mobility should be tested passively.

Patient: The patient is supine.

Practitioner: Take up a position beside the patient at the level of the shoulder.

Hand position:
- Position your thumbs inside the mouth on the rows of lower teeth, on each side.
- Position the other fingers on the body of the mandible. With your middle fingers, grasp the angle of the mandible on both sides (Figure 2.78).

Method:
- Testing of mouth opening.
- Testing of craniocaudal mobility in joint play: apply pressure in the cranial direction and traction in the caudal direction.
- Testing of anteroposterior mobility: apply traction in the posterior and in the anterior direction.
- Testing of ventromedial translation in joint play: administer traction in the ventral and medial direction.
- Testing of rotation: induce rotation to the right and to the left.
- Testing of lateral displaceability: induce lateral displacement to the right and to the left.

Compare the ease, amplitude, end feel, and symmetry of the movements of the mandible.

Normal end feel is sensed as a hard, ligamentous resistance; i.e., passive mobility is stopped by the increasing tension of the joint capsule and ligaments (see Table 2.4).

Interpretation:
- A light, resilient resistance at the end of mouth opening: **disk**.
- A solid resistance at the end of mouth opening: **muscle cramp**.
- Hard resistance in joint play on **caudal traction**: indication of **capsulitis**.
- Resistance in joint play on anteromedial translation: indication of dysfunction of the posterior parts of the capsule, stylomandibular ligament, and sphenomandibular ligament.
- Limited lateral displaceability to the right: **CMD on the left** (arthrogenous, muscular, etc.).
- A positive test result (= limitation of mobility), but a negative test result in the isometric test: **arthrogenous dysfunction**.
- A negative test result: probably **myogenic dysfunction**.

Other indications:
- Arthrogenous disturbance
  - If lateral mobility is severely limited (unilaterally or bilaterally), with reduced or almost normal mouth opening.
  - When an existing pain changes as a result of passive motion, in contrast with isometric testing.
- Probably no arthrogenous dysfunction
  - If mouth opening is reduced, with normal or almost normal lateral mobility.
  - When an existing pain does not change as a result of passive motion.
  - When an existing restriction does not change as a result of passive testing (possible disturbance of muscle innervation).
- Myogenic dysfunction: when an existing pain changes as a result of passive motion, in accordance with isometric testing.

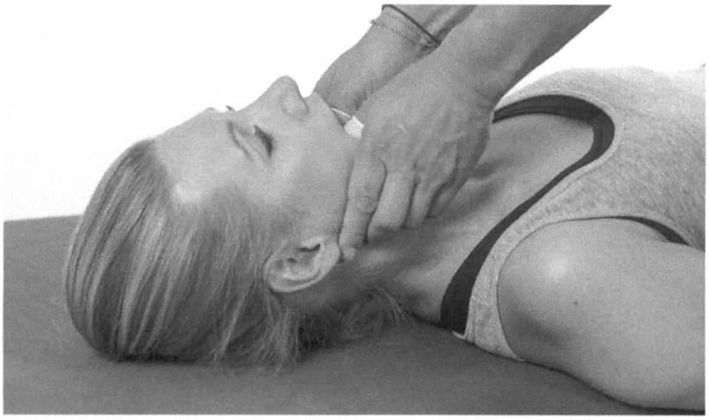

Figure 2.78 Testing the passive mobility of the TMG

Passive compression test

Passive compression tests enable further differentiation of a disturbance of articular surfaces or of the bilaminar zone.

- Passive compression test in the **dorsal direction**
  - No pain: negative result.
  - Painful: traumatic, or inflammation in the region of the bilaminar zone.
- Passive compression test in the **dorsocranial direction**
  - Possible unevenness or rubbing sounds (because traversing the condylar path under compression): disturbance of articular surfaces.
  - Sound of terminal clicking (on passing beyond the articular tubercle): hypermobility or subluxation of condyle. Subluxation is visibly evidenced on mouth opening. Mouth closing may also be restricted until the compression is released.

Test of the motion of the retrodiscal tissue according to Langendoen-Sertel and Hamouda, modified

This test [250] differentiates disturbances of the retrodiscal tissue (Figure 2.79).

Table 2.4 Differential diagnosis of the end feel

End feel	With pain	With reduced amplitude	With normal amplitude
Sudden resistance	Sudden muscle contraction	Muscle cramp	
Softer resistance as compared with the end feeling of ligamentous resistance	Slow muscle contraction; possibly shortening of muscle	Muscle inhibition	Muscle inhibition
Harder resistance than end feel of ligamentous resistance	Connective-tissue obstruction, possibly shrinkage of the capsule	Connective-tissue obstruction, possibly shrinkage of the capsule	Connective-tissue obstruction
Osseous resistance		Osseous obstruction	
Elastic resistance		Displacement of the disk without repositioning	

Mouth opening with cranial compression at the TMJ according to Sebald and Kopp, modified

This test is indicated when clicking occurs on active mouth opening. It enables further differentiation of the clicking.[397:39–41] It is also used to examine the disk.

Hand position (Figure 2.78):

- Position your thumbs intraorally, resting on the row of lower teeth each side.
- Your other fingers should lie on the body of the mandible. Grasp the angle of the mandible each side with your middle fingers.

Method: Ask the patient to actively open the mouth. At the same time, you should apply equal cranial compression to both temporomandibular joints. Differentiate the joint sounds that occur (Table 2.5). If pain occurs, this may indicate discopathy; if there is reduction in mouth opening at the same time, this points to disk displacement.

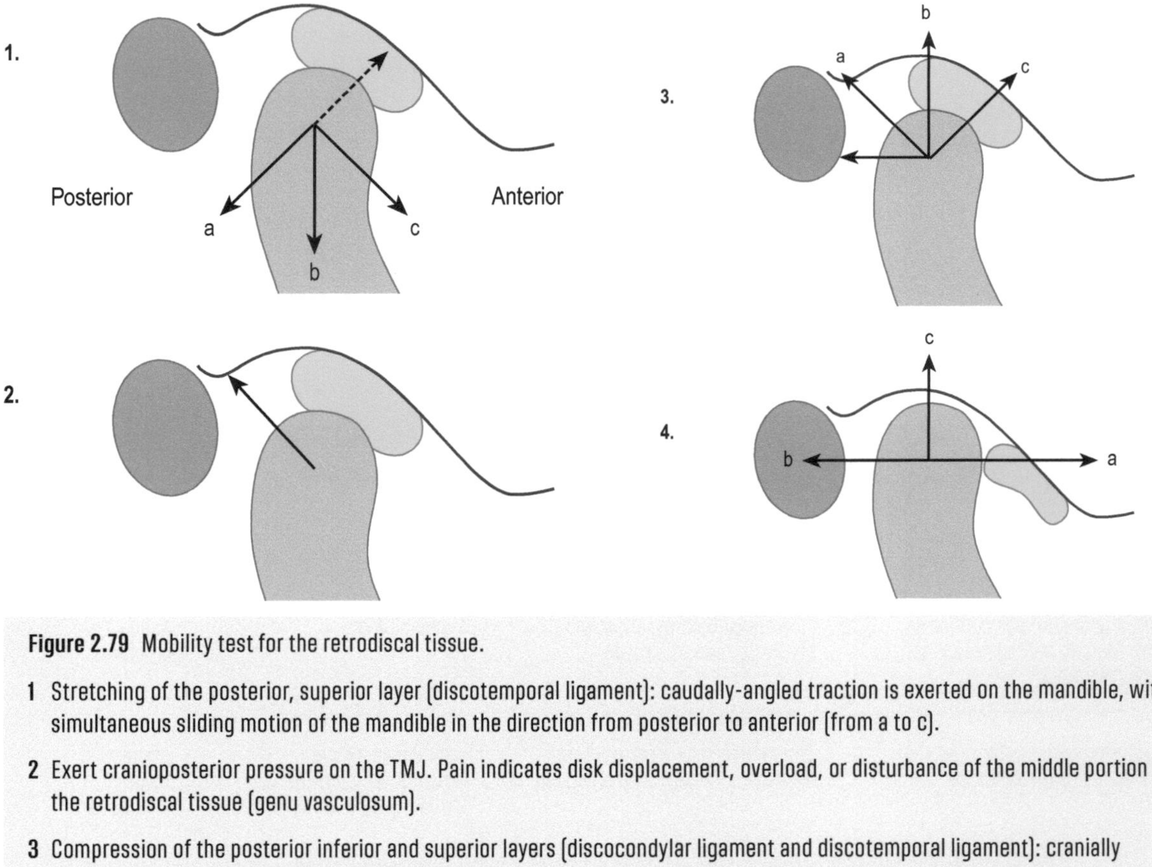

Figure 2.79 Mobility test for the retrodiscal tissue.

1 Stretching of the posterior, superior layer (discotemporal ligament): caudally-angled traction is exerted on the mandible, with simultaneous sliding motion of the mandible in the direction from posterior to anterior (from a to c).

2 Exert cranioposterior pressure on the TMJ. Pain indicates disk displacement, overload, or disturbance of the middle portion of the retrodiscal tissue (genu vasculosum).

3 Compression of the posterior inferior and superior layers (discocondylar ligament and discotemporal ligament): cranially angled, with simultaneous sliding motion of the mandible in the direction from anterior to posterior (from c to a).

4 Diagnosis of an anterior displacement of the disk in static occlusion: **a** a postero-anterior sliding motion of the mandible causes stretching of the retro-articular tissue, with pain; **b** an antero-posterior sliding motion of the mandible leads to compression of the inferior layer (discocondylar ligament); **c** a purely cranial movement of the mandible will compress the posterior inferior and superior layers (discocondylar and discotemporal ligaments)

Table 2.5 Differentiation of joint sounds

Active mouth opening	Without cranial compression	Initial I	Initial / intermediate II	Intermediate III	Terminal IV
On active mouth opening with cranial compression	Clicking at the same place as on mouth opening without cranial compression	No clicking	Clicking later in the course of mouth opening[2] and louder	Clicking at the same place, but louder and brighter[4] or duller sound (possibly crepitation)	Clicking louder or with a duller sound
Possible causes	Articular surface	Tension of lateral ligament or incipient hypermobility of the disk;[1] with reduced mouth opening: total displacement of disk without repositioning	Partial or total displacement of disk[3]	Restriction ("stuck disk") or cartilage defect	Total displacement of disk or cartilage defect

[1] In the case of initial clicking, lateral translation should also be tested. If clicking occurs again, hypermobility of disk.

With your thumb, ease the jaw of the side to be tested in a lateral direction, and on active mouth opening with cranial compression, tension of the lateral ligament results in no clicking; in the case of disk hypermobility, clicking would initially be somewhat louder.

[2] If clicking occurs later in the course of mouth opening than it does on mouth opening without cranial compression, but there is no clicking on closing and then re-opening the mouth, this indicates a good prognosis.

[3] On account of the reduced joint space, under compression, anterior displacement of the disk with repositioning does not occur until later, usually with deflexion.

[4] Restricted ("stuck") disk: disk displacement occurs, but the disk remains "stuck" on the condylar path and cannot be shifted. Under compression, there is delayed clicking, but it is a brighter and louder sound.

General testing of the capsule

Practitioner: Take up a position at the head of the patient, on the side opposite to the one to be tested.

Hand position:

- Cranial hand: five-finger temporal bone technique (Figure 2.80).
  - Grasp the zygomatic process with your thumb and index finger.
  - Place your middle finger in the external acoustic meatus.

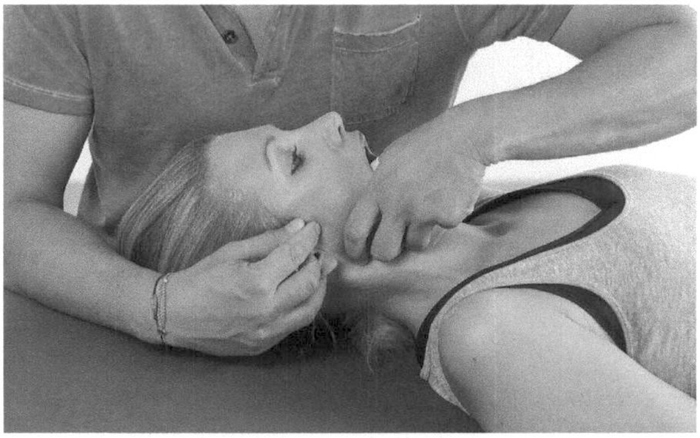

Figure 2.80 General testing of the capsule

  - Place your ring finger in front of the mastoid process.
  - Place your little finger behind the mastoid process.
- Caudal hand: position your thumb on the biting surface of the back molar of the opposite side. With your fingers, grasp the angle of the mandible.

Method:

- Administer traction in the caudal, anterior direction with the thumb on the back molar. Hold the temporal bone in position with your other hand.
- Pain indicates a "locked," restricted capsule; the effect of this is to restrict rotation of the temporomandibular joint.

Testing lateral parts of the capsule

Hand position: As above.

Method:

- Administer traction in the caudal and anterior direction, and induce mediotrusion. Meanwhile hold the temporal bone in position with your other hand (Figure 2.81).
- Pain indicates restriction of the lateral parts of the capsule.

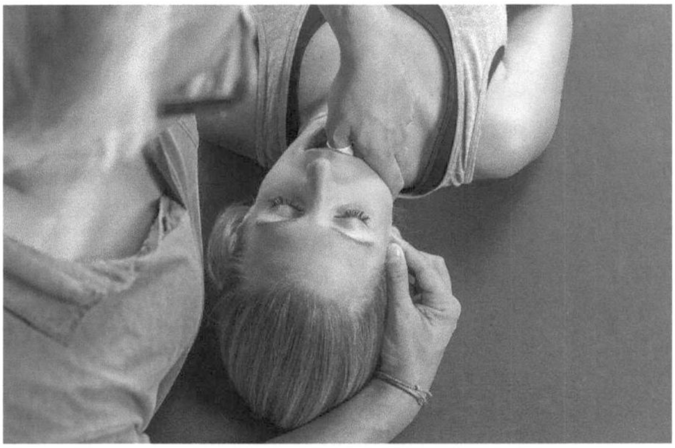

Figure 2.81 Testing lateral parts of the capsule

Testing the stylomandibular ligament

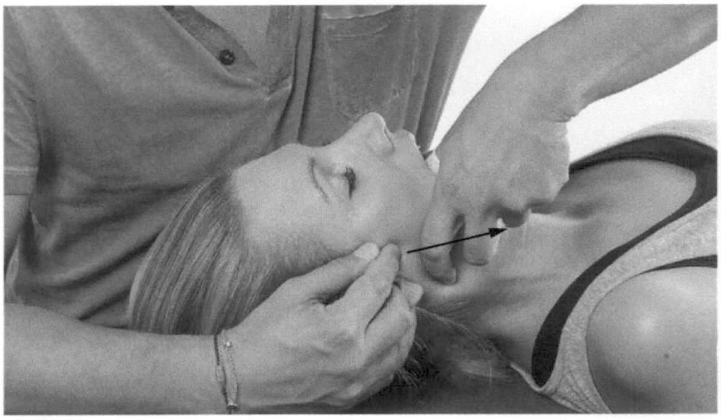

Figure 2.82 Testing the stylomandibular ligament

Hand position: As above.

Method: With your thumb, move the lower jaw diagonally in a caudal, anterior, and slightly lateral direction (corresponding to the course of the ligament). With your other hand, register the reaction along the course of the ligament, or a possible movement of the temporal bone (Figure 2.82). If there is an abnormal increase in tension of the stylomandibular ligament, increased tissue resistance may be sensed along the course of the ligament. According to Frymann, there is a pull on the temporal bone of the tested side.

Sequelae: See section 2.6.3.

Testing the sphenomandibular ligament

Hand position:

- Cranial hand: with your thumb and middle or index finger, grasp the greater wings.
- Caudal hand: as above.

Method: With your thumb, ease the lower jaw in a caudal direction. Register the movement at the greater wings with your other hand (Figure 2.83). If there is an abnormal increase in tension of the sphenomandibular ligament, increased tissue

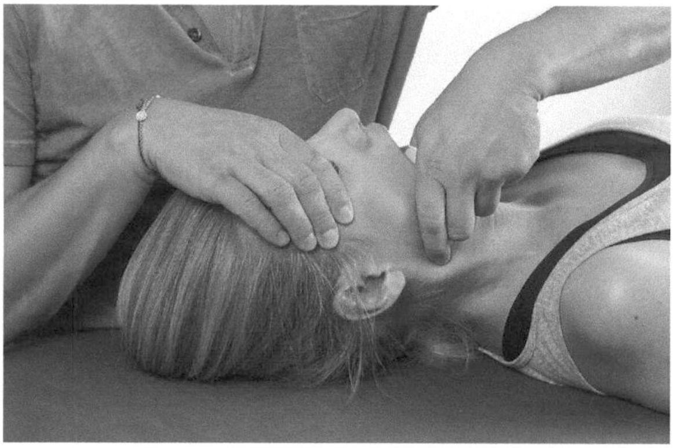

Figure 2.83 Testing the sphenomandibular ligament

resistance may be sensed along the course of the ligament. According to Frymann, there is superior movement of the greater wing of the tested side.

FURTHER INFORMATION The sphenomandibular ligament arises on the spine of the sphenoid. This lies posterior to the flexion/extension axis of the SBS; it is this that gives rise to Viola Frymann's view that an increase in tension or fibrosis of the ligament leads to a caudal pull on the base of the sphenoid, with movement of the ipsilateral greater wing in the superior direction.

Sequelae: See section 2.6.3.

Palpation of the masticatory muscles

The investigation and successful treatment of the masticatory and associated muscles are extremely important for successful treatment of CMD. Take care always to apply an equal degree of pressure during testing. In the case of any uncertainty during palpation, gently biting together can make it easier to differentiate the masticatory muscle in question.

Check whether any pain is caused, and look for tension, myogelosis, and any activated trigger points (see below). The main difference between tenderness to pressure and trigger points is the presence of referred pain. The degree of sensitivity or pain on palpation of the TMJ muscles (Figure 2.84) provides an indication of the severity of the TMJ disturbance, and of hyperactivity or hypoactivity of the neuromuscular system. Apart from searching for the underlying cause, if the TMJ muscles are hypoactive they should be toned, and if they are hyperactive they should be relaxed. It is helpful if you always palpate the masticatory muscles, hyoid muscles, and selected neck muscles in the same order and note any differences between sides. Further investigation of the interrelationship with occlusion is essential.

- **Masseter muscle**: between the zygomatic arch and the angle of the mandible.
- **Temporalis muscle**
  - Posterior part: above the ears and behind the ears.
  - Medial part: above the ears.
  - Anterior part: above and in front of the ears.
  - Point of attachment medial, on the coronoid process: intraoral, between the cheek and the maxillary tuberosity toward the back in the direction of the coronoid process, at the level of the first molar on the buccal side.
- **Lateral pterygoid muscle**
  - Intraorally, between the maxillary tuberosity and the ascending mandibular ramus, in the direction of the external acoustic meatus. Position your finger in the first instance so that the palmar surface faces medially, toward the gingivae, and turns to the side on the mandibular ramus. Move the finger in a posterior, cranial direction until the tip of the finger meets the tissue directly anterior to the muscle.
  - This muscle cannot be palpated directly.
- **Medial pterygoid muscle**

Figure 2.84
Palpation of the masticatory muscles.

1 Temporalis muscle.

2 Temporalis muscle, intraoral.

3 Masseter muscle.

4 Medial pterygoid muscle, intraoral.

5 Lateral pterygoid muscle, intraoral

- Intraorally:
  - * Medially on the mandibular ramus, extending from the maxillary tuberosity to the angle of the mandible. (For palpation and listening tests of the mouth floor, see also section 3.3.4.)
  - * Ask the patient to open the mouth wide.
- Extraorally: position the finger medially on the angle of the mandible, and apply pressure in a superior direction.

- **Digastric muscle:** with head extension
  - Posterior belly: posterior to the angle of the mandible, in front of the sternocleidomastoid muscle, in the direction of the ear. (Meanwhile, apply inward pressure with the finger.)
  - Anterior belly: beneath the tip of the chin, extending along the floor of the mouth on both sides of the midline.
- **Zygomaticus major muscle (Figure 2.85)**

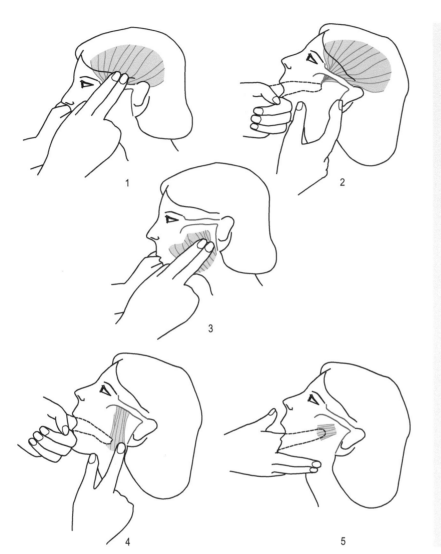

- Origin: zygomatic bone, anterior to the zygomaticotemporal suture.
- Insertion: medial and caudal to the modiolus (knot of muscle at the angle of the mouth), extending to the upper lip and merging with skin.
- Function: raises corner of mouth; laughing (together with risorius).

- **Zygomaticus minor muscle** (Figure 2.85)
  - Origin: zygomatic bone, immediately posterior to the zygomaticomaxillary suture.
  - Insertion: medially and caudally, extending to the upper lip, merging with skin.
  - Function: raises the upper lip.
  - Palpation of the zygomaticus major and minor: slide your index finger between the upper lip and teeth, under the zygomaticus major and minor, and administer outward pressure on these; meanwhile palpate the muscles from exterior with a finger of the other hand.
  - Treatment would involve administering pressure and following the myofascial tensions.
- **Modiolus**

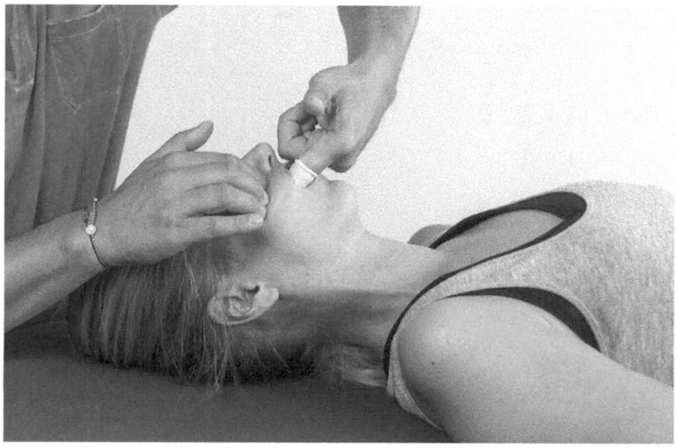

Figure 2.85
Palpation of the zygomaticus major and minor muscles

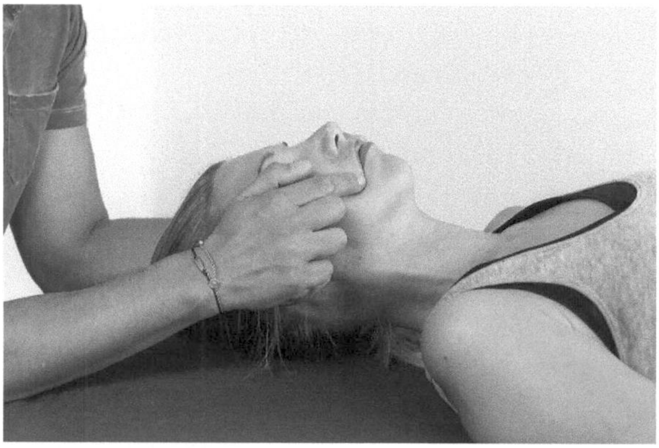

Figure 2.86
Modiolus

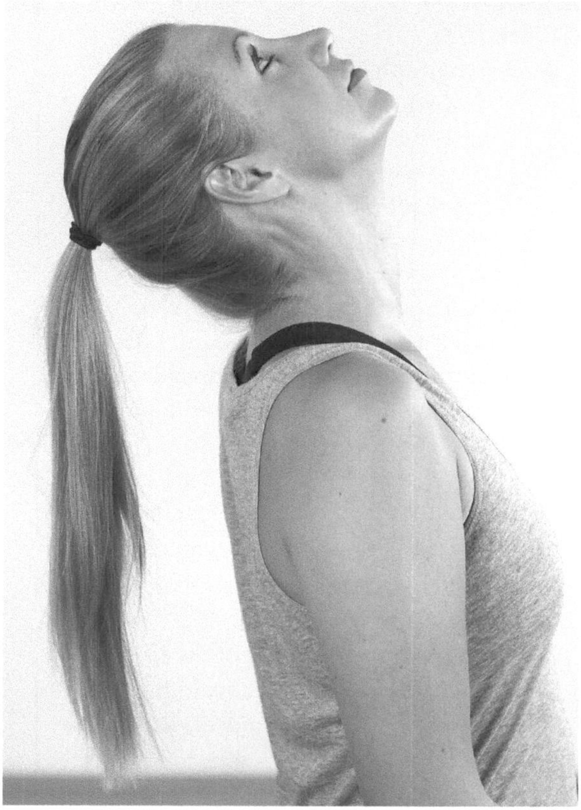

Figure 2.87
Testing of the suprahyoid and retrohyoid muscles

- Palpation of the knot of muscle at the corner of the mouth (Figure 2.86), the point where the following facial muscles meet: orbicularis oris, levator anguli oris, depressor anguli oris, buccinator, risorius, zygomaticus major.
- Treatment would involve administering pressure in the region of the modiolus and following the myofascial tensions. Depending on the myofascial dysfunction, gentle stretching of the muscles involved can also be applied.

- **Testing of suprahyoid and retrohyoid muscles**

Ask the patient to bring the teeth into contact, and extend the neck back (Figure 2.87). The test is positive if contact between the teeth is lost (Figure 2.88).

- **Further palpation**
  - Palpation of the muscles of the floor of the mouth and of the hyoid (section 3.4.4).
  - Palpation of the muscles of facial expression (mimetic muscles), e.g., modiolus, zygomaticus major and minor (see above).
  - Palpation of the muscles of the neck and shoulder, especially the sternocleidomastoid and scalenes. These last often exhibit increased tone; for successful treatment, these muscles should be relaxed.
  - In addition, palpation of facial (mimetic) muscles, especially the mentalis, orbicularis oris, and buccinator muscles (see also section 3.1.1).
  - Palpation and testing of the infrahyoid, suprahyoid, and retrohyoid muscles.
  - Palpation of the craniocervical fasciae.

Trigger points

A trigger point is a hypersensitized/hyperstimulated region in a tissue (myofascial, cutaneous, ligamentous, fascial, periosteal). When pressure is applied, the effect is localized sensitivity to touch. Referred pain and referred contact sensitivity are generally encountered (Table 2.6).

Autonomic symptoms or proprioceptive disturbances may also occur.

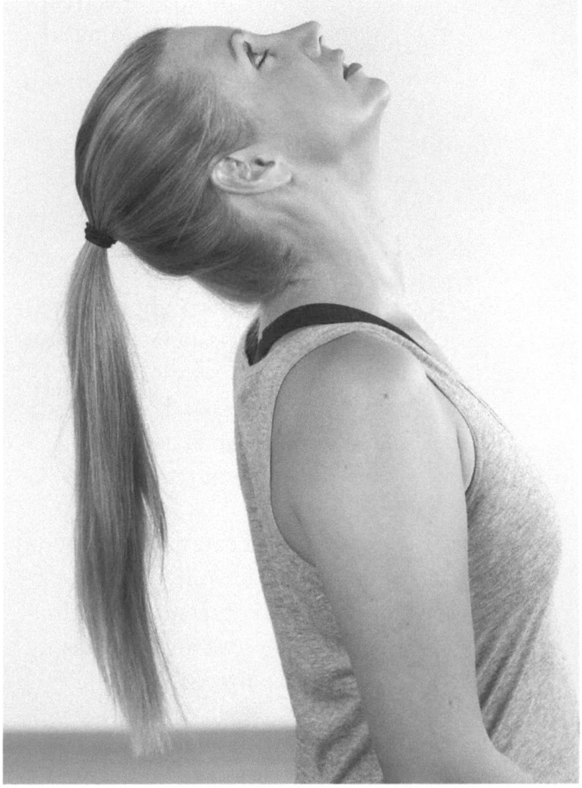

Figure 2.88
Testing of the suprahyoid and retrohyoid muscles, loss of tooth contact

Isometric muscle test according to Sebald and Kopp, after Winkel

The force and the duration of contraction are tested. Isometric contraction should normally be strong and pain-free.[397:117–132,475:373f.] The isometric testing of the masticatory muscles is seen as significant in differential diagnosis and should always be used if the result from palpation is uncertain.

Table 2.6 Trigger points (Travell and Simmons 1983:202, 219, 236, 249, 260, 273)

Muscles	Location and palpation	Referred to	Trigger
Temporalis	• Mouth opened 2–3 cm • Extraoral: move one finger in a horizontal line from the zygomatic arch on each of the anterior, middle (Figure 2.89), and posterior (Figure 2.90) portions of the muscle • Intraoral: index finger on the insertion at coronoid process and on neighboring region at ramus of mandible	Temporal region, eyebrow, upper teeth, more rarely maxilla and TMJ	Immobilization of the TMJ, grinding of the teeth, disturbance of occlusion, effect of cold or injury on the muscle, whiplash injury
Masseter	• With the mouth slightly opened for preliminary muscle stretch • Superficial part (Figure 2.91): press the muscle against the ramus of the mandible, or squeeze the muscle together with two fingers • Deep part (Figure 2.92): press the muscle against the posterior part of the ramus and along the lower margin of the zygomatic bone (pressure posterior, superior on trigger points may possibly trigger tinnitus)	• Superficial part: eyebrow, maxilla, mandible, upper and lower molars • Deep part: TMJ and deep into the ear	Traumatic injury, grinding of the teeth, overload, malocclusion, disturbance of occlusion
Lateral pterygoid	• Anterior part of the inferior head (Figure 2.93): mouth opened 2 cm; mandible laterally displaced toward the test side. Intraoral: finger between maxilla and coronoid process, pressure on the pterygoid process (lateral plate) • Posterior part of the inferior head and superior head (Figure 2.94): mouth opened 3 cm; extraoral: via the masseter muscle beneath the zygomatic bone in the mandibular notch	TMJ, maxilla	Disturbance of occlusion

Continued

Table 2.6 Trigger points (Travell and Simmons 1983:202, 219, 236, 249, 260, 273) *Continued*

Muscles	Location and palpation	Referred to	Trigger
Medial pterygoid	• Mouth wide open • Extraoral (Figure 2.95): finger medially on angle of the mandible, upward pressure • Intraoral (Figure 2.96): slide the finger along the molars to the ramus of the mandible; the muscle is immediately posterior to the anterior border of the ramus	Back of the mouth and pharynx, beneath and behind the TMJ, deep in the ear	Usually secondary to dysfunction of the lateral pterygoid muscle or disturbance of occlusion
Digastric	• Extension of the head • Posterior belly (Figure 2.97): finger posterior to angle of the mandible; slide it in front of the sternocleidomastoid in the direction of the ear while pressing inwards with the finger • Anterior belly (Figure 2.98): fingers on the tissue beneath the chin tip, on both sides of the midline	• Posterior belly: upper part of the sternocleidomastoid (pseudo-pain of the sternocleidomastoid) • Anterior belly: lower incisors • Note: pain becomes distinct when the sternocleidomastoid muscle is relaxed	Secondary to dysfunction of the masseter muscle, overload of the muscle when grinding the teeth, retrusion of the mandible (associated with mouth breathing)
Stylohyoid	As posterior belly of digastric muscle: press with the finger toward the styloid process	Neck region, larynx, region of digastric muscle	
Buccinator	With the thumb from exterior and with the index finger intraorally, press the region between the masseter muscle and the mouth	Upper palate	Diffuse pain on chewing and swallowing
Sternocleidomastoid	On the sternal and clavicular parts	• Sternal part: vertex, occiput, cheek, eye (atypical facial neuralgia), pharynx, sternum • Clavicular part: forehead, ear with dizziness, disturbance of balance	Overload of the muscle due to structural dysfunctions of the body; breathing problems

TMJ, temporomandibular joint.

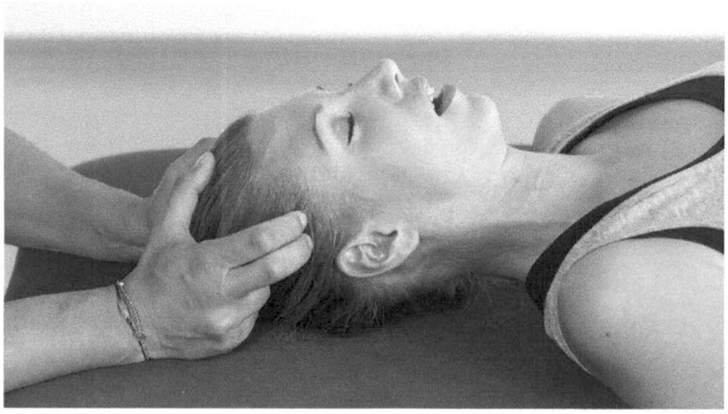

Figure 2.89
Trigger point of the temporalis muscle (anterior and medial parts)

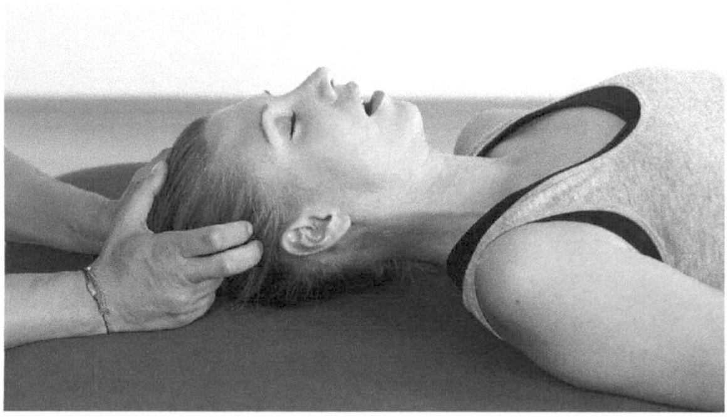

Figure 2.90
Trigger point of the temporalis muscle (posterior part)

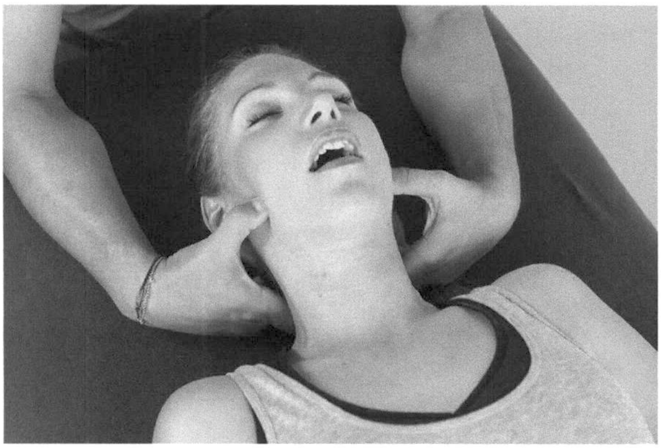

Figure 2.91
Trigger point of the masseter muscle (superficial part)

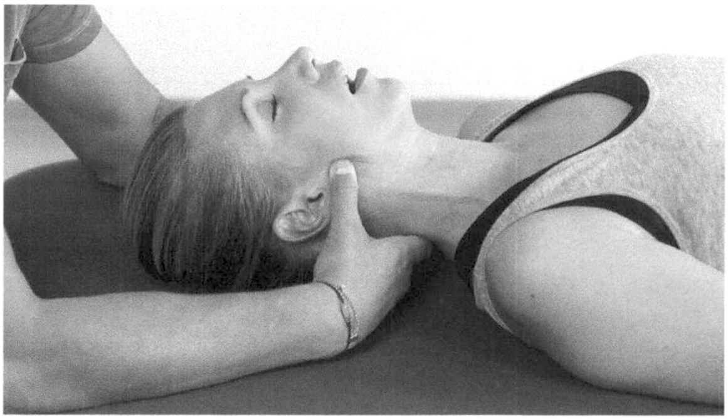

Figure 2.92
Trigger point of the masseter muscle (deep part)

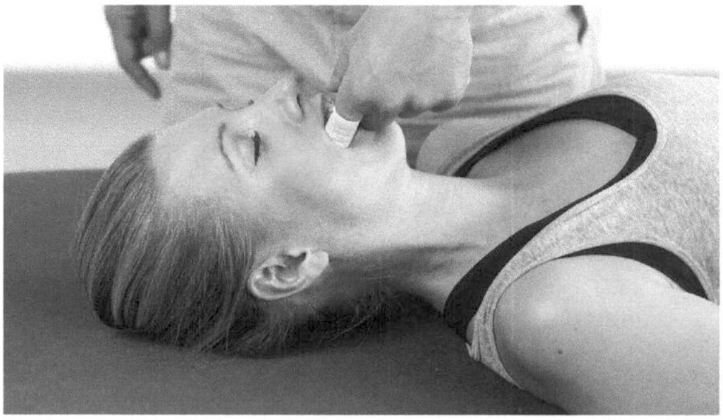

Figure 2.93
Trigger point of the lateral pterygoid muscle (anterior part of inferior head)

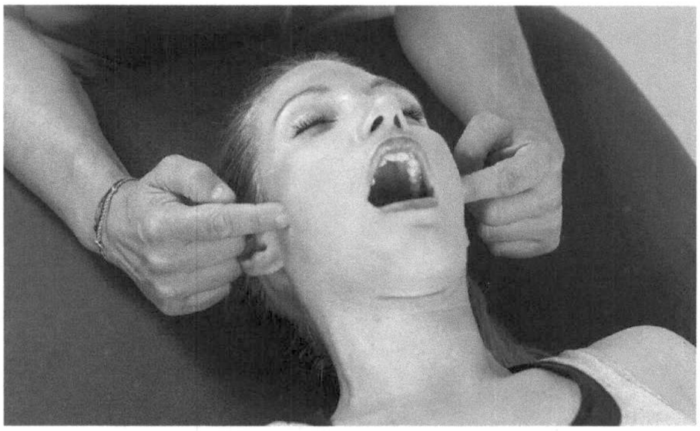

Figure 2.94
Trigger point of lateral pterygoid muscle (posterior part of inferior head and superior head)

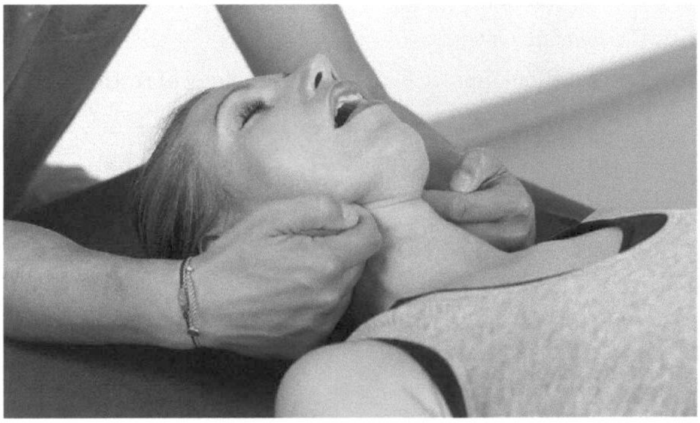

Figure 2.95
Trigger point of the medial pterygoid muscle (extraoral)

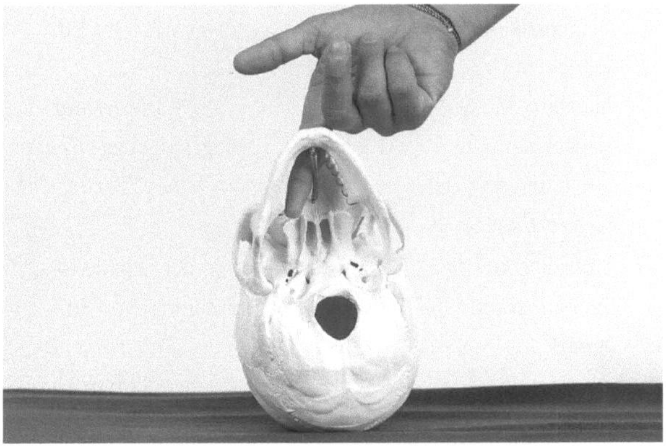

Figure 2.96
Trigger point of the medial pterygoid muscle (intraoral)

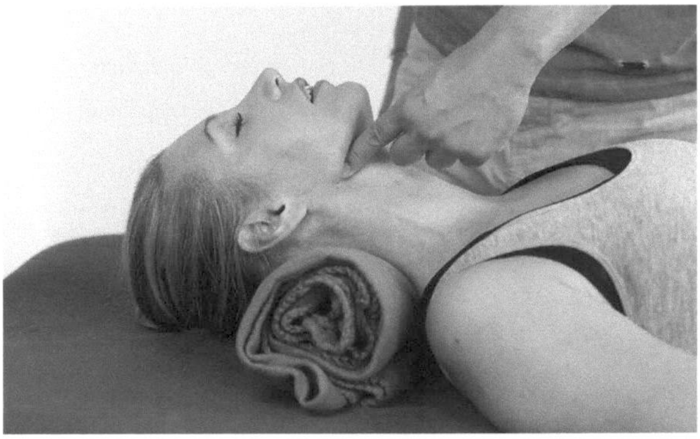

Figure 2.97
Trigger point of the digastric muscle, posterior belly

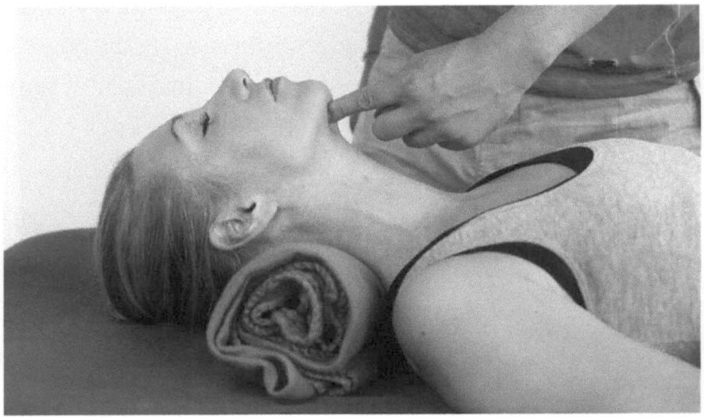

Figure 2.98
Trigger point of the digastric muscle, anterior belly

Patient: The patient is seated.

Hand position: Take up a position in front of the patient and grasp the jaw bilaterally with your thumbs and thenar eminences outside on the alveolar part of the mandible and with your index fingers on the angle of the mandible, whilst positioning the middle fingers on the underside of the mandible.

- For isometric contraction of the muscles responsible for mediotrusion (Table 2.8), the thumb and thenar eminence are positioned on the opposite side from the mediotrusion on the outside of the mandible (as described above). Place the other hand on the temple on the mediotrusion side.
- For isometric contraction of the muscles that close the mouth (Table 2.8), the palmar surfaces of the thumbs are placed intraorally on the chewing surface of the lower teeth.

Alternative hand position for all tests V-grip: grasp the chin from the front with your thumb and index finger. The middle finger is bent under the chin.

Method:

- Ask the patient to relax the jaw joints, with the tongue lying relaxed in the mouth and the mouth slightly opened.
- Apply pressure in a given direction, while the patient resists this pressure (Table 2.7).

- No movement should occur in the TMJ (isometric muscle contraction).
- Increase the pressure slowly (approximately for a period of not more than 10 s).
- Then hold the pressure for about 10 s, and slowly release it again over a period of up to 5 s.

Tip for practitioners

If only one muscle is being tested, less force should be exerted than when testing muscle groups.

Table 2.7 Isometric testing

Isometric test	Initial position of the patient	Direction of pressure applied by practitioner
Muscles that open the mouth in centric relation	Mouth opened slightly	Cephalad
Muscles that open the mouth in protrusion	Protrusion of the mandible 3–4 mm when the mouth is slightly open	Cephalad
Muscles that open the mouth in mediotrusion	Mediotrusion of the mandible until the tips of the canines are opposite one another, with the mouth slightly open	Cephalad
Protractor muscles	Slight protrusion with the mouth slightly open	In a posterior direction
Muscles that produce mediotrusion, e.g., to the right	Mandible to the left, until the tips of the canines on the left are opposite one another, with the mouth slightly open	To the right
Muscles that close the mouth in centric relation	Mouth slightly open	Caudad
Muscles that close the mouth in protrusion	Protrusion of the mandible 3–4 mm when the mouth is slightly open	Caudad
Muscles that close the mouth in mediotrusion	Mediotrusion of the mandible until the tips of the canines are opposite one another, with the mouth slightly open	Caudad

Table 2.8 Muscles involved

Isometric test	Muscles tested
Muscles that open the mouth	Digastric, mylohyoid, geniohyoid, stylohyoid, suprahyoid, and lateral pterygoid muscles
Protractor muscles	Lateral pterygoid, masseter (superficial part)
Muscles that produce mediotrusion	Lateral pterygoid, medial pterygoid
Muscles that close the mouth	Temporalis, masseter, medial pterygoid

Table 2.9 Interpretation of isometric testing, according to Sebald and Kopp (1996:131)

Isometric test	Possible disturbance in cases where pain is changed or triggered	Follow-on investigation
Muscles that open the mouth in centric relation	Dysfunction of muscles that open the mouth	Isometric test of muscles that open the mouth in protrusion
Muscles that open the mouth in protrusion	Dysfunction of muscles that open the mouth	Isometric test of muscles that open the mouth in mediotrusion
Muscles that open the mouth in mediotrusion	Joint effusion, osteoarthritis, anterior dislocation of disk	• Isometric test of muscles that produce mediotrusion • Test for arthrogenous disturbance
Protractor muscles	Dysfunction of protractor muscles	Isometric test of muscles that produce mediotrusion
Muscles that produce mediotrusion	Muscles of floor of mouth	Passive motion testing
Muscles that close the mouth in centric relation	Muscles that close the mouth	Isometric test of muscles that close the mouth in protrusion
Muscles that close the mouth in protrusion	Muscles that close the mouth	Isometric test of muscles that close the mouth in mediotrusion
Muscles that close the mouth in mediotrusion	Joint effusion, osteoarthritis, anterior dislocation of disk	• Passive motion testing • Test for arthrogenous disturbance

Interpretation

- The test is negative if normal force is exerted and there is no pain: no myogenic dysfunction.
- The test is positive if the force is less and pain is triggered: myogenic or arthrogenous dysfunction.
    - Reduced force gives an indication of a disturbance of innervation (neurogenic origin).
    - Pain; location of pain:
        - Pain in the muscles tends to indicate myogenic disturbance.
        - Pain in the joint tends to indicate an arthrogenous disturbance.
        - Pain in various positions of the joint tends to indicate a myogenic disturbance.
        - Pain in only one position of the joint tends to indicate an arthrogenous disturbance (differentiate further by passive motion testing).

Isometric testing may be accompanied by a change in pain or may trigger pain (Table 2.9), or there may be no change and no pain triggered (Table 2.10). The interpretation of isometric tests serves merely

Table 2.10 Interpretation of isometric testing according to Sebald and Kopp (1996: 131)

Isometric test	Pain unchanged or not triggered	Follow-on investigation
Muscles that open the mouth in centric relation	Muscles that open the mouth not involved	Isometric test of muscles that close the mouth at rest
Muscles that open the mouth in protrusion	Muscles that open the mouth not involved	• Isometric test of muscles that close the mouth at rest • Isometric test of protractor muscles
Muscles that open the mouth in mediotrusion	Muscles that open the mouth not involved	Isometric test of muscles that close the mouth at rest
Protractor muscles	Protractor muscles not involved	Isometric test of muscles that close the mouth at rest
Muscles that produce mediotrusion	Dysfunction of lateral and medial pterygoid muscles	Passive motion testing
Muscles that close the mouth in centric relation	Muscles that close the mouth not involved	Passive motion testing
Muscles that close the mouth in protrusion	Muscles that close the mouth not involved	Passive motion testing
Muscles that close the mouth in mediotrusion	Muscles that close the mouth not involved	Passive motion testing

as a diagnostic guide and should be confirmed by further investigations.

Palpation of the trigeminal nerve exit points

- Pressure on the nerve exit points of the trigeminal branches, comparing both sides (Volume 2, section 7.5.2).
- The test is positive if there is tenderness to pressure and disturbances of sensitivity.
- Heat and warmth at the nerve exit points of the trigeminal nerve.

Paradoxical sensations are possible in cases of bruxism. Total absence of anything perceived is an indication of neurological or neoplastic disease. Further neurological investigation and examination of the paranasal sinuses are indicated.

Masseteric reflex

This reflex involves the masseter (and the temporalis muscle). The mandibular nerve (CN V_3) innervates these muscles and is thus part of the monosynaptic reflex arc.

Method

- The patient's mouth should be slightly open.
- Place your index finger on the patient's chin. Tap your finger with the reflex hammer.
- A slight tap is followed by closure of the mouth.
- The reflex is weaker if there is disease along the course of the trigeminal nerve (CN V), or bulbar paralysis.
- The reflex is stronger if there is a lesion of the first motor neuron, or pseudo-bulbar paralysis.

Neurodynamic test of the mandibular nerve

See Volume 2, section 7.5.2.

Auscultation

A double stethoscope is very useful for diagnosing jaw sounds (Table 2.11). (See also section 2.7.2.) For the analysis of TMJ joint clicking, see section 2.6.1.

Table 2.11 Diagnosis of joint sounds

Sounds	Diagnosis
Rubbing sounds	Possibly due to cartilaginous and osseous structures
Rubbing sounds without radiographic findings	Disturbances of occlusion
Clicking, general	Discopathy
Reciprocal clicking	Discopathy
Terminal clicking on closure, intensified when pressure applied cephalad on the angle of the jaw	Dislocation in centric position
Terminal clicking on opening and initial clicking on closing	Hypermobility, subluxation
Intermediate clicking	Localized thickening of cartilage
Bright, loud clicking	Ligamentous, when the disk slides along the lateral and medial ligament

Reciprocal clicking = initial clicks on opening and terminal clicks on closure.

Intermediate clicking = intermediate clicks on opening and closure.

What to do next

- Besides the mandible, temporal bone, and maxilla, the osteopathic examination also includes the other cranial bones (sutural, intraosseous), especially the palatine and zygomatic bones, vomer, sphenoid, and occipital bone.

- Account should also be taken of the dural folds, dural venous sinuses, and fasciae of the head and neck, and the integral examination of the rest of the body.
- If the findings are arthrogenous, an imaging technique is indicated.
- Investigation of static and primary dysfunction in other regions of the body.
- It is fundamentally important to distinguish central from peripheral sensitization (see also section 2.6.6), and to differentiate sensitization of the mandibular nerve and that of the entire trigeminal nerve.

Other investigations Function analysis (in the case of pain of unclear origin in the craniomandibular system or recurrent trouble, in the case of orthodontic interventions and treatment using braces, following traumatic injury in the region of cranium and neck, etc.), radiography, MRI (less often, CT), functional MRI, etc.

Differential diagnosis in CMD is presented in Table 2.12. That of ascending and descending dysfunctions can be found in Table 2.13.

Table 2.12 Differential diagnosis in cases of craniomandibular dysfunction

	Myogenic	Arthrogenous	Occlusal
History-taking	First indication of presence of CMD		
• Visual assessment • Teeth • Soft tissues	Bruxism (grinding, clenching)		Bruxism (grinding, clenching)
Deviation of chin tip	Indication of the side of the dysfunction		
Active mouth opening and closure	Indication of the side of the dysfunction and prognosis		
Discoordination	Probably myogenic		
Deviation	Probably myogenic	Less often, unilateral dysfunction	
Deflection		Unilateral dysfunction, discopathy, ankylosis	
3-finger test	Indication of CMD		
Palpation of TMJ: position and tenderness		Arthrogenous or bilaminar zone	

Continued

Table 2.12 Differential diagnosis in cases of craniomandibular dysfunction *Continued*

	Myogenic	Arthrogenous	Occlusal
Palpation of PRM rhythm	Indication of dysfunctions of widely varying origins, e.g., mandible, temporal bone, sutural, membranous, ligamentous, etc.		
Test of TMJ movement	Indication of side of dysfunction and prognosis		
Test of passive mobility of TMJ positive, but isometric finding negative		Arthrogenous	
Test of passive mobility of TMJ	Probably myogenic		
Differential diagnosis of jaw clicking with TMJ compression cephalad		Disk, joint surface, ligament	
Mobility testing for the retrodiscal tissue		Retrodiscal, dislocation of disk	
Palpation of masticatory and hyoid muscles	Myogenic		
Trigger points	Myogenic, pain referral zones		
Isometric muscle testing	Associated with reduced strength* and pain in the muscles and while the joint is in various positions	Associated with reduced strength and pain in the joint, and in only one joint position	
Auscultation		Arthrogenous	Occlusal
Nerve palpation/reflex	Neurogenic; disorder of the paranasal sinuses		
Inconsistent findings with psychological signs	Possibly psychosomatic		
Radiographic investigation		Arthrogenous	

* Reduced strength without pain indicates a disturbance of innervation (neurogenic origin).

CMD, craniomandibular dysfunction; TMJ, temporomandibular joint; PRM, primary respiratory mechanism/movement.

Table 2.13 Differential diagnosis of ascending and descending functions

Investigation	Interpretation
Palpation of the muscles of the neck and shoulder	Parietal involvement
Investigation of body posture, positional: • Static signs of CMD • Vertical test according to Barre	Differential diagnosis of ascending and descending dysfunction
Investigation of body posture, dynamic: • Fascial organization according to Zink • Meersseman test • Fukuda test • See Table 2.2	Differential diagnosis of ascending and descending dysfunction
Contradictory findings with psychological signs	Possibly psychosomatic

CMD, craniomandibular dysfunction.

2.8 Treatment of craniomandibular dysfunctions

The osteopathic treatment should always be conducted in a **multimodal, interdisciplinary** way, in consultation and cooperation with an orthodontic or dental specialist, or specialist from another discipline.

There are different treatment approaches for adults and children (regarding the treatment of children, see section 2.10.12). In adults, osteopathic treatment particularly involves the normalization of the jaw, masticatory, and associated muscles and occlusion, including ascending and descending chains. In cases involving inflammatory changes of the TMJ, extreme mouth opening should be avoided.

NOTE

Prophylaxis

Parents should be pointed to the fact that breastfeeding can be seen as a preventative functional treatment for the jaw. Breastfeeding promotes a physiological, anteriorly directed development of the jaw, and if possible it should be carried out exclusively for at least six months.[343]

In cases of peripheral sensitization, emphasis is on **local treatment** of the affected regions: TMJ, local myofascial, orofacial, neurocranial, and craniocervical structures, and affected cranial nerves/centers, especially of the trigeminal nerve (esp. mandibular nerve). Besides these, the focus here should be directed to movement therapy/exercises, sport, and functional activities.

In the case of central sensitization, the therapeutic measures indicated are those that reduce the nociceptive influences on the trigeminal system and all other dysfunctional afferent influences on the function of the affected structures. Here, a **multimodal approach** is extremely important in treatment.

Normally, to achieve and maintain satisfactory positioning of the teeth following successful orthodontic treatment, long-term (sometimes lifelong) use of a retainer is indicated.[320,369] In such cases, osteopathic approaches can be used to try to reduce or prevent relapses, for example by treating associated dysfunctional body patterns or damaging habits/dyskinesias.

FURTHER INFORMATION Steinfurth[426] conducted a randomized study of the effect of osteopathic dysfunctions of the temporal bones on maximum mouth opening.

It involved 50 trial participants (44 women and 6 men, average age 36.06 years). The criteria for inclusion in the study were deviation of the midline, joint sounds, a temporarily existing barrier, hypermobility or hypomobility of the TMJ, and orthopedic treatment or treatment with occlusal appliances. In addition to at least one of the listed criteria, at least one osteopathic dysfunction of the temporal bones was found. Following osteopathic examination and treatment based on the principles of Sutherland and Magoun, maximum active mouth opening in the treatment group increased significantly compared to the control group.

A systematic review by List and Axelsson in 2010 showed that the following approaches can improve **pain symptoms in CMD**.[269] In addition to manual treatment approaches, there should be combined use of occlusal appliances (especially using occlusal splints), acupuncture, behavioral therapy, active, specific exercises, movement therapy, and pharmacological treatments. However, considerable caution should be used in prescribing active movements in the case of central sensitization with orofacial pain, because these can lead to hyperalgesia.[309]

Further treatment methods are orthodontics, arthroscopy of the TMJ,[206] discectomy, condylectomy, arthrotomy, sclerotherapy, pain-response training, psychosomatic therapy, repair of a disk perforation, arthrocentesis, soft splints, and transcutaneous nerve stimulation. Long-term studies[372] found no influence of orthodontic treatment in youth on TMJ disturbances in later life. Of 300 TMJ disturbances with displacement of the disk (usually anteromedially to the condyle), 270 cases could be successfully treated with the aid of splints.[473]

Evidence for the effect of electrophysical modalities and surgical interventions is insufficient, and occlusal adjustment appears to have no effect on CMD pain.[269]

Therapeutic interventions should also take account of the patient's subjective views. This includes such considerations as suitable passive and active strategies, active listening, empathy, and the integration of related psychosocial matters,[123,266] and also exercise therapies. Psychotherapy can sometimes be indicated. A change in diet, treatment of dental foci, etc. may possibly also be needed to ensure success of treatment.

Ultimately holistic treatment of mouth/jaw function is guided by the underlying causes.

Tip for practitioners

Treatment methods

- Treatment of all underlying muscular, fascial, osseous, and visceral dysfunctions in the body that impair the function of the temporomandibular joint and the postural patterns.
- Treatment of the occipital bone and temporal bone (section 2.8.2).
- Intraosseous treatment (section 2.8.3).
- Treatment of the masticatory muscles (section 2.8.1).
- Treatment of the hyoid and hyoid muscles.[265]
- Treatment of the nuchal muscles, atlanto-occipital joint, and T4 (according to Littlejohn).
- Treatment of the craniocervical fasciae.[265]
- Treatment of the facial (mimetic) muscles and fasciae, e.g., zygomaticus major/minor, modiolus, superficial musculoaponeurotic system (SMAS), paratideomasseteric fascia, buccopharyngeal fascia, and pterygomandibular raphe (Volume 2, section 4.6.5).
- Treatment of the condyles and disks (bilaterally). As a general rule, a reduction in the intensity of pain in the facilitated segment should be achieved before normalizing the alignment of the TMJ locally.
- Auditory tube technique (Volume 2, section 6.4.2).
- Improvement of nasal breathing: treatment of the paranasal sinuses and tonsils (Volume 2, section 6.4.2).

- Treatment of the mandibular ligaments: capsule/lateral ligament, sphenomandibular ligament, stylomandibular ligament (section 2.8.4).
- Treatment of sphenopetrosal ligament at the sphenopetrosal synchondrosis (Volume 2, section 2.5).
- Improvement of nasal breathing: treatment of the paranasal sinuses and tonsils (Volume 2, section 2.5).
- Techniques for the cranial nerves (Volume 2, section 7.5.2): mandibular nerve, auriculotemporal nerve, etc.
- Technique for the external carotid artery/maxillary artery.
- Treatment of venolymphatic structures (section 2.8.5): internal jugular vein, external jugular vein, jugular foramen.
- Treatment of mouth/pharynx/larynx function (section 3.4).
- Self-help techniques: stretching and relaxation (section 2.9.1), coordination exercises (section 2.9.2), strengthening exercises (section 2.9.3), chewing exercises (section 2.9.4), and if/as appropriate, tongue, swallowing, and lip exercises and myofascial relaxation (section 3.4.13).
- Specific treatment approaches (section 2.10).

2.8.1 Treatment of the masticatory muscles

Temporalis muscle and tendon of insertion

Indication: Pain in the maxillary sinus, at the parietal, temporal, or occipital bone, hypersensitivity and pain of the upper teeth, disturbance of occlusion, teeth-grinding, centric teeth-clenching, limited mouth opening, compression in the TMJ with disk dysfunction, muscle spasm, temporal bone in anterior rotation or external rotation, referred pain in the larynx, disturbance of venous drainage of the cranium.

Practitioner: Take up a position at the head of the patient.

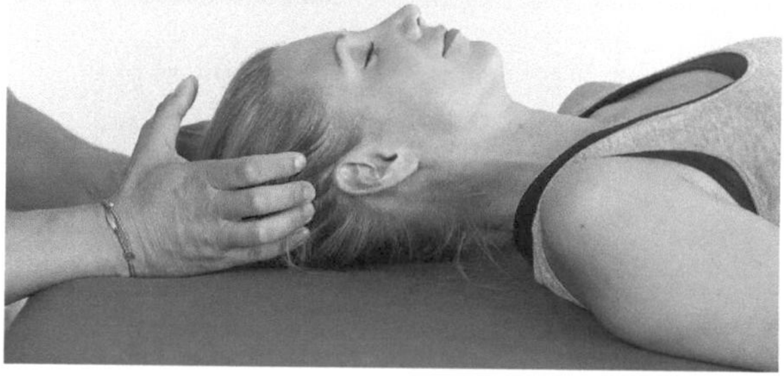

Figure 2.99 Temporalis muscle technique

Hand position:

- For the posterior muscle fibers, position your hands on the muscles, above and posterior to the ears.
- For the medial muscle fibers, position your hands above the ears.
- For the anterior muscle fibers, position your hands above and anterior to the ears, approximately 1 cm posterior to the lateral ocular margins.

Method: At the particular position, administer gentle traction in a cranial direction to relax the muscle (Figure 2.99).

To treat the tendon of the temporalis muscle, position your index finger intraorally, on the medial side of the coronoid process. Confirmation that you are palpating the tendon of the temporalis can be provided by asking the patient to close the mouth slightly against resistance. The tendon can be stretched obliquely across. Bear in mind that the tendon can extend far down, sometimes even as far as the angle of the mandible.

Tip for practitioners

In cases of chronic tension of the temporalis muscle, the increased transverse tension of the epicranial aponeurosis may also need to be treated.

Masseter muscle

Indication: Muscle hypertonicity, grinding of teeth (protrusive bruxism), pain in the upper jaw, lower molars, or mid-facial region, in the maxillary sinus and behind the eyeball, limited mouth opening, compression of TMJ, unilateral tinnitus, frontal headache. Where there is unilateral hypertonicity, the mandible may deviate to the ipsilateral side.

Practitioner: Take up a position at the head of the patient.

Hand position: Position your hands on the masseter muscle of each side, in the region between the zygomatic process of the temporal bones and the zygomatic bones and the muscle attachments at the angles of the mandible.

Method:

- For the muscle **fascia**, administer very gentle pressure and follow the fascial tensions of the muscle until the tension is balanced (Figure 2.100).
- For the **superficial part of the muscle**, slowly stroke the muscle on one side, using slightly firmer pressure, from the anterior two-thirds of the zygomatic arch obliquely to the angle of the mandible (Figure 2.101). While you are doing this, grasp the chin with the other hand and ask the patient to open the mouth slightly against gentle resistance (stretching the muscle).
- For the **deep part of the muscle**, stroke the masseter muscle with firmer pressure from the posterior third of the zygomatic arch almost vertically toward the masseteric tuberosity of the ramus (Figure 2.102). Then gently release the tensions in the muscle, focusing locally on the points affected, with small rotatory movements.
- Note No compression should be applied to the parotid plexus (CN VII, between the superficial and deep parts of the parotid gland; motor innervation of the facial muscles).

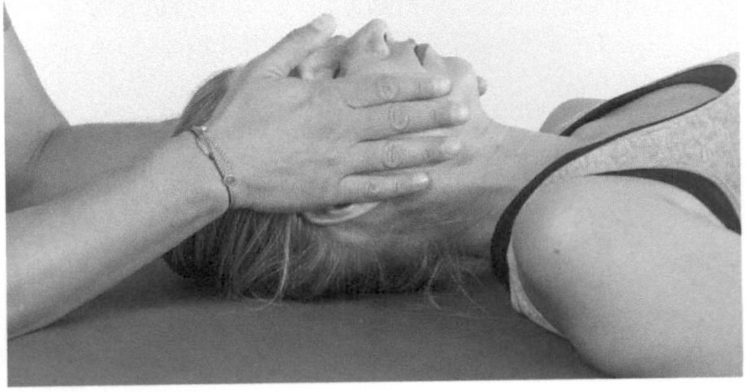

Figure 2.100 Masseter muscle technique (fascia)

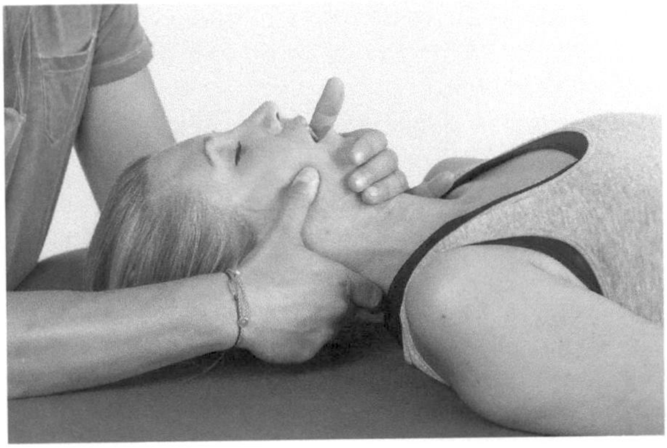

Figure 2.101 Masseter muscle technique (superficial part)

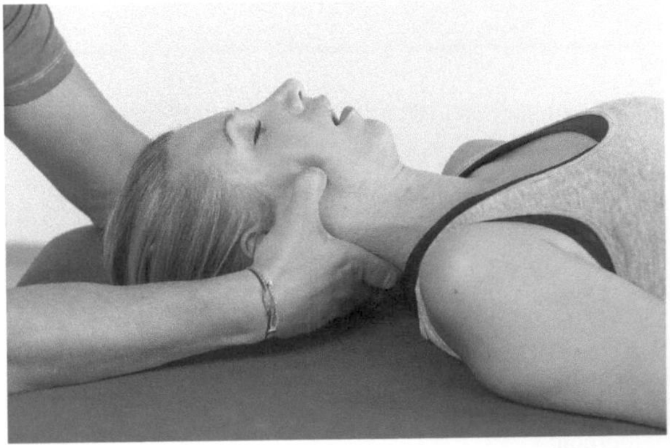

Figure 2.102 Masseter muscle technique (deep part)

Lateral pterygoid muscle

Indication: Bruxism and clenching the teeth, pain in the TMJ, maxilla, floor of the mouth, or ear, protrusion of the lower jaw with slightly reduced mouth opening, reduced medial movement of the lower jaw, occlusal disturbance, muscle hypertonicity (inferior head: condyle anterior → premature contact of contralateral front teeth and malocclusion of the ipsilateral back teeth; superior head: disk anterior → joint clicking), deviation of the midline of the incisors on mouth opening, dysfunction of the pterygopalatine ganglion, dysfunction of the anterior ligament of the malleus.

Practitioner: Take up a position beside the patient's head, on the opposite side to the dysfunction.

Hand position:

- Place the index finger or little finger of your caudal hand intraorally
  - ▸ Guide it along the outer surface of the alveolar process of the maxilla, in the direction of the external acoustic meatus. The palmar surface of the finger faces medially toward the gingiva (Figure 2.103).
  - ▸ When the finger comes into contact with the ascending ramus of the mandible, rotate it so that its palmar surface touches the cheek (Figure 2.104).
  - ▸ It may be necessary to ask the patient to move the mandible slightly toward the ipsilateral side for you to be able to move your finger through medially to the ramus of the mandible.
  - ▸ Move your finger posterior and cephalad sufficiently far for the tip to meet the tissue situated anterior to the muscle.
  - ▸ Grasp the greater wings with the middle finger and thumb of your cranial hand.

Method:

- With your cranial hand, stabilize the sphenoid without blocking the PRM.
- Caudal hand
  - ▸ With the tip of your index finger or little finger, apply gentle pressure on the muscle in the direction of the external acoustic meatus.
  - ▸ The pressure should be maintained until you sense a release of the tonicity of the muscle.
  - ▸ The pressure should induce no pain.
  - ▸ With each release of the tissue, seek the new limit of motion.
  - ▸ At the end of the technique, administer somewhat firmer pressure on the muscle 3 to 4 times to stimulate the tendon-receptor activity.

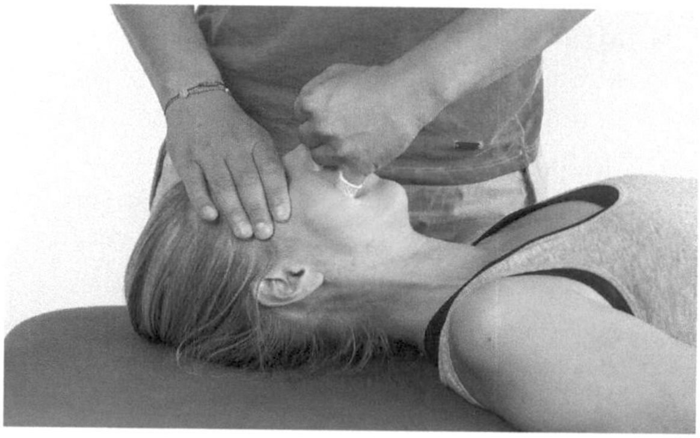

Figure 2.103 Technique for the lateral pterygoid muscle, palmar surface of finger toward gingiva

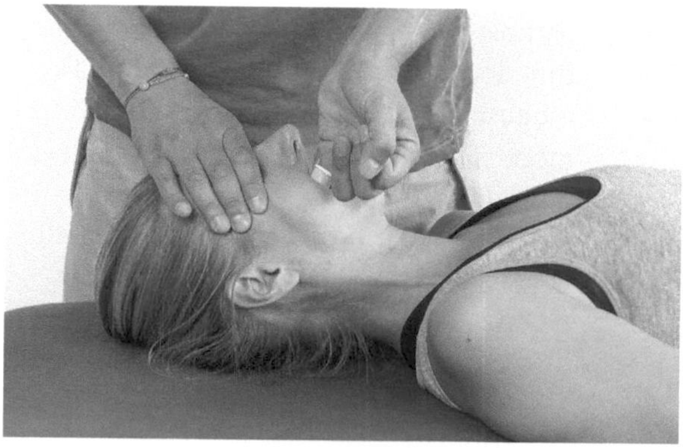

Figure 2.104 Technique for the lateral pterygoid muscle, palmar surface of finger toward cheek

Medial pterygoid muscle

Indication: Pain in the TMJ and floor of the mouth, reduced, painful mouth opening, disturbances of swallowing, deviation of the midline of the incisors, muscle spasm (condyle toward anterior and cranial), dysfunction of the pterygopalatine ganglion.

Practitioner: Take up a position beside the patient's head, on the side to be treated.

Hand position: Position the index finger of your caudal hand intraorally. Inside the mouth, guide it along the row of teeth as far as the angle of the mandible, where it meets the medial pterygoid muscle.

Method:

- If possible, hook it round the muscle cord from posterior (Figure 2.105). If this induces retching, another possibility is to apply the gentle pressure to the muscle with the tip of the index finger without hooking it round.
- The pressure should be maintained until a release of the muscle tonicity can be felt.
- The pressure should induce no pain.
- With each release of the tissue, seek the new limit of motion.
- At the end of the technique, administer somewhat firmer pressure on the muscle 3 to 4 times to stimulate the tendon-receptor activity.

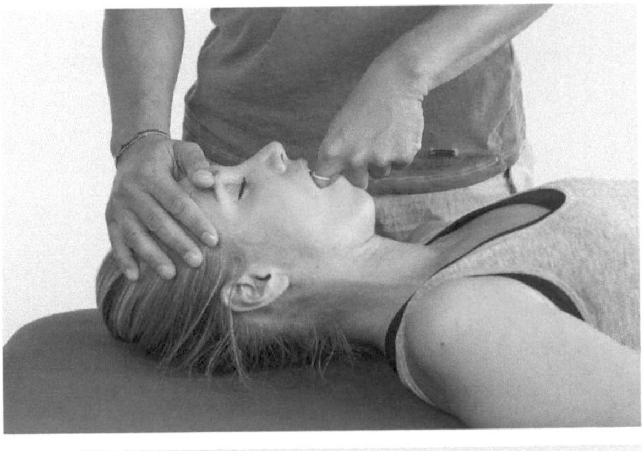

Figure 2.105 Technique for the medial pterygoid muscle

Modified inhibition technique for the medial and lateral pterygoid muscles according to Alexander

Inhibition techniques for the pterygoid muscles[7] can be painful and should be performed in a way suited to the pain tolerance of the patient.

Practitioner: Take up a position beside the patient's head, on the side to be treated.

Hand position:

- Cranial hand: in the region of C0/C1/C2 and the rest of the cervical spine.
- Caudal hand: with your little finger, follow the lower molars to the medial pterygoid muscle.

Method:

- Apply pressure to the belly of the medial pterygoid muscle until the muscle relaxes (Figure 2.106).
- The pressure should be applied in the direction of the muscle fibers.
- Following the release, you can gently increase the pressure.
- At the same time, with your cranial hand, administer a fluid technique between the splenius and the pterygoid muscles.
- Then perform the same technique for the lateral pterygoid. To do this, position the tip of your little finger laterally past the alveolar part in the direction of the ear.

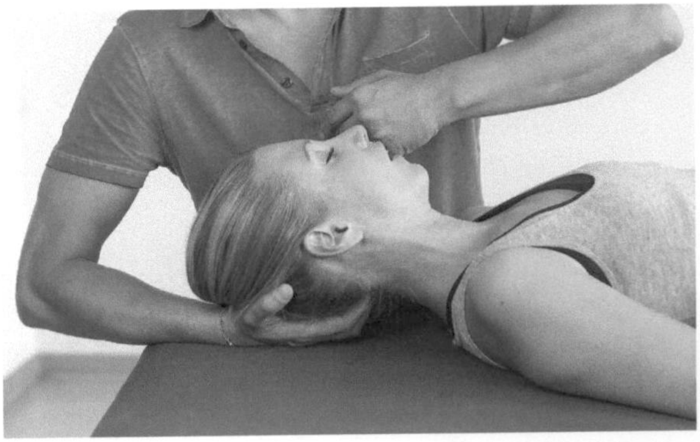

Figure 2.106 Modified inhibition technique for the medial and lateral pterygoid muscles according to Alexander

Technique to release tension of the interpterygoid aponeurosis

Hand position: With the index finger of one hand, palpate the pterygoid process posterior to the last molar (Figure 2.107).

Method: Release the aponeurosis obliquely between the lateral and medial pterygoid muscles.

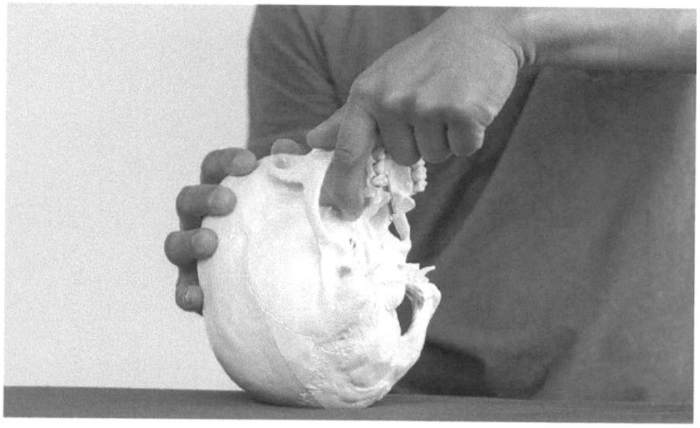

Figure 2.107 Technique to release tension of the interpterygoid aponeurosis (shown on model)

Isometric muscle contraction

Indication: Joint sounds, muscle spasm with limitation of mouth opening, and asymmetric mouth-opening motion and muscle activity.

Hand position: Place your hands on the mandible in such a way that the patient can resist the particular movement of the jaw (Figure 2.108).

Method: For example, opening of the jaw

- The patient relaxes the jaw joints, with the tongue lying relaxed in the mouth and the mouth slightly opened.
- Ask the patient to exert gentle contraction of the masticatory muscles in the direction of jaw opening. With your fingers, resist the muscular contraction so that no movement can take place in the TMJ (isometric muscular contraction).
- The force of muscle contraction should be only minimal and be exerted for about 6 s.
- Follow each contraction phase with a short relaxation phase.
- Each contraction/pause sequence should be repeated about three times.
- The technique is then performed accordingly for the movements of mouth closure, protrusion, retrusion, and laterotrusion.

Isometric contraction of the muscles that open the mouth

Hand position: Position your index and middle fingers against the base of the mouth, enclosing the chin.

Method: Contraction in the mouth-opening direction against resistance (Figure 2.108).

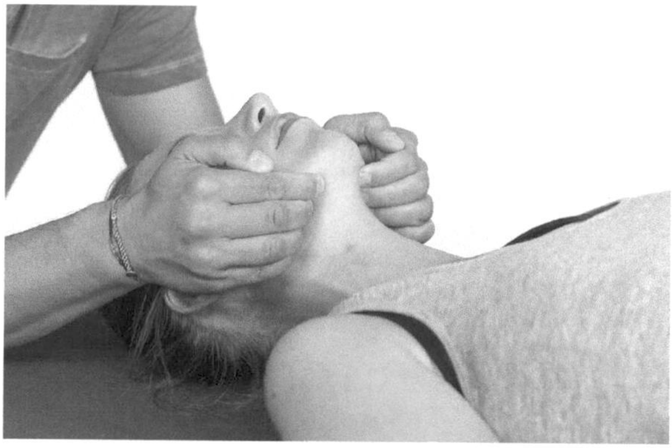

Figure 2.108 Isometric contraction of muscles that open the mouth

Isometric contraction of muscles that close the mouth

Hand position: Place the thumb of one hand anterior on the mandibular symphysis, above the mental protuberance, while the other fingers grasp the lower jaw. The other hand is passive.

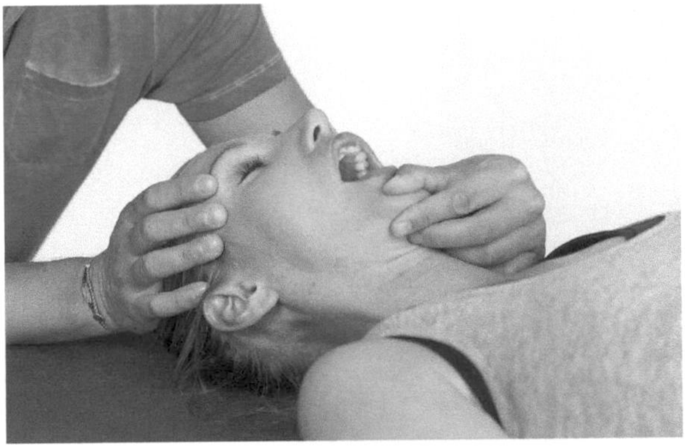

Figure 2.109 Isometric contraction of muscles that close the mouth

Method: Contraction in the direction of mouth closure against resistance (Figure 2.109).

Isometric contraction of the protractor muscles

Hand position: Place the thumb of one hand anterior on the mandibular symphysis above the mental protuberance. The other hand is passive.

Method: Contraction in the direction of protrusion against resistance (Figure 2.110).

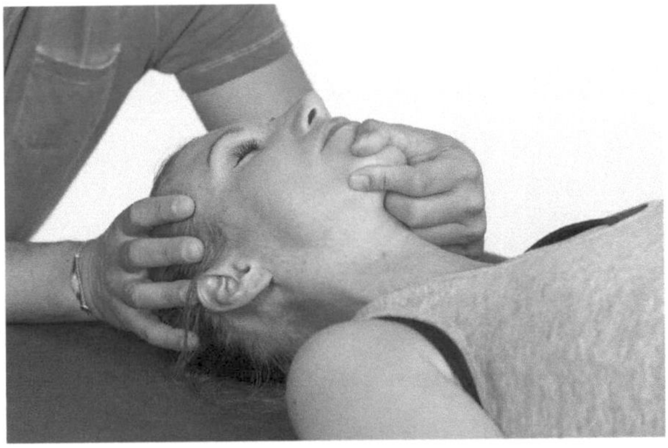

Figure 2.110 Isometric contraction of the protractor muscles

Isometric contraction of the retractor muscles

Hand position: Place your index and middle fingers against the base of the mouth, posterior to the mental protuberance.

Method: Contraction in the direction of retrusion against resistance (Figure 2.111).

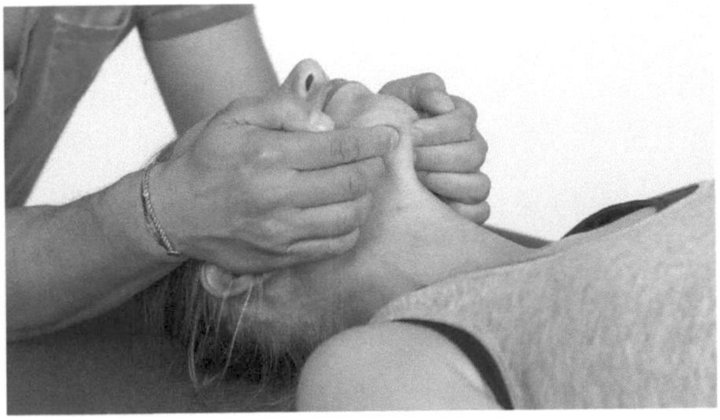

Figure 2.111 Isometric contraction of the retractor muscles

Isometric contraction of the laterotractor muscles

Hand position: Position the hand on the laterotrusion side against the side of the mandible. Place the other hand on the opposite temple.

Method: Contraction in the direction of laterotrusion against resistance (Figure 2.112).

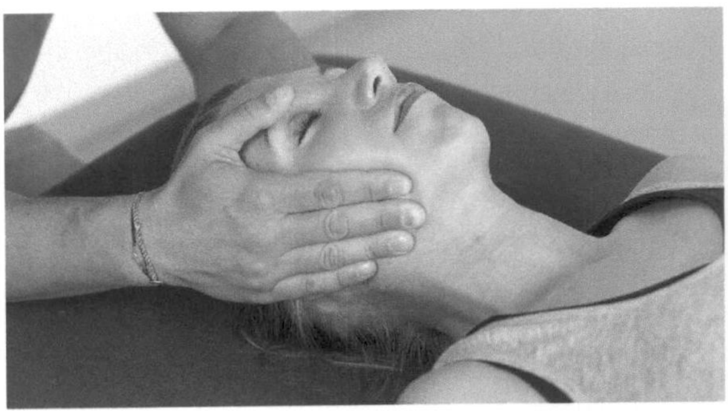

Figure 2.112 Isometric contraction of the laterotractor muscles

Stroking (effleurage) of connective tissue/fasciae

Establishing the finding: Ask the patient to indicate with their finger where there is a painful line in the region of the masticatory muscles; alternatively, palpate linear tissue tensions in the myofascial structures. The course of these may also run across several muscles.

Method:

- Bend your thumb and draw it slowly and firmly along the line indicated by the patient, or which you have palpated (Figure 2.113).
- At a speed of about 2–5 mm/s and using medium-firm pressure of your thumb, focus on incorporating the viscoelastic "give" of the tissue.
- Possibly, you may work in a more pronounced way, additionally bringing about microdistortions of the muscle fibers to induce matrix remodeling,[385] at a speed of about 10–20 mm/s and using extremely firm pressure of your thumb, such as is used, for example, in the fascial distortion model (FDM).

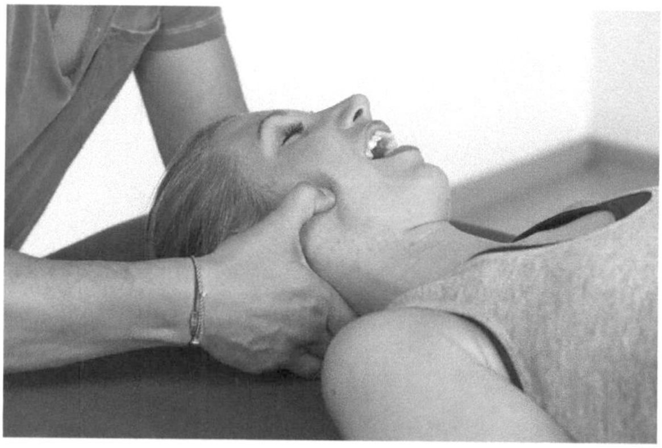

Figure 2.113 Stroking/effleurage of connective tissue/fasciae

Treating trigger points

Treatment of trigger points, manual therapy, or dry needling are successful approaches to treating the masticatory and associated muscles.[269]

Myofascial release techniques/reciprocal inhibition techniques

Indication: Marked dislocation and deviation, as the next step following on from mobilization techniques in the context of treatment for osteoarthritis, to balance the muscles at the end of treatment of children, before taking an impression or carrying out an instrumental functional analysis. (Following the technique, a water-cushioned dental splint should be worn until the consultation with the dentist or orthodontist.)

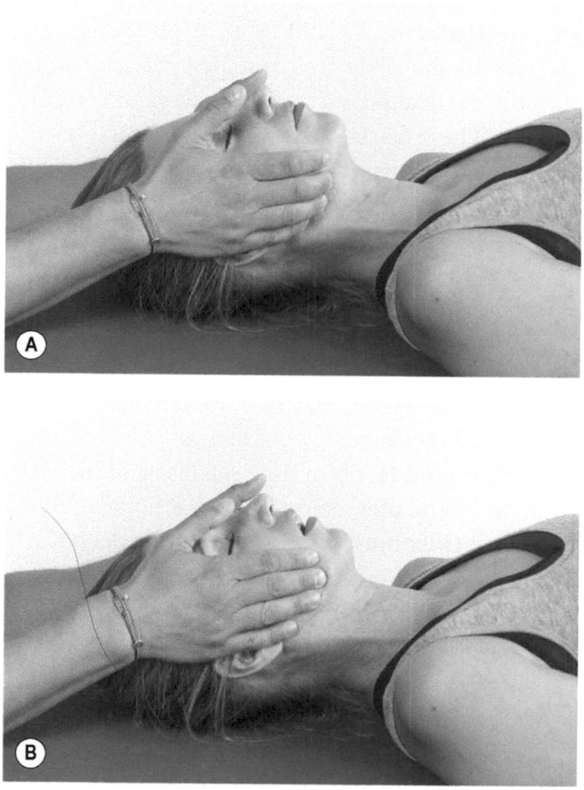

Figure 2.114 Release technique for the temporomandibular joint: compression release technique **A** with contact of the teeth and jaw closed (compression), and **B** without contact of the teeth and with jaw open (decompression)

The patient first drinks a mouthful of water in order to activate the neurosensory aspect of jaw and mouth function.
Method: Then carry out release techniques for the following muscles. Perform them first with the patient's teeth in contact and then with mouth open. For each release technique, observe a slight break during the changeover from the technique performed with teeth in contact and that without contact of the teeth.

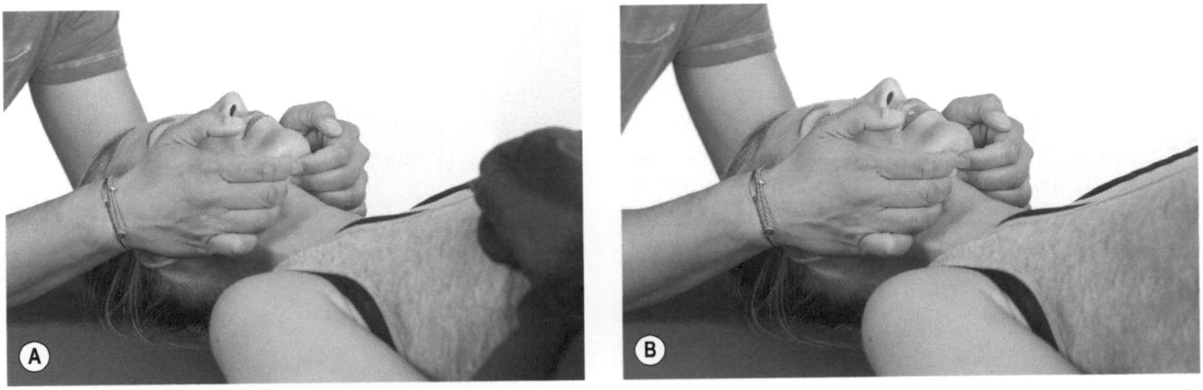

Figure 2.115 Release technique for the floor of the mouth, digastric muscle, anterior belly **A** with contact of the teeth and jaw closed, and **B** without contact of the teeth and with jaw open

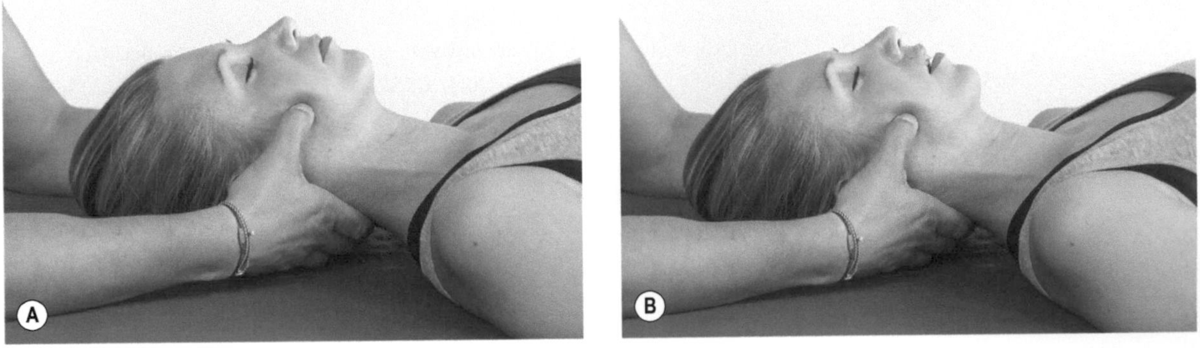

Figure 2.116 Release technique for the masseter and medial pterygoid muscles **A** with contact of the teeth and jaw closed, and **B** without contact of the teeth and with jaw open

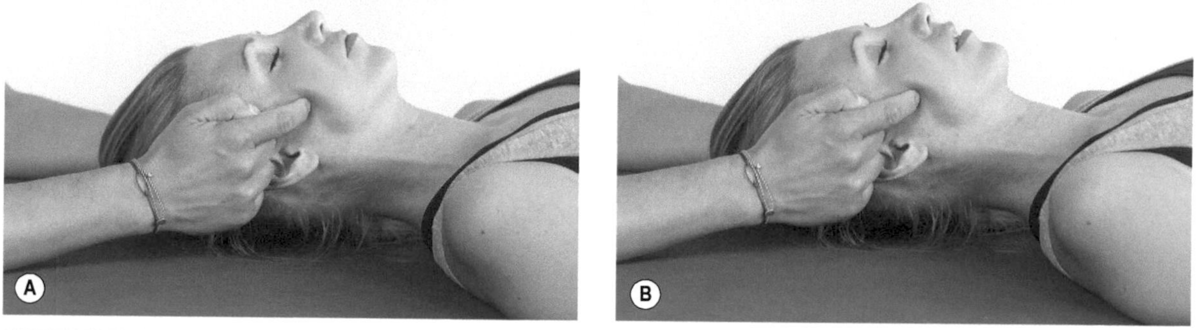

Figure 2.117 Release technique for the lateral pterygoid **A** with contact of the teeth and jaw closed, and **B** without contact of the teeth and with jaw open

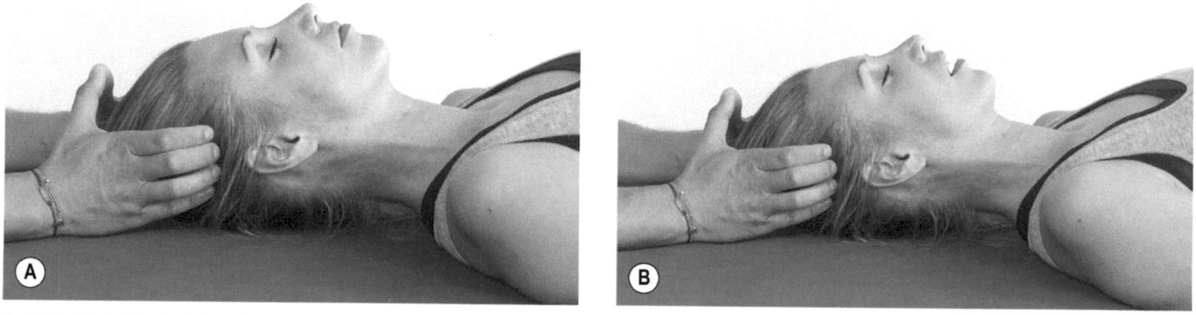

Figure 2.118 Release technique for the temporalis muscle **A** with contact of the teeth and jaw closed, and **B** without contact of the teeth and with jaw open

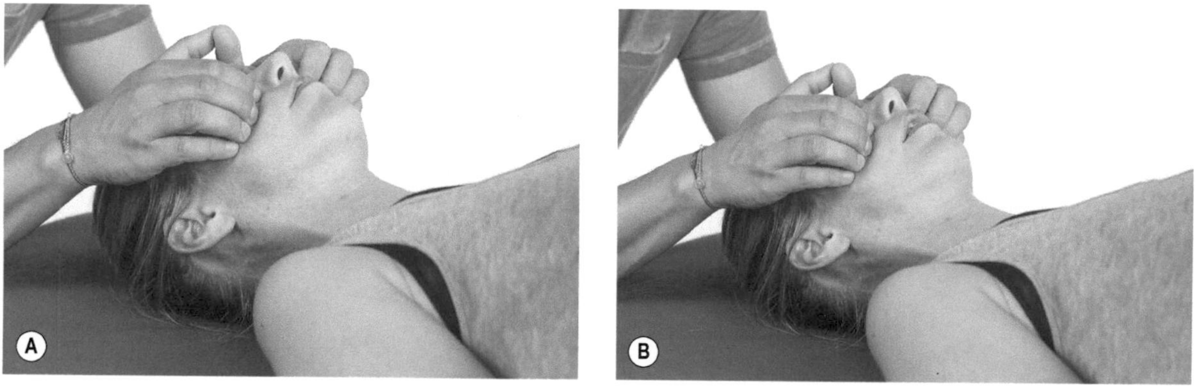

Figure 2.119 Release technique for the zygomaticus major and minor **A** with contact of the teeth and jaw closed, and **B** without contact of the teeth and with jaw open

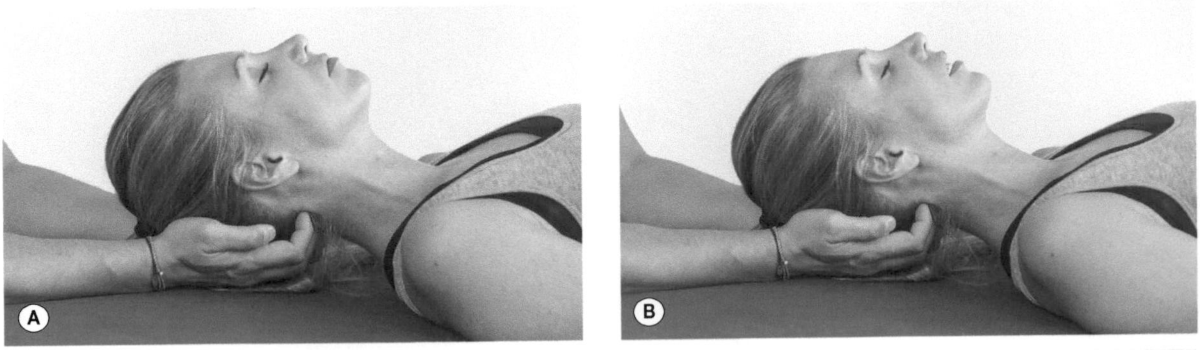

Figure 2.120 Occiput-atlas release technique **A** with contact of the teeth and jaw closed, and **B** without contact of the teeth and with jaw open

NOTE It is not necessary to release the hypertonous tension in the muscle completely. Carry out each release technique just until there is symmetry between the two sides.

- **Compression release technique for the TMJ** (with contact of the teeth)/**decompression release technique for the TMJ** (without contact of the teeth [Figure 2.114])
    - Hand position: place your index, middle, and ring fingers on the angle and ramus of the mandible on both sides.
    - Method: for the compression, apply pressure in a cranial direction; for decompression, traction in a caudal direction.
- **Release technique for the floor of the mouth**, in particular the anterior belly of the digastric muscle (with contact of the teeth; then without tooth contact [Figure 2.115])
    - Hand position: place your index and middle fingers, and if appropriate your ring fingers, paramedially on the base of the mouth.
    - Method: administer pressure in the cranial direction to the base of the mouth.
- **Release technique for the masseter and medial pterygoid** (with contact of the teeth; then without tooth contact [Figure 2.116])
    - Hand position: place your thumbs on the ramus of both sides. If appropriate you can also place your index fingers medially on the angle of the mandible of both sides.
    - Method: administer pressure in the medial direction with your thumbs. With your index fingers, apply pressure in the cranial direction.
- **Release technique for the lateral pterygoid** (with contact of the teeth; then without tooth contact [Figure 2.117])
    - Hand position: place your index fingers in the region of the mandibular notch on both sides.
    - Method: with your index fingers, administer pressure in the medial direction.
- **Release technique for the temporalis muscle** (with contact of the teeth; then without tooth contact [Figure 2.118])
    - Hand position: place your index, middle, and ring fingers on the temporalis muscle, in a line above the pinna of the ear on both sides.
    - Method: with your fingers, administer pressure in a medial direction and gentle cephalad traction.

- **Release technique for the zygomaticus major and minor** (with contact of the teeth; then without tooth contact [Figure 2.119])
  - Hand position: place your index and middle fingers, if appropriate also your ring fingers, on the inferior border of the zygomatic bone on both sides.
  - Method: administer pressure in a medial and cranial direction with your fingers.
- **Occiput-atlas release technique** (with contact of the teeth; then without tooth contact [Figure 2.120])
  - Hand position: place your index, middle, and ring fingers immediately under the occiput.
  - Method: release is achieved with the aid of the finger contact through the weight of the head.

Where there is marked discoordination and deviation, the myofascial release techniques should be followed by having the patient practice symmetrical mouth opening and closing in front of a mirror. (See Exercise with a mirror, section 2.9.2.)

Before doing this, the patient should also carry out one or two self-administered release exercises. Choose the release techniques where the greatest asymmetry appeared while you were performing the techniques.

2.8.2 Treatment of the condyles

Compression and decompression of the TMJ

The technique described below produces both the release of restrictions at the TMJ and squamous suture, and the release of tension of the intracranial membranes.

Practitioner: Take up a position at the head of the patient.

Hand position:

- Position your arms on the table beside the patient's head.

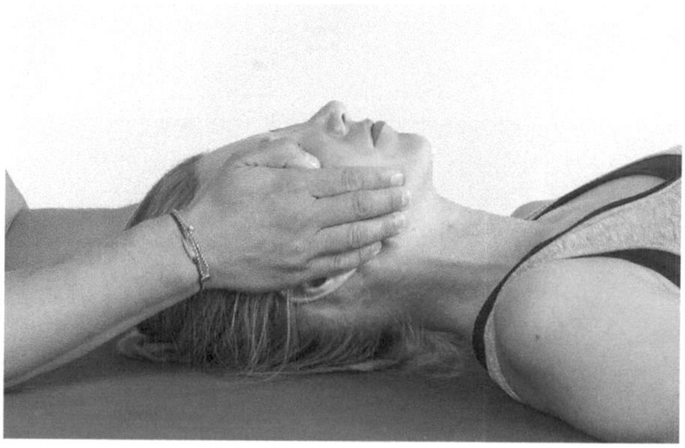

Figure 2.121 Compression and decompression of the temporomandibular joint

- Hook your middle fingers beneath the angles of the mandible.
- The basal joints of the fingers cover the temporomandibular joints, while the palms of the hands cover the ears and temporal regions (Figure 2.121).

Method: Ask the patient to relax the TMJ, and tell them not to allow the teeth to touch.

Compression (see Figure 2.122)

- With your hands, apply cranially directed pressure on the mandible.
- Permit any movements of the mandible, without releasing the pressure cephalad.
- As soon as the restrictions of the mandible have been released, the temporal bones will also execute a rocking motion.
- The temporal bones move in a cranial direction, and at the same time exert a cranially directed pull on the tentorium. When the squamoparietal suture is released, the superior border of the temporal bone tends to incline laterally.
- The parietal bones also move in a cranial direction, drawing the falx cerebri with them.
- The falx prevents any further cranial movement of the parietal and temporal bones, so causing these bones to rotate externally.

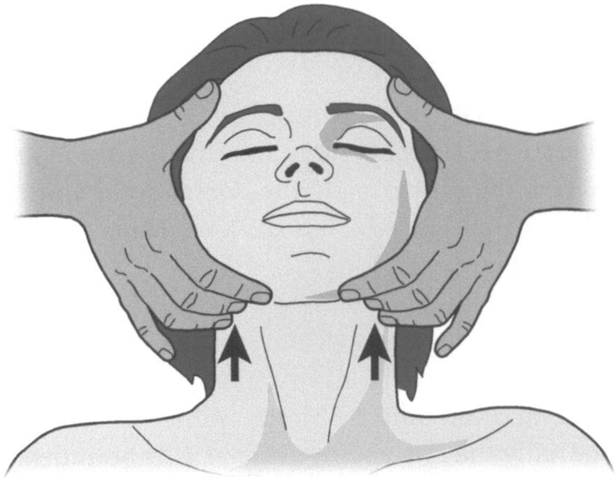

Figure 2.122
Compression of the temporomandibular joint

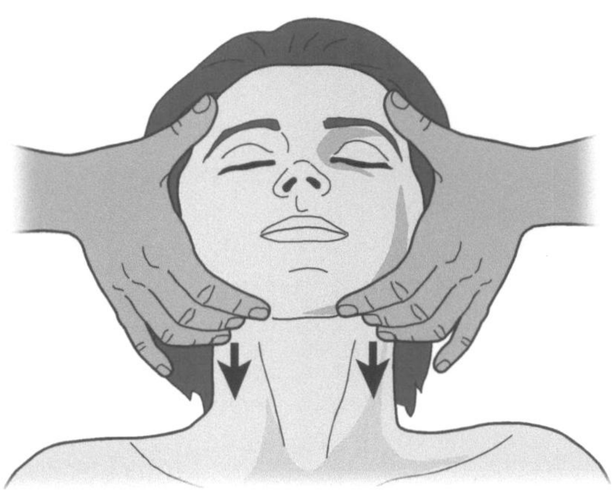

Figure 2.123
Decompression of the temporomandibular joint

- Due to the external rotation of the temporal bones, the tentorium cerebelli is stretched between the two superior borders of the petrous part.
- During the ensuing release of the intracranial membrane, you will be able to perceive membrane tensions at the foramen magnum and in the dural sheath, right down to the sacrum.
- Note all motions of the bones and membranes without preventing them and without reducing the gentle pressure cephalad.
- When no further relaxation can be perceived, gently reduce the pressure on the mandible and start to induce decompression by administering traction in a caudal direction.

Decompression (Figure 2.123)

- Now administer caudally directed traction on the mandible.
- The TMJ is freed, and the temporal bones move in a caudal direction.
- This draws the tentorium cerebelli caudad, resulting in a caudal displacement of the straight sinus and falx cerebri.
- The squamoparietal suture is released from restrictions, and the parietal bone also moves caudad.
- With increasing relaxation of the structures, the tiny movements of the bones and membranes involved come to a standstill, so that the traction can be gently reduced.

Establishing the PBMT, PBLT Hold this position until a release at the joints and an improvement in the mobility occur.

Compression of the TMJ (Figure 2.124)

- Administer pressure in the cranial direction.
- Very slight compression is produced at the TMJ.
- Temporal bones: move in a cranial direction.
- Shear force at the squamoparietal suture. On release of the suture, the superior border of the temporal bone moves laterally.
- Parietal bones: move in a cranial direction, drawing the falx with them.
- From a certain moment the falx prevents cephalad movement of the parietal bones.
- External rotation of the parietal bones.
- External rotation of the temporal bones.
- This causes stretching of the tentorium cerebelli.

Decompression of the TMJ (Figure 2.124)

- Administer traction in the caudal direction.

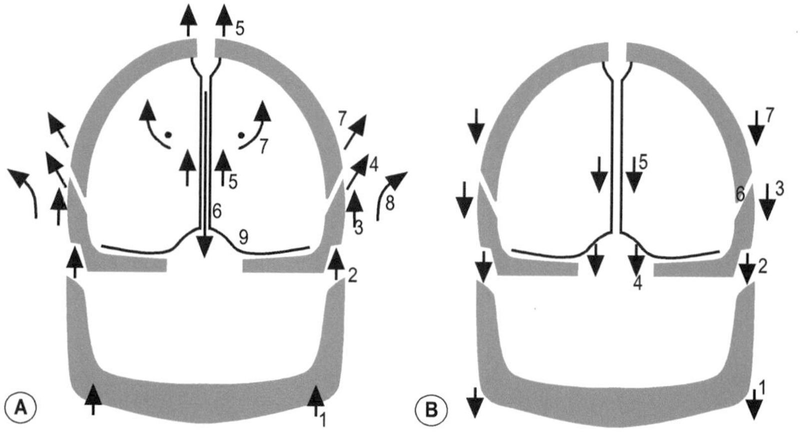

Figure 2.124
Schematic representation of the effects of the technique [based on data from reference 449]

- Release of the TMJ.
- The temporal bones move in a caudal direction.
- As a result the tentorium cerebelli is drawn in a caudal direction.
- Shifting of straight sinus and falx cerebri.
- Squamoparietal suture is freed.
- The parietal bones move in a caudal direction.

Global treatment of the TMJ

Practitioner: Take up a position at the head of the patient.

Hand position:

- Support your elbows on the treatment table.
- Position your middle or index fingers on the angle of the mandible.
- Rest your hands on the treatment table (Figure 2.125).

Method:

- Ask the patient to relax the TMJ; tell them not to allow the teeth to touch.
- Balance the angle of the mandible via your middle or index finger.
- Establish a PBLT, PBFT at the TMJ via your middle or index finger.
- Maintain this until a relaxation at the joints and an improvement in the mobility occur.

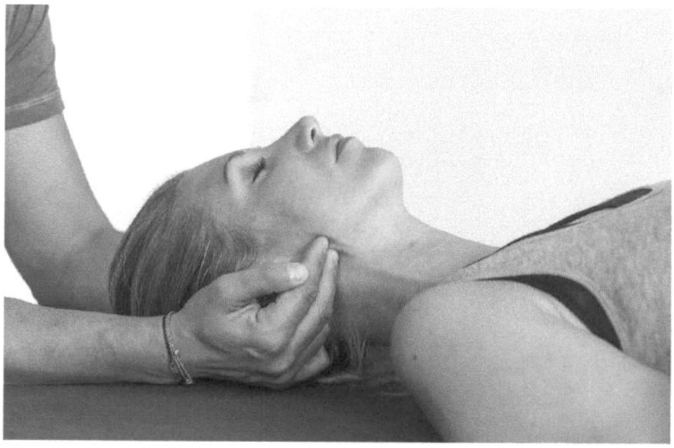

Figure 2.125 Global treatment of the temporomandibular joint

Global treatment of the TMJ, intraoral

Practitioner: Take up a position beside the patient at the level of the shoulder.

Hand position:

- Position your thumbs intraorally on the chewing surfaces of the lower rows of teeth.
- Hook the middle and index fingers behind the angles of the mandible.
- For the torsion and lateral movement, position your index fingers on the maxillae (Figure 2.126).

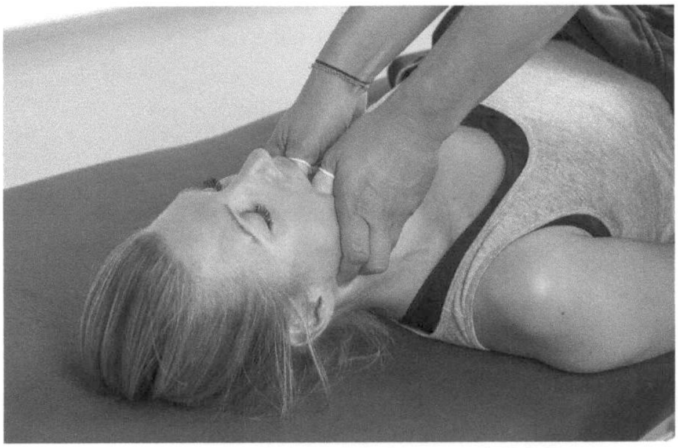

Figure 2.126 Global treatment of the temporomandibular joint, intraoral

Method: Posterior/anterior release

- With your hands, apply a posteriorly directed pressure on the mandible.
- Permit any movements of the mandible, without ceasing the posteriorly directed pressure.
- When you can sense no further release, gently reduce the pressure on the mandible and administer traction in the anterior direction.

Torsion movement

- With your hands, apply a torsion movement to the mandible, while your index fingers stabilize the cranium via the maxillae.
- The mandible is first of all rotated in the direction of the dysfunction, i.e., in the direction of greater mobility (of ease).
- Permit any movements of the mandible, without ceasing the rotation.
- When you can sense no further release, rotate the mandible in the direction of the motion restriction.

Lateral movement

- With your hands, apply a lateral movement to the mandible, while your index fingers stabilize the cranium via the maxillae.
- Now, first induce a lateral movement of the mandible in the direction of the dysfunction, i.e., in the direction of greater mobility (of ease).
- Permit any movements of the mandible, without ceasing induction of the lateral movement.
- When you can sense no further release, induce a lateral movement of the mandible in the direction of the motion restriction.

Compression/decompression

- With your hands, apply cranially directed pressure to the mandible.
- Permit any movements of the mandible, without reducing the pressure cranially.
- When you can sense no further release, gently reduce the pressure on the mandible and begin decompression by administering a traction caudally and anterior (at an angle of 45°).
- Once again, permit all movements that occur.

NOTE It is also possible to establish a PBLT, PBFT of all directions of movement on the mandible.

Treatment of the TMJ according to Blagrave
Dysfunction of the right temporomandibular joint I

Indication: Restriction of protrusion and/or mediotrusion of the right TMJ.

Patient: The patient is supine, with a cushion under the upper thoracic spine to bring the cervical spine into slight extension. The patient's head should be rotated to the left.

Practitioner: Take up a position at the head of the patient.

Hand position:

- Right hand: place your index and middle fingers on the body of the mandible, with the fingers pointing anterior. Position the ring finger

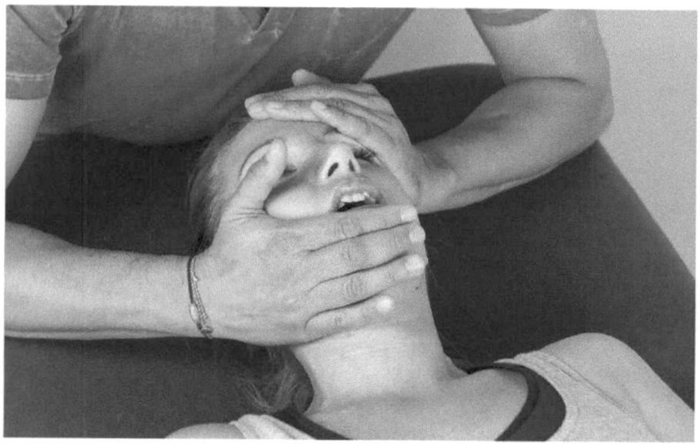

Figure 2.127 Treatment of the temporomandibular joint according to Blagrave.[102] Dysfunction of the right temporomandibular joint I

and little finger on the inferior border of the mandible.

- Left hand: the left hand is on the forehead, with the fingers pointing toward the ear.

Method: Ask the patient to open the mouth slightly. At the same time, move your hands in parallel but opposite directions. The right hand on the mandible is moved in an anterior, inferior direction and the left hand on the forehead is moved posterior and superior (Figure 2.127).

Dysfunction of the right temporomandibular joint II

Indication: Restriction of protrusion or opening of the right TMJ.

Patient: The patient is supine, head slightly rotated to the left.

Practitioner: Take up a position beside the patient's head, on the opposite side to the dysfunction.

Hand position:

- Cranial hand: place your cranial hand on the forehead to hold the head firmly in position.
- Caudal hand: position your thumb intraorally on the posterior lower molars. With your other fingers, grip the mandible from the outside.

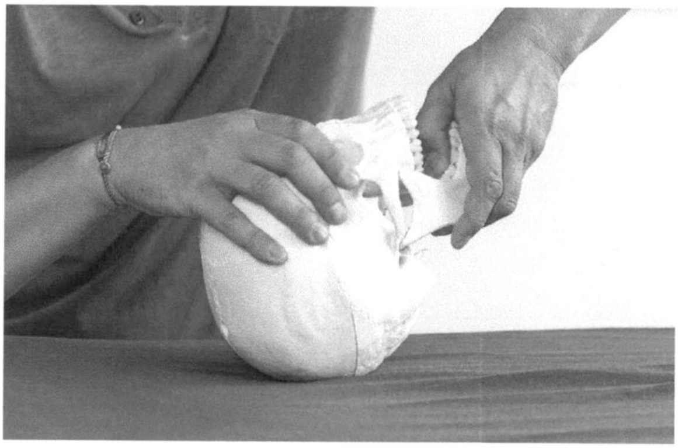

Figure 2.128 Treatment of the temporomandibular joint according to Blagrave. Dysfunction of the right temporomandibular joint II

Method:

- Ask the patient to close the mouth sufficiently for the posterior part of the thumb to come into contact with the upper molars.
- Flex the terminal joint of your thumb, so that the TMJ is passively mobilized against the upper molars by a lever movement of the thumb (Figure 2.128).
- In addition, with your caudal hand you may administer traction in the anterior direction, in order to strengthen the movement.

Manipulation (impulse technique) of the TMJ according to Herbert, patient seated

Indication: Limitation of mouth opening.

Patient: The patient is seated.

Practitioner: Take up a position beside the patient, on the opposite side to the dysfunction.

Hand position:

- Anterior arm: your lower arm is positioned on the mandible, in the region of body and ramus.
- Posterior hand: position your middle finger posterior to the head of the mandible and hold it firmly in position in the posterior direction.

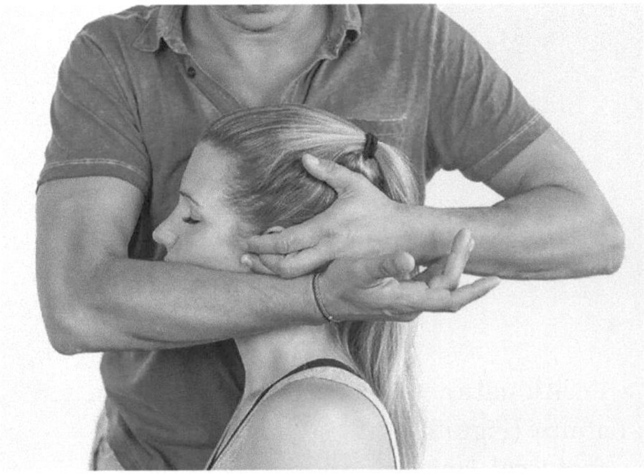

Figure 2.129 Manipulation (impulse technique) of the temporomandibular joint according to Herbert, patient seated

Method:

- Hold the patient's head between your hands and your ribcage.
- Doing so holds the patient's head firmly in position; at the same time you also induce ipsilateral side-bending toward the dysfunction of the TMJ.
- Apply the impulse by means of **anterior traction**. The impulse is delivered less by the anterior arm than with your entire body (Figure 2.129).

Manipulation (impulse technique) of the TMJ according to Herbert, patient supine

Indication: Limitation of mouth opening, without pain on rotating the head and without dysfunction of C0, C1, C2.

Patient: The patient is supine, head rotated to the right (with a support under the patient's head so that it is in line with the body).

Practitioner: Take up a position at the patient's head, on the left-hand side and at a slight angle.

Hand position:

- Caudal hand: place this hand with the thenar eminence on the angle of the mandible.

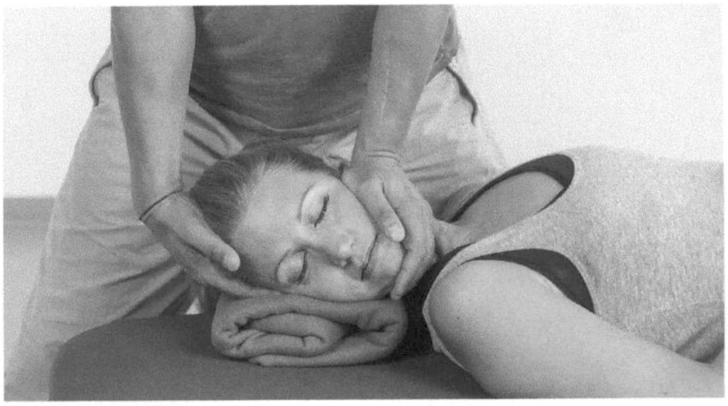

Figure 2.130 Manipulation (impulse technique) of the temporomandibular joint according to Herbert, patient supine

- Cranial hand: position this hand under the patient's head. With your middle finger, palpate the right TMJ.

Method:

- With the thenar eminence of your caudal hand, administer an impulse (traction) in the **anteroinferior** or **inferior** direction. Your arms should be only slightly bent. Administer the impulse with your whole body.
- As you do so, hold the patient's head firmly in place with your cranial hand.
- Alternatively, you can administer an impulse with your caudal hand **inferiorly and down into the table**, in order to release a motion restriction in the contralateral TMJ (Figure 2.130).
- Whichever impulse you choose, it should be delivered using your whole body.

Repositioning an anteromedial disk displacement by a modification of the Kaluza/Goering method

Technique: Articulation.

> **NOTE** Before performing the technique, you should first reduce the facilitation intensity of the affected segment, using myofascial and strain/counterstrain techniques.

Indication: Joint sounds (clicking, crepitation), motion restrictions, pain; condylar head displaced slightly laterally and more prominent.

Patient: Supine.

Practitioner: Take up a position at the head of the patient.

Hand position: Place one hand on the side of the head to stabilize it. Position your other hand on the opposite angle and ramus of the mandible.

Method:

- Ask the patient to open the mouth as wide as possible.
- Once the mouth is opened to the maximum, apply a continuous, lateral translation force with the hand that is on the mandible. This should be directed toward the opposite TMJ (Figure 2.131).
- The hand positioned on the side of the head acts as a stabilizer and counterbalances the force from the other hand, so that no head movements occur.
- Maintain the forces exerted by the hands, while the patient slowly closes the mouth again.
- The aim is to achieve an opening between the mandibular condyle and the cranium.
- When the treatment is successful, a palpable and sometimes audible change in the joint can usually be heard or sensed.
- The technique is then repeated on the other side.
- The number of repetitions is variable, but as a rule 4 to 8 repetitions are performed per side. The applied force may be increased as required.

NOTE The signs of successful normalization are: normalization of the disk position, increased radius of movement, and pain and associated symptoms are reduced or disappear altogether.
The repetitions are intended to reset the stretch receptors in the superior part of the lateral pterygoid muscle.
If there is no clear improvement, the treatment may be repeated at weekly or fortnightly intervals.

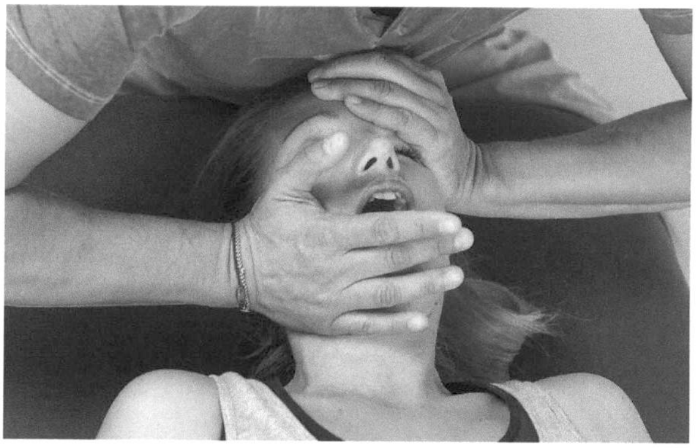

Figure 2.131 Repositioning of an anteromedial disk displacement according to Kaluza and Goering[203]

Repositioning an anterolateral disk displacement according to Kaluza

This largely corresponds to the treatment for dysfunction of the right TMJ II (see above), since the trismus associated with anterolateral disk displacement does not allow the mouth to be opened sufficiently wide to use an articulatory technique. In some cases, however, the use of greater force is necessary than in the above-named technique.

Repositioning an anteromedially displaced disk according to Farrar

Restriction of a TMJ of no longer than 3–4 weeks' duration is usually relatively easy to release.

Hand position: With both hands, grasp the mandible firmly by positioning your thumbs on the posterior region of the lower row of teeth, while the other fingers enclose the inferior border of the anterior mandible from the outside.

Method: On the side of the displaced disk, use your thumb to apply pressure in the caudal direction on the condyle, while administering cranially directed pressure with your fingers. Then the condyle on the affected side is moved in an anterior, medial direction (Figure 2.132).

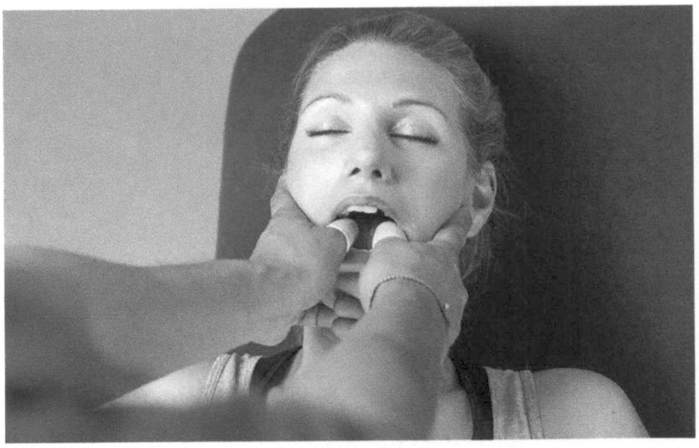

Figure 2.132 Repositioning an anteromedially displaced disk using Farrar's technique[118,119,120,121]

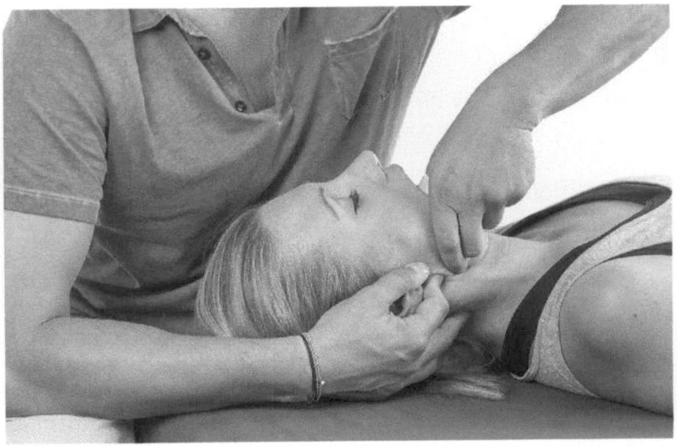

Figure 2.133 Unilateral treatment of the condyles, decompression

Repositioning an anteromedially displaced disk, alternative hand position

Hand position, unilateral: With your caudal hand, grasp the mandible firmly by positioning your thumb on the posterior region of the lower row of teeth, and enclosing the inferior border of the anterior mandible from the outside with your other fingers. Place the index and middle finger of your cranial hand lightly on the temporomandibular joint and palpate its motion.

Method: As above.

Unilateral treatment of the condyles

Practitioner: Take up a position beside the patient's head on the opposite side to the dysfunction.

Hand position:

- Cranial hand: grip the angle of the mandible on the affected side with your thumb and index finger.
- Caudal hand
  - ▸ Position the thumb intraorally, on the chewing surfaces of the lower teeth on the affected side. Place it on the last molars.
  - ▸ Place the index finger outside on the inferior border of the horizontal part of the mandible.
  - ▸ With your thumb and index finger, grip the horizontal part of the mandible.

Method:

- Administer traction in a caudal and anterior direction (at an angle of 45°) with the thumb and index finger of the caudal hand (Figure 2.133).
- Support this traction with your cranial hand.
- In addition, with your cranial hand, you can administer gentle translation of the condyle in the anterior direction.
- Note all movements of the mandible that arise, without preventing them and without relaxing the gentle traction caudad and anterior.
- When no further release of the tissue (capsule, ligaments, muscles) can be sensed, the traction on the mandible can be stopped.
- Establish the PBLT, PBFT.
- A fluid impulse may be used to direct energy from the opposite occipitomastoid suture.

Harmonization of the temporal bone

Hand position:

- Caudal hand: with your thumb and index finger, maintain a grip on the angle of the mandible on the affected side.

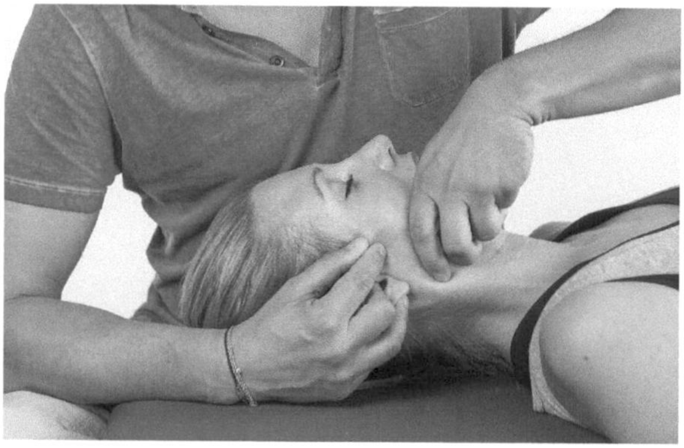

Figure 2.134 Harmonization of the temporal bone

- Cranial hand: with your cranial hand, grasp the temporal bone with the five-finger temporal bone technique (Figure 2.134).
  - The thumb and index finger grasp the zygomatic process.
  - Position your middle finger in the external acoustic meatus.
  - Place your ring finger on the tip of the mastoid process.
  - The little finger will be on the mastoid part.

Method: After the TMJ has been decompressed, establish the PBMT, PBFT of the temporal bone.

Auditory tube technique according to Magoun and Galbreath

See Volume 2, section 6.4.2.

Indication and effect:
Release of the jaw joint, medial pterygoid muscle, and myofascial structures of the nasopharyngeal space, etc.

Multiple hand technique

Practitioners: Practitioner 1 stands at the head of the patient. Practitioner 2 stands beside the patient's head.

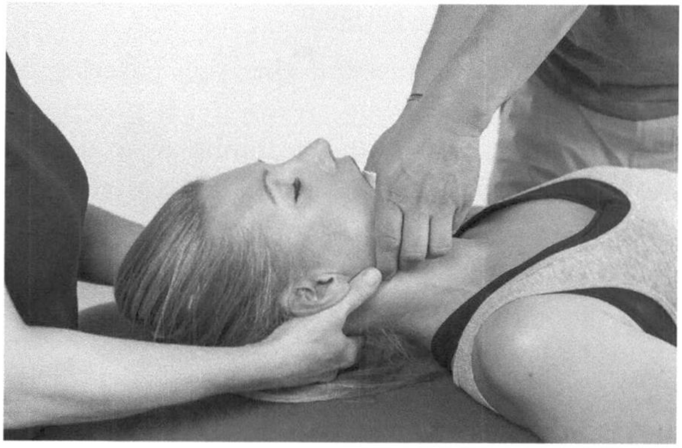

Figure 2.135 Multiple hand technique for the temporomandibular joint

Hand position (Figure 2.135):

Practitioner 1:

- Position your thenar eminences bilaterally on the mastoid parts.
- Position your thumbs on the anterior points of the mastoid process.
- Place the palms of your hands on the occiput.
- Clasp the fingers of your two hands.
- Position the elbows of both arms on the table.

Practitioner 2:

- Position the thumbs intraorally, on the chewing surfaces of the lower teeth.
- Hook the middle fingers behind the angles of the mandible.

Method:

- Practitioner 1 holds the occiput and temporal bones firmly in position.
- Practitioner 2 administers caudally and anteriorly directed traction (at an angle of 45°) on the mandible.
- Permit any movements of the mandible without reducing the traction caudad.
- When you can sense no further release, gently reduce the traction on the mandible.
- Then, via the hand contact, establish a PBT between the mandible and the cranium.

2.8.3 Intraosseous treatment

The chewing pressure and the "pull" exerted by the masticatory muscles are the most prominent mechanical forces in the cranium. Special constructions absorb these forces, to the greatest extent damping any shock; their structure is fundamental to the way this absorption of force functions. At the same time that structure is an expression of the forces operating.[see also 70]

Intraosseous dysfunctions, in the form of increased density and resistance, reduced bony viscoelasticity and bone resilience, and strain of the mandible, maxilla, temporal bone, palatine bone, and other bones of the cranium—torsion, transverse, lateral and flexion strain—can be palpated. In respect of treatment of the cranial base, see Volume 2, section 4.6.2.

Apart from palpatory findings, the following are indications for intraosseous treatments: symptoms relating to associated nerve and vessel pathways in the bones, e.g., in the mandible, relating to the inferior alveolar nerve, pain and hypersensitivity in the teeth of the lower jaw or in the bone.

Treatment of the dysfunctional pressure trajectories running from the mandibular head to the ramus

Pressure trajectories run from the head of the mandible, along the posterior portion of the ramus, and in an arc from posterior inferior to the anterior, superior region of the body of the mandible.

Effects of pressure on the course of the trajectories

1. The upward, posteriorly directed pull of the temporalis muscle.
2. The upward and anterior direction of pull of the masseter and medial pterygoid.
3. The downward and anteriorly directed pull of the lateral pterygoid in interaction with the activity of the temporalis (posterior portion).
4. Directions of pull of the suprahyoid and infrahyoid muscles.

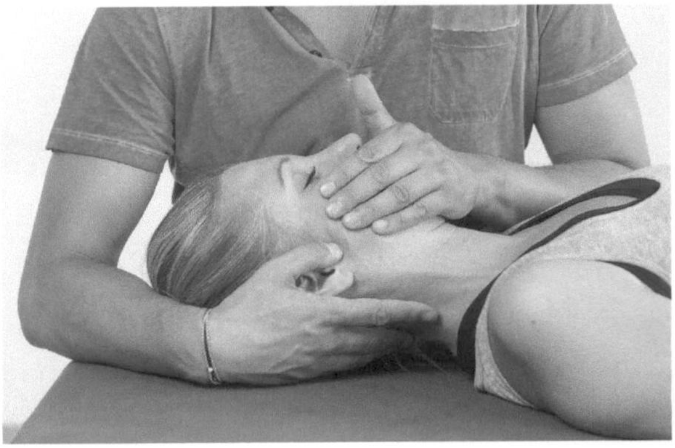

Figure 2.136 Treatment of the dysfunctional pressure trajectories running from the mandibular head to the ramus

Practitioner: Take up a position at the head of the patient.

Hand position (Figure 2.136):

- Place the base of both hands on the head and the neck of the mandible.
- Place the index fingers of both hands on the alveolar part.

Method: Compression of the head of the mandible and alveolar part, and establishing a point of balance.

Treatment of the dysfunctional pressure trajectories running from the coronoid process to the body of the mandible

The pressure trajectories at the anterior border of the coronoid process run in an arc to the body of the mandible.

Hand position: Place your index fingers and thumbs on the ramus of the mandible on both sides (Figure 2.137).

Method: Compression delivered with both fingers, and establishing a point of balance.

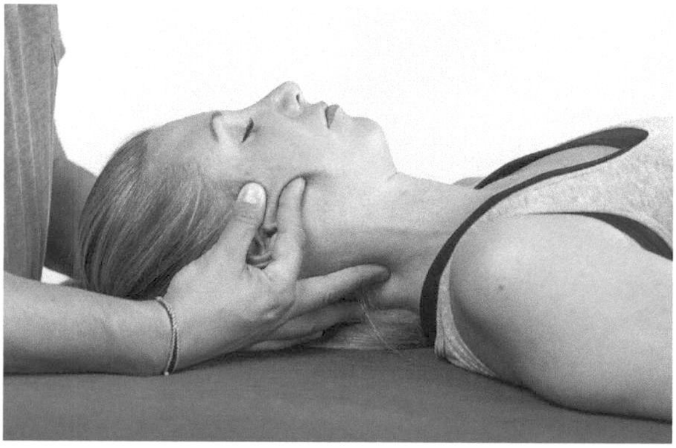

Figure 2.137 Treatment of the dysfunctional pressure trajectories running from the coronoid process to the body of the mandible

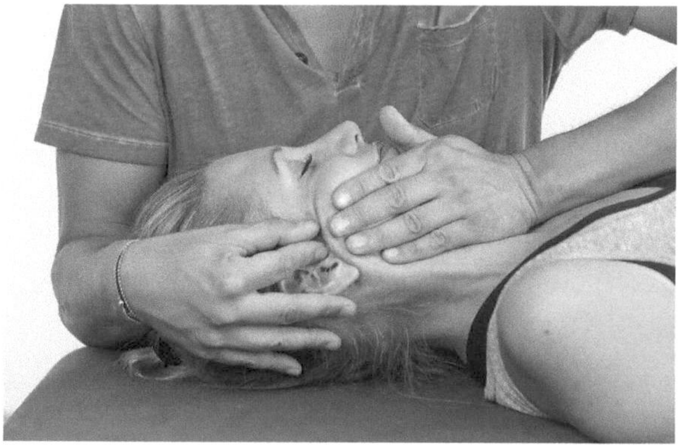

Figure 2.138 Treatment of the dysfunctional trajectories of pull running from the head and neck of the mandible

Treatment of the dysfunctional trajectories of pull running from the head and neck of the mandible

The trajectories of pull run from the posterior region of the head and neck of the mandible to the anterior part of the angle of the jaw and into the alveolar part of the mandible. One portion of the trajectories of pull runs in a caudal direction to the inferior border of the body of the mandible, crossing the trajectories of pressure at right angles. At the coronoid process, the trajectories of pull run parallel to the course of the muscle, combining at the angle of the jaw with the trajectories of the main system of tension.

Practitioner: Take up a position beside the patient's head, on the opposite side to the dysfunction.

Hand position (Figure 2.138):

- Cranial hand: position the thumb of your hand on the coronoid process and the index finger on the posterior border of the head and neck of the mandible.
- Grasp the inferior border of the body of the mandible with your thumb, index, and middle finger.

Method: Apply divergent traction of your two hands, and establish a point of balance.

You should include the intraosseous treatment of the reinforcing buttresses of the viscerocranium and neurocranium (Volume 2, section 4.6.2).

2.8.4 Treatment of the capsule and the ligaments of the lower jaw

Technique for the capsule and lateral ligament

Practitioner: Take up a position beside the patient's head, opposite the side to be treated.

Hand position:

- Cranial hand: five-finger temporal bone technique:
  - Grasp the zygomatic process with your thumb and index finger.
  - Position your middle finger in the external acoustic meatus.
  - Position your ring finger in front of the mastoid process.
  - Your little finger lies behind the mastoid process.
- Caudal hand: place your thumb on the chewing surface of the last molar on the side opposite. With your fingers, grasp the angle of the lower jaw.

Method (Figure 2.139):

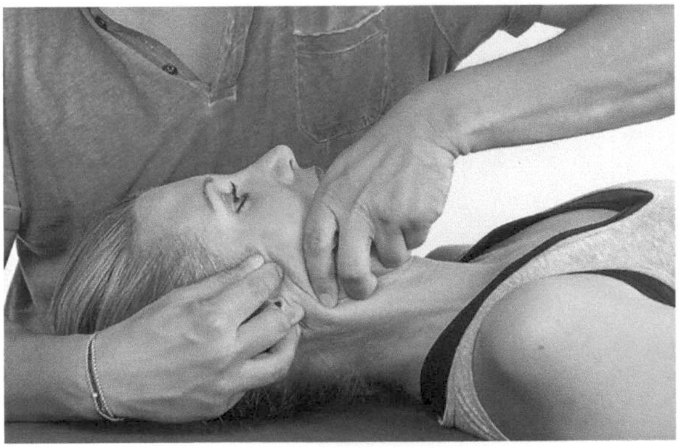

Figure 2.139 Technique for the capsule and lateral ligament

- Hold the temporal bone firmly in position.
- For the capsule, begin by applying traction in a cranial and posterior direction (to produce direct relaxation), followed by traction in the caudal and anterior direction using the thumb on the last molar, and for the lateral parts of the capsule, caudad, anterior traction, and medi-otrusion, until the tension has been reduced.
- To treat the lateral ligament, first apply compression in the temporomandibular joint and follow this with caudad traction applied to the joint. At the same time use your thumb on specific restricted or tender places on the lateral ligaments to assist the release of the ligament.

Technique for the sphenomandibular ligament according to Frymann, modified

Indication: Visual disturbance (CN VI), facial pain (CN V, trigeminal ganglion), disturbances of blood outflow in this region, tinnitus.

Practitioner: Take up a position beside the patient's head, opposite the side to be treated.

Hand position:

- Cranial hand: span the greater wings with your thumb and middle or index finger.

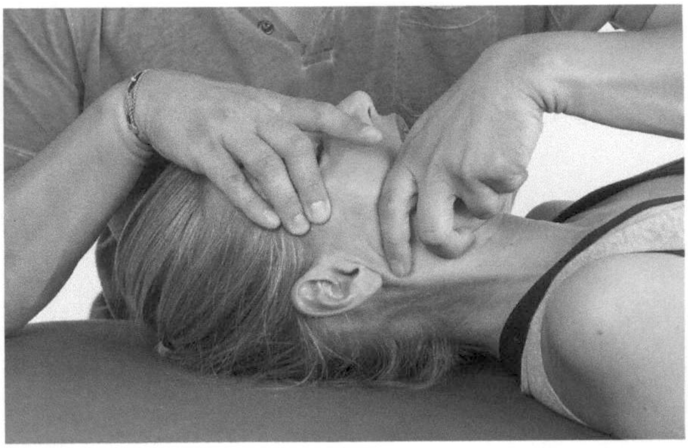

Figure 2.140 Technique for the sphenomandibular ligament according to Frymann, modified

- Caudal hand: place your thumb on the chewing surface of the last molar on the side opposite. With your other fingers, grasp the angle of the lower jaw from outside.

Method:

- Move the mandible in a caudal direction with your thumb (Figure 2.140). At the same time, apply gentle caudad traction to the greater wings.
- Continue until you sense a release of the sphenomandibular ligament.

Technique for the stylomandibular ligament according to Frymann, modified

Indication: Neuralgia, dysphonia, earache, dysphagia, and carotodynia; also tenderness at the styloid process.

Practitioner: Take up a position beside the patient's head, opposite the side to be treated.

Hand position:

- Cranial hand: five-finger temporal bone technique (see above).
- Caudal hand: place your thumb on the chewing surface of the last molar on the opposite side. With your fingers, grasp the angle of the lower jaw.

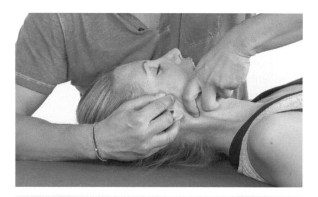

Figure 2.141 Technique for the stylomandibular ligament according to Frymann, modified

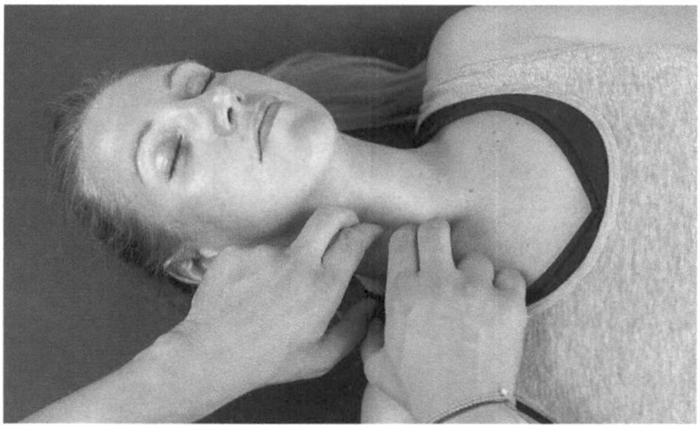

Figure 2.142 Technique for the common carotid artery according to Pappas, modified

Method:

- Move the mandible in a caudal, anterior, and lateral direction with your thumb (Figure 2.141). As you do so, hold the temporal bone firmly in position.
- Continue until you sense a release of the stylomandibular ligament.

NOTE The sphenomandibular and stylomandibular ligaments can also be treated using the V-spread technique.

2.8.5 Treating the arteries, veins, and nerves

Treatment is directed toward possible narrowing or hindrances to transmission, and looks at the capacity of the particular structure to glide. In the case of arteries, the vessel wall should also be treated if possible.

Technique for the common carotid artery according to Pappas, modified

Indication: To improve arterial supply to the head regions served by the common carotid artery.

Practitioner: Take up a position on the side to be treated.

Hand position:

- With the fingertips of both hands, seek the artery from anterior.
- Your fingers lie along the course of the common carotid artery, in the region a little above the clavicle to below C3 (Figure 2.142).
- Alternatively, place just your two middle fingers here, and rest your caudal finger at the level of C5/C6 and your cranial finger below C3.

Method:

- Begin by palpating the pulsation of the artery and then release the pressure to the point where you no longer sense the pulsation as prominently but do more clearly sense the contact surface between the artery and the surrounding fascia.
- Carefully apply divergent longitudinal traction to the artery with your fingers or middle fingers.
- To test the restriction, perform a caudal and cranial gliding movement, maintaining the divergent traction as you do so.
- Gently hold the artery in place on the opposite side to the restriction (side of ease) while you apply gentle traction in the direction of the restriction.
- As you do this, follow the micromotions of the artery and gently reinforce them.
- Continue this until you sense a softening and an inherent motion of the surrounding tissue.
- Then you can apply gentle pressure on the tissue of the artery. During the expanding expression of tissue elasticity and as you gently release the pressure, follow all the tissue dynamics you sense.

Technique for the common carotid artery/external carotid artery

Patient: Supine, with head in a neutral position.

Practitioner: Take up a position on the side to be treated.

Hand position (Figure 2.143):

- The middle fingers of your two hands are both medial to the sternocleidomastoid.
- Caudal hand: position the tip of the middle finger on the external carotid artery at the level of the thyroid cartilage.
- Cranial hand: position the tip of the middle finger on the external carotid artery at the level of the hyoid or just above it.

Method: According to the technique for the common carotid artery (see above).

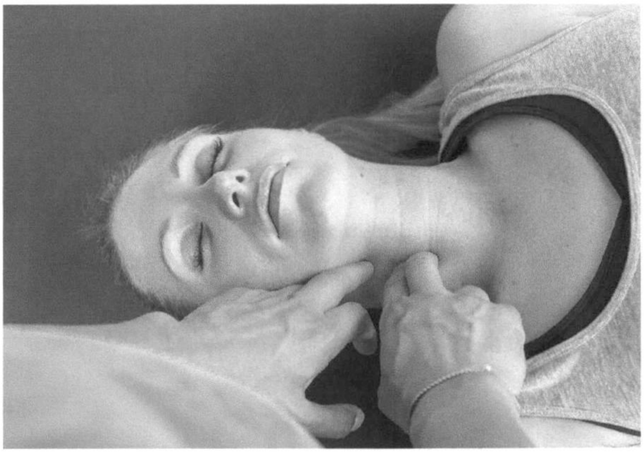

Figure 2.143 Technique for the common carotid artery/ external carotid artery

Technique for the external carotid artery/ maxillary artery

The location treated is the point where the maxillary artery branches off the external carotid.

Aim: To improve arterial supply to the temporomandibular joint.

Patient: Head turned contralaterally to the treatment side.

Practitioner: At the head of the patient.

Hand position (Figure 2.144):

- Your index and/or middle finger should lie posterior to the ramus of the mandible (posterior and slightly below the neck of the mandible), where the maxillary artery branches off.
- With your caudal hand, grasp the occipital bone. Position the index and/or middle finger directly under the angle of the jaw.

Method:

- The build-up of tension at the tissue barrier is created by slight sidebending of the head toward the contralateral side.
- Continue according to the technique for the common carotid artery (see above).

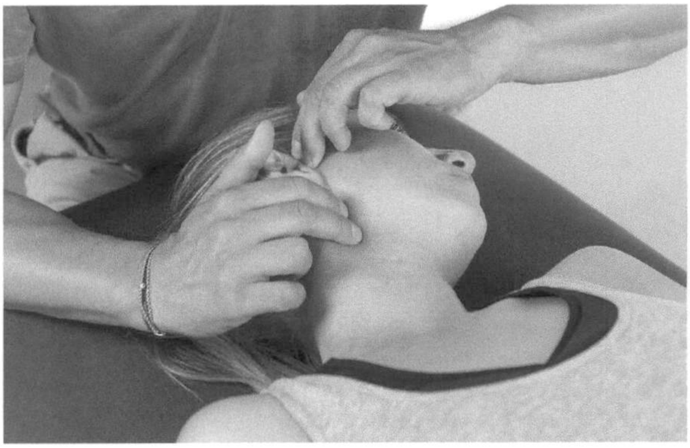

Figure 2.144 Technique for the external carotid artery/ maxillary artery

The internal jugular vein

The internal jugular vein is located in the carotid sheath, beneath the medial border of the sternocleidomastoid. A good place to palpate it is beside or between the sternal and clavicular attachments of the muscle. It drains the region within the cranium, in the brain and the facial region.

Hand position: Place the pads of the middle fingers of both hands medial to the sternocleidomastoid, posterior to the clavicle and lateral to the sterno-clavicular joint (Figure 2.145). The vein is lateral to the common carotid artery.

Method:

- Apply divergent longitudinal traction until you sense the tissue barrier.
- Another possible approach is to hold in position with your cranial finger and use the caudal finger to apply traction.
- Maintain the tension and permit micromotions between the internal jugular vein and the surrounding tissue/area around it, until release occurs and you sense an improvement in the capacity of the vein to glide.

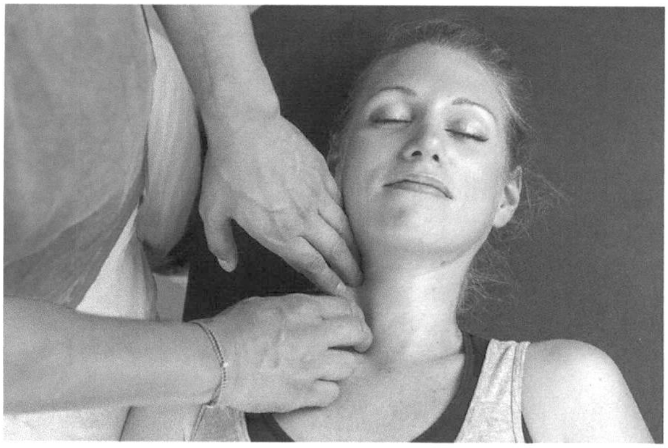

Figure 2.145 Internal jugular vein

The external jugular vein

The external jugular vein, which is easily visible and runs epifascially, is visible inside the parotid gland, near the angle of the mandible. It receives blood from the superficial posterior region of the head. It runs parallel to the great auricular nerve, amid the platysma, crossing the sternocleidomastoid from craniomedial to caudolateral. At the mid-clavicular point it passes through the prevertebral layer of cervical fascia. Anterior or lateral to the scalenus anterior muscle, it runs into the subclavian vein. There is a sinus with a venous valve about 4 cm (1½ inches) above the clavicle.

NOTE Important to note for palpation: the position of the head affects the filling of the vein—when lying down, the vein is full; when standing or sitting, it is empty.

Hand position:

- Position one middle finger posterior to the angle of the mandible, on the vein.
- Place the other middle finger above the middle of the clavicle, in the caudal region of the vein (Figure 2.146).

Method: According to the technique for the internal jugular vein (see above).
Further veins, such as the anterior jugular or facial veins, may be treated.[see 265]

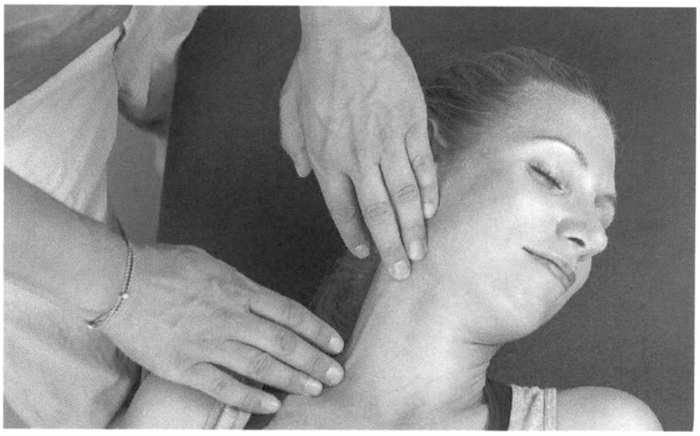

Figure 2.146 External jugular vein

Technique for the jugular foramen

Practitioner: Take up a position at the head of the patient.

Hand position:

- Grasp the occipital bone with the hand on the side opposite that to be treated. Your index, middle, and ring fingers should be immediately posterior to the occipitomastoid suture.
- Caudal hand: position your middle finger in the external acoustic meatus, your ring finger on the tip of the mastoid process, and your little finger on the mastoid part. With your thumb and index finger, grasp the zygomatic process.

Method:

- Carry out a disengagement between the temporal bone and occipital bone, focusing in particular on the jugular foramen. To do this, apply gentle traction to the temporal bone in an anterior superior direction, and gentle traction in a posterior inferior direction on the occipital bone (Figure 2.147).
- At the same time, establish a balance of tension at the temporal bone, between external rotation (posteromedial pressure with your ring finger) and internal rotation (posteromedial pressure with your little finger) and anterior and posterior rotation.
- At the occipital bone, establish a balance between flexion and extension.
- Induce this disengagement actively during the inhalation phase; as you do this, you gently reinforce dysfunctional tension patterns.
- During the exhalation phase, you should either simply passively follow the parameters of tension, or administer gentle compression.
- PBT or PBFT.
- Usually, a fulcrum is established between the regions.
- Additionally you can use the ball of your cranial hand on the occipital bone to deliver a gentle fluid impulse in the direction of the jugular foramen.

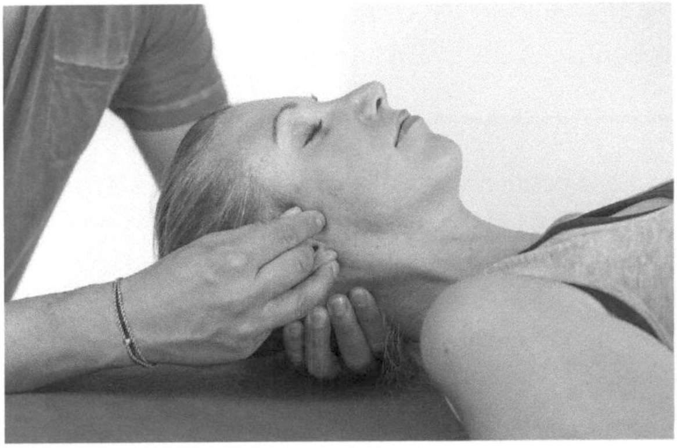

Figure 2.147 Technique for the jugular foramen

Technique for the cranial nerves

The following techniques for the cranial nerves are given in Volume 2, section 7.5.2:

- Technique for the trigeminal ganglion.
- Technique for the infraorbital nerve and branches of the maxillary nerve: in the case of disturbances of sensitivity of the lips or palate (also the vault of the pharynx and auditory tube).
- Technique for the superior alveolar nerve.
- Technique for the mandibular nerve.
- Technique for the mental nerve and its branches.
- Technique for the auriculotemporal nerve.
- Technique for the lingual nerve.

2.9 Self-help techniques, exercise programs for CMD and other disturbances

Most exercise programs for the treatment of myogenic CMD were developed to reduce pain, spasms, and hyperactivity of the muscles, to promote the muscular coordination of the masticatory muscles and tissue healing and regeneration, and to re-establish original muscle length.[312] It also appears helpful for the patient to learn ways to deal with stress, e.g., in cases of grinding, gnashing, or clenching the teeth.

Exercise programs appear to have a positive effect in myogenic CMD, although scientific proof is limited by the fact that therapeutic exercises are never used as the sole treatment approach, but always in combination with other conservative procedures, and there are no randomized clinical studies available. Further study is needed, especially regarding questions of intensity, repetition, frequency, and duration.[312]

If there is pain, stretching and relaxation exercises should be the first prescribed. In the case of asymmetrical movements of the mouth, coordination exercises are indicated, and strengthening exercises may be prescribed to prevent relapse.

In addition to local exercise programs, postural exercises or training for the cervical spine and for the body as a whole can play a significant role.[299] Similarly, breathing exercises and help in enabling better sleep should be considered.

If the exercise regimens are to be followed successfully, it is important for the exercises to be described in detail and to have feedback or, if necessary, correction of the procedure.[303]

Alongside these, decompression of inflamed temporomandibular joints can assist head posture, with the use of oral orthotic appliances.[335]

2.9.1 Stretching and relaxation

Indication: Pain in the craniomandibular region, in the case of reduced amplitude,[139,299] to reduce the tension of muscle fibers,[76] and to promote local perfusion.

Method:

- Active and/or passive.
- Stretching using reciprocal inhibition techniques, by isometric contraction of antagonist muscles.[283]
- Contraction/relaxation techniques can be used to stretch shortened muscle fibers. Contraction of a shortened muscle is followed by relaxation by passive stretching.[359]

Several established stretching and relaxation exercises are given below.

Decompression of the TMJ

Indication: To release the tension in the joint in cases of muscle hypertonicity, inflammation of the joint, hardening of the tissue, pain, etc.

Patient: Seated.

Hand position: Patient: your two hands cover the angles and the ascending rami of the mandible. Do not support the elbows.

Method: Relax the joints of the jaw and the mouth as much as possible, allow the tongue to lie relaxed in your mouth, with mouth slightly open. A slight decompression is exerted on the temporomandibular joints simply by the weight of the arms (Figure 2.148).

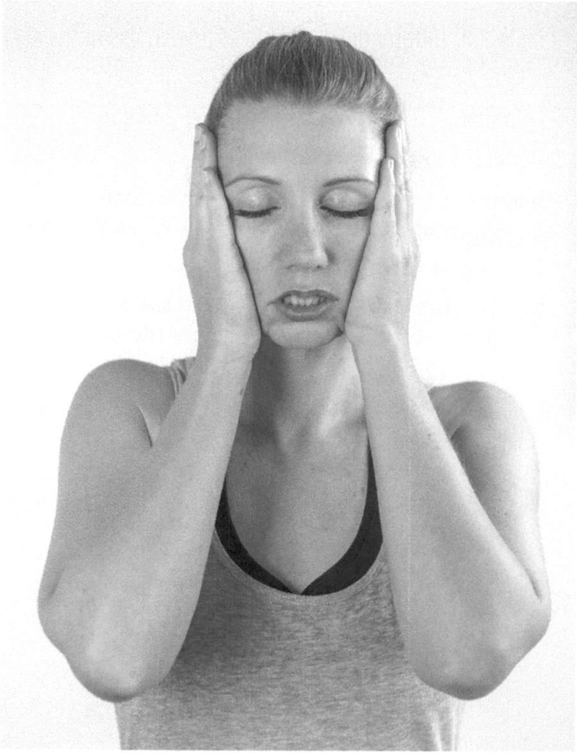

Figure 2.148 Self-help technique. Decompression of the temporomandibular joint

Decompression of the TMJ, alternative technique

Patient: Seated, with a roll of cotton wool between the back molars on each side.

Hand position: Place one hand on top of your head, on the roof of the skull, and the other under the chin on the mandible.

Method: Relax the temporomandibular joints and masticatory muscles as much as possible. With the hand that is on the chin, administer gentle upward pressure. At the same time, the other hand on the roof of the skull stabilizes the head. Decompression of the TMJ occurs through the fulcrum of the cotton wool roll.

Relaxing the masticatory muscles with traction or pressure

The techniques described below should be performed gently and should never cause pain.

Patient: Seated.

Method:

- **Temporalis muscle** Position your fingers on the muscles above the ears. Relax the mouth and jaw joints as best you can. Release the anterior, middle, and posterior parts of the muscle by gentle traction in a cranial direction (Figure 2.149).

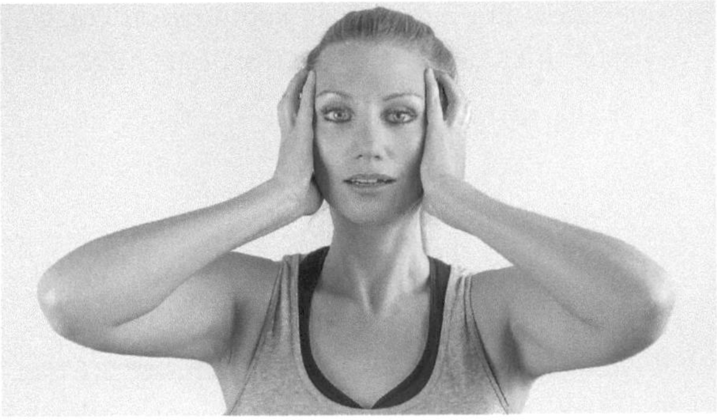

Figure 2.149 Self-help technique. Relaxation of the temporalis muscle

- **Masseter muscle** Place your index and middle fingers on the masseter muscle each side. Relax the mouth and jaw joints as best you can. With your fingers, administer gentle pressure on the muscles, particularly on the hard areas in the muscles (Figure 2.150).
- **Lateral pterygoid muscle** Guide your index finger or little finger intraorally along the outer margin of the alveolar process of the maxilla in the direction of the opening of your ear (external acoustic meatus). If it is difficult to take your finger past the ramus of the mandible, it usually helps to turn your index finger so that the palmar surface of the finger faces toward the cheek. Move the finger in a posterior and cranial direction, sufficiently far for the tip to come up against the muscle. Apply gentle pressure to the muscle with your finger (Figure 2.151).

Active mouth opening and closing with the tongue placed against the incisors/palate

Indication:

- Slowly, and repeatedly, open and close the mouth.
- Position the tip of your tongue against the lingual surface of your upper front teeth.

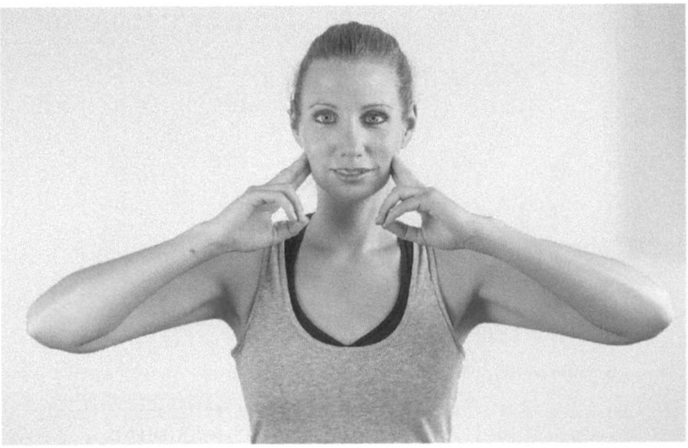

Figure 2.150 Self-help technique. Relaxation of the masseter muscle

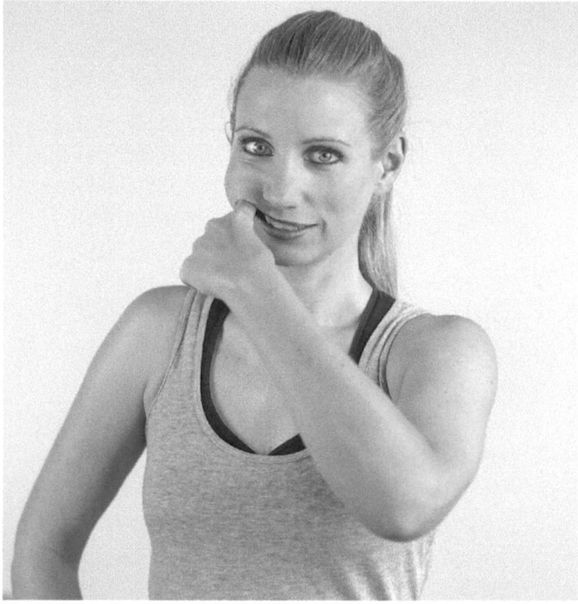

Figure 2.151 Self-help technique. Relaxation of the lateral pterygoid muscle

- It can help to say the letter "N" with your mouth closed.[139]
- Carry out this exercise several times a day.

2.9.2 Coordination exercises

Coordination exercises include controlled mouth opening and closing, and isotonic exercises.[302,325]

Indication: Disturbances of coordination in opening and closing the mouth (discoordination, deviation), for joint sounds,[291] and in order to improve joint muscle function and mobility.

Exercise with a mirror

Draw a straight, vertical line on the mirror.

Method:

- As you open and close your mouth, try to keep the midline of the lower jaw (in the middle, between the front teeth) parallel to the line on the mirror.[302,325]
- It is also helpful to mark a dot above your upper lip and another under your lower lip, in the middle. (Alternatively, you might fix a toothpick between the middle front teeth of your upper and lower jaw.) Now try to open and close your mouth in such a way that the marks (or tip of the toothpick) on the upper and lower jaw follow the line on the mirror throughout.
- As you do this, you can place your index fingers on the condyles each side to assist the movement.
- Repeat 20 times. Carry out the exercise three times a day.
- In addition, gentle isometric contractions of the opposite movement (see below) can be carried out.

Improving the protrusion and sideways movement

This self-help technique can be used where protrusion and sideways movement are restricted due to increased tension of the capsule. It also teaches coordination and proprioceptive perception in the TMJ.

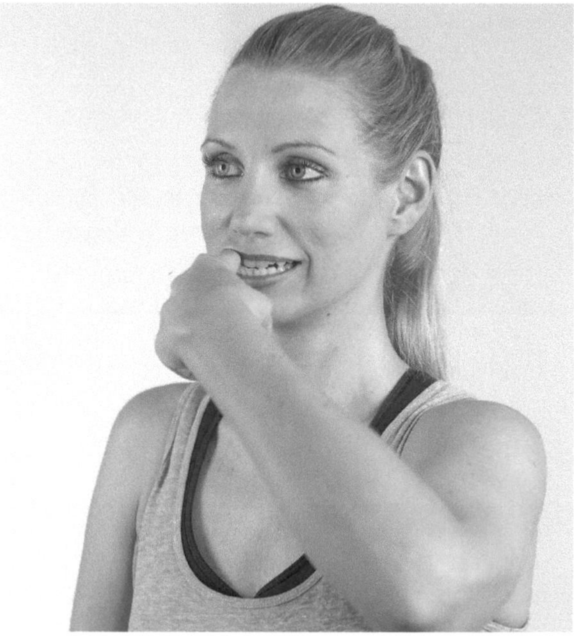

Figure 2.152 Self-help technique. Practicing the sideways movement

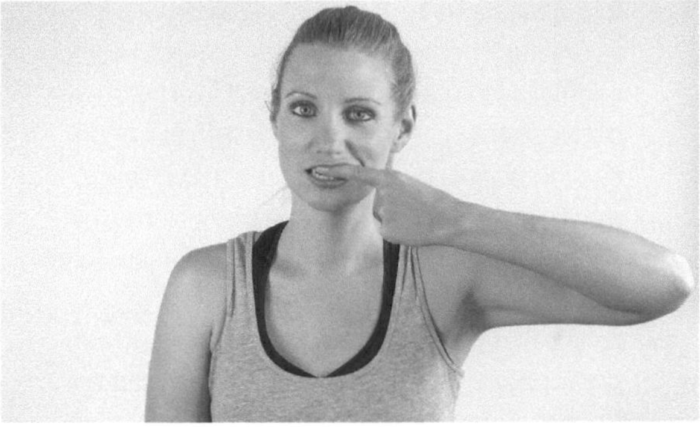

Figure 2.153 Self-help technique. Practicing the protrusive movement

Patient: Seated or lying down.

- **Practicing the sideways movement:** Place your index finger on the canine tooth of the upper jaw, on the side opposite to the dysfunction. Try to bite onto this finger (Figure 2.152).
- **Practicing the protrusive movement:** Position your index finger on the front incisors of the upper jaw. Try to bite onto this finger (Figure 2.153).

2.9.3 Strengthening exercises

Isometric exercises in particular can be used as strengthening exercises; concentric and eccentric isotonic[325] and isokinetic exercises can also be used to achieve this.

Indication: Especially in order to prevent relapse.

Isometric muscle contraction

Indication: Hypermobility of the TMJ, joint sounds, muscle spasm with limited mouth opening, and asymmetric mouth opening and muscle activity.

Hand position: Place your hands on each side of the mandible with the heel of your hands either side of the tip of the chin (Figure 2.154).

Method:

- The joints of the jaw should be relaxed, and the tongue lies relaxed in the mouth. The mouth is slightly open.
- Perform gentle contraction of your masticatory muscles in the direction of mouth opening (Figure 2.154) against resistance. No movement of the TMJ should take place (isometric muscle contraction).
- The force of muscle contraction should be extremely slight, and held for about 6 s.
- Each phase of muscle contraction should be followed by a brief one of relaxation.
- Each contraction/relaxation sequence should be repeated about three times.
- Then repeat the same technique in the appropriate way for mouth closure, protrusion, retrusion, and laterotrusion.
- The exercise should be performed several times a day.

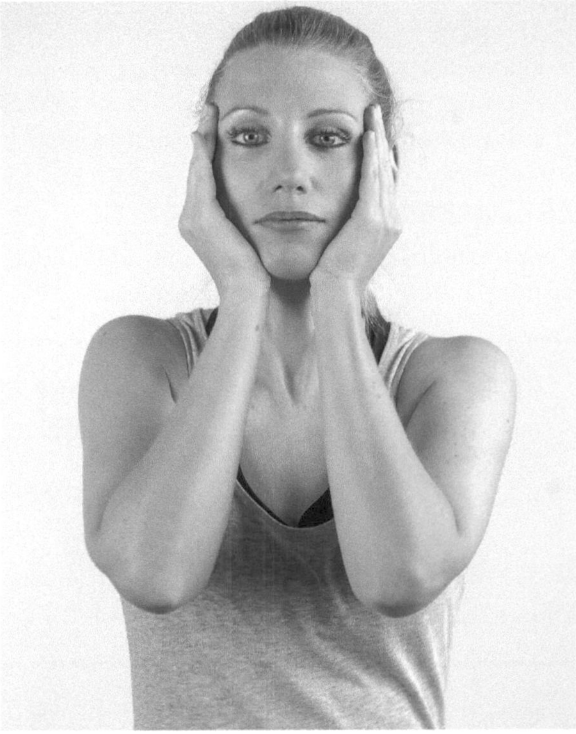

Figure 2.154 Isometric muscle contraction; example shown here: mouth opening movement

Alternative method:
- Patient: apply gentle pressure to the chin in the direction of mouth closure.
- The muscles of the jaw should contract to counteract this gentle pressure, so that there is no movement of the jaw (isometric muscle contraction).
- The method continues as above.
- This method has the advantage that patients learn better control of their muscle activity.

Tip for practitioners

Avoid using excessive counterpressure, as this could evoke reciprocal inhibition.[374]

2.9.4 Chewing exercises

Good myofascial and myocentric balance, and symmetrical action, are needed for harmonious mastication. The mandibular nerve is the most important cranial nerve involved. Chewing exercises are also indicated in cases of CMD. The following are taken from a course given by Philip van Caille (OSD, Hamburg, 2014).

- **Bilateral chewing using a chewy tube** (encourages myocentricity, inhibition of masticatory muscles) (Figure 2.155)
    - The tongue should be above the chewy tube.
    - Position the chewy tube as far back as possible on the molars.
    - Bite onto this.
    - Shift the chewy tube in the anterior direction, continuing forward to the fullest extent.
    - Then shift it backward again in the posterior direction.
    - The process of shifting forward and back should be performed in about five steps.
    - Carry out the exercise (both forward and back) ten times.

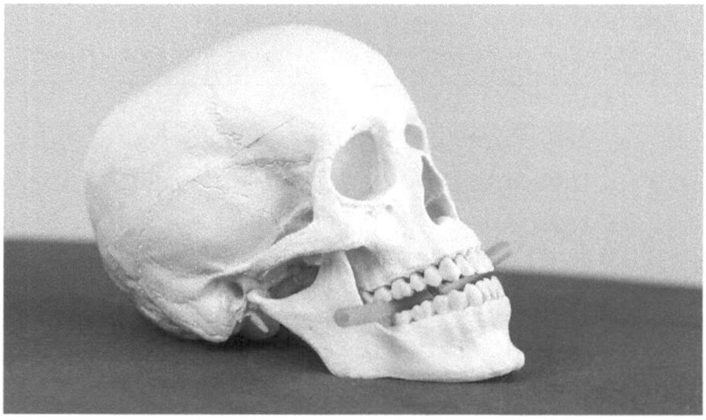

Figure 2.155
Bilateral chewing using a chewy tube

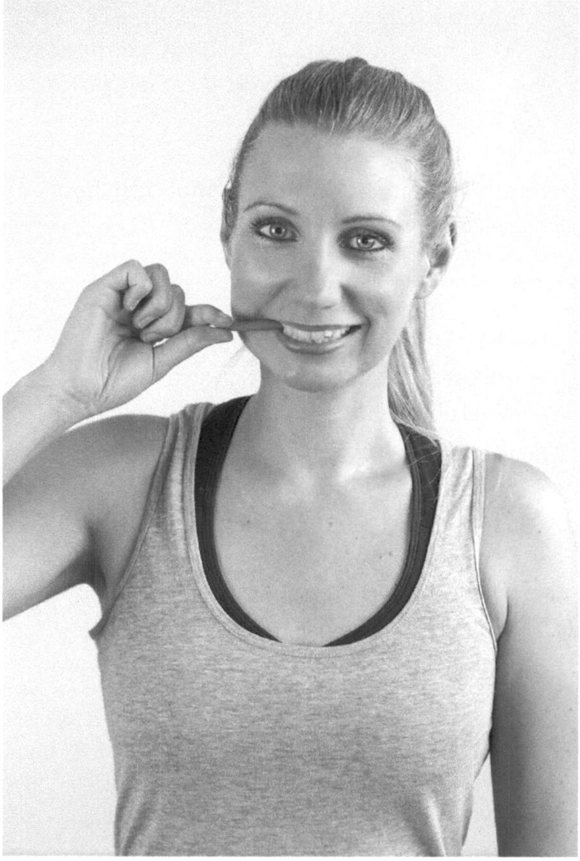

Figure 2.156
Unilateral chewing with a chewy tube

- **Unilateral chewing using a chewy tube** (exercise in laterotrusion and mediotrusion) (Figure 2.156)
  - Hold the chewy tube with one hand and bite onto it on one side, working forward from the back. As you shift the chewy tube gradually forward with your hand, you are performing a "translation" movement.
  - When you reach the middle, change sides (and change to the other hand).
  - Carry out this sequence twice.
- **Free chewing on a chew tool** (Figure 2.157)
  - Attach a cord to the chew tool to prevent you from swallowing it.
  - Bite on the chew tool, working forward from the back as you do so and moving it gradually forward.
  - When you arrive at the front, continue via the front teeth to make the changeover to the other side.

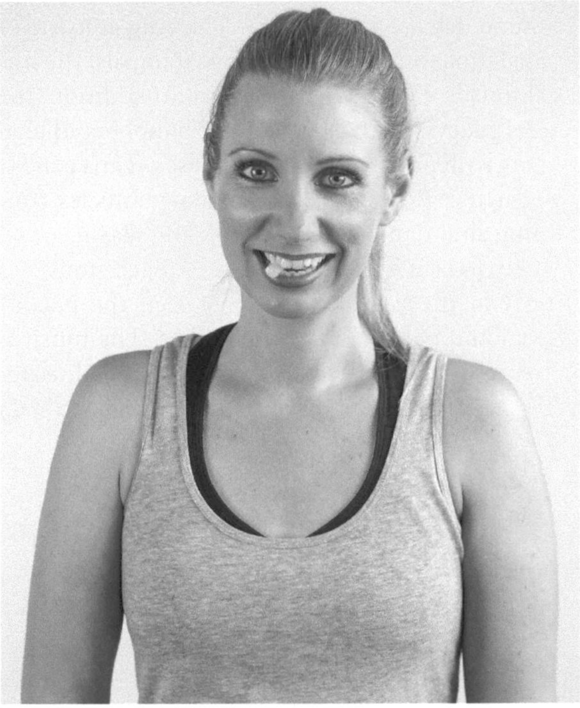

Figure 2.157
Free chewing on a chew tool

  - At the molars, bring the chew tool over to the other side again.
  - Carry out this exercise sequence twice.
- **Chewing with open bite, using a chewy tube**
  - At the location of the open bite, chew on a chewy tube that has been folded double.
  - Doing this stimulates the teeth to emerge further, so increasing the height.
  - Chew 30 times onto the chewy tube, anteriorly or at the side (with chewy tube).
  - In cases of anterior open bite, lip training should also be carried out.
  - If there is a gap in the teeth—but only if the tooth is already visible—the chewy tube can also be placed in the gap and chewed on.
  - In the case of unilateral crossbite, the patient can chew on a chewy tube on one side only, the side of the normal bite.

2.10 Treatment approaches for specific disturbances of the temporomandibular joint

2.10.1 Disturbances resulting from traumatic injury

Treatment methodology

- Release of fascial "pull," treatment of trigger points.
- Decompression or compression techniques in the case of pain in the joint (the patient should indicate using three fingers on the joint, or grasp the joint)
  - Compression techniques are indicated if the patient experiences biting as comfortable, but experiences it as unpleasant to let the jaw hang loosely.
  - Decompression techniques are indicated if the patient experiences biting the teeth together as unpleasant, but finds it comfortable to allow the jaw to hang loosely.
- Psychoemotional integration.[264]

2.10.2 Osteoarthritis and degenerative processes

Symptoms Loss of movement in mouth opening, crepitation, pain on excitation or irritation, positive radiological findings.

Treatment approach

- Muscular: treatment of trigger points, fascial stroking.
- Thrust technique
  - 10–20 impulses in the direction of the restrictions, given to the connective tissue in the region of the joint.
  - Impulse technique, seated or lying down.
- Intraosseous and periosteal technique on the bone and at the transition between bone and cartilage: flexion with traction, compression/traction, low thrust, recoil, locally focused pressure technique on specific points, balancing at the end.
- Mobilization: in rotation, translation, and/or global; slowly intensifying from one treatment session to the next.
- Release of the bilaminar zone: moving the TMJ anteriorly and inferiorly and then posteriorly.
- Reciprocal inhibition techniques (myofascial release techniques).
- Further approaches to reduce inflammation processes: dietary: avoiding consumption of short chain carbohydrates, especially fizzy drinks, confectionery, and products made with white flour; taking preparations containing glucosamine sulfate, chondroitin, omega-3 fatty acids, and frankincense.

Treatment sequence Once a week for the first four weeks, then slowly increasing the time between treatments (every two weeks, every four weeks). Treatment should be maintained over a period of at least a year.

2.10.3 Resistant occlusal stress

Cause Of dental origin, and disturbance of jaw position.

Symptom Worse in the morning, improving during the day.

Treatment approach

- Treatment of the TMJ and descending myofascial chain.
- Wearing a dental splint of the Aqualizer type for a specific time.
- Using an occlusal splint/nightguard to relieve stress on the TMJ.
- Treatment in cooperation with the dentist.

NOTE In all therapy using splints, it is important to readjust the splint after each osteopathic treatment session.

2.10.4 Types of transverse deviation: crossbite; scissorbite (non-occlusion)

In the case of **laterognathia**, there is no centering on opening or closing the mouth. If the joints are on one level in the sagittal and horizontal plane, the cause is traumatic injury with unilateral or bilateral total anterior disk displacement. The consequence is to hinder growth.

In the case of **lateral forced bite**, the mandible is centered on mouth opening. Disturbances of the masticatory muscles or TMJ or asymmetries of the face and body can occur.

Treatment approach

- Mobilization of the maxilla and palatine bone.
- Treatment of the upper cervical region.
- Treatment of ascending dysfunctions and of body posture.
- Treatment of somatic dysfunctions of the thoracic spine and lumbar spine.
- Treatment of disturbances of the tongue.
- Where necessary, reducing hypertonicity of the buccinator muscle.
- Very important: treatment of mouth breathing, if present.
- Training to discontinue visceral swallowing patterns and other dyskinesias: breathing exercises, tongue, swallowing, lip, and cheek exercises.
- Use of myofunctional devices (e.g., myobrace).

2.10.5 Dysgnathias characterized by mandibular protrusion

Cause A skeletal malformation (usually genetically determined) causes inhibition of the sagittal growth of the maxilla and potentially to impairment of the periodontium or teeth.

Differential diagnosis to distinguish a hypoblastic maxilla from a hyperblastic mandible requires a lateral cephalogram.

In cases of a hypoblastic maxilla or mixed form in which a hypoblastic maxilla predominates, therapy is possible in children who have their milk teeth or are in the process of acquiring their secondary dentition (up to around the age of nine years).

> *i* **FURTHER INFORMATION** Mandibular prognathia is described as true mandibular protrusion; maxillary retrognathia is pseudomandibular protrusion.

Treatment approach

- Supportive use of osteopathy, especially in the case of headache arising in the course of orthodontic work.
- Treatment of the viscerocranium and SBS.
- Treatment of tongue position and muscles of the lips and face.

Posture Self-help exercises, e.g., balancing a book on the head while walking, or exercises using a balance board.

2.10.6 Retrusive occlusion

This is one of the most frequent types of malocclusion. Treatment has a good prognosis.

Cause Particularly, reduced mandibular growth.

Symptoms

- Chin posterior.
- Lower front teeth posteriorly displaced.
- Upper incisors anterior.

Sequelae Impairment of the temporomandibular joint, which can lead to clicking, pain on chewing, osteoarthritis, and further hindrance to the sagittal development of the mandible.

Treatment approach

- Very important: treatment of mouth breathing, if present.
- Training to discontinue visceral swallowing patterns and other dyskinesias
  - Breathing exercises, tongue, swallowing, lip, and cheek exercises.
  - Use of myofunctional devices (e.g., myobrace); possibly use of face shaper/lip trainer.
  - Stretching the suprahyoid muscles.
- Treatment of body posture (frequent anterior displacement of head).
- Reduction of upper cervical kyphosis and mid-cervical lordosis, and stabilization of a hypermobile mid-cervical region.
- Treatment of a flattened thoracic spine and lordosed lumbar spine.

2.10.7 Open bite

Symptoms

- Frontal open bite is seen in the region of the front teeth: limits speaking and taking a bite.
- Lateral open bite is seen in the lateral dental region: limits chewing.
- Those with a dolichofacial (vertical) facial pattern tend to a skeletal open bite.

Causes

- Thumb-sucking; placing a finger being sucked, or the tongue, between the front teeth.
- Malposition of the jaw or of the teeth in the jaw and irregular tooth growth.
- Abnormal stress on teeth, bones, and muscles.
- Developmental malformation of the jaw, e.g., inhibition of growth of maxilla in the case of split palate/jaw/lips.

- Malformation of the jaw or facial muscles.
- Oversized tongue.
- Infectious diseases.
- Chronic vitamin deficiency.

Treatment approach

- Training to discontinue orofacial dyskinesias or habits, e.g., sucking thumb or dummy/pacifier
  - Breathing exercises, tongue, swallowing, lip, and cheek exercises.
  - Use of face shaper/lip trainer, myofunctional devices (e.g., myobrace), oral screen.
- Thumb-sucking chart.

2.10.8 Extreme deep bite

Where there is an enlarged overbite of the upper incisors over the lower, there can be inhibition of mandibular growth, dysfunctions of the TMJ, and possibly retrodisplacement or compression of the TMJ, as well as frequent headaches and dysfunctions of the upper cervical spine in consequence. Deep bite is often associated with malposition of the tongue.

Treatment approach

- Tongue exercises (tongue anterior on the palate).
- Treatment of orofacial dyskinesias.
- Muscle energy technique (MET): resistance against mouth opening.
- Stretching, release, and/or trigger point treatment for the masseter and temporalis muscles (see section 2.7.3 and Table 2.6).
- Mobilization techniques for the neurocranium.
- Normalizing posture, especially in the region of the cervical spine.
- Possibly use of myofunctional devices (e.g., myobrace).

2.10.9 Dry lips

How the condition develops May indicate any of several causes: mouth breathing, incompetent mouth closing, dental brace, dry air in heated indoor environments, cold winter air temperatures, inadequate intake of liquids, vitamin/mineral deficiency (vitamin B2, iron, zinc, vitamin C), digestive disturbances, infections (esp. herpes simplex), colds, stress-related hypersympathetic state (leads to reduced production of saliva), associated condition in autoimmune diseases, chemotherapy, chronic overuse of cosmetics, allergies.

Treatment Depending on etiology: Vaseline®, stopping mouth breathing (e.g., using face shapers; lip and tongue exercises), taking vitamin B2, vitamin C, iron, or zinc supplements, drinking adequate amount of liquid, healthy diet.

2.10.10 Rhagades at corner of mouth

How the condition develops Incompetent mouth closing, dental brace, poorly fitting dentures, dampness at corner of mouth (frequently moistening or chewing the lips), dry skin, infections, allergies to cosmetics, nodding off, metabolic disorders, e.g., diabetes mellitus, associated condition in Down's syndrome, Parkinson's.

Sequelae Breeding ground for pathogens (viruses, bacteria, fungal infection).

Treatment Stopping mouth breathing (e.g., using face shapers; lip and tongue exercises); according to etiology.

2.10.11 Bruxism

There are two types of bruxism: awake and sleep bruxism. In **awake bruxism**, the person can consciously tell when they are clamping the jaw. Awake bruxism is mainly associated with nervous tics and with reactions to stress. **Sleep bruxism** is seen as a sleep-associated movement disturbance.[256,334]

Prevalence Prevalence of awake bruxism in the adult population is 20%.[334] According to a systematic review, prevalence of sleep bruxism among children lies between 5.9% and 49.6%.[279] A number of authors found an increased occurrence mainly among anxious children.[156,191] Bruxism is found to occur more frequently in children (51.3%) when bruxism on the part of one parent is reported than in children where there is no bruxism in the family (30.6%).[273] In children of separated parents the risk of sleep bruxism and primary headaches is significantly increased.[45] There is no correlation between anatomical, structural factors and sleep bruxism.[270]

Genotypic factors Polymorphisms of the 2A serotonin receptor gene (HTR2A) lead to a higher risk of sleep bruxism[2,273,337,338] or of stress and anxiety,[104,136,215,469] via serotonergic pathways.

Risk factors

- The physiology and pathology of awake bruxism are unknown, although stress and anxiety are seen as risk factors.[256]
- Post-traumatic stress disorders,[52] anxiety, stress, alcohol consumption, smoking, consumption of more than six cups of caffeinated coffee,[329] and anxiety states.[52,156,339]
- Passive smoking, sleep disturbances in children.[69]
- Sudden brief waking reactions (microarousal), which occur in the brain on account of obstruction to the respiratory pathways during sleep, cause an increase in heart rate, which in turn stimulates rhythmic masticatory muscle activity and grinding of the teeth. The increase in activity of the masticatory muscles activates the trigeminocardiac reflex; that then leads to a slowing of the heart rate.[74]
- Bruxism seems to be associated with anterior and inferior head posture and pathological tooth wear.[453]
- Occlusal factors appear to play hardly any role in the etiology of sleep bruxism.[256]

Pathophysiological factors Sleep bruxism is mainly centrally, not peripherally regulated (e.g., dento-occlusal factors).[274,479] A distinction has to be made here between pathophysiological and psychosocial factors. In the case of sleep bruxism, there may be abnormal excitability of the central motor innervation of the jaw, on account of impaired modulation of brainstem inhibitory switching mechanisms. Cranial nerves V and X are also involved here, as well as subcortical structures.[146]

During sleep, **rhythmic activity of the masticatory muscles** occurs in up to 60% of normal study subjects; this involves slow (1 Hz) masticatory-like movements without any wear of the teeth. If rhythmic masticatory muscle activity occurs frequently during sleep, or if this is associated with tooth wear, it is referred to as sleep bruxism. In patients with sleep bruxism, the occurrence of rhythmic masticatory muscle activity is three times higher compared to normal study subjects, and up to 30% more intensive.[254] Rhythmic masticatory muscle activity during sleep occurs in association with transient activation of cortical, limbic, and autonomic switching circuits.[51] The motor response of the jaw is preceded by cortical, autonomic cardiac activation. Alongside this, sympathetic cardiac activity was recorded.[295] Activation of the temporal lobe and the limbic system accompanies tension of the jaw and occurs in clamping of the jaw.[51]

Figure 2.158 illustrates the neuronal influences in sleep bruxism.

Sleep bruxism in preverbal, healthy infants can be an expression of fear or anger.[51] Bracha[49] infers that clamping of the jaw in acute stress leads to increased pumping of blood through the veins leaving the temporal bone, with the effect of increasing blood flow to structures of the anterior temporal lobe. This mechanism could represent a potential survival advantage in threatening situations (fight or flight).[49,50] In addition, masticatory movements (e.g., non-nutritive chewing) were found to have an effect on the function of the hippocampus.[51]

Bruxism caused by emotional stress is accompanied by a rise in the **neurotransmitters** noradrenaline (norepinephrine), adrenaline (epinephrine),[77,400] glutamate, dopamine,[255,434] and gamma-aminobutyric acid (GABA).[255] Thus, on clenching the jaws, a higher signal effect of norepinephrine-producing neurons of the brainstem was registered, especially together with a situation in which receptors were not yet non-downregulated.[51] In this connection a particular role is accorded to some serotonin receptor subtypes.[51] This means that the release of serotonin as a neurotransmitter is important for reactions to environmental stimuli (especially in the social environment), and is associated with mood, sleep, the circadian rhythm, thermoregulation, and social behavior; also the regulation of stress reactions and managing stress,[469,215] and the maintenance of excitation and regulation of muscle tone and respiration. So there might be seen to be a link between serotonin and the pathogenesis of sleep bruxism.[337] Serotonin reuptake inhibitors (SSRIs) could cause episodes of sleep bruxism in susceptible persons.[271]

Neuroevolutionary and paleoanthropological perspectives Between 2 million and 200,000 years ago, bruxism strengthened the masseter and temporalis muscles and thus biting force; especially before the discovery of fire, that would have aided the required nutrition intake and so the survival of early humans.[52] A forceful bite would also have been useful in defense, and the human oral flora meant that bites were often fatal.[356] Sleep bruxism would have kept teeth sharp.[52,114,216,315]

Possible further advantages of bruxism

- Protective function during sleep, e.g., maintaining patent airway in sleep:[272,210] for example, the masseter muscle assists the genioglossus in widening the upper respiratory pathways,[247] and stimulates the flow of saliva to lubricate the oropharynx;[305] by doing so it protects the upper digestive tract.[439,255,305,306]
- Improving performance during sport: both moderate and maximum activity of the masseter muscle increased significantly during the golf swing with the distance aimed at. Clenching the jaw could be a physiological strategy to increase the neuronal activity of distal body segments and so improve performance.
- Improvement of occlusion.
- Biting as a form of self-defense in response to physical or sexual attack.[356]

Phenotypic factors

- Clenching and grinding could in the first instance be a manifestation of acute fear or chronic emotional stress.[52]

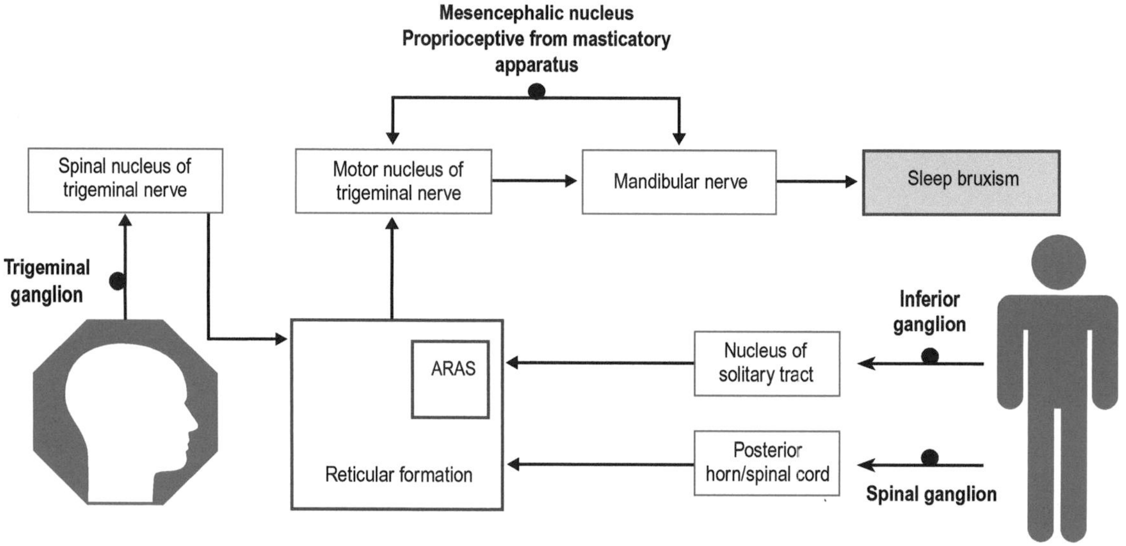

Figure 2.158
Neuronal influences in sleep bruxism (ARAS = ascending reticular activation system)

- Sleep bruxism has been associated with characteristic personality traits such as anxiety,[9,71,88,128,159,170,333,338,346,364] stress,[128] and neuroticism.[88]
- Changes in neurotransmitters were recorded.[338]

Sequelae Sleep bruxism in children is self-limiting; intervention is seldom required,[288] and normally it has no serious effects.[362] The most important consequences of bruxism are damage to teeth, tooth loss, pain in the temporomandibular joint and muscles of the jaw or restrictions of jaw movement, and headaches.[20,205,222,365] In children with sleep bruxism, headaches were recorded in 59.2% of cases, whereas in children without sleep bruxism headaches were recorded in only 31.4% of cases.[45]

There are comorbidities with other stress-induced disturbances such as chronic fatigue syndrome and fibromyalgia.[1] Connections were also demonstrated between gastroesophageal reflux disease and bruxism, and these are possibly associated with depression, anxiety disturbances, and reduced sleep quality. The causal connections are however unclear.[263]

Diagnosis

- Sleep bruxism should be differentiated from awake bruxism.
- Tenderness to pressure and/or visible hypertrophy of the temporalis and masseter muscles.[52]
- Worn teeth/impressions on soft tissue.
- Tooth-grinding: distinct wear faceting of the teeth and wear of chewing surfaces; low premolars.
- Teeth-clenching: no wear faceting, and little wear of chewing surfaces.
- Possibly biting or sucking the cheeks.
- Possibly cracks/splits in tooth enamel.

Treatment According to several review studies, there is little or no connection between sleep bruxism and negative consequences for health.[287,289,290] Treatment is only indicated if problems emerge on account of the bruxism.[26] Manual therapeutic treatment for sleep bruxism in children is a matter of controversy.[375]

Treatment approaches

- Reducing muscle hyperactivity by
  - Massaging masticatory and nuchal muscles.
  - Stretching exercises to increase range of movement, reduce pain, and improve resting position of lower jaw.[455]
  - Controlled cycles of relaxation and contraction of various muscle groups.
- Training in diaphragmatic breathing.
- Employing the power of imagination (constructing mental pictures and relaxing activities).
- Relaxation therapy techniques aimed at promoting awareness of muscle tenseness.[336]

2.10.12 Treatment of children

When treating disturbances of the mouth and jaw in children, particular attention should be paid to the following influences, which should be differentiated:

- Genetic components.
- Fields of growth (synchondroses, sutures of the visceral cranium, maxillary tuberosities, alveolar processes).
- Facial development.
- Pattern of swallowing.
- Breathing.
- Tongue position.
- Positioning of lips.
- Orofacial dyskinesias/habits.
- Autonomic nervous system: sympathetic stresses.
- Diet/nutrition.
- Anabolic and catabolic hormone activity.
- Ascending and descending chains; somatic dysfunctions.
- Body posture.

The **examination** and recording of findings includes position of the teeth, shape of the arch, occlusion, and possibly radiological examination (orthopantomogram [OPG] and lateral cephalogram).

The aim of **treatment** is to promote the health of the child as a whole person. The further focus of treatment is directed to the following aspects:

- The fields of growth (synchondroses, especially the SBS, but also the sphenofrontal and sphenoethmoid synchondroses, sutures of the viscerocranium, maxillary tuberosities, and alveolar processes) are stimulated and brought into balance.
- Normal development of the face: stimulation of the facial sutures and intraosseous treatment, sucking exercises, exercises in nasal breathing, etc.
- Normal swallowing procedures (without involvement of the mentalis muscle).
- Promoting nasal breathing.
- Normal position of tongue and lips, by means of exercise therapy.
- Assisting neutral bite and straight teeth.
- Release of dysfunctional, associated tensions of the nape of the neck on swallowing.
- Treating orofacial dyskinesias/habits: here, too, the child's cooperation is decisive.
- Autonomic nervous system: reducing sympathetic stresses.
- Regulating anabolic and catabolic hormonal activity.
- Treating ascending and descending chains, somatic dysfunctions, reducing or releasing related dysfunctional patterns.
- Reducing relapses and the need for the (possibly lifelong) use of a retainer.
- Diet: reduction of sugar and carbohydrate intake in particular.
- Treatment for body posture.

NOTE After the first consultation, but before treatment begins, the patient should undergo a complete examination by an orthodontist.

Photographs should be taken every four weeks to **monitor progress during the course of treatment**.

2.10.13 Interdisciplinary cooperation in the production of occlusal splints and splint correction

The osteopathic treatment of the patient is carried out taking account of ascending and descending myofascial chains/continuities as well as central and peripheral sensitization; particular focus is placed on the functional unit of mouth and jaw. Treatment should include reciprocal inhibition of tension of the relevant masticatory muscles, mimetic, hyoid, and upper cervical muscles (section 2.8.1).

Ideally, the fitting and adjustment of the occlusal splint should be done immediately following the osteopathic treatment. If this is not possible for reasons of appointment time or location, it is important to preserve the bite at the end of the treatment session so as to maintain the myofascial and osseous balance of the mouth and jaw region that has been achieved. The following provide means of **preserving the bite**:

- Aqualizer-type: the advantage of this is that it is reusable, and preserves the relaxed state of the masticatory muscles. The patient should be advised not to eat or chew if at all possible, until the fitting and adjustment of the occlusal splint, as doing so may alter the bite.
- Silicone impression material: this is mixed with a paste hardener and pressed onto the teeth of the lower jaw. The patient is then asked to close the bite to shape the silicone material to the occlusion. The remaining material at the sides is removed. This means of preserving the bite holds for about five hours.
- Cotton wool roll or chewy tube: a cotton wool roll or chewy tube is placed on the lateral teeth on each side. This means of preserving the bite is only suitable for short-term use: 10–30 minutes at most. The patient should be warned to expect considerable production of saliva.

2.10.14 Occlusal splints

Oliver Prätorius

Today, occlusal splints (bite splints) are the most frequently used therapy option for patients with muscle- and joint-related pain. The aim of treatment for patients with CMD symptoms is in the first instance a reversible approach; that is, to decouple the positions of forced bite and occlusion, based on professional dental advice as to indication and intraoral "fine-tuning," using a splint judged to be individually suited to the patient. Ideally, this should be complemented by collaboration with practitioners from the fields of human medicine, osteopathy, and physiotherapy.

Various different occlusal splints are recommended, according to the author and working group. Ultimately, a highly important step is the "fine-tuning," to ensure that the chosen model of splint individually accords with the particular need of the individual patient. A further important point in the care of CMD patients is that, following fitting, the patient should continue to return for regular follow-up, to check the occlusal contacts on the splint surface, and carry out any necessary adjustment, should this be needed, by grinding away points of occlusal disturbance as splint therapy progresses.

Regarding the symptoms and occurrence of articular pain, the model concept is that of nociceptor pain.[384] Local ischemia due to muscular overstrain (especially by parafunctions of the masticatory system) and microtrauma provide a systemic explanatory model. One of the effects caused by the release of inflammatory mediators in the tissues involved in CMD is to activate nociceptors. Splints that maintain a low turning moment of the teeth as they bite down could reduce the stress on nociceptors in the periodontium.

In principle, all occlusal splints decouple the current forced bite situation and, with correct placing and individual grinding adjustments, produce a rebalancing of neuromuscular stimuli (trigeminal afferent fibers—CNS—efferent fibers serving masticatory muscles). Accounts in the literature of the association between occlusion with therapeutic occlusal splints and the resultant reduction in tension/pain in the masticatory muscles are predominantly positive.

Care of occlusal splints

In order to achieve **spontaneous occlusal decoupling** and speedy reduction of pain on first contact with a patient, the method that immediately recommends itself is to provide the patient with a temporary, ready-made splint (which should be worn as continuously as possible for a few days) (e.g., MIClancer [Figure 2.159] or Aqualizer).

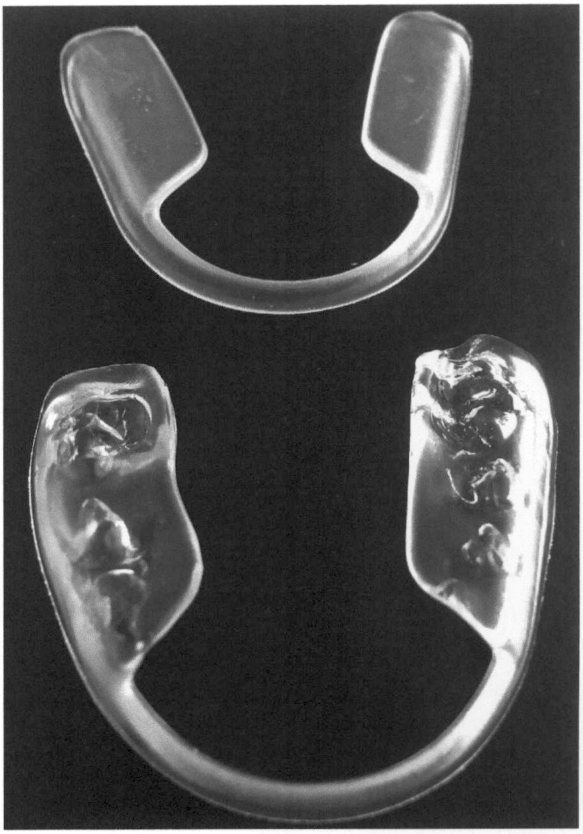

Figure 2.159
MIClancer, before and after warming and adjustment (©Dentale Orthopädie)

This approach should be linked as close to immediately as possible with cautious osteopathic expansion of the soft tissue structures involved in mouth opening, and complemented by initial home exercises to reduce the tone of the masticatory muscles.[383] Other treatment philosophies reduce the time recommendation for wearing an occlusal splint to nighttime only.

In order to achieve more effective treatment, a **laboratory-made splint** should be provided as soon as possible. This is made on the basis of the functional diagnosis made by the individual practitioner/treatment team in the particular case and the aspects on which they wish to focus regarding measurement and fitting. In this respect considerations that to a degree play a role are those that determine centric jaw relations, as important target parameters. The first step is always to make models of the patient's upper jaw and lower jaw. These are then placed in an articulator (laboratory apparatus that simulates simplified jaw movement) to provide a rough impression of the clinical bite relations.

Many splints are made on the basis of a computer assisted analysis of the movement of the lower jaw; this produces a theoretical centric condylar position. This diagnostic method offers the prospect of a set occlusal situation for the occlusal splint that is to be made which will be as disturbance-free as possible.[185] The aim is to reduce the necessity for subsequent grinding of faulty occlusal contacts, to achieve the right vertical dimension (splint height) and as a result better patient compliance. Many CMD experts accord considerable importance to the "correct" position of the condyle with a physiological disk–condyle relation and position in both temporomandibular joints in habitual occlusion. They believe that, by doing so, troublesome afferent impulses from the stomatognathic tissue can be kept to a minimum.

The next step in production is to determine the target position of the bite that the splint will subsequently have, i.e., the final occlusal situation in habitual intercuspation in the occlusal splint. Depending on the practitioner's preferred approach, this is recorded—with much experience, sensitivity, and skill—as centric registration; or, for example, as "mushbite" registration using a wax plate or silicone-based material to capture the occlusion. The registration is then placed between the models in the articulator.

Examples of occlusal splints

The **COPA splint** (craniomandibular orthopedic positioning appliance, Figure 2.160) is placed reversibly in the lower jaw; it does not cover the anterior teeth and has a sublingual strap. Some practitioners also firmly adhere the splint to the lateral teeth of the lower jaw. Prior to this, a construction bite is used to arrive at the desired mandibular position in the subsequent splint. This recording of the bite is done following whole-body diagnosis plus preliminary treatment by the physiotherapist and/or osteopath, together with a neuromuscular coherence test.[42]

The **Michigan occlusal splint** (Figure 2.161), with planar relief and a single centric row of cusps, has been shown in numerous studies to be well suited for treating myoarthropathies in the masticatory musculature. It can also help to reduce

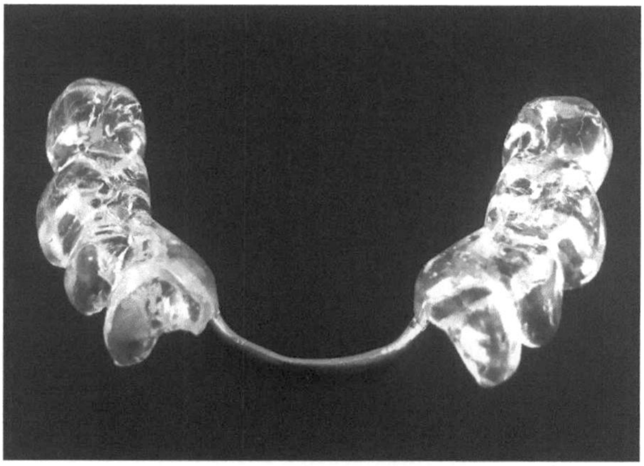

Figure 2.160
COPA occlusal splint (©Dentale Orthopädie)

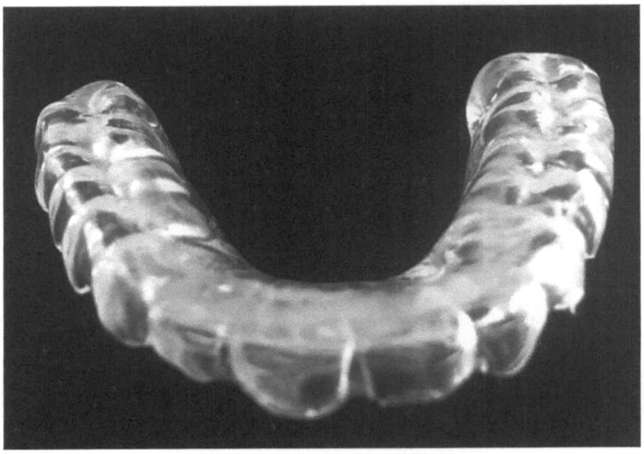

Figure 2.161
Michigan occlusal splint (©Dentale Orthopädie)

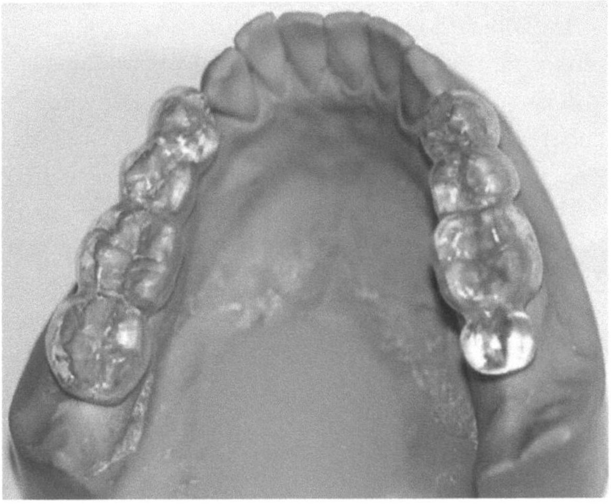

Figure 2.162
Our occlusal splint, "Flügel," in the lateral dental region of the lower jaw (©Dentale Orthopädie)

stresses on teeth and temporomandibular joints. It is made either for the upper jaw or the lower jaw. For patients whose teeth are sometimes considerably abraded and may have vertical loss, it provides effective, inexpensive protection from further tooth attrition. It can also be used as a mouthguard to protect against bruxism. Here too, close follow-up is important; the occlusal contacts of the splint should be monitored in the desired, supporting zones of the dental arch and malocclusions promptly ground if this is found necessary.[16]

In addition to the examples given here, many other types of occlusal splints can be made in order to treat CMD and the associated painful functional disturbances (Figure 2.162). With individual close follow-up and adjustment these serve well in achieving the desired reduction of pain symptoms related to CMD.

FURTHER INFORMATION In the case of all products that are to be placed in a patient, whether fixed or removable, we recommend first testing the tolerance of the patient's immune system. Laboratory tests such as the basophil degranulation test (BDT, type I hypersensitivity immediate type reaction) and the lymphocyte transformation test (LTT, type IV delayed type reaction) can reveal possible intolerances to the foreign material to be processed or employed in the oral cavity, and so help prevent chronic inflammation in the body system as a whole. These environmentally and medically focused tests can be used both preventively and curatively.

Areas of application

One of the explanatory models given in the current literature regarding the accommodation of an occlusal splint that seeks to explain possible therapeutic effects is a reorganization of intramuscular and intraarticular functional patterns. The effects of malocclusion on the body as a whole, with postural changes and consequent orthopedic symptoms, has been described for many years by numerous authors.[225]

Initial study results obtained by our team—which to a great extent remain unpublished—point to plumbline postural changes brought about by malocclusion, in which a primary descending influence from the incisors bringing a weakening effect to the muscles of the foot (neuromuscular coupling) could lead to a secondary ascending problem in the articular planes of the knee and hip joints. Systemically investigated connections of tooth–muscle pairs leave a demanding complex of symptoms to be worked through; this can call for osteopathic treatment to support the process.[355]

While disagreement remains over the connections between dentistry and a person's posture, and bearing in mind that it is still standard practice to use occlusal splints almost exclusively in dentistry, there is a need for further study if we are to be able to incorporate treatment with occlusal splints much more often as being indicated in therapy regimes of human medicine, especially orthopedics.

2.11 References

1 Aaron, L. A. and Buchwald, D. (2001) 'A review of the evidence for overlap among unexplained clinical conditions.' *Ann. Intern. Med. 134*, 9/2, 868–881.

2 Abe, Y., Suganuma, T., Ishii, M. et al. (2012) 'Association of genetic, psychological and behavioral factors with sleep bruxism in a Japanese population.' *J. Sleep Res. 21*, 289–296.

3 Aerni, F. (1988) *Lehrbuch der Menschenkenntnis*. Zürich: Kalos, p. 363.

4 Äkerman, S., Kopp, S. and Rohlin, M. (1986) 'Histological changes in temporomandibular joints from elderly individuals. An autopsy study.' *Acta Odontol. Scand. 44*, 231–239.

5 Ahlers, M. and Jakstat, H. (2007) *Klinische Funktionsanalyse*. Hamburg: DentaConcept Verlag GmbH.

6 Albe-Fessard, D., Cordes-Lara, M., Sanderson, P. et al. (1984) 'Advances in pain, research and therapy.' In: Kruger, L. and Liebeskin, J. C. (Ed.) *Neural Mechanisms of Pain*, Vol. 6. New York: Raven Press, pp. 167–182.

7 Alexander, J. (2017) 'OMT for tinnitus: evidence based applications.' Presented at AAO *Convocation the balance point: bridging the science and art of osteopathic medicine together*; March 24, 2017; Colorado Springs.

8 Alonso-Blanco, C., Fernández-de-Las-Peñas, C., de-la-Llave-Rincón, A. I. et al. (2012) 'Characteristics of referred muscle pain to the head from active trigger points in women with myofascial temporomandibular pain and fibromyalgia syndrome.' *J. Headache. Pain. 13*, 6, 625–623.

9 Alves, A. C., Alchieri, J. C. and Barbosa, G. A. (2013) 'Bruxism. Masticatory implications and anxiety.' *Acta Odontol. Latinoam. 26*, 1, 15–22.

10 Amigues, J. P. (1991) *L'A.T.M. Une Articulation Entre l'Osteopathe et le Dentiste*. Aix en Provence: Editions de Verlaque, pp. 52, 54.

11 An, J., Jeon, D., Jung, W. et al. (2015) 'Influence of temporomandibular joint disc displacement on craniocervical posture and hyoid bone position.' *Am. J. Orthod. Dentofacial. Orthop. 147*, 72–79.

12 Antczak-Boukoms, A. (1995) 'Epidemiology of research for temporomandibular disorders.' *J. Orofacial Pain. 9*, 226–234.

13 Apkarian, A. V., Baliki, M. N. and Geha, P. Y. (2009) 'Towards a theory of chronic pain.' *Prog. Neurobiol. 87*, 2, 81–97.

14 Arbuckle, B. E. (1994) *The Selected Writings of Beryl E. Arbuckle, D.O., F.A.C.O.P.* Indianapolis: American Academy of Osteopathy.

15 Arendt-Nielsen, L., Svensson, P., Sessle, B. J. et al. (2008) Interactions between glutamate and capsaicin in inducing muscle pain and sensitization in humans. *Eur. J. Pain. 12*, 5, 661–670.

16 Ash Major, M. (2006) *Schienentherapie, Evidenzbasierte Diagnostik und Behandlung bei TMD und CMD*. 3rd Ed. München: Urban and Fischer, pp. 266–278.

17 Augthun, M., Müller-Leisse, C., Bauer, W., Roth, A. and Spiekermann, H. (1998) 'Anteriore Verlagerung des Discus articularis des Kiefergelenks.' *J. Orofac. Orthop./Fortschr. Kieferorthop. 59*, 39–46.

18 Aumüller, G. (1985) 'Gestaltungsfaktoren der Schädelform.' In: Staubesand, J., Fleischhauer, K. and Zenker, W. (Ed.) *Benninghoff, Anatomie. Makroskopische und mikroskopische Anatomie des Menschen*, Vol. 1. München: Urban and Schwarzenberg, p. 96.

19 Baba, A., Okuyama, Y., Ojiri, H. et al. (2017) 'Eagle syndrome.' *Clin. Case Rep. 17*, 5, 2, 201–202.

20 Bader, G. and Lavigne, G. (2000) 'Sleep bruxism—an overview of an oromandibular sleep movement disorder: review article.' *Sleep Med. Rev. 4*, 1, 27–43.

21 Bahnemann, F. (Ed.) (1993) *Der Bionator in der Kieferorthopädie. Grundlagen und Praxis*. Heidelberg: Haug.

22 Bahnemann, F. (1992) *Anthropologische Grundlagen einer Ganzheitsmedizin aus kieferorthopädischer Sicht*. Heidelberg: Haug, p. 84.

23 Barbenel, J. C. (1974) 'The mechanics of the temporomandibular joint—a theoretical and electromyographical study.' *J. Oral Rehabil. 1*, 19–27.

24 Bauer, A. and Gutowski, A. (1975) *Gnathologie. Einführung in Theorie und Praxis*. Berlin: Quintessenz, p. 83.

25 Baumann, J. (1951) 'Contribution à l'étude de l'innervation de l'articulation temporomandibulaire.' *C.R.A.A. 2*, 120.

26 Beddis, H., Pemberton, L. and Davies, S. (2018) 'Sleep bruxism: an overview for clinicians.' *Br. Dent. J. 225*, 6, 497–501.

27 Beek, M., Koolstra, J. H., van Ruijven, L. J. et al. (2000) 'Three-dimensional finite element analysis of the human temporomandibular joint disc.' *J. Biomechan. 33*, 307–316.

28 Beek, M., Koolstra, J. H., van Ruijven, L. J. et al. (2001) 'Three-dimensional finite element analysis of the cartilaginous structures in the human temporomandibular joint.' *J. Dent. Res. 80*, 10, 1913–1918.

29 Bell, W. E. (1977) 'Management of masticatory pain.' In: von Alling, C. C. and Mahan, P. E. *Facial Pain*. Philadelphia: Lea and Febiger, p. 185.

30 Bell, W. E. (1969) 'Nonsurgical management of the pain-dysfunction syndrome.' *J. Am. Dent. Assoc. 79*, 161–170.

31 Bell, W. E. (1969) 'Clinical diagnosis of the pain-dysfunction syndrome.' *J. Am. Dent. Assoc. 79*, 154.

32 Benjamin, S., Barness, Dd., Berger, S. et al. (1988) 'The relationship of chronic pain, mental illness and organic disorders.' *Pain. 32*, 185.

33 Benner, K. U. (1993) 'Bau, Innervation und rezeptive Strukturen des Kiefergelenks.' In: Benner, K., Fanghänel, J., Kowalewski, R., Kubein-Meesenburg, D. and Ranzio, J. (Ed.) *Morphologie, Funktion und Klinik des Kiefergelenks*. Berlin: Quintessenz, 43–60.

34 Bennett, N. G. (1908, reprinted 1958) 'A contribution to the study of the movements of the mandible.' *J. Prosthét. Dent. 8*, 41–54.

35 Benninghoff, A. and Staubesand, J. (Ed.) (1985) *Anatomie des Menschen*, Vol. 1, 14th Ed. München: Urban and Schwarzenberg.

36 Berger, M., Szalewski, L. and Szkutnik, J. (2017) 'Different association between specific manifestations of bruxism and temporomandibular disorder pain.' *Neurol. Neurochir. Pol. 51*, 1, 7–11.

37 Bergsmann, O. (1979) *Bioelektronische Funktionsdiagnostik*. Heidelberg: Haug.

38 Bernhardt, O., Gesch, D., Schwahn, C. et al. (2005) 'Risk factors for headache, including TMD signs and symptoms, and their impact on quality of life. Results of the Study of Health in Pomerania (SHIP).' *Quintessence. Int. 36*, 1, 55–64.

39 Berrett, A. (1983) 'Radiology of the temporomandibular joint.' *Dent. Clin. North Am. 27*, 3, 527–540.

40 Blackwood, H. J. J. (1969) 'Pathology of the temporomandibular joint.' *J. Am. Dent. Assoc. 79*, 118.

41 Blood, S. D. (1986) 'The craniosacral mechanism and the temporomandibular joint.' *J. Am. Osteopath. Assoc. 1986*, 8.

42 Boisserée, W. and Schupp, W. (2012) *Kraniomandibuläres und Muskuloskelettales System. Funktionelle Konzepte in der Zahnmedizin, Kieferorthopädie und Manualmedizin*. Berlin: Quintessenz, pp. 258–277.

43 Bonato, L. L., Quinelato, V., De Felipe Cordeiro, P. C. et al. (2017) 'Association between temporomandibular disorders and pain in other regions of the body.' *J. Oral Rehabil. 44*, 1, 9–15.

44 Boobennova, M. A. (1950) 'Innervation of the capsule of temporo-mandibular joint.' *Stomatolog. 2*, 3–13.

45 Bortoletto, C. C., Salgueiro, M. D. C. C., Valio, R. et al. (2017) 'The relationship between bruxism, sleep quality, and headaches in schoolchildren.' *J. Phys. Ther. Sci. 29*, 11, 1889–1892.

46 Bousema, E. J., Koops, E. A., van Dijk, P. et al. (2018) 'Association between subjective tinnitus and cervical spine or temporomandibular disorders. A systematic review.' *Trends Hear.* 2018; 22: 2331216518800640.

47 Bowbeer, G. (1993) *Facial Beauty and the TMJ, Part III*. Isle of Wight: Cranio-View.

48 Boyd, R. L., Gibbs, C. H., Mahan, P. E. et al. (1990) 'Temporomandibular forces measured at the condyle of macaca arctoides.' *Am. J. Orthod. Dentofacial. Orthop. 97*, 472–474.

49 Bracha, H. S. (2004) 'Freeze, fight, flight, fright, faint: adaptionist perspectives on the acute stress response spectrum.' *CNS Spectr. 9*, 679–685.

50 Bracha, H. S., Ralston, T. C., Matsukawa, J. M. et al. (2004) 'Does "fight or flight" need updating?' *Psychosomatics. 45*, 448–449.

51 Bracha, H. S., Bracha, A. S., Williams, A. E. et al. (2005a) 'The human fear-circuitry and fear-induced fainting in healthy individuals: the paleolithic threat hypothesis.' *Clin. Auton. Res. 15, 3*, 238–241.

52 Bracha, H. S., Ralston, T. C., Williams, A. E. et al. (2005b) 'The clenching-grinding spectrum and fear circuitry disorders: clinical insights from the neuroscience/paleoanthropology interface.' *CNS Spectr. 10*, 4, 311–318.

53 Brandini, D. A., Benson, J., Nicholas, M. K. et al. (2011) 'Chewing in temporomandibular disorder patients: an exploratory study of an association with some psychological variables.' *J. Orofac. Pain. 25*, 1, 56–67.

54 Brehnan, K., Boyd, R. L., Laskin, J. et al. (1981) 'Direct measurement of loads at the temporomandibular joint in macaca arctoides.' *J. Dent. Res. 60*, 1820–1824.

55 Breiner, M. (1999) *Whole Body Dentistry*. Fairfield: Quantum Health Press.

56 Breul, R., Mall, G., Landgraft, J. et al. (1999) 'Biomechanical analysis of stress distribution in the human temporomandibular-joint.' *Ann. Anat. 181*, 55–60.

57 Breul, R. (2002) 'Bau und Funktion des Kiefergelenks.' *Osteopath. Med. 1*, 12–16.

58 Breul, R. (1993) 'Die stellungsabhängige Beanspruchung des Kiefergelenks des Menschen. Eine biomechanische Analyse.' In: Benner, K., Fanghänel, J., Kowalewski, R., Kubein-Meesenburg, D. and Ranzio, J. (Ed.) *Morphologie, Funktion und Klinik des Kiefergelenks*. Berlin: Quintessenz, pp. 111–119.

59 Broich, I. (1999) 'Kieferorthopädie und Orthopädie: Fehlfunktionen im Mund-Kiefer-Bereich ganzheitlich diagnostizieren und behandeln.' *Manuelle Therapie. 3*, 32, 34.

60 Cahill, C. M. and Stroman, P. W. (2011) 'Mapping of neural activity produced by thermal pain in the healthy human spinal cord and brain stem: a functional magnetic resonance imaging.' *J. Magn. Reson. Imaging*. 29, 342–352.

61 Cailliet, R. (1992) *Head and Face Pain Syndromes*. Philadelphia, PA: F. A. Davis Co.

62 Caldas, W., Conti, A. C., Janson, G. and Conti, P. C. (2016) 'Occlusal changes secondary to temporomandibular joint conditions: a critical review and implications for clinical practice.' *J. Appl. Oral Sci. 24*, 4, 411–419.

63 Cardonnet, M. and Clauzade, M. (1987) 'Diagnostic différentiel des dysfonctions de l'ATM.' *Les Cahiers de Prothèse. 58*, 125–169.

64 Carlson, G. E. (1999) 'Epidemiology and treatment need for temporomandibular disorders.' *J. Orofac. Pain. 13*, 4, 232–237.

65 Carlsson, G. E., Kopp, S. and Öberg, T. (1979) 'Arthritis and allied diseases of the temporomandibular joint.' In: Zarb, G. A., Carlsson, G. E. (Ed.) *Temporomandibular Joint. Function and Dysfunction*. Copenhagen: Munksgaard, pp. 269–320.

66 Carlsson, G. E. and Öberg, T. (1974) 'Remodelling of the temporomandibular joint.' *Oral Sci. Rev. 6*, 53–86.

67 Castrillon, E. E., Ernberg, M., Cairns, B. E. et al. (2010) 'Interstitial glutamate concentration is elevated in the masseter muscle of myofascial temporomandibular disorder patients.' *J. Orofac. Pain. 24*, 2, 350–360.

68 Castrillon, E. E., Cairns, B. E., Wang, K. et al. (2012) 'Comparison of glutamate-evoked pain between the temporalis and masseter muscles in men and women.' *Pain. 153*, 4, 823–829.

69 Castroflorio, T., Bargellini, A., Rossini, G. et al. (2015) 'Risk factors related to sleep bruxism in children: a systematic literature review.' *Arch. Oral Biol. 60*, 11, 1618–1624.

70 Chauffour, P. and Prat, E. (2002) *Mechanical Link*. Florida: North Atlantic Books.

71 Cheifetz, A. T., Osganian, S. K., Allred, E. N. et al. (2005) 'Prevalence of bruxism and associated correlates in children as reported by parents.' *J. Dent. Child. 72*, 67–73.

72 Choi, J. K. (1992) 'A study on the effects of maximal voluntary clenching on the tooth contact points and masticatory muscle activities in patients with temporomandibular disorders.' *J. Craniomand. Disord. 6*, 41–46.

73 Choukas, N. C. and Sicher, H. (1960) 'The structure of the temporomandibular joint.' *Oral Surg. 12*, 1203–1213.

74 Chowdhury, T., Bindu, B., Singh, G. P. et al. (2017) 'Sleep disorders: is the trigemino-cardiac reflex a missing link?' *Front. Neurol. 8*, 63.

75 Chun, D. S. and Koskinen-Moffett, L. (1990) 'Distress, jaw habits and connective tissue laxity as predisposing factors to TMJ sounds in adolescents.' *J. Craniomand. Disord. 4*, 165–176.

76 Clark, G. T. (2008) 'Classification, causation and treatment of masticatory myogenous pain and dysfunction.' *Oral Maxillofac. Surg. Clin. North. Am. 20*, 145–157.

77 Clark, G. T., Rugh, J. D. and Handelman, S. L. (1980) 'Nocturnal masseter muscle activity and urinary catecholamine levels in bruxers.' *J. Dent. Res. 59*, 1571–1576.

78 Clark, G., Solberg, W. and Monteiro, A. A. (1988) 'Kiefergelenkbeschwerden. Neue Entwicklung in der klinischen Behandlung, in Forschung und Lehre.' In: Clark, G. and

Solberg, W. (Ed.) *Perspektiven der Kiefergelenkstörungen.* Berlin: Quintessenz, p. 17.

79 Clark, G. T., Seligman, D. A., Solberg, W. K. et al. (1989) 'Guidelines for the examination and diagnosis of temporomandibular disorders.' *J. Craniomandib. Disord. 3*, 7–14.

80 Colicchia, G. and Wiesner, H. (2000) 'Statik des Kauapparats von Reptilien und Säugetieren.' In: *Der mathematisch-naturwissenschaftliche Unterricht (MNU). 53*, 3, 158–163.

81 Contreras, E. F. R., Fernandes, G., Ongaro, P. C. J. et al. (2018) 'Systemic diseases and other painful conditions in patients with temporomandibular disorders and migraine.' *Braz. Oral Res. 32*, e77.

82 Costen, J. B. (1934) 'A syndrome of ear and sinus symptoms dependent upon disturbed function of the temporomandibular joint.' *Ann. Otol., Rhinol. and Laryngol. 18*, 1–15.

83 Couly, G., Brocheriou, C. and Vaillant, J. M. (1975) 'Les ménisques temporo-mandibulaires.' *Rev. Stomat. (Paris). 4*, 303–310.

84 Couly, G., Guilbert, F., Cernéa, P. et al. (1976) 'The temporomandibular joint in the newborn infant. Oto-meniscal relations.' *Rev. Stomatol. Chir. Maxillofac. 77*, 4, 673–684.

85 Couly, G., Hureau, J. and Vaillant, J. M. (1975) 'The dynamic complex of the temporomandibular meniscus.' *Rev. Stomatol. Chir. Maxillofac. 76*, 8, 597–605.

86 Couly, G. (1976) 'Articulations temporo-mandibulaires et interrelations fonctionnelles masticatrices.' *Actualités Odonto-Stomat. 50*, 233–252.

87 Craft, R. M. (2007) 'Modulation of pain by estrogens.' *Pain. 132*, Suppl. 1, 3–12.

88 Cruz-Fierro, N., Martínez-Fierro, M., Cerda-Flores, R. M. et al. (2018) 'The phenotype, psychotype and genotype of bruxism.' *Biomed. Rep. 8*, 3, 264–268.

89 Cunali, P. A., Almeida, F. R., Santos, C. D. et al. (2009) 'Prevalence of temporomandibular disorders in obstructive sleep apnea patients referred for oral appliance therapy.' *J. Orofac. Pain. 23*, 339–344.

90 Da Silva, C. G., Pachêco-Pereira, C., Porporatti, A. L. et al. (2016) 'The prevalence of temporomandibular disorders in children and adolescents.' *J. Am. Dent. Assoc. 147*, 1, 10–18.

91 De Boever, J. A. (1979) 'Functional disturbance of the temporomandibular joint.' In: Zarb, G. and Carlsson, G. (Ed.) *Temporomandibular Joint—Function and Dysfunction.* Copenhagen: Munksgaard, pp. 194–195.

92 De Laat, A., van Steenberghe, D. and Sesaffre, E. (1986) 'Occlusal relationships and temporo-mandibular joint dysfunction. Part II: Correlations between occlusal and articular parameters and symptoms of TMJ dysfunction by means of stepwise logistic regression.' *J. Prosthet. Dent. 55*, 116–121.

93 De Wijer, A., Lobbezzo-Scholte, A. M., Steenks, M. H. et al. (1995) 'Reliability of clinical findings in temporomandibular disorders.' *J. Orofac. Pain. 9*, 2, 181–191.

94 Delaire, J. et al. (1974) 'Considération sur la physiologie du ménisque temporo-mandibulaire.' *Rev. Stomat. 2*, 447–454.

95 Delaire, J. (1978) 'L'analyse architecturale et structurale cranio-faciale (de profil).' *Rev. Stomatol. 79*, 8.

96 Delattre, A. and Fenart, R. (1960) *L'Hominisation du crâne.* Paris: Centre National de la Recherche Scientifique.

97 Deutsche Gesellschaft für Zahnbehandlungsphobie: Fragen and Antworten. *Die häufigsten Fragen zum Thema Zahnarztphobie.* Internet: http://www.dgzp.de/faq.html. Accessed: 05.10.2018.

98 Diatchenko, L., Anderson, A. D., Slade, G. D. et al. (2006) 'Three major haplotypes of the b2 adrenergic receptor define psychological profile, blood pressure, and risk for development of a common musculoskeletal pain disorder.' *Am. J. Med. Gen. Neuropsychiatr. Gent. 141B*, 5, 449–461.

99 Diatchenko, L., Nackley, A. G., Tchivileva, I. E., Shabalina, S. A. and Maixner, W. (2007) 'Genetic architecture of human pain perception.' *Trends. Genet. 23*, 12, 605–613.

100 Dibbets, J. M. H. (1991) 'Wachstum und craniomandibuläre Dysfunktion.' In: Steenks, M. H. and Wijer, A. (Ed.) *Kiefergelenkfehlstellungen aus physiotherapeutischer und zahnmedizinischer Sicht: Diagnose und Therapie.* Berlin: Quintessenz.

101 DiGiovanna, E. L. and Schiowitz, S. (1997) *An Osteopathic Approach to Diagnosis and Treatment.* Philadelphia: Lippincott-Raven, p. 369.

102 Dobler, T. (2002) 'Diagnostik und Behandlung der Art. temporomandibularis.' In: Liem, T. and Dobler, T. (Ed.) *Leitfaden Osteopathie.* München: Urban and Fischer.

103 Doepel, M., Söderling, E., Ekberg, E. L. et al. (2009) 'Salivary cortisol and IgA levels in patients with myofascial pain treated with occlusal appliances in the short term.' *J. Oral Rehabil. 36*, 3, 210–216.

104 Donnelan, M. B., Burt, S. A., Levendosky, A. A. et al. (2008) 'Genes, personality, and attachment in adults: a multivariate behavioral genetic analysis.' *Pers. Soc. Psychol. Bull. 34*, 3–16.

105 Du Brul, E. L. (1964) 'Evolution of the temporomandibular joint.' In: Sarnat, B. G. (Ed.) *The Temporomandibular Joint*, 2nd Ed. Springfield: Charles C. Thomas, pp. 3–27.
106 Dworkin, S. F. and LeResche, L. (1992) 'Research diagnostic criteria for temporomandibular disorders: review, criteria, examinations and specifications, critique.' *J. Craniomandib. Disord. 6*, 4, 301–355.
107 Edwards, R. R., Grace, E., Peterson, S. et al. (2009) 'Sleep continuity and architecture: associations with pain-inhibitory processes in patients with temporomandibular joint disorder.' *Eur. J. Pain. 13*, 10, 1043–1047.
108 Effat, K. G. (2016) 'Otological symptoms and audiometric findings in patients with temporomandibular disorders: Costen's syndrome revisited.' *J. Laryngol. Otol. 130*, 12, 1137–1141.
109 van Eijden, T. M. G. J. and Koolstra, J. H. (1998) 'A model for mylohyoid muscle mechanics.' *J. Biomechan. 31*, 1017–1024.
110 End, E. (2005) *Die physiologische Okklusion des menschlichen Gebisses. Diagnostik und Therapie.* München: Neuer Merkur.
111 Ernberg, M. and Gerdle, B. (2014) 'Peripheral algesic substances in musculoskeletal pain assessed by microdialysis.' In: Graven-Nielsen, T. and Arendt-Nielsen, L. (Ed.) *Musculoskeletal Pain: Basic Mechanisms and Implications.* Washington, DC: IASP Press.
112 Eschler, J. (1970) 'L'influence des muscles masséter et ptérygoïdien interne sur le développement et la croissance de la mandibule.' *Actualités Odonto-Stomat. 89*, 7.
113 Escoto, M., O'Shaughnessy, T. and Yerkes, I. (2000) 'Functional Forum.' *Funct. Orthod. 17*, 32–34.
114 Every, R. G. (1975) 'Significance of tooth sharpness for mammalian, especially primate, evolution.' In: Szalay, F. S. (Ed.) *Approaches to Primate Paleobiology: Contributions to Primatology.* Basel: Karger, pp. 293–325.
115 Falla, D. (2004) 'Unravelling the complexity of muscle impairment in chronic neck pain.' *Manuelle Therapie. 9*, 3, 125–133.
116 Farella, M., Michelotti, A., Steenks, M. H. et al. (2000) 'The diagnostic value of pressure algometry in myofascial pain of the jaw muscles.' *J. Oral Rehabil. 27*, 1, 9–14.
117 Farrar, W. and McCarty, W. L. Jr. (1982) *A Clinical Outline of Temporomandibular Joint Diagnosis and Treatment.* Montgomery: Normandie Publications.
118 Farrar, W. (1978) 'Characteristics of the condylar path in internal derangements of the TMJ.' *J. Prosthet. Dent. 39*, 3, 319–323.
119 Farrar, W. (1971) *Diagnosis and Treatment of Anterior Dislocation of the Articular Disc.* New York: *J. Dent. 41*, 348.
120 Farrar, W. (1972) 'Differentiation of temporomandibular joint dysfunction to simplify treatment.' *J. Prosthet. Dent. 28*, 629.
121 Farrar, W. (1976) 'Dysfunctional centric relation of the jaw associated with dislocation and displacement of the disc.' *Compendium Amer. Equil. Soc. 13*, 272.
122 Faulkner, M. G., Hatcher, D. C. and Hay, A. (1987) 'A three-dimensional investigation of temporomandibular joint loading.' *J. Biomechan. 20*, 997–1002.
123 Fernandez-de-las-Peñas, C. and Svensson, P. (2016) 'Myofascial temporomandibular disorder.' *Curr. Rheumatol. Rev. 12*, 1, 40–54.
124 Fernández-de-las-Peñas, C., Galán del Río, F., Fernández Carnero, J. et al. (2009) 'Bilateral widespread mechanical pain sensitivity in myofascial temporomandibular disorder: evidence of impairment in central nociceptive processing.' *J. Pain. 10*, 11, 1170–1178.
125 Fernández-de-Las-Peñas, C., Galán-Del-Río, F., Alonso-Blanco, C. et al. (2010) 'Referred pain from muscle trigger points in the masticatory and neck-shoulder musculature in women with temporomandibular disorders.' *J. Pain. 11*, 12, 1295–1304.
126 Ferrario, V. F. and Sforza, C. (1994) 'Biomechanical model of the human mandible in unilateral clench: distribution of temporomandibular joint reaction forces between working and balancing sides.' *J. Prosthet. Dentistry. 72*, 169–176.
127 Ferré, J. C., Chevalier, C., Lumineau, J. P. et al. (1990) 'L'Ostéopathie crânienne, leurre ou réalité? Les Instantanés médicaux.' *Actual. Odontostomatol. (Paris). 44*, 171, 481–494.
128 Ferreira-Bacci Ado, V., Cardoso, C. L. and Díaz-Serrano, K. V. (2012) 'Behavioral problems and emotional stress in children with bruxism.' *Braz. Dent. J. 23*, 3, 246–251.
129 Fillingim, R. B., Ohrbach, R., Greenspan, J. D. et al. (2011) 'Potential psychosocial risk factors for chronic CMD: descriptive data and empirically identified domains from the OPPERA case-control study.' *J. Pain. 12*, Suppl. 11, T46–T60.
130 Fischer, L., Clemente, J. T. and Tambeli, C. H. (2007) 'The protective role of testosterone in the development of temporomandibular joint pain.' *J. Pain. 8*, 5, 437–442.
131 Fischer, L., Torres-Chávez, K. E., Clemente-Napimoga, J. T. et al. (2008) 'The influence of sex and ovarian hormones on temporomandibular joint nociception in rats.' *J. Pain. 9*, 7, 630–638.

132 Florencio, L. L., Oliveira, A. S., Carvalho, G. F. et al. (2017) 'Association between severity of temporomandibular disorders and the frequency of headache attacks in women with migraine. A cross-sectional study.' *J. Manipulative Physiol. Ther. 40*, 4, 250–254.

133 Fonder, A. (1990) *Dental Distress Syndrome.* Rock Falls: Medical Dental Arts.

134 Fonder, A. (1977) *The Dental Physician.* Blacksburg: University Publications.

135 Fossum, C. (2002) 'Allgemeine Diagnostik.' In: Liem, T. and Dobler, T. (Ed.) *Leitfaden Osteopathie.* München: Urban and Fischer.

136 Fraley, R. C., Roisman, G. I., Booth-LaForce, C. et al. (2013) 'Interpersonal and genetic origins of adult attachment styles: a longitudinal study from infancy to early adulthood.' *J. Pers. Soc. Psychol. 104*, 817–838.

137 France, R. D., Urban, B. J., Pelton, S. et al. (1987) 'CSF monoamine metabolites in chronic pain.' *Pain. 31*, 189.

138 Freimann, R. (1954) 'Untersuchungen über Zahl und Anordnung der Muskelspindeln in den Kaumuskeln des Menschen.' *Anat. Anz. 100*, 258–264.

139 Fricton, J. (2007) 'Myogenous temporomandibular disorders: diagnostic and management considerations.' *Dent. Clin. North. Am. 51*, 1, 61–83.

140 Fryette, H. H. (1994) *Principles of Osteopathic Technic.* California: AAO, pp. 234–241.

141 Gabutti, M. and Draper-Rodi, J. (2014) 'Osteopathic decapitation: why do we consider the head differently from the rest of the body? New perspectives for an evidence-informed osteopathic approach to the head.' *Int. J. Osteopath. Med. 17*, 4, 256–262.

142 Gallo, L. M., Airoldi, G. B., Airoldi, R. L. et al. (1997) 'Description of mandibular finite helical axis pathways in asymptomatic subjects.' *J. Dent. Res. 76*, 704–713.

143 Gallotta, S., Bruno, V., Catapano, S. et al. (2017) 'High risk of temporomandibular disorder in irritable bowel syndrome. Is there a correlation with greater illness severity?' *World. J. Gastroenterol. 23*, 1, 103–109.

144 Garliner, D. (1980) *Myofunktionelle Diagnose und Therapie der gestörten Gesichtsmuskulatur.* München: Zahnärztlich-Medizinisches-Schrifttum, p. 83.

145 Garry, J. F. (1985) 'Frühe iatrogene Dysfunktionen von orofazialen Muskeln, des Skeletts und des Kiefergelenks.' In: Morgan, D., House, L., Hall, W. and Vamvas, J. (Ed.) *Das Kiefergelenk und seine Erkrankungen.* Berlin: Quintessenz, pp. 94, 96.

146 Gastaldo, E., Quatrale, R., Graziani, A. et al. (2006) 'The excitability of the trigeminal motor system in sleep bruxism: a transcranial magnetic stimulation and brainstem reflex study.' *J. Orofac. Pain. 20*, 2, 145–155.

147 Gelb, H. and Goodheart, G. (1977) *Clinical Management of Head, Neck and TMJ Pain and Dysfunction.* Philadelphia: W. B. Saunders.

148 Gerstner, G. E., Gracely, R. H., Deebajah, A. et al. (2012) 'Posterior insular molecular changes in myofascial pain.' *J. Dent. Res. 91*, 5, 485–490.

149 Gerstner, G., Ichesco, E., Quintero, A. et al. (2011) Changes in regional gray and white matter volume in patients with myofascial-type temporomandibular disorders: a voxel-based morphometry study. *J. Orofac. Pain. 25*, 2, 99–106.

150 Gesch, D., Bernhardt, O., Alte, D. et al. (2004) 'Malokklusionen und klinische Zeichen sowie subjektive Symptome craniomandibulärer Dysfunktionen bei Erwachsenen. Ergebnisse der bevölkerungsrepräsentativen Study of Health in Pomerania (SHIP).' *Fortschr. Kieferorthop./J. Orofac. Orthop. 65*, 2, 88–103.

151 Gesch, D., Bernhardt, O., Mack, F. et al. (2005) 'Association of malocclusion and functional occlusion with subjective symptoms of TMD in adults: results of the Study of Health in Pomerania (SHIP).' *Angle. Orthod. 75*, 2, 183–190.

152 Gharaibeh, T. M., Jadallah, K. and Jadayel, F. A. (2010) 'Prevalence of temporomandibular disorders in patients with gastroesophageal reflux disease: a case-controlled study.' *J. Oral Maxillofac. Surg. 68*, 7, 1560–1564.

153 Giannakopoulos, N. N., Keller, L., Rammelsberg, P. et al. (2010) 'Anxiety and depression in patients with chronic temporomandibular pain and in controls.' *J. Dent. 38*, 5, 369–761.

154 Gibbs, C. H., Messerman, T., Reswick, J. B. and Derda, H. J. (1971) 'Functional movements of the mandible.' *J. Prosthet. Dent. 26*, 604–620.

155 Gill, H. I. (1971) 'Neuromuscular spindles in human lateral pterygoid muscles.' *J. Anat. 109*, 157–167.

156 Giraki, M., Schneider, C., Schafer, R. et al. (2010) 'Correlation between stress, stress-coping and current sleep bruxism.' *Head Face Med. 6*, 2.

157 Gonçalves, D. A. G., Bigal, M. E., Jales, L. C. F. et al. (2010) 'Headache and symptoms of temporomandibular disorder. An epidemiological study.' *Headache. 50*, 2, 231–241.

158 Goodson, J. M. and Johansen, E. (1975) 'Analysis of human mandibular movement.' *Monogr. Oral Sci. 5*, 1–80.

159 Gorayeb, M. A. M. and Gorayeb, R. (2002) 'Headache associated with indicators of anxiety in a sample of schoolchildren of Ribeirão Preto, SP, Brazil.' *Arq. Neuropsiquiatr. 60*, 764–768.

160 van Gorp, J. and Stöcker, D. (2017) 'Kraniozervikomandibulär bedingte Gleichgewichtsstörungen.' *Deutsche Zeitschrift für Osteopathie. 15*, 3, 13–18.

161 Graber, G. (1985) 'Was leistet die funktionelle Therapie und wo findet sie ihre Grenzen?' *Dtsch. Zahnärztl. Zeitschr. 40*, 165.

162 Graber, G. (1989) 'Der Einfluss von Psyche und Stress bei dysfunktionsbedingten Erkrankungen des stomatognathen Systems.' In: Hupfauf, L. (Ed.) *Funktionsstörungen des Kauorgans*, 2nd Ed. München: Urban and Schwarzenberg.

163 Graber, T. (1967) *Orthodontics: Principles and Practice*, 2nd Ed. Philadelphia: W. B. Saunders, p. 481.

164 Graven-Nielsen, T. and Mense, S. (2001) 'The peripheral apparatus of muscle pain: evidence from animal and human studies.' *Clin. J. Pain. 17*, 2–10.

165 Greenfield, B. E. and Wyke, B. (1966) 'Reflex innervation of the temporomandibular joint.' *Nature. 211*, 940–941.

166 Greenspan, J. D., Slade, G. D., Bair, E. et al. (2011) 'Pain sensitivity risk factors for chronic CMD: descriptive data and empirically identified domains from the OPPERA case control study.' *J. Pain. 12*, Suppl. 11, T61–T74.

167 Greenwood, L. F. (1987) 'Is temporomandibular joint dysfunction associated with generalized joint hypermobility.' *J. Prosthet. Dent. 58*, 6, 701–703.

168 Griffin, C. J. and Sharpe, C. J. (1960) 'The structure of the human temporomandibular meniscus.' *Austr. Dent. J. 6*, 35–39.

169 Guillaume, P. (1988) *Vision et posture II*. Paris: Agréssologie-Spei médical.

170 Gungormus, Z. and Erciyas, K. (2009) 'Evaluation of the relationship between anxiety and depression and bruxism.' *J. Int. Med. Res. 37*, 547–550.

171 Haberfellner, H. (1981) 'Wechselwirkung zwischen Gesamtkörperhaltung und Gesichtsbereich.' *Pädiatrie and Pädologie. 16*, 2, 203–225.

172 Hack, G. D., Dumm, G. and Toh, M. Y. (1998) 'The anatomist's new tools.' In: *Encyclopaedia Britannica Medical and Health Annual*. Chicago: NCMIC Insurance Co., pp. 16–29.

173 Häggman-Henrikson, B., List, T., Westergren, H. T. et al. (2013) 'Temporomandibular disorder pain after whiplash trauma. A systematic review.' *J. Orofac. Pain. 27*, 3, 217–226.

174 Hatala, M. P., Westesson, P. L., Tallents, R. H. et al. (1991) 'TMJ disc displacement in asymptomatic volunteers detected by MR imaging.' *J. Dent. Res. 70*, 278.

175 Hatcher, D. C., Faulkner, M. G. and Hay, A. (1986) 'Development of mechanical and mathematical models to study temporomandibular joint loading.' *J. Prosthet. Dent. 55*, 377–384.

176 Hellsing, G. and Holmlund, A. (1985) 'Development of anterior disk displacement in the temporomandibular joint: an autopsy study.' *J. Prosthet. Dent. 53*, 397–401.

177 Helluy, L. (1962) 'Étude cinématique et dynamique du jeu mandibulaire dans l'abaissement et l'élévation simples.' *Actual. Odonto-Stomat. 58*, 147–180.

178 Hesse, J. and Hansson, T. L. (1988) 'Factors influencing joint mobility in general and in particular respect of the craniomandibular articulation: a literature review.' *J. Craniomand. Disord.*, p. 1.

179 Hoffmann, E., Räder, C., Fuhrmann, H. and Maurer, P. (2013) 'Styloid-carotid artery syndrome treated surgically with Piezosurgery: a case report and literature review.' *J. Craniomaxillofac. Surg. 41*, 2, 162–166.

180 Honee, G. L. J. M. (1966) 'An investigation on the presence of muscle spindles in the human lateral pterygoid muscle.' *Ned. Tijdschr. Tandheilkd.* 73, Suppl. 3, 43–48.

181 Horst, O. V., Cunha-Cruz, J., Zhou, L. et al. (2015) 'Prevalence of pain in the orofacial regions in patients visiting general dentists in the Northwest Practice-based Research Collaborative in Evidence-based Dentistry research network.' *J. Am. Dent. Assoc. 146*, 10, 721–728.

182 Hruby, R. J. (1985) 'The total body approach to the osteopathic management of temporo-mandibular joint dysfunction.' *J. Am. Osteopath. Assoc. 8*.

183 Huang, G. J., LeResche, L., Critchlow, C. W. et al. (2002) 'Risk factors for diagnostic subgroups of painful temporomandibular disorders (TMD).' *J. Dent. Res. 81*, 4, 284–288.

184 Hülse, M. (2005) 'Die Bedeutung vertebragener Störungen im HNO-Bereich.' In: Hülse, M., Neuhuber, W. and

Wolff, H. D. (Ed.) *Die obere Halswirbelsäule*. Springer: Heidelberg, pp. 111–164.

185 Hugger, A. and Kordaß, B. (2018) *Handbuch Instrumentelle Funktionsanalyse und funktionelle Okklusion, Wissenschaftliche Evidenz und klinisches Vorgehen*. Berlin: Quintessenz, pp. 201–209.

186 Huguenin, L. (2004) 'Myofascial trigger points: the current evidence.' *Phys. Ther. Sport. 5*, 2–12.

187 Huijbers, A. J. M. (1991) 'Schienentherapie und Okklussionskorrekturen.' In: Steenks, M. H. and Wijer, A. de (Ed.) *Kiefergelenkfehlfunktionen aus physiotherapeutischer und zahnmedizinischer Sicht*. Berlin: Quintessenz, p. 47.

188 Hupfauf, L. (1989) 'Einführung in die Problematik funktionsbedingter Erkrankungen.' In: Hupfauf, L. (Ed.) *Funktionsstörungen des Kauorgans*, 2nd Ed. München: Urban and Schwarzenberg, p. 6.

189 Hylander, W. I. and Bays, R. (1979) 'An in vivo strain-gauge analysis of the squamosal-dentary joint reaction force during mastication and incisal biting in macaca mulatta and macaca fasciculans.' *Arch. Oral Biol. 24*, 689–697.

190 Ingelhard, M. R., Habil, P., Patel, M. H. et al. (2016) 'Self-reported temporomandibular joint disorder symptoms, oral health, and quality of life of children in kindergarten through grade 5.' *J. Am. Dent. Assoc. 147*, 131–141.

191 Insana, S. P., Gozal, D., McNeil, D. W. et al. (2013) 'Community based study of sleep bruxism during early childhood.' *Sleep Med. 14*, 183–188.

192 International Headache Society, IHS, ICD-10: G44.846. Internet: http://www.ihs-klassifikation.de/de/02_klassifikation/03_teil2/11.06.00_cranial.html. Accessed: 05.10.2018.

193 Isberg, A. and Isacsson, G. (1985) 'TMJ tissue reactions following retrusive guidance of the mandible.' *J. Dent. Res. 4*, 764.

194 Isberg, A., Widmalm, S. E. and Ivarsson, R. (1985) 'Clinical radiographical and electromyographical study of patients with internal derangement of the TMJ.' *J. Dent. Res. 4*, 764.

195 Isberg, A. M., Isacsson, G., Williams, W. N. et al. (1987) 'Lingual numbness and speech articulation deviation associated with temporomandibular joint disc displacement.' *Oral Surg. Oral Medic. Oral Pathol. 1*, 9–14.

196 Jasim, H., Louca, S., Christidis, N. et al. (2014) 'Salivary cortisol and psychological factors in women with chronic and acute orofacial pain.' *J. Oral Rehabil. 41*, 2, 122–132.

197 Jecmen, J. (1994) *Cranial Osteopathy—Sidebend and Dentistry*. Isle of Wight: Cranio-View.

198 Jensen, R., Rasmussen, B. K., Pedersen, B. et al. (1993) 'Prevalence of oromandibular dysfunction in a general population.' *J. Orofac. Pain. 7*, 2, 175–182.

199 John, M., Hirsch, C. and Reiber, T. (2003) 'Häufigkeit, Bedeutung und Behandlungsbedarf craniomandibularer Dysfunktionen (CMD).' *Z. Gesundh. Wiss. 9*, 136–155.

200 Jones, D. A., Rollman, G. and Brooke, R. (1997) 'The cortisol response to psychological stress in temporo-mandibular dysfunction.' *Pain. 72*, 1–2, 171–182.

201 Jull, G., Sterling, M., Kenardy, J. et al. (2007) 'Does the presence of sensory hypersensitivity influence outcomes of physical rehabilitation for chronic whiplash? A preliminary RCT.' *Pain. 129*, 1–2, 28–34.

202 Kahle-Nieke, B. (2009) *Einführung in die Kieferorthopädie: Diagnostik, Behandlungsplanung, Therapie*. Köln: Deutscher Zahnärzte Verlag.

203 Kaluza, C. L., Goering, E. K. and Kaluza, K. N. (2002) 'Osteopathischer Ansatz bei TMG-Dysfunktion.' *Osteopath. Med. 1*, 4–7.

204 Kampe, T. and Hannerz, H. (1991) 'Five-year longitudinal study of adolescents with intact and restored dentitions: signs and symptoms of temporomandibular dysfunction and functional recordings.' *J. Oral Rehabil. 18*, 387–398.

205 Kato, T. J. and Lavigne, G. J. (2010) 'Sleep bruxism: a sleep-related movement disorder.' *Sleep Med. Clin. 5*, 1, 9–35.

206 Katzenberg, R. W., David, A. K., Ten Eick, W. R. and Guralnick, W. C. (1983) 'Internal derangements of the temporomandibular joint: an assessment of condylar position in centric occlusion.' *Journal of Prosthetic Dentistry 49*, 2, 250–254.

207 Keith, D. A. (1982) 'Development of the human temporomandibular joint.' *Br. J. Oral Surg. 20*, 217–224.

208 Khan, H. S. and Stroman, P. W. (2015) 'Inter-individual differences in pain processing investigated by functional magnetic resonance imaging of the brainstem and spinal cord.' *Neuroscience. 307*, 231–241.

209 Khandelwal, S., Hada, Y. S. and Harsh, A. (2011) Eagle's syndrome—a case report and review of the literature. *Saudi. Dent. J. 23*, 4, 211–215.

210 Khoury, S., Rouleau, G. A., Rompre, P. H. et al. (2008) 'A significant increase in breathing amplitude precedes sleep bruxism.' *Chest. 134*, 332–337.

211 Kiehn, C. L. (1952) 'Meniscectomy for internal derangement of temporomandibular joint.' *Amer. J. Surg. 83*, 364.

212 Kikuchi, M., Watanabe, M. and Hattori, Y. 'Three dimensional bite force and associated masticatory muscle activities.'

213 Kindler, S., Samietz, S., Houshmand, M. et al. (2012) 'Depressive and anxiety symptoms as risk factors for temporomandibular joint pain: a prospective cohort study in the general population.' *J. Pain. 13*, 12, 1188–1197.

214 Kirk, W. S. Jr. (1989) 'Diagnostic disk dysfunction and tissue changes in the temporomandibular joint with magnetic resonance imaging.' *JADA. 119*, 527ff.

215 Kiser, D., Steemers, B., Branchi, I. et al. (2012) 'The reciprocal interaction between serotonin and social behaviour.' *Neurosci. Biobehav. Rev. 36*, 786–798.

216 Kleinberg, I. (1994) 'Bruxism: aetiology, clinical signs and symptoms.' *Aust. Prosthodont. J. 8*, 9–17.

217 Kleinknecht, R. A., Mahoney, E. R. and Alexander, L. D. (1987) 'Psychosocial and demographic correlates of temporomandibular disorders and related symptoms: an assessment of community and clinical findings.' *Pain. 29*, 173.

218 Klineberg, I. J. and Ash, M. M. (1980) 'Some temporomandibular articular reflex effects on jaw muscles.' *J. Dent. Res. 57*, 130.

219 Klineberg, I. J., Greenfield, B. E. and Wyke, B. (1970) 'Afferent discharges from temporomandibular articular mechanoreceptors: an experimental study in the cat.' *Arch. Oral Biol. 15*, 935–952.

220 Klineberg, I. J. (1980) 'Influences of temporomandibular articular mechanoreceptors on functional jaw movements.' *J. Oral Rehabil. 7*, 307–317.

221 Klobas, L., Tegelberg, A. and Axelsson, S. (2004) 'Symptoms and signs of temporomandibular disorders in individuals with chronic whiplash-associated disorders.' *Swed. Dent. J. 28*, 1, 29–36.

222 Knutson, G. A. (2003) 'Vectored upper cervical manipulation for chronic sleep bruxism, headache, and cervical spine pain in a child.' *J. Manipulative Physiol. Ther. 26*, 6, E1.

223 Kobayashi, Y. and Hansson, T. L. (1988) 'Auswirkungen der Okklusion auf den menschlichen Körper. Philip.' *J. Restaur. Zahnmed. 5*, 255–263.

224 Köhler, A. A., Hugoson, A. and Magnusson, T. (2013) 'Clinical signs indicative of temporomandibular disorders in adults: time trends and associated factors.' *Swed. Dent. J. 37*, 1, 1–11.

225 Köneke, C. (2010) *Craniomandibuläre Dysfunktion. Interdisziplinäre Diagnostik und Therapie.* Berlin: Quintessenz, pp. 187–196.

226 Koolstra, J. H., van Eijden, T. M. G. J., Weijs, W. A. et al. (1988) 'A three-dimensional mathematical model of the human masticatory system predicting maximum possible bite forces.' *J. Biomechan. 21*, 563–576.

227 Koolstra, J. H. and van Eijden, T. M. G. J. (1995) 'Biomechanical analysis of jaw closing movements.' *J. Dent. Res. 74*, 1564–1570.

228 Koolstra, J. H. and van Eijden, T. M. G. J. (1996) 'Influence of the dynamical properties of the human masticatory muscles on jaw closing movements.' *Europ. J. Morphol. 34*, 11–18.

229 Koolstra, J. H. and van Eijden, T. M. G. J. (1997) 'The jaw open-close movements predicted by biomechanical modelling.' *J. Biomechan. 30*, 943–950.

230 Koolstra, J. H. and Van Eijden, T. M. G. J. (1999) 'Three-dimensional dynamical capabilities of the human masticatory muscles.' *J. Biomechan. 32*, 145–152.

231 Kopp, S. (1989) 'Die Bedeutung der oberen Kopfgelenke bei der Ätiologie von Schmerzen im Kopf-, Hals-, Nackenbereich. Dtsch.' *Zahnärztl. Zeitschr. 44*, 12, 966–967.

232 Kopp, S. (2001) 'Neuroendocrine, immune, and local responses related to temporomandibular disorders.' *J. Orofac. Pain. 15*, 1, 9–28.

233 Korsun, A., Young, E. A., Singer, K., Carlson, N. E., Brown, M. B. and Crofford, L. (2002) 'Basal circadian cortisol secretion in women with temporomandibular disorders.' *J. Dent. Res. 81*, 4, 279–283.

234 Kraus, M., Lilienfein, W., Reinhart, E. et al. (1998) 'Das Kiefergelenk in der zahnärztlich-physiotherapeutischen Kombinationsbehandlung.' *Zeitschr. Physioth. 9*, 1545–1551.

235 Kroening, R. (1988) 'Die Leitungsanästhesie zur Differenzierung von craniofacialem Schmerz.' In: Clark, G. and Solberg, W. (Ed.) *Perspektiven der Kiefergelenkstörungen.* Berlin: Quintessenz, p. 137.

236 Krogh-Poulsen, W. (1967) 'Zusammenhänge zwischen Lokalisation von Abrasionsfacetten und Schmerzen in der Kaumuskulatur und deren Bedeutung für Diagnostik und Behandlung.' *Österr. Z. Stomatol. 64*, 402–404.

237 Krogh-Poulsen, W. and Troest, T. (1989) 'Form und Funktion im stomatognathen System.' In: Hupfauf, L. (Ed.)

Funktionsstörungen des Kauorgans. 2nd Ed. München: Urban and Schwarzenberg, p. 15.

238 Kubein-Meesenburg, D., Nägerl, H. and Fanghänel, J. (1991) 'Elements of a general theory of joints.' *Anat. Anz. 172*, 309–321.

239 Kummer, B. (1985) 'Anatomie und Biomechanik des Unterkiefers.' *Fortschr. Kieferorthop. 46*, 335–342.

240 Kurita, H. (2000) 'The relationship between the degree of disk displacement and ability to perform disk reduction.' *Oral Surg. Oral Med. Oral Pathol. 90*, 16–20.

241 Kurita, K., Westesson, P. L., Tasaki, M. et al. (1992) 'Temporomandibular joint: diagnosis of medial and lateral disk displacement with anteroposterior arthrography correlation with cryosections.' *Oral Surg. Oral Med. Oral Pathol. 73*, 364–368.

242 Lafrenière, C. M. (1997) 'The role of the lateral pterygoid muscles in TMJ disorders during static conditions.' *J. Craniomandib. Pract. 15*, 38–51.

243 Lai, W. F., Bowley, J. and Burch, J. G. (1998) 'Evaluation of shear stress of the human temporomandibular joint disc.' *J. Orofac. Pain. 12*, 2, 153–159.

244 Landeweer, G. G. (2001) 'Funktionelle Anatomie der Kaumuskeln.' *Update. 2*, 2, 20–24.

245 Landeweer, G. G. (2001) 'Können Spannungen im Tentorium cerebelli einen Einfluss auf die Diskusposition im Kiefergelenk haben?' *Update. 2*, 1, 21–23.

246 Landeweer, G. G. (2001) 'Untersuchungsmethoden zur Beurteilung von Funktionsveränderungen im Kausystem.' *Update. 2*, 2, 25–29.

247 Landry, M. L., Rompré, P. H., Manzini, C. et al. (2006) 'Reduction of sleep bruxism using a mandibular advancement device: an experimental controlled study.' *Int. J. Prosthodont. 19*, 549–556.

248 Landzberg, G., El-Rabbany, M., Klasser, G. D. et al. (2017) 'Temporomandibular disorders and whiplash injury. A narrative review.' *Oral Surg. Oral Med. Oral Pathol. Oral Radiol. 124*, 2, e37–e46.

249 Lang, J. (1995) *Clinical Anatomy of the Masticatory Apparatus and Peripharyngeal Spaces*. New York: Thieme.

250 Langendoen-Sertel, J. and Hamouda, M. (1998) 'Die Bedeutung des retrodiskalen Gewebes bei temporo-mandibulären Arthropathien.' *Manuelle Therapie. 19*, 1, 8–14.

251 von Lanz, T. and Wachsmuth, W. (1985) *Praktische Anatomie*, Vol. 1, Part A. Berlin: Springer, pp. 126, 215.

252 Laskin, D. M. (1969) 'Etiology of the pain dysfunction syndrome.' *J. Am. Dent. Assoc. 79*, 147.

253 Laughlin, J. D. (2002) 'Bodywide Influences of Dental Procedures. Part I.' *J. Bodywork and Movement Therapies. 1*, 9–16.

254 Lavigne, G. J., Rompré, P. H., Poirier, G. et al. (2001) 'Rhythmic masticatory muscle activity during sleep in humans.' *J. Dent. Res. 80*, 443–448.

255 Lavigne, G. J., Kato, T., Kolta, A. et al. (2003) 'Neurobiological mechanisms involved in sleep bruxism.' *Crit. Rev. Oral Biol. Med. 14*, 30–46.

256 Lavigne, G. J., Khoury, S., Abe, S. et al. (2008) 'Bruxism physiology and pathology: an overview for clinicians.' *J. Oral Rehabil. 35*, 7, 476–494.

257 Lawrence, E. S. and Razook, S. J. (1994) 'Nonsurgical management of mandibular disorders.' In: Kraus, L. S. (Ed.) *Temporomandibular Disorders*, 2nd Ed. New York: Churchill Livingstone, p. 130.

258 Lechner, J. (2002) *Armlängenreflex-Test und systemische Kinesiologie*. Kirchzarten: VAK.

259 Lejoyeux, J. (1987) 'Aspect comportemental morphologique et typologique du syndrôme algodysfonctionnel de appareil manducateur.' *Rev. Orthop. Dent. Facial. 21*, 561–578.

260 LeResche, L. (1997) 'Epidemiology of temporomandibular disorders: implications for the investigation of etiologic factors.' *Crit. Rev. Oral Biol. Med. 8*, 3, 291–305.

261 Levy, P. H. (1981) 'Physiologic response to dental malocclusion and misplaced mandibular posture: the keys to temporomandibular joint and associated neuromuscular disorders.' *Basal. Facts. 4*, 4, 103–122.

262 Lewit, K. (2010) *Manipulative Therapy*. Edinburgh: Elsevier.

263 Li, Y., Yu, F. N. L. and Long, Y. (2018) 'Association between bruxism and symptomatic gastroesophageal reflux disease. A case-control study.' *J. Dent. 77*, 51–58.

264 Liem, T. (2017) 'An osteopathic approach to the treatment of trauma and emotional integration.' In: Liem, T. and Van den Heede, P. (Ed.) *Foundations of Morphodynamics in Osteopathy*. Edinburgh: Handspring.

265 Liem, T. (2018) *Kraniosakrale Osteopathie. Ein praktisches Lehrbuch*, 7th Ed. Stuttgart: Thieme.

266 Liem, T. and Heede, P. (2017) *Foundations of Morphodynamics in Osteopathy*. Edinburgh: Handspring.

267 Lin, C. S. (2014) 'Brain signature of chronic orofacial pain: a systematic review and meta-analysis on neuroimaging research of trigeminal neuropathic pain and temporo-mandibular joint disorders.' *PLoS One. 9*, 4, e94300.

268 Linder-Aronson, S. (1970) 'Adenoids. Their effect on mode of breathing and nasal airflow and their relationship to characteristics of the facial skeleton and the dentition.' *Acta Otolaryngol. 1970*, 265.

269 List, T. and Axelsson, S. (2010) 'Management of TMD: evidence from systematic reviews and meta-analyses.' *J. Oral Rehabil. 37*, 6, 430–451.

270 Lobbenzoo, F., Rompré, P. H., Soucy, J. P. et al. (2001a) 'Lack of associations between occlusal and cephalometric measures, side imbalance in striatal D2 receptor binding, and sleep-related oromotor activities.' *J. Orofac. Pain. 15*, 64–71.

271 Lobbenzoo, F., van Dendersen, R. J., Verheij, J. G. et al. (2001b) 'Reports of SSRI-associated bruxism in the family physician's office.' *J. Orofac. Pain. 15*, 340–346.

272 Lobbenzoo, F., Ahlberg, J., Glaros, A. G. et al. (2013) 'Bruxism defined and graded: an international consensus.' *J. Oral Rehabil. 40*, 2–4.

273 Lobbenzoo, F., Visscher, C. M., Ahlberg, J. et al. (2014) 'Bruxism and genetics: a review of the literature.' *J. Oral Rehabil. 41*, 709–714.

274 Lobbenzoo, F., Ahlberg, J., Raphael, K. G. et al. (2018) 'International consensus on the assessment of bruxism: report of a work in progress.' *J. Oral Rehabil. 45*, 11, 837–844.

275 Long, J. A., Mark-Kurik, E. and Johanson, Z. (2015) 'Copulation in antiarch placoderms and the origins of gnathostome internal fertilization.' *Nature. 517*, 196–199.

276 Losert-Bruggner, B., Hülse, M. and Hülse, R. (2018) 'Fibromyalgia in patients with chronic CCD and CMD—a retrospective study of 555 patients.' *Cranio. 36*, 5, 318–326.

277 Louis, T. K., Douglas, A. O., Alexander, S. M. et al. (1987) 'Magnetic resonance imaging of the TMJ disc in asymptomatic volunteers.' *J. Oral Maxillofac. Surg. 45*, 852–854.

278 Lückerath, W. (1991) 'Die Bennettbewegung.' *Dtsch. Zahnärztl. Zeitschr. 46*, 189–193.

279 Machado, E., Dal-Fabbro, C., Cunali, P. A. et al. (2014) 'Prevalence of sleep bruxism in children: a systematic review.' *Dental Press J. Orthod. 19*, 6, 54–61.

280 Maghsudi, M. (2000) 'Untersuchung zur Validitat und diagnostischen Aussagekraft der ‚kleinen Funktionsanalyse' nach Krogh-Poulson als Screening-Test für kraniomandibulare Dysfunktionen.' Unpublished dissertation. Hamburg: University of Hamburg.

281 Magni, G. and Merskey, H. (1987) 'A simple examination of the relationships between pain, organic lesions and psychiatric illness.' *Pain. 29*, 295.

282 Magni, G. (1987) 'On the relationship between chronic pain and depression when there is no organic lesion.' *Pain. 31*, 1.

283 Magnusson, T. and Syrén, M. (1999) 'Therapeutic jaw exercises and interocclusal appliance therapy.' *Swed. Dent. J. 23*, 1, 27–37.

284 Magoun, H. I. (1976) *Osteopathy in the Cranial Field*, 3rd Ed. Kirksville, MO: Journal Printing Company, pp. 162f., 202.

285 Maixner, W., Fillingim, R., Booker, D. et al. (1995) 'Sensitivity of patients with painful temporo-mandibular disorders to experimentally evoked pain.' *Pain. 63*, 3, 341–351.

286 Manfredini, D., Guarda-Nardini, L., Winocur, E. et al. (2011) 'Research diagnostic criteria for temporomandibular disorders: a systematic review of axis I epidemiologic findings.' *Oral Surg. Oral Med. Oral Pathol. Oral Radiol. Endod. 112*, 4, 453–462.

287 Manfredini, D. and Lobbezoo, F. (2010) 'Relationship between bruxism and temporomandibular disorders: a systematic review of literature from 1998 to 2008.' *Oral Surg. Oral Med. Oral Pathol. Oral Radiol. Endod. 109*, e26–e50.

288 Manfredini, D., Restrepo, C. and Diaz-Serrano, K. (2013) 'Prevalence of sleep bruxism in children: a systematic review of the literature.' *J. Oral Rehabil. 40*, 8, 631–642.

289 Manfredini, D., Poggio, C. E. and Lobbezoo, F. (2014) 'Is bruxism a risk factor for dental implants? A systematic review of the literature.' *Clin. Implant. Dent. Relat. Res. 16*, 460–469.

290 Manfredini, D., Ahlberg, J., Mura, R. et al. (2015) 'Bruxism is unlikely to cause damage to the periodontium: findings from a systematic literature assessment.' *J. Periodontol. 86*, 546–555.

291 Marbach, J. J. (1996) 'Temporomandibular pain and dysfunction syndrome. History, physical examination, and treatment.' *Rheum. Dis. Clin. North Am. 22*, 3, 477–498.

292 Marguelles-Bonnet, R., Yung, J. P., Carpentier, P. et al. (1989) 'Temporomandibular joint serial sections made with mandible in intercuspal position.' *J. Cranio-mandib. Pract. 2*, 7, 97–106.

293 Marini, I., Paduano, S., Bartolucci, M. et al. (2013) 'The prevalence of temporomandibular disorders in patients with late whiplash syndrome who experience orofacial pain: a case-control series study.' *J. Am. Dent. Assoc. 144*, 5, 486–490.

294 Maronneaud, P. (1952) 'La constitution du squelette branchial méckelien primordial, ses variations phylogénétiques, les processus invoevolutifs observés à son niveau chez l'homme.' *Arch. Anat. Hist. Embryo. 34*, 285–295.
295 Marthol, H., Reich, S., Jacke, J. et al. (2006) 'Enhanced sympathetic cardiac modulation in bruxism patients.' *Clin. Auton. Res. 16*, 4, 276–280.
296 May, A. (2008) 'Chronic pain may change the structure of the brain.' *Pain. 137*, 1, 7–15.
297 McCormack, T. and Mansour, J. M. (1998) 'Reduction in tensile strength of cartilage precedes surface damage under repeated compressive loading in vivo.' *J. Biomechan. 31*, 55–61.
298 McNamara, J. A. (1976) 'The independent functions of the two heads of the lateral pterygoid muscle.' *Am. J. Anat. 138*, 197–206.
299 McNeely, M. L., Armijo Olivo, S. and Magee, D. J. (2006) 'A systematic review of the effectiveness of physical therapy interventions for temporomandibular disorders.' *Phys. Ther. 86*, 5, 710–725.
300 McNeill, C. (1997) *Science and Practice of Occlusion.* Chicago: Quintessence.
301 Messerman, T. (1967) 'A means for studying mandibular movements.' *J. Prosthet. Dent. 17*, 36–43.
302 Michelotti, A., Steenks, M. H., Farella, M. et al. (2004) 'The additional value of a home physical therapy regimen versus patient education only for the treatment of myofascial pain of the jaw muscles: short-term results of a randomized clinical trial.' *J. Orofac. Pain. 18*, 2, 114–125.
303 Michelotti, A., De Wijer, A., Steenks, M. et al. (2005) 'Home exercises regimes for the management of non-specific temporomandibular disorders.' *J. Oral Rehabil. 32*, 11, 779–785.
304 Michelotti, A., Farella, M., Stellato, A. et al. (2008) 'Tactile and pain thresholds in patients with myofascial pain of the jaw muscles: a case-control study.' *J. Orofac. Pain. 22*, 2, 139–145.
305 Miyawaki, S., Lavigne, G. J., Pierre, M. et al. (2003a) 'Association between sleep bruxism, swallowing-related laryngeal movement, and sleep positions.' *Sleep. 26*, 461–465.
306 Miyawaki, S., Tanimoto, Y., Araki, Y. et al. (2003b) 'Association between nocturnal bruxism and gastroespohageal reflux.' *Sleep. 26*, 888–892.
307 Moffett, B. (1957) 'The prenatal development of the human temporomandibular joint.' *Contr. Embryol. 36*, 21–28.
308 Mohl, N. D. and Davidson, R. M. (1990) *Okklusionskonzepte. Lehrbuch der Okklusion.* Berlin: Quintessenz.
309 Mohn, C., Vassend, O. and Knardahl, S. (2008) 'Experimental pain sensitivity in women with temporomandibular disorders and pain-free controls: the relationship to orofacial muscular contraction and cardiovascular responses.' *Clin. J. Pain. 24*, 4, 343–352.
310 Molitor, J. (1991) 'Untersuchungen über die Beanspruchung des Kiefergelenks.' *Z. Anat. Entw. Gesch. 129*, 109–140.
311 Mongini, F., Ciccone, G., Ceccarelli, M. et al. (2007) 'Muscle tenderness in different types of facial pain and its relation to anxiety and depression: a cross-sectional study on 649 patients.' *Pain. 131*, 1–2, 106–111.
312 Moraes, A. R., Sanches, M. L., Ribeiro, E. C. et al. (2013) 'Therapeutic exercises for the control of temporomandibular disorders.' *Dental. Press. J. Orthod. 18*, 5, 134–139.
313 Müller, J., Schmid, C. H., Bruckner, G. et al. (1992) 'Morphologisch nachweisbare Formen von intraartikulären Dysfunktionen der Kiefergelenke.' *Dtsch. Zahnärztl. Zeitschr. 47*, 416–423.
314 Mundt, T., Mack, F., Schwahn, C. et al. (2005) 'Gender differences in associations between occlusal support and signs of temporomandibular disorders: results of the population-based Study of Health in Pomerania (SHIP).' *Int. J. Prosthodont. 18*, 3, 232–239.
315 Murray, C. G. and Sanson, G. D. (1998) 'Thegosis—a critical review.' *Aust. Dent. J. 43*, 192–198.
316 Myers, T. W. (2001) *Anatomy Trains.* Edinburgh: Churchill Livingstone.
317 Nadendla, L. K., Meduri, V., Paramkusam, G. et al. (2014) 'Evaluation of salivary cortisol and anxiety levels in myofascial pain dysfunction syndrome.' *Korean J. Pain. 27*, 1, 30–34.
318 Nägerl, H., Kubein-Meesenburg, D., Fanghänel, J. et al. (1991) 'Die posteriore Führung der Mandibula als neuromuskulär gegebene innere Gelenkkette.' *Dtsch. Stomat. 41*, 279–283.
319 Nägerl, H. and Kubein-Meesenburg, D. (1990) 'Comparative examination of the determination of the individual contour-curve from the incisors and from the premolar region.' *Anat. Anz. 170*, 163–170.
320 Nanda, R. S. and Nanda, S. K. (1992) 'Considerations of dentofacial growth in long-term retention and stability: is

active retention needed?' *Am. J. Orthod. Dentofacial. Orthop. 101*, 4, 297–302.

321 Nell, A., Niebauer, W., Sperr, W. et al. (1994) 'Special variations of the lateral ligament of the human TMJ.' *Clin. Anat. 7*, 267–270.

322 Newberry, W. N., Mackenzie, C. D. and Haut, R. C. (1998) 'Blunt impact causes changes in bone and cartilage in a regularly exercised animal model.' *J. Orthop. Res. 16*, 348–354.

323 Nickel, J. C., McLachlan, K. R. and Smith, D. M. (1998) 'A theoretical model of loading and eminence development of the postnatal human temporomandibular joint.' *J. Dent. Res. 67*, 903–910.

324 Nickel, F. T., Seifert, F., Lanz, S. et al. (2012) 'Mechanisms of neuropathic pain.' *Eur. Neuropsychopharmacol. 22*, 2, 81–91.

325 Nicolakis, P., Erdogmus, B., Kopf, A. et al. (2002) 'Effectiveness of exercise therapy in patients with myofascial pain dysfunction syndrome.' *J. Oral Rehabil. 29*, 4, 362–368.

326 Nijs, J. and Van Houdenhove, B. (2009) 'From acute musculoskeletal pain to chronic widespread pain and fibromyalgia: application of pain neurophysiology in manual therapy practice.' *Manuelle Therapie. 14*, 1, 3–12.

327 Nilner, M. (1992) 'Epidemiologic studies in TMD.' In: McNeill, C. (Ed.) *Current Controversies in Temporomandibular Disorders*. Chicago: Quintessence, pp. 21–26.

328 Oeconomos, O. (1932) 'Le ménisque et les surfaces articulaires temporo-mandibulaires chez quelques animaux domestiques.' *C.R.A.A.*, p. 427.

329 Ohayon, M. M., Li, K. K. and Guilleminault, C. (2001) 'Risk factors for sleep bruxism in the general population.' *Chest. 119*, 53–61.

330 Ohlendorf, D., Pusch, K. and Kopp, S. (2008) 'Beinlängendifferenz versus zentrische Lage des Unterkiefers.' *Man. Med. 46*, 6, 418–423.

331 Ohrbach, R. and Dworkin, S. F. (2016) 'The evolution of TMJ diagnosis: past, present, future.' *J. Dent. Res. 95*, 10, 1093–1101.

332 Ojima, K., Watanabe, N., Narita, N. et al. (2007) 'Temporomandibular disorder is associated with a serotonin transporter gene polymorphism in the Japanese population.' *Biopsychosocial. Med. 1*, 3.

333 Oliveira, M. T., Bittencourt, S. T., Marcon, K. et al. (2015) 'Sleep bruxism and anxiety level in children.' *Braz. Oral Res. 29*, 1, 1–5.

334 Olmos, S. R. (2016) 'Comorbidities of chronic facial pain and obstructive sleep apnea.' *Curr. Opin. Pulm. Med. 22*, 570–575.

335 Olmos, S. R., Kritz-Silverstein, D., Halligan, W. et al. (2005) 'The effect of condyle fossa relationships on head posture.' *Cranio. 23*, 48–52.

336 Ommerborn, M. A., Schneider, C., Giraki, M. et al. (2007) 'Effects of an occlusal splint compared with cognitive-behavioral treatment on sleep bruxism activity.' *Eur. J. Oral Sci. 115*, 7–14.

337 Oporto, G. H., Lagos, J. D., Bornhardt, T. et al. (2012) 'Are there genetic factors involved in bruxism?' *Int. J. Odontostomat. 6*, 249–254.

338 Oporto, G. H., Bornhardt, T., Iturriaga, V. et al. (2016) 'Genetic polymorphisms in the serotonergic system are associated with circadian manifestations of bruxism.' *J. Oral Rehabil. 43*, 11, 805–812.

339 Ortiz, M. I., Rangel-Barragan, R. O., Contreras-Ayala, M. et al. (2014) 'Procedural pain and anxiety in pediatric patients in a Mexican dental clinic.' *Oral Health Dent. Manag. 13*, 495–501.

340 O'Ryan, F. and Epker, B. N. (1984) 'Temporomandibular joint function and morphology: observations on the spectra of normalcy.' *Oral Surg. 58*, 272–279.

341 Ostry, D. J. and Flanagan, J. R. (1989) 'Human jaw movement in mastication and speech.' *Arch. Oral Biol. 34*, 685–693.

342 Paesani, D., Westesson, P. L., Hatala, M. et al. (1992) 'Prevalence of temporomandibular joint internal derangement in patients with craniomandibular disorders.' *Am. J. Orthod. Dentofac. Orthop. 101*, 41–47.

343 Page, D. C. (2001) 'Breastfeeding is early functional jaw orthopedics (an introduction).' *Funct. Orthod. 18*, 3, 24–27.

344 Perl, E. R. (1984) 'Advances in pain research and therapy.' In: Kruger, L. and Liebeskind, J. C. (Ed.) *Neural Mechanisms of Pain*, Vol. 6. New York: Raven Press, pp. 23–51.

345 Perlemuter, L. and Waligora, J. (1980) *Cahiers d'anatomie 1, système nerveux central*. Paris: Masson.

346 Petit, D., Touchette, E., Tremblay, R. E. et al. (2007) 'Dyssomnias and parasomnias in early childhood.' *Pediatrics. 119*, 1016–1025.

347 Petrovic, A. and Charlier, J. P. (1967) 'La synchondrose sphéno-occipitale de jeune rat en culture d'organes: mise en

évidence d'un potentiel de croissance indépendant.' Paris: C. R. Acad. Sc., pp. 1511–1513.
348 Pfau, D. B., Rolke, R., Treede, R. D. et al. (2009) 'Somatosensory profiles in subgroups of patients with myogenic temporomandibular disorders and fibromyalgia syndrome.' *Pain. 147*, 1–3, 72–83.
349 von Piekartz, H. J. M. (2001) 'Vorschlag für einen neurodynamischen Test des N. mandibularis Reliabilität und Referenzwerte.' *Manuelle Therapie. 5*, 56–66.
350 Plato, G. and Kopp, S. (1996) 'Das Dysfunktionsmodell: Gedanken zum Therapieansatz in der Manuellen Medizin.' *Man. Med. 34*, 1–8.
351 Posselt, U. (1968) *Physiology of Occlusion and Rehabilitation*, 2nd Ed. Oxford: Blackwell Scientific Publications.
352 Krogh-Poulsen, W. (1966) 'Die Bewegungsanalyse.' *Dtsch. Zahnärztl. Zeitschr. 21*, 877–880.
353 Poveda Roda, R., Díaz Fernández, J. M., Hernández Bazán, S. et al. (2008) 'A review of temporomandibular joint disease—Part II: Clinical and radiological semiology. Morbidity processes. *Med. Oral Patol. Oral Cir. Bucal. 13*, 2, E102–E109.
354 Poveda-Roda, R., Bagan, J. V., Sanchis, J. M. et al. (2012) 'Temporomandibular disorders: a case-control study.' *Med. Oral Patol. Oral Cir. Bucal. 17*, 5, 794–800.
355 Prätorius, O. (2015) 'Die Einflüsse der Kieferorthopädie auf die Haltung des Menschen aus orthopädisch/osteopathischer Sicht.' *Umwelt Medizinische Gesellschaft. 28*, 172–178.
356 Pretty, I. A. and Hall, R. C. (2002) 'Forensic dentistry and human bite marks: issues for doctors.' *Hosp. Med. 63*, 476–482.
357 Price, W. A. (1997) *Nutrition and Physical Degeneration*. Connecticut: Price-Pottenger Nutrition Foundation Keats.
358 Pringle, J. (1918) 'Displacement of the mandibular meniscus and its treatment.' *Brit. J. Surg. 6*, 385.
359 Quinn, J. H. (1995) 'Mandibular exercises to control bruxism and deviation problems.' *J. Craniomandibular Pract. 13*, 1, 30–34.
360 Ralli, M., Altissimi, G., Turchetta, R. et al. (2016) 'Somatosensory tinnitus. Correlation between cranio-cervico-mandibular disorder history and somatic modulation.' *Audiol. Neurootol. 21*, 6, 372–382.
361 Rantala, M. A. (2003) 'Temporomandibular joint related painless symptoms, orofacial pain, neck pain, headache, and psychosocial factors among non-patients.' *Acta. Odontol. Scand. 61*, 4, 217–222.
362 Reddy, S. V., Kumar, M. P., Sravanthi, D. et al. (2014) 'Bruxism: a literature review.' *J. Int. Oral Health. 6*, 6, 105–109.
363 Rees, L. A. (1954) 'The structure and function of the mandibular joint.' *Br. Dent. J. 96*, 125–133.
364 Restrepo, C. C., Vásquez, L. M., Alvarez, M. et al. (2008) 'Personality traits and temporomandibular disorders in a group of children with bruxing behaviour.' *J. Oral Rehabil. 35*, 585–593.
365 Restrepo, C., Gomez, S. and Manrique, R. (2009) 'Treatment of bruxism in children: a systematic review.' *Quintessence Int. 40*, 10, 849–855.
366 Ricketts, R. (1969) 'Occlusion—the medium of dentistry.' *J. Prostmet. Dent. 21*, 154.
367 Riley, J. L., Benson, M. B., Gremillion, H. A. et al. (2002) 'Sleep disturbance in orofacial pain patients: pain-related or emotional distress?' *TMD. Sleep. 19*, 2, 106–113.
368 Ringhof, S., Hellmann, D., Meier, F. et al. (2015) 'The effect of oral motor activity on the athletic performance of professional golfers.' *Front. Psychol. 6*, 750.
369 Robert, M., Little, R. M., Riedel, R. A. et al. (1988) 'An evaluation of changes in mandibular anterior alignment from 10 to 20 years postretention.' *Am. J. Orthod. Dentofacial. Orthop. 93*, 423–428.
370 Rohen, J. W. (1988) *Anatomie für Zahnmediziner*, 2nd Ed. Stuttgart: Schattauer, pp. 113–114.
371 Rohen, J. W. (2002) *Morphologie des menschlichen Organismus*, 2nd Ed. Stuttgart: Verlag Freies Geistesleben, pp. 368f.
372 Sadowsky, C. (1984) 'Temporomandibular disorders and functional occlusion after orthodontic treatment: results of two long-term studies.' *Amer. J. Orthod. 5*, 86, 386ff.
373 Sanders, A. E., Essick, G. K., Fillingim, R. et al. (2013) 'Sleep apnea symptoms and risk of temporomandibular disorder: OPPERA cohort.' *J. Dent. Res. 92*, 70S–77S.
374 Santiesteban, J. (1989) 'Isometric exercises and a simple appliance for temporomandibular joint dysfunction: a case report.' *Phys. Ther. 69*, 6, 463–466.
375 Santos Miotto Amorim, C., Firsoff, E. F., Vieira, G. F. et al. (2014) 'Effectiveness of two physical therapy interventions, relative to dental treatment in individuals with bruxism: study protocol of a randomized clinical trial.' *Trials. 15*, 8.

376 Santos Silva, R. S., Conti, P. C., Lauris, J. R. et al. (2005) 'Pressure pain threshold in the detection of masticatory myofascial pain: an algometer-based study.' *J. Orofac. Pain. 19*, 4, 318–324.

377 Sarlani, E. and Greenspan, J. (2003) 'Evidence for generalized hyperalgesia in temporo-mandibular disorders patients.' *Pain. 102*, 3, 221–226.

378 Sarlani, E., Grace, E. G., Reynolds, M. A. et al. (2004) 'Evidence for up-regulated central nociceptive processing in patients with masticatory myofascial pain.' *J. Orofac. Pain. 18*, 1, 41–55.

379 Sarnat, B. (1964) *The Temporomandibular Joint*. Springfield: Charles C. Thomas, pp. 133–184.

380 Scapino, R. P., Canham, P. B., Finlay, H. M. et al. (1996) 'The behaviour of collagen fibers in stress relaxation and stress distribution in the jaw-joint disc of rabbits.' *Archives of Oral Biology. 41*, 1039–1052.

381 Schiffman, E. L., Fricton, J. R. and Haley, D. (1992) 'The relationship of occlusion, parafunctional habits and recent life events to mandibular dysfunction in a non-patient population.' *J Oral Rehabil. 19*, 3, 201–223.

382 Schiffman, E., Ohrbach, R., Truelove, E. et al. (2014) 'Diagnostic Criteria for Temporomandibular Disorders (DC/CMD) for clinical and research applications: recommendations of the International RDC/CMD Consortium Network and Orofacial Pain Special Interest Group.' *J. Oral Facial. Pain. Headache. 28*, 1, 6–27.

383 Schindler, H. J. and Türp, J. C. (2017) *Konzept Okklusionsschiene. Basistherapie bei schmerzhaften kraniomandibulären Dysfunktionen*. Berlin: Quintessenz, pp. 91–107.

384 Schindler, H. J., Hugger, A., Hellmann, D. et al. (2013) 'Die Schienentherapie bei Myoarthropathien des Kausystems.' *Quintessenz Zahntech. 39*, 11, 1505–1516.

385 Schleip, R. Persönliche schriftliche Kommunikation mit Robert Schleip, 10.04.2017.

386 Schmitter, M., Rammelsberg, P. and Hassel, A. (2005) 'The prevalence of signs and symptoms of temporomandibular disorders in very old subjects.' *J. Oral Rehabil. 32*, 7, 467–473.

387 Schmolke, C. (1994) 'The relationship between the temporomandibular joint capsule, articular disc and jaw muscles.' *J. Anat. 184*, 2, 335–345.

388 Schöttl, W. (1991) *Die cranio-mandibuläre Regulation*. Heidelberg: Hüthig.

389 Schroeder, H., Siegmund, H. and Santibánez, H. (1991) 'Causes and signs of temporomandibular joint pain and dysfunction: an electromyographical investigation.' *J. Oral Rehabilit. 18*, 301–310.

390 Schumacher, G. H. (1997) *Anatomie für Zahnmediziner*. Heidelberg: Hüthig.

391 Schumacher, G. H. (1991) *Anatomie: Lehrbuch und Atlas. 1. Kopf, orofaziales System, Auge, Ohr, Leitungsbahnen*, 2nd Ed. Leipzig: J. A. Barth.

392 Schwartz, L. L. and Tausig, D. P. (1954) 'Temporomandibular joint pain—treatment with intramuscular infiltration of tetracaine hydrochloride: a preliminary report.' *NY State Dent. J. 20*, 219–223.

393 Schwartz, L. L. (1958) 'Conclusions of the temporomandibular joint clinic at Columbia.' *J. Periodontol. 5*, 210–212.

394 Schwarz, L. and Chayes, C. M. (Ed.) (1968) *Facial Pain and Mandibular Dysfunction*. Philadelphia: Saunders.

395 Schwarz, L. (1968) 'The pain-dysfunction syndrome.' In: Schwarz, L. and Chayes, C. M. (Ed.) *Facial Pain and Mandibular Dysfunction*. Philadelphia: Saunders.

396 Sebald, W. G. (2000) 'Cranio-mandibuläre Dysfunktion. Versuch einer bewertenden Übersicht.' *Z. Bay. 9*, 35–40.

397 Sebald, W. G. and Kopp, S. (1996) *Funktionsstörungen und Schmerzphänomene des craniomandibulären Systems (CMS). Grundlagen und Basisdiagnostik*. Jena: Silvia Kopp.

398 Seider, R. (1999) 'Der Einfluss von kraniosakraler Therapie auf den Bewegungsumfang entfernt liegender großer Gelenke, bei Zustand nach kieferorthopädischer Zahnstellungskorrektur mittels Zahnspange.' Diplomarbeit. Hamm.

399 Seligmann, D. A. and Pullinger, A. G. (1991) 'The role of intercuspal occlusal relationships in temporomandibular disorders: a review.' *J. Craniomandib. Disord. Facial Oral Pain. 5*, 96–106.

400 Seraidarian, P., Seraidarian, P. I., das Neves Cavalcanti, B. et al. (2009) 'Urinary levels of catecholamines among individuals with and without sleep bruxism.' *Sleep Breath. 13*, 85–88.

401 Shah, J. P. (2008) 'Integrating dry needling with new concepts of myofascial pain, muscle physiology, and sensitization.' In: Audette, J. F. and Bailey, A. (Ed.) *Integrative Pain Medicine: The Science and Practice of Complementary and Alternative Medicine in Pain Management*. Totowa, NJ: Humana Press, pp. 107–121.

402 Shaper, E. P. (1985) 'Aspekte bei der Behandlung von Muskelspasmen.' In: Morgan, D., House, L., Hall, W. and Vamvas, J. *Das Kiefergelenk und seine Erkrankungen*. Berlin: Quintessenz.

403 Sheldrake, R. (1988, updated and revised 2012) *The Presence of the Past: Morphic Resonance and the Habits of Nature*. New York: Times Books.

404 Shore, N. (1959) *Occlusal Equilibration and Temporomandibular Joint Dysfunction*. Philadelphia: J. B. Lippincott.

405 Sicher, H. and Dubral, L. E. (1970) *Oral Anatomy*, 5th Ed. St. Louis: Mosby.

406 Silver, C. M., Simon, S. D. and Savastano, A. A. (1956) 'Meniscus injuries of the temporomandibular joint.' *J. Bone Surg. 38*, 54.

407 Silver, C. M. and Simon, S. D. (1963) 'Meniscus injuries of the temporomandibular joint: further experience.' *J. Bone and Joint. Surg. 45*, 113.

408 Silverman, J. L., Rodriquez, A. A. and Agre, J. C. (1991) 'Quantitative cervical flexor strength in healthy subjects and in subjects with mechanical neck pain.' *Arch. Phys. Med. Rehabil. 72*, 9, 679–681.

409 Slade, G. D., Fillingim, R. B., Sanders, A. E. et al. (2013) 'Summary of findings from the OPPERA prospective cohort study of incidence of first-onset temporomandibular disorder: implications and future directions.' *J. Pain. 14*, Suppl. 12, T116–T124.

410 Slavicek, R. (1982) 'La "soi-disant" relation centrée.' *Rev. Orthop. Dento. Fac. 16*, 413–415.

411 Slavicek, R. (1983) 'Les principes de l'occlusion.' *Rev. Orthop. Dento. Faciale. 17*, 449–490.

412 Slegter, R. and Azouman, M. (1993) 'Observation of the anterior loop of the inferior alveolar canal.' *International J. Oral Maxillofac. Implants. 7*, 295–300.

413 Smith, D. M., McLachlan, K. R. and McCall, W. D. (1986) 'A numerical model of temporomandibular joint loading.' *J. Dent. Res. 65*, 1046–1052.

414 Smith, M. R., Wickwire, E. M., Grace, E. G. et al. (2009) 'Sleep disorders and their association with laboratory pain sensitivity in temporomandibular joint disorder.' *Sleep. 32*, 779–790.

415 Smith, M. T., Wickwire, E. M., Grace, E. G. et al. (2009) 'Sleep disorders and their association with laboratory pain sensitivity in temporomandibular joint disorder.' *Sleep. 32*, 6, 779–790.

416 Smith, R. D. and Marcarian, H. Q. (1967) 'The neuromuscular spindles of the lateral pterygoid muscle.' *Anat. Anz. 120*, 47–53.

417 Smith, S. B., Mir, E., Bair, E. et al. (2013) 'Genetic variants associated with development of TMD and its intermediate phenotypes: the genetic architecture of TMD in the OPPERA prospective cohort study.' *J. Pain. 14, Suppl. 12*, T91–T101.

418 Smith, S. D. (1981) 'Structural and facial influences on TMJ apparatus.' *J. Am. Osteopath. Assoc. 10*.

419 Solberg, W. K. and Clark, G. T. (Ed.) (1983) *Kiefergelenk—Diagnostik und Therapie*. Berlin: Quintessenz, p. 152.

420 Solberg, W. K. and Clark, G. T. (1985) *Kiefergelenkfunktion. Diagnostik und Therapie*. Berlin: Quintessenz.

421 Solberg, W. K., Hansson, T. L. and Nordstroem, B. (1985) 'The temporomandibular joint in young adults at autopsy: a morphologic classification and evaluation.' *J. Oral Rehab. 12*, 303.

422 Solow, B. and Siersbaek-Nielsen, S. (1986) 'Growth changes in head posture related to craniofacial development.' *Am. J. Orthod. 89*, 132–140.

423 Spadaro, A., Ciarrocchi, I., Masci, C. et al. (2014) 'Effects of intervertebral disc disorders of low back on the mandibular kinematic. Kinesiographic study.' *BMC Res. Notes*. 2014; 7: 569.

424 Sperber, G. H. (1992) *Embryologie des Kopfes*. Berlin: Quintessenz, p. 370.

425 Starck, D. (1987) *Embryologie*, 3rd Ed. Stuttgart: Thieme.

426 Steinfurth, G. (2002) 'Einfluss osteopathischer Dysfunktionen der Ossa temporalia auf die maximale aktive Mundöffnung. Diplom SKOM, DAO, Düsseldorf, 2001.' *Osteop. Med. 4*, 16–21.

427 Stelzenmüller, W. and Wiesner, J. (2010) *Therapie von Kiefergelenkschmerzen: ein Behandlungskonzept für Zahnärzte*. Stuttgart: Thieme, pp. 253, 264.

428 Stepan, L., Shaw, C. L. and Oue, S. (2017) 'Temporomandibular disorder in otolaryngology: systematic review.' *J. Laryngol. Otol. 131*, S1, 50–56.

429 Still, A. T. (1992) *Osteopathy, Research and Practice*. Seattle: Eastland Press, pp. 199–200.

430 Strachan, F. and Robinson, M. J. (1965) 'Short leg linked to malocclusion.' *Osteopath. News, 1965*, 4.

431 Strauss, F., Christen, A. and Weber, W. (1960) 'The architecture of the disc of the human temporomandibular joint.' *Helv. Odontol. Acta. 4*, 1–4.

432 Sutherland, W. G. (1939) *The Cranial Bowl*. Monkato, Minnesota: Free Press Company, pp. 99–100.

433 Svensson, P., List, T. and Hector, G. (2001) 'Analysis of stimulus-evoked pain in patients with myofascial temporomandibular pain disorders.' *Pain. 92*, 3, 399–409.

434 Tan, E. K. (2003) 'Severe amphetamine-induced bruxism: treatment with botulinum toxin.' *Acta Neurol. Scand. 107*, 161–163.

435 Tanaka, T. T. (1992) 'TMJ microanatomy: an anatomy approach to current controversies. An educational videotape.' Chula Vista, CA: Clinical Research Foundation.

436 Tanaka, T. T. (1988) 'Advanced dissection of the temporomandibular joint. An educational videotape.' Chula Vista, CA: Clinical Research Foundation.

437 Tasaki, M., Westesson, P. L., Isberg, A., Ren, Y. F. and Tallents, R. (1996) 'Classification and prevalence of temporomandibular joint disk displacement in patients and symptom-free volunteers.' *Am. J. Orthod. Dentofac. Orthop. 109*, 3, 249–296.

438 Teutsch, S., Herken, W., Bingel, U., Schoell, E. and May, A. (2008) 'Changes in brain gray matter due to repetitive painful stimulation.' *Neuroimage. 42*, 2, 845–849.

439 Thie, N. M. R., Kato, T., Bader, G. et al. (2002) 'The significance of saliva during sleep and the relevance of oromotor movements.' *Sleep Med. Rev. 6*, 213–227.

440 Thoma, K. H. (1958) *Oral Surgery*. St. Louis: Mosby, pp. 705f.

441 Throckmorton, G. S. and Dechow, P. C. (1994) 'In vitro measurements in the condylar process of the human mandible.' *Arch. Oral Biology. 39*, 853–867.

442 Tillmann, B. (1997) *Farbatlas der Anatomie. Zahnmedizin-Humanmedizin*. Stuttgart and New York: Thieme.

443 Travell, J. G. and Simons, D. G. (1983) *Myofascial Pain and Dysfunction*, Vol. 1. Baltimore: Williams and Wilkins.

444 von Treuenfels, H. (1984) 'Kopfhaltung, Atlasposition und Atemfunktion beim offenen Biss.' *Fortschritte der Kieferorthopädie. 45*, 111–121.

445 von Treuenfels, H. (1985) 'Orofaziale Dyskinesien als Ausdruck einer gestörten Wechselbeziehung von Atmung, Verdauung und Bewegung.' *Fortschritte der Kieferorthopädie. 46*, 191–208.

446 von Treuenfels, H. (2012) 'Kindesentwicklung, Kieferanomalien und Kieferorthopädie.' In: Liem, T., Schleupen, A., Altmeyer, P. and Zweedijk, R. (Ed.) *Osteopathische Behandlung von Kindern*, 2nd Ed. Stuttgart: Haug.

447 Türp, J. C. and Schindler, H. C. (2006) 'Gibt es eine Beziehung zwischen craniomandibulären Dysfunktionen und Kopfschmerzen?' *Dtsch. Zahnärztl. Zeitschr. 61*, 3, 124–130.

448 Türp, J. C., Kowalski, C. J., O'Leary, N. et al. (1998) 'Pain maps from facial pain patients indicate a broad pain geography.' *J. Dent. Res. 77*, 6, 1465–1472.

449 Upledger, J. E. and Vredevoogd, J. D. (1983) *Craniosacral Therapy*. Seattle, WA: Eastland Press.

450 Vathrakokoilis, K., Liem, T., Aetopoulos, I. et al. (2018) 'The efficacy of an osteopathic treatment protocol on pain and function in patients with TMJ disorders.' *Int. J. Oral Maxillofac. Surg. 2*, 125–138.

451 Vedolin, G. M., Lobato, V. V., Conti, P. C. et al. (2009) 'The impact of stress and anxiety on the pressure pain threshold of myofascial pain patients.' *J. Oral Rehabil. 36*, 85, 313–321.

452 Velly, A. M., Gornitsky, M. and Philippe, P. (2003) 'Contributing factors to chronic myofascial pain: a case-control study.' *Pain. 104*, 3, 491–499.

453 Velz, A. L., Restrepo, C. C., Pelaez-Vargas, A. et al. (2007) 'Head posture and dental wear evaluation of bruxist children with primary teeth.' *J. Oral Rehabil. 34*, 663–670.

454 Vignolo, V., Vedolin, G. M., de Araujo Cdos, R. et al. (2008) 'Influence of the menstrual cycle on the pressure pain threshold of masticatory muscles in patients with masticatory myofascial pain.' *Oral Surg. Oral Med. Oral Pathol. Oral Radiol. Endod. 105*, 3, 308–315.

455 Visscher, C. M., Lobbenzoo, F. and Naeije, M. (2000) 'Treatment of bruxism: physiotherapeutic approach.' *J. Ned. Tijdschr. Tandheelkd. 107*, 293–296.

456 Vivaldi, D., Di Giosia, M., Tchivileva, I. E. et al. (2018) 'Headache attributed to TMD is associated with the presence of comorbid bodily pain. A case-control study.' *Headache. 58*, 10, 1593–1600.

457 Wakeley, C. (1929) 'The causation and treatment of displaced mandibular cartilage.' *Lancet. 2*, 543.

458 Walker, N., Bohannon, R. W. and Cameron, D. (2000) 'Discriminant validity of temporomandibular joint range of motion measurements obtained with a ruler.' *J. Orthop. Sports Phys. Ther. 30*, 8, 484–492.

459 Walczyńska-Dragon, K., Baron, S., Nitecka-Buchta, A. et al. (2014) 'Correlation between TMD and cervical spine pain and mobility. Is the whole body balance TMJ related?' *BioMed Res. Int. 2014*, 582414.

460 Weinberg, L. A. (1976) Posterior bilateral condylar displacement: its diagnosis and treatment. *J. Prosthet. Dent. 36*, 272.

461 Weinberg, L. A. (1980) 'The etiology, diagnosis and treatment of TMJ dysfunction-pain syndrome.' *J. Prosthet. Dent. 43*, 186–196.

462 Weinberg, L. A. and Lager, L. A. (1980) 'Clinical report on the etiology and diagnosis of TMJ dysfunction-pain syndrome.' *J. Prosthet. Dent. 44*, 6, 642–653.

463 Wernham, J. (1996) *Lectures on Osteopathy.* Maidstone: John Wernham College of Classical Osteopathy.

464 Wernham, J. (1956) *Mechanics of the Spine.* Yearbook of Institute of Applied Osteopathy. Maidstone: John Wernham College of Classical Osteopathy.

465 Wernham, J. (1985) *Mechanics of the Spine.* Yearbook of Maidstone College of Osteopathy. Maidstone: John Wernham College of Classical Osteopathy.

466 Westesson, P. L. (1998) 'Posterior disc displacement in the temporomandibular joint.' *J. Oral Maxillofacial. Surg. 56*, 1266–1273.

467 Westling, L. (1989) 'Craniomandibular disorders and general joint mobility.' *Acta Odontol. Scand. 47*, 293–299.

468 Wickwire, E., Bellinger, K., Kronfli, T. et al. (2008) 'Relations between objective sleep data, sleep disorders, and signs and symptoms of temporomandibular joint disorder' (TMD). *J. Pain. 9*, Suppl. 2, 14.

469 Wilhelm, K., Siegel, J. E., Finch, A. W. et al. (2007) 'The long and the short of it: associations between 5-HTT genotypes and coping with stress.' *Psychosom. Med. 69*, 614–620.

470 Willard, F. (2008) 'Basic mechanisms of pain.' In: Audette, J. F. and Bailey, A. (Ed.) *Integrative Pain Medicine: The Science and Practice of Complementary and Alternative Medicine in Pain Management.* Totowa, NJ: Humana Press, pp. 19–61.

471 Williams, P. L., Warwick, R., Dyson, M. and Bannister, L. H. (1995) *Gray's Anatomy*, 37th Ed. New York: Churchill Livingstone.

472 Williams, P. L., Bannister, L. H., Berry, M. M., Collins, P., Dyson, M., Dussek, J. E. and Ferguson, M. W. (1995) *Gray's Anatomy*, 38th Ed. New York: Churchill Livingstone, p. 579.

473 Williamson, E. H. and Sheffield, J. W. (1985) 'The non-surgical treatment of internal derangement of the temporomandibular joint: a survey of 300 cases.' *Facial Orthop. Temporomandibular Arthrol. 2*, 10, 18–20.

474 Williamson, P. C. (1999) 'Horizontal condylar angulation and condyle position associated with adolescent TMJ disk status.' *J. Craniomandib. Pract. 17*, 101–107.

475 Winkel, D. (1993) *Nichtoperative Orthopädie, Part 4/2: Diagnostik und Therapie der Wirbelsäule.* Stuttgart: Fischer, pp. 341, 373f.

476 Wittlinger, H. and Wittlinger, G. (1992) *Lehrbuch der manuellen Lymphdrainage nach Dr. Vodder*, Vol. 1, 10th Ed. Heidelberg: Haug, p. 51.

477 Witzig, J. and Spahl, T. (1987) *Clinical Management of Basic Maxillofacial Orthopedic Appliances.* Littleton: Mosby.

478 Woolf, C. J. (2011) 'Central sensitization: implications for the diagnosis and treatment of pain.' *Pain. 152*, 3, S2–S15.

479 Yap, A. U. and Chua, A. P. (2016) 'Sleep bruxism: current knowledge and contemporary management.' *J. Conserv. Dent. 19*, 5, 383–389.

480 Yeler, D. Y., Yılmaz, N. and Koraltan, M. (2017) 'A survey on the potential relationships between TMD, possible sleep bruxism, unilateral chewing, and occlusal factors in Turkish university students.' *Cranio. 35*, 5, 308–314.

481 Yemm, R. (1976) 'Neurophysiological studies of temporomandibular joint dysfunction.' *Oral Sci. Rev. 7*, 31.

482 Yoshihara, T., Shigeta, K., Hasegawa, H. et al. (2005) 'Neuroendocrine responses to psychological stress in patients with myofascial pain.' *J. Orofac. Pain. 19*, 3, 202–208.

483 Younger, J. W., Shen, Y. F., Goddard, G. et al. (2010) 'Chronic myofascial temporo-mandibular pain is associated with neural abnormalities in the trigeminal and limbic systems.' *Pain. 149*, 222–228.

484 Yunus, M. B. (2008) 'Central sensitivity syndromes: a new paradigm and group nosology for fibromyalgia and overlapping conditions and the related issue of disease versus illness.' *Semin. Arthritis. Rheum. 37*, 6, 339–352.

485 Zarb, G. A. and Carlsson, G. E. (1999) 'Temporomandibular disorders: osteoarthritis.' *J. Orofacial. Pain. 13*, 294–306.

486 Zarb, G. A. and Mock, D. (1999) 'On emphasizing a scientifically prudent approach to the management of temporomandibular disorders.' *J. Orofacial. Pain. 13*, 220–222.

487 Zeines, V. (2002) *Healthy Mouth, Healthy Body.* New York: Kensington Books.

488 Zimny, M. L. (1988) 'Mechanoreceptors in articular tissues.' *Am. J. Anat. 182*, 16–32.

489 Zubieta, J. K., Heitzeg, M. M., Smith, Y. R. et al. (2003) 'Val158 met genotype affects μ-opioid neurotransmitter responses to a pain stressor.' *Science. 299*, 5610, 1240–1243.

3.1	Anatomy of the orofacial, pharyngeal, and laryngeal structures	198
3.1.1	The oral cavity	198
3.1.2	The pterygopalatine fossa	211
3.1.3	The pterygopalatine ganglion	211
3.1.4	The pharynx	212
3.1.5	The larynx	220
3.2	The causes of dysfunction in orofacial, pharyngeal, and laryngeal structures	221
3.2.1	Potential dysfunctions of the orofacial system, with particular reference to swallowing disorders	222
3.2.2	Potential dysfunctions of the tongue	223
3.2.3	Potential dysfunctions involving the teeth/periodontal ligament	225
3.2.4	Potential dysfunctions of the pharynx	226
3.2.5	Potential dysfunctions in laryngeal disorders	226
3.3	Diagnostic investigations for orofacial, pharyngeal, and laryngeal structures	227
3.3.1	History-taking	227
3.3.2	Inspection	228
3.3.3	Larynx questionnaire	228
3.3.4	General test	228
3.4	Treatment of the orofacial structures	232
3.4.1	Treating the periodontal ligament	234
3.4.2	Disorders which are sequelae of dental trauma	235
3.4.3	Treatment of the tongue	235
3.4.4	Treatment of the floor of the mouth and the omohyoid muscle	236
3.4.5	Treatment of the hyoid bone	238
3.4.6	Technique for the pharynx	241
3.4.7	General laryngeal mobilization	242
3.4.8	Techniques for the cranial nerves	245
3.4.9	Treatment of the arteries, veins, and lymph vessels	246
3.4.10	Treatment of venous structures	248
3.4.11	Further procedures for chronic inflammation of the tonsils and also of the oral cavity, pharynx, and larynx	249
3.4.12	Procedures in the case of a dysfunctional microbiome of the oral cavity	249
3.4.13	Self-help techniques, exercise programs	249
3.5	References	256

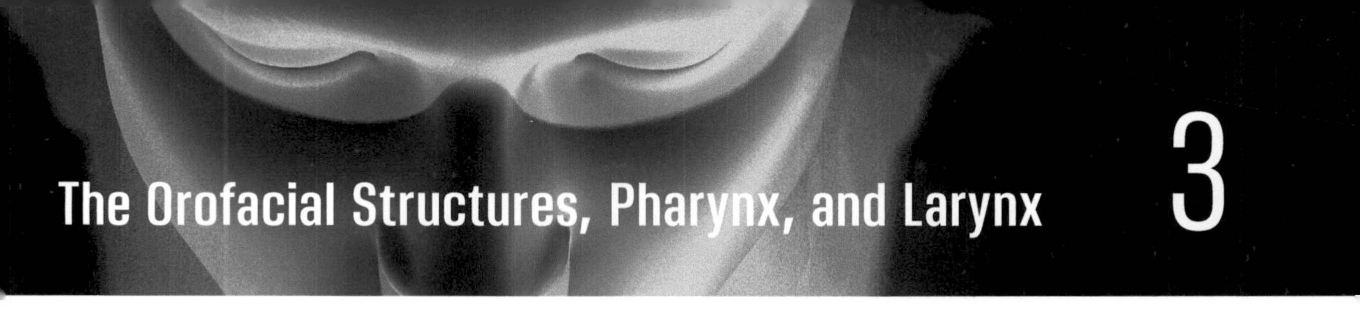

The Orofacial Structures, Pharynx, and Larynx 3

The German term for "baby," *Säugling* (literally "suckling"), clearly illustrates the great significance of the oral functions even at this early phase of human development. A normal sucking and swallowing function requires the morphodynamic development of all the structures in the oral cavity. The treatment of the oral structures during childhood is essential to healthy development. In these first years of life especially, the mouth, as the entrance area to the body, acts as a kind of control room, and many problems in the locomotor and nervous systems originate in this early period.[45] The mouth and its expressive movements also have important social and communicative elements which decisively influence the way in which emotions are put across.

3.1 Anatomy of the orofacial, pharyngeal, and laryngeal structures

The orofacial system comprises the following structures:

- Bones: the palatine bone, maxilla, mandible, and temporomandibular joints.
- The teeth and periodontal ligament.
- Muscles: the muscles controlling mouth opening and closure, the muscles of the tongue, floor of the mouth, palate, and palatopharyngeal arch, and those governing facial expression.
- Soft tissues: the cheeks, lips, mucosa of the mouth and pharynx, salivary glands, (palatine) tonsils, pharyngeal tonsils (adenoids), etc.
- Nerves and vessels supplying this region.
- Taste receptors.
- Pharynx: connecting the oral cavity, nasal cavity, and esophagus.
- Larynx: this consists of an articulated cartilaginous framework, muscles, and a mucosal lining. Among other things, the larynx is involved in phonation.
- Functions of the orofacial system: mastication, sucking, swallowing, respiration, articulation, sensory perception of taste, temperature, pain, and depth, expression of emotions, etc.

3.1.1 The oral cavity

The oral cavity is the central feature of the orofacial system. It is subdivided into the oral vestibule, which is the area outside the dental arch, and the oral cavity proper, which is the area inside the dental arch (Figures 3.1 and 3.2).

The oral cavity is bounded below by the suprahyoid muscles (floor of the mouth), above by the hard palate (maxilla and palatine bone) and soft palate, and laterally by the mandible and cheeks (especially the buccinator muscle). It is bounded in front by the lips and behind by the oropharyngeal isthmus.

The teeth and tongue are important organs in the oral cavity.

The posterior part of the roof of the mouth depends in particular on the tone of the levator and tensor veli palatini muscles, the palatopharyngeus muscle, and the tongue, and on the orientation of the pterygoid process of the sphenoid.

Functions of the oral cavity

- The digestive process starts in the mouth.
- Chewing is the means by which mechanical digestion takes place in the mouth.
- Salivary production is 0.5–1.5 L/day.
- The secretion of α-amylase in the mouth initiates carbohydrate digestion. It exerts its optimum effect at a pH of around 7.4. An adequate chewing and salivation process is important. Gastric juice denatures the α-amylase. Excessive fruit acid hinders digestion.

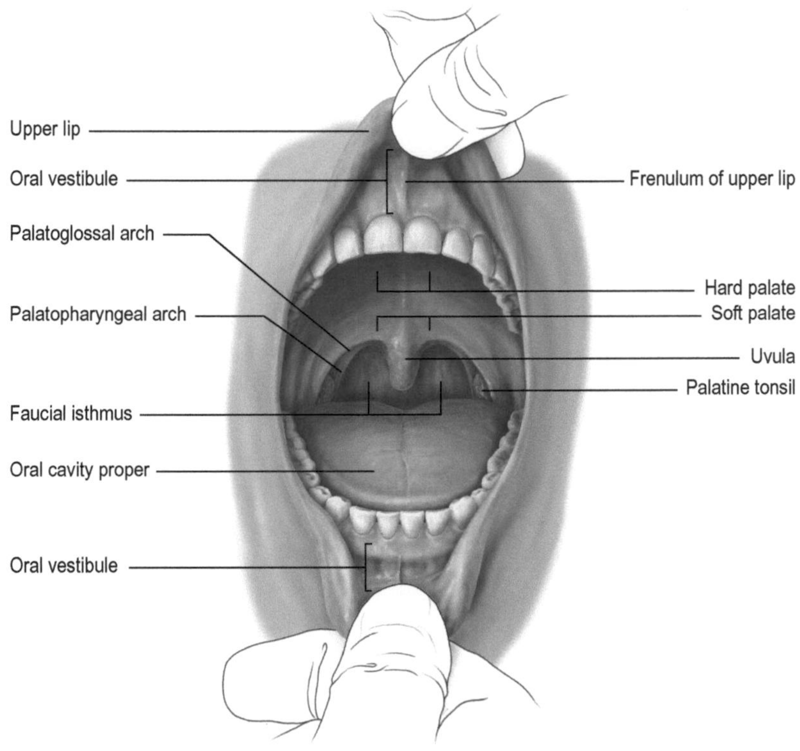

Figure 3.1
Oral cavity, ventral view. [Schünke, M., Schulte, E., Schumacher, U. [2015] *Prometheus LernAtlas der Anatomie. Kopf, Hals und Neuroanatomie.* Illustrations by M. Voll and K. Wesker, 4th ed. Stuttgart: Thieme]

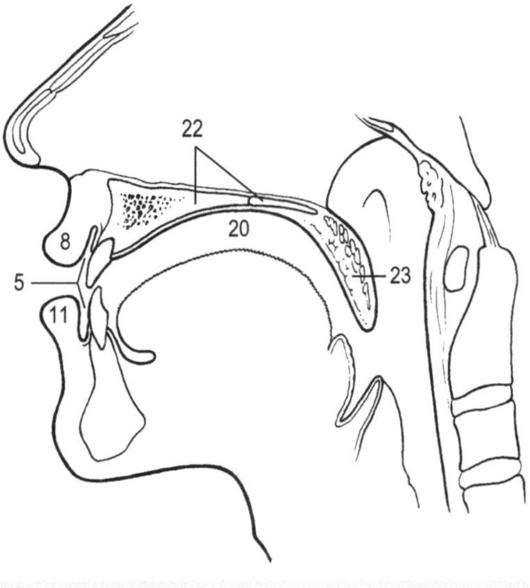

Figure 3.2
Sagittal section through the oral cavity. **5** Oral vestibule. **8** Upper lip. **11** Lower lip. **20** Oral cavity proper. **22** Hard palate. **23** Soft palate. [From: Dauber, W. [2008] *Feneis' Bild-Lexikon der Anatomie*, 10th ed. Stuttgart: Thieme]

- The saliva contains many salivary proteins which demonstrate antibacterial, antiviral, and fungicidal properties, e.g., immunoglobulin A, immunoglobulin G, lactoferrins, lysozymes, or histatins (these last aid in wound healing).
- The most important part of dental remineralization takes place through a layer of saliva around the teeth. This protective dental layer, called pellicle, counteracts wear from the opposing teeth and also serves to protect the teeth and gums by preventing bacterial adhesion.
- Haptocorrin promotes vitamin B12 uptake via the oral mucosa. It also binds vitamin B12 and thus protects it from the acid gastric juice. Fluorides cause impairments to absorption, e.g., of vitamin B12.
- There are about 5×10^8 bacteria per ml of saliva. The microbiomes of related people (mother and child) resemble each other more

closely than do those of unrelated people. The placenta contains microorganisms of the flora of the mouth. The microbiome of a neonate's intestine resembles that of the mother's vaginal flora.
- Opiorphin, an opioid, can have an analgesic effect and inhibit the breakdown of opiates.
- Hormones are also detectable in the saliva, e.g., cortisol, testosterone, estradiol, progesterone, and melatonin.
- Salivary lipases are also present in the mouth but cannot exert their optimum effect there (pH 4).

Salivary gland innervation

In sensory terms the salivary glands are innervated by the mandibular nerve (CN V_3) (Figure 3.3).

For secretory purposes, the parotid gland is innervated by the glossopharyngeal nerve (CN IX) via the otic ganglion, and the submandibular and sublingual glands are innervated by the intermedius nerve (CN VII) via the submandibular ganglion.

The otic ganglion

The parasympathetic ganglion (Figure 3.4) is situated below the foramen ovale, medial to the mandibular nerve (CN V_3), and lateral to the tensor veli palatini muscle. The preganglionic fibers come from the glossopharyngeal nerve (CN IX), and pass via the lesser petrosal nerve to arrive at the ganglion. Here are located the perikarya of the postganglionic parasympathetic fibers. These fibers pass by communicating branches to

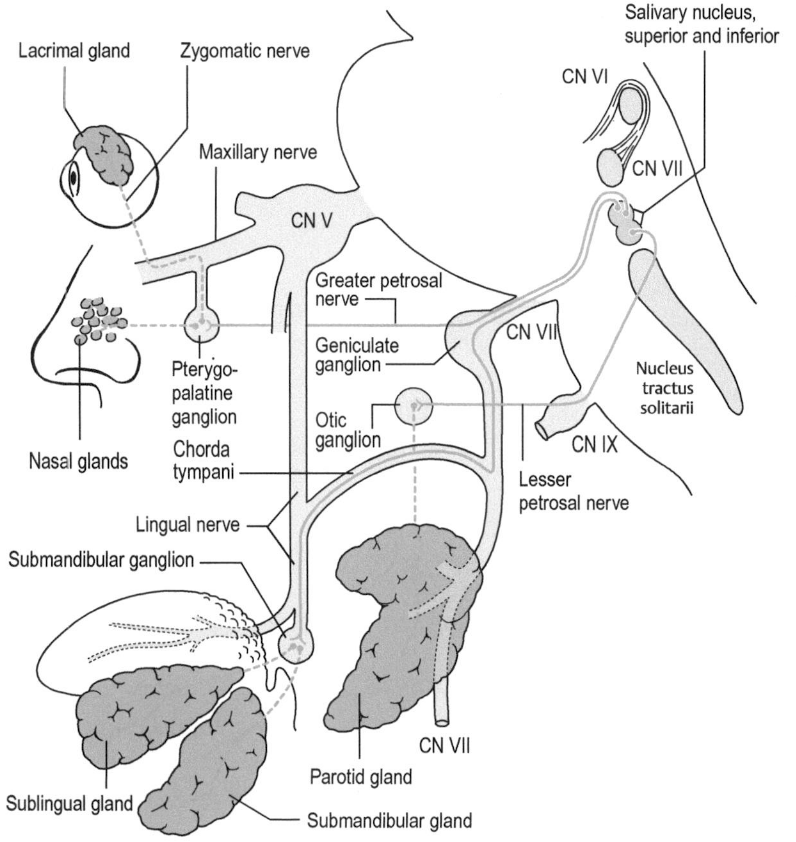

Figure 3.3
Innervation of the salivary glands. [From Bähr, M., Frotscher, M. [2014] *Neurologisch-topische Diagnostik*, 10th ed. Stuttgart: Thieme]

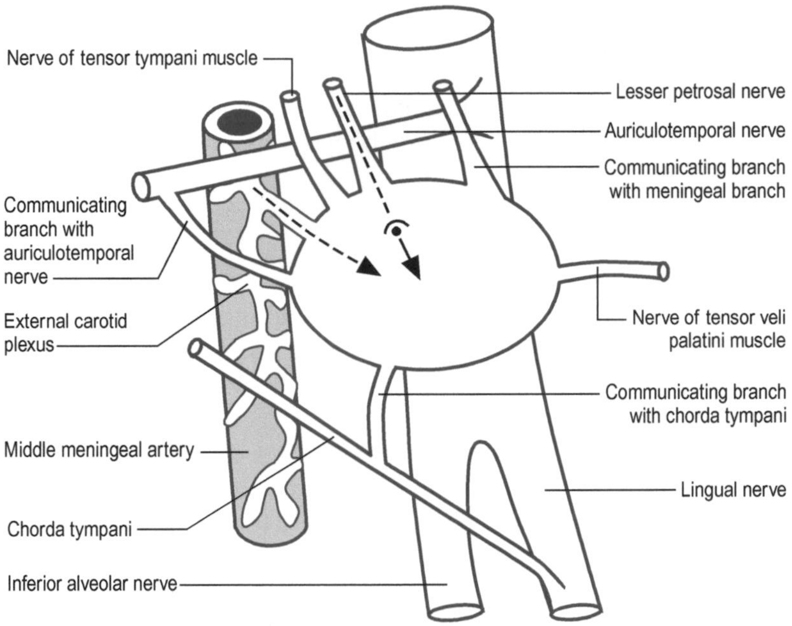

Figure 3.4
The otic ganglion

the auriculotemporal nerve, by which they are conveyed to the parotid gland (secretory innervation of the parotid gland).

Connects with the:

- Tensor veli palatini nerve, which supplies the tensor veli palatini muscle.
- Tensor tympani nerve, which supplies the tensor tympani muscle.
- Meningeal branch of the mandibular nerve via the communicating branch of the same name.
- Sympathetic nervous system: arising in the superior cervical ganglion, fibers from the external carotid plexus of the middle meningeal artery also pass through the ganglion without being interrupted.
- Chorda tympani nerve: via the communicating branch of the same name. Instead of relaying them via the chorda tympani nerve through the middle ear, this branch sometimes sends gustatory fibers from the anterior two-thirds of the tongue via the lesser petrosal nerve (CN IX) and via the nerve of the pterygoid canal to the geniculate ganglion of the facial nerve.

NOTE The connections to the ganglion listed above do not form synapses within the ganglion.

The submandibular ganglion

The ganglion (Figure 3.5) is located superior to the submandibular gland and below the lingual nerve (CN V_3). The preganglionic fibers pass via the chorda tympani nerve from the intermedius nerve (CN VII) to enter the ganglion. Here are located the perikarya of the postganglionic parasympathetic fibers which pass to the submandibular and sublingual glands (secretory innervation of the submandibular and sublingual glands).

Connects with the:

- Sympathetic nervous system: commencing in the superior cervical ganglion, fibers from the sympathetic plexus of the facial artery pass through the ganglion without being interrupted. These supply the vascular smooth muscle in the submandibular and sublingual glands.

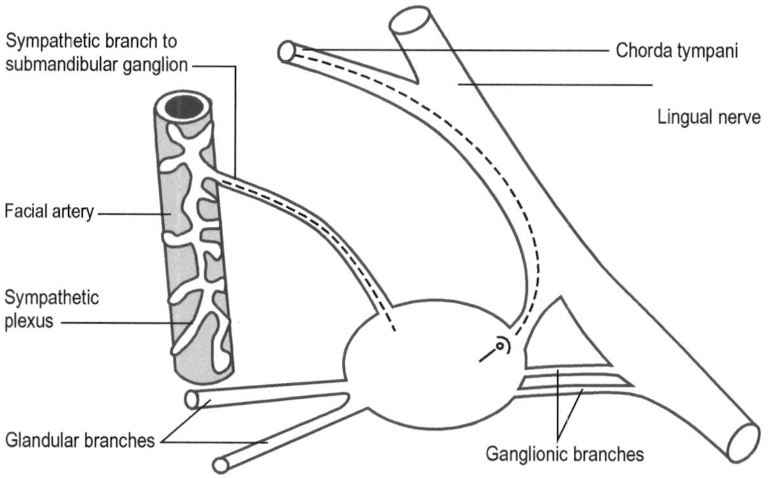

Figure 3.5
The submandibular ganglion

18	17	16	15	14	13	12	11	21	22	23	24	25	26	27	28
48	47	46	45	44	43	42	41	31	32	33	34	35	36	37	38

Figure 3.6
Adult dentition code

- Submandibular and sublingual glands: postganglionic parasympathetic and sympathetic as well as sensory fibers pass through the glandular branches to supply these glands.
- Lingual nerve: via ganglionic branches. As well as sensory fibers, postganglionic parasympathetic and sympathetic ganglionic fibers are carried in the lingual nerve to the glands of the oral mucosa.

The teeth

Adults have a full complement of 32 teeth. Each quadrant of the mouth contains 2 incisors, 1 canine, 2 premolars, and 3 molars (dental formula: 2-1-2-3). Deciduous teeth include no molars (dental formula: 2-1-2).

Adult dentition code (Figure 3.6) The first digit (1–4) identifies the quadrant of the mouth: 1 right upper, 2 left upper quadrant, 3 left lower, and 4 right lower quadrant.

The second digit (1–8) denotes the position of the tooth in the jaw: incisors (1 and 2), canine (3), premolars (4 and 5), and molars (6 to 8).

Positional and orientation terms used in dental anatomy (Figure 3.7)

- Buccal, labial: side of the cheek or lip.
- Lingual, palatal: side of the tongue or palate.
- Mesial: toward the anterior adjacent tooth.
- Distal: toward the posterior adjacent tooth.
- Occlusal: pertaining to the chewing surfaces of the teeth.

Dental structure Teeth consist of three hard tissues: dentin, enamel, and cementum (Figure 3.8).

Dentin forms the bulk of the tooth: it is harder than bone because it contains more inorganic substances. The odontoblasts are located only at the margin of the dentin and they send cellular processes into the interior of the tooth.

The **enamel** forms an external layer coating the dentin. It is the hardest substance in the human body and is designed to protect the dentin. The enamel-forming cells are located at the outer surface of the enamel and are worn away rapidly by chewing after the teeth erupt. When the enamel is damaged (caries), it cannot therefore regenerate itself.

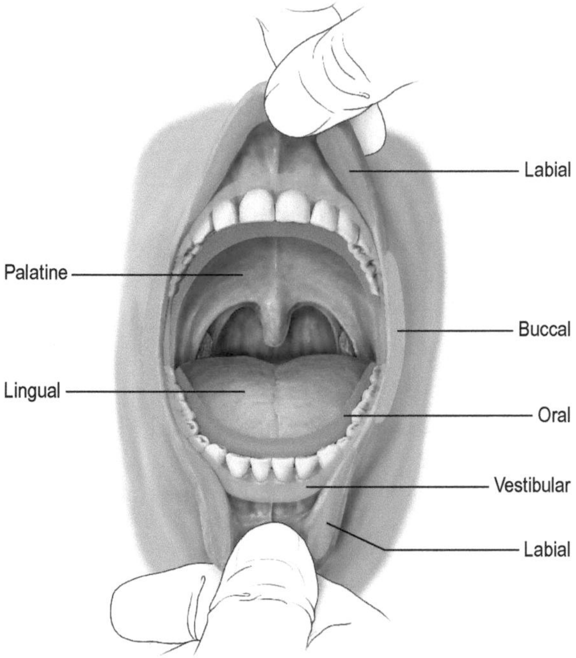

Figure 3.7
Positional and orientational terminology. [Schünke, M., Schulte, E., Schumacher, U. [2015] *Prometheus LernAtlas der Anatomie. Kopf, Hals und Neuroanatomie.* Illustrations by M. Voll and K. Wesker, 4th ed. Stuttgart: Thieme]

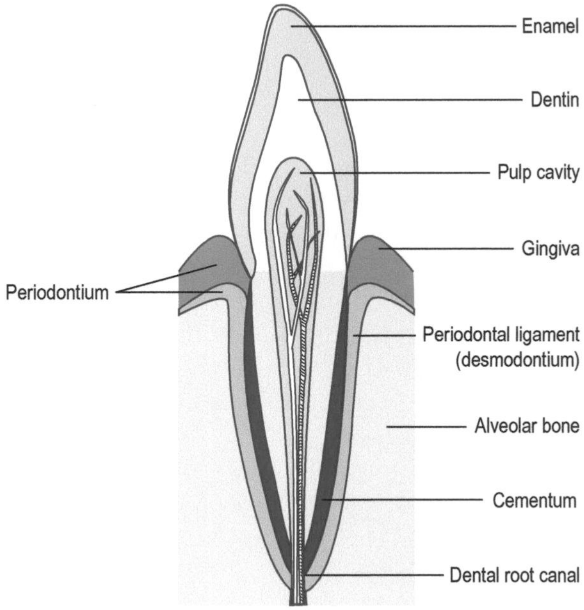

Figure 3.8
Sagittal section through tooth

The woven bone-like dentin in the alveolar bone is surrounded by **cementum** instead of by enamel. From the cementum, ligamentous fibers travel to the alveolar bone, anchoring the tooth in the bone.

Other parts of the tooth:

- Crown: coated with enamel.
- Root: coated with cementum.
- Neck: border between the enamel and the cementum.
- Pulp cavity: the space within the dentin containing the blood vessels and nerves of the tooth; it extends from the root to the crown.
- Pulp: the tissue inside the pulp cavity (blood vessels, nerves, loose connective tissue, etc.).

The periodontal ligament The periodontal ligament (desmodontium) is a fibrous joint (syndesmosis) that connects the root of each tooth to the alveolar bone. The periodontal ligament fibers are anchored in the cementum layer of the tooth and in the alveolar bone. The periodontal ligament (Figure 3.8) holds the teeth in sprung suspension, with the result that each tooth is capable of small movements within its alveolar bone socket. Blood vessels and nerves are also found at the junction between the dental root and alveolar bone. The nerves there transmit proprioceptive information via the periodontal ligaments, enabling the teeth to use the periodontal ligaments to adapt to the prevailing forces and to reposition themselves to a limited extent.

In this area in particular, manual treatment can correct abnormal tensions in the ligamentous connections so as to positively influence the further transmission of proprioceptive information and

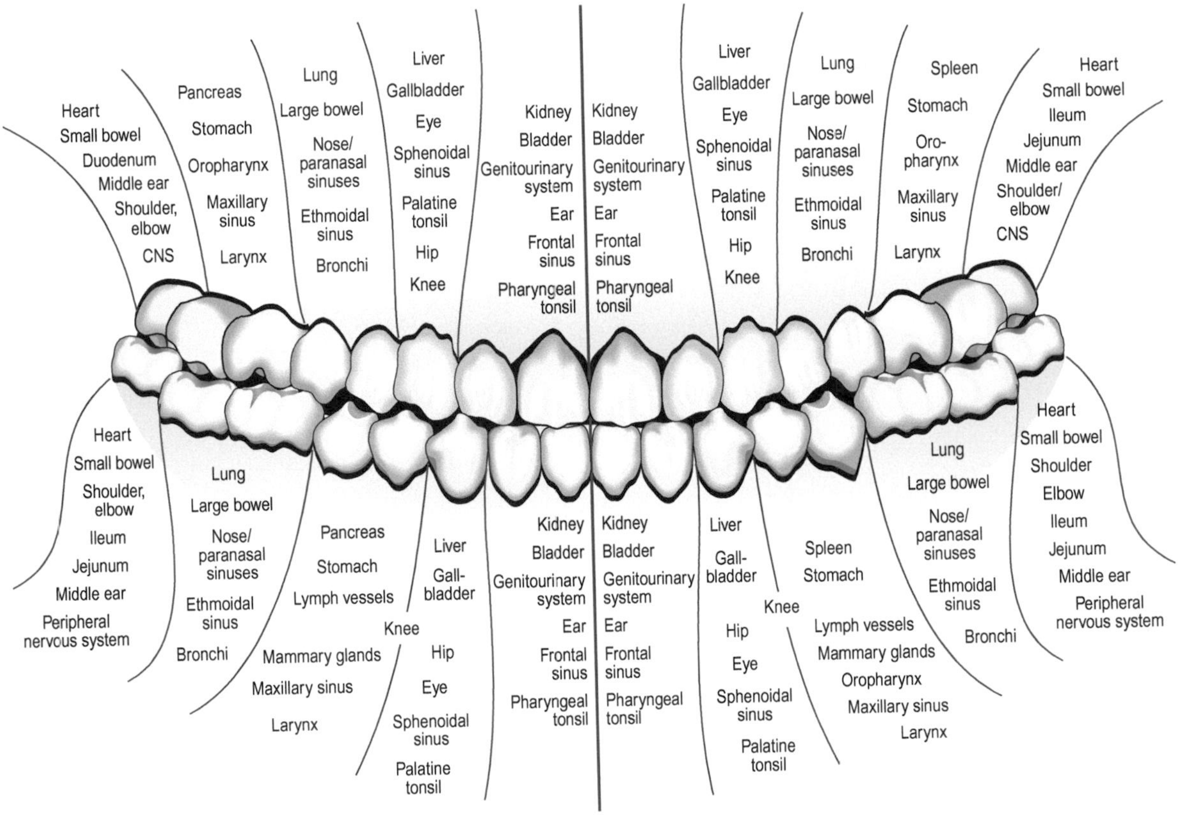

Figure 3.9
Interactions between teeth and organs

pain and the arterial blood supply to the teeth.[46] Influence can also be brought to bear on any reflex connections with other organ systems (Figure 3.9).

Nerves and blood vessels The dental nerves in the mandible (inferior alveolar nerves) arise from the mandibular nerve (CN V_3), and the dental nerves in the maxilla (superior alveolar nerves) arise from the maxillary nerve (CN V_2). Dental pain may be felt as far down as the level of the second spinal cord segment due to the segmental interconnections of the trigeminal nerve.

The vascular supply of the teeth is provided by the inferior alveolar artery (mandible) and by the posterior superior alveolar artery and the anterior superior alveolar arteries (maxilla). These arise from the maxillary artery, a terminal branch of the external carotid artery.

The nerves follow the same path as the blood vessels (Figures 3.10 and 3.11).

The influence of muscle forces on tooth development The teeth are exposed to the outward pressure of the tongue and the inward pressure of the buccinator and orbicularis oris muscles. In normal circumstances, the pressure of the tongue during the processes of mastication, swallowing, and articulation is compensated for by the peribuccal muscles. Any imbalance between the tongue and peribuccal muscles has repercussions for the positioning of the teeth (Figure 3.12). From the spiral dynamic viewpoint, the orbicularis

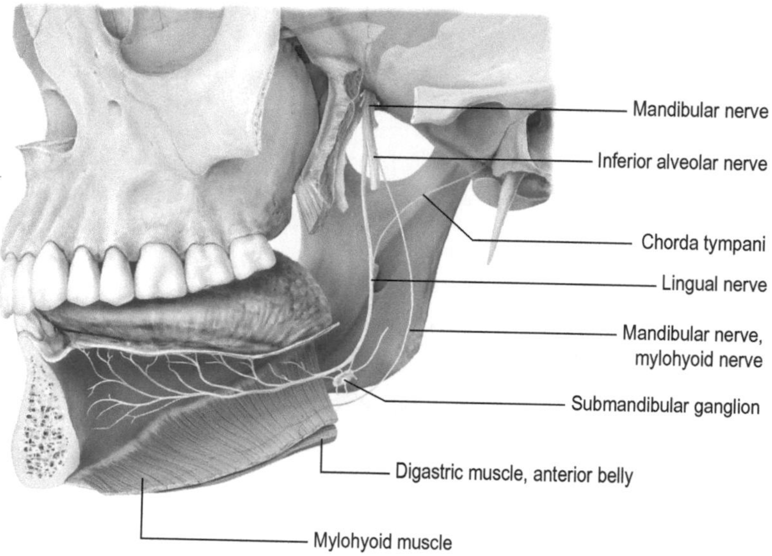

Figure 3.10
Innervation of the muscles of the floor of the mouth. Viewed from the left (medial view of the right half of the mandible). (From: Schünke, M., Schulte, E., Schumacher, U. [2015] *Prometheus LernAtlas der Anatomie. Kopf, Hals und Neuroanatomie.* Illustrations by M. Voll and K. Wesker, 4th ed. Stuttgart: Thieme)

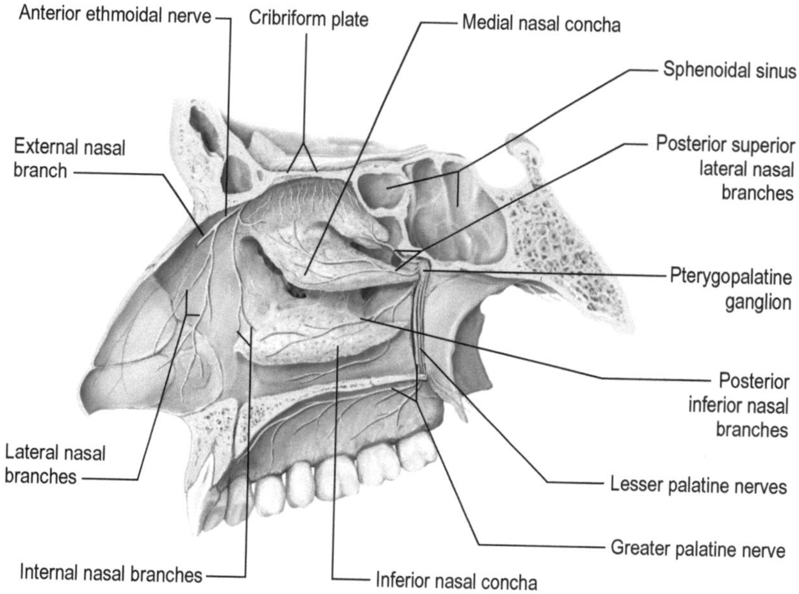

Figure 3.11
Innervation of the maxilla. (From: Schünke, M., Schulte, E., Schumacher, U. [2015] *Prometheus LernAtlas der Anatomie. Kopf, Hals und Neuroanatomie.* Illustrations by M. Voll and K. Wesker, 4th ed. Stuttgart: Thieme)

oris muscle is also thought to be important for head alignment and coordination of the muscles of facial expression.[18]

Dental contact during swallowing Dental contact occurs during the act of swallowing, at the moment when the tongue presses against the palate. There is no dental contact during biting and chewing.

The tongue

The tongue is a muscular organ that is coated with highly differentiated mucosa. Its root rests on the floor of the mouth, with which it is fused (Figure 3.13).

Origin of the tongue

- The brain (and with it the head) arches **anterobasally upward and forward.**

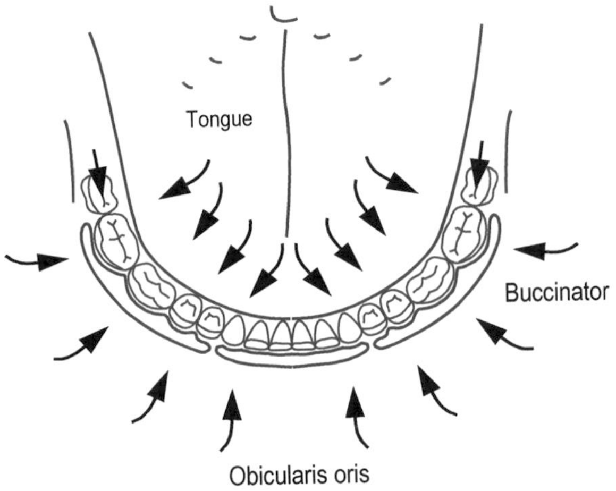

Figure 3.12
The influence of muscle forces on dental development

- The weak endodermal oropharyngeal tube adapts to these growth dynamics, **arching** convexly upward and **widening transversely**.
- At its more strongly arched basal aspect, the oropharyngeal tube forms the anlage of the tongue.
- The muscles follow this and take shape within the stroma of the anlage of the tongue. They form in three main orientations, **longitudinal, transverse, and vertical**, of the anlage of the tongue.
- Rich innervation.
- The tongue is visible at about the fourth week of intrauterine life.
- The anterior two-thirds of the tongue forms within the uterus by fusion of the two lateral swellings and of a swelling in the midline (tuberculum impar).

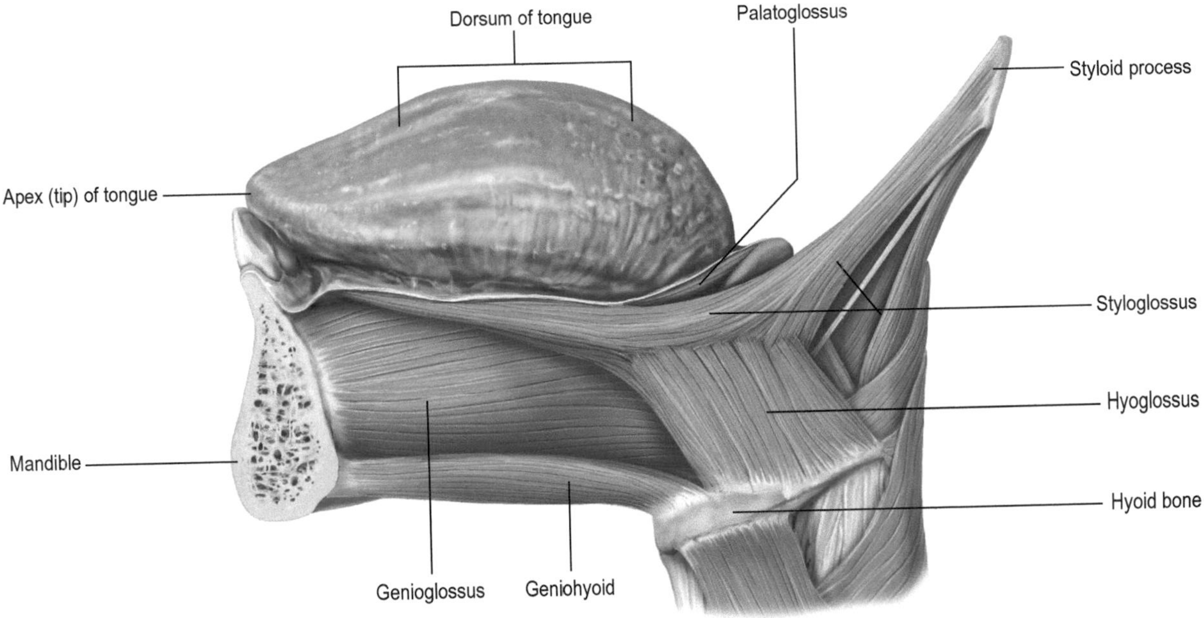

Figure 3.13
The muscles of the tongue. (From: Schünke, M., Schulte, E., Schumacher, U. [2015] *Prometheus LernAtlas der Anatomie. Kopf, Hals und Neuroanatomie*. Illustrations by M. Voll and K. Wesker, 4th ed. Stuttgart: Thieme)

- The lateral swellings unite and grow across the tuberculum impar.
- These structures originate from the first branchial arch.
- The posterior portions of the tongue originate from the second and third branchial arches.
- Taste buds appear around the eighth week via the inductive interactions of epithelial cells and inward migration of gustatory cells from the chorda tympani, the glossopharyngeal nerve, and the vagus nerve.
- Fetal facial reactions to bitter substances are detectable from the 26th to 28th week, indicating the presence of reflex patterns between the facial muscles and the taste buds.

Function Bolus propulsion (initiation of the act of swallowing by pressure of the tongue against the roof of the mouth), food-grinding (propulsion of the bolus onto the teeth in conjunction with the buccinator), receptor for tactile, thermal, and gustatory stimuli, sucking, articulation, and organ of defense (lymphoid tissues at the root of the tongue). The normal activity of the tongue is also important for the development of teeth and maxilla.

Tongue position Except when engaged in chewing, swallowing, and sucking, in coughing or articulation, the tongue is normally located in a neutral position in the oral cavity. In this resting position the anterior upper part of the tip of the tongue is located immediately behind the upper incisors at the roof of the mouth. The posterior part of the tongue is in contact with the soft palate, i.e., it completely fills the oral cavity when the mouth is closed. In this position the tongue exerts an outward force on dental development. It counterbalances the inward force from the buccinator and the other muscles of mastication. This is important to normal dental development. The resting position of the tongue induces a resting tone for the muscles controlling jaw closure, as well as for the lingual muscles.

Anatomical relations of the tongue While the tongue is suspended on the cranial base via muscles and ligaments, it has anterior and inferior attachments to the mandible and hyoid bone. The cranial base (via the temporal bone), the mandible, and the hyoid bone influence the tension balance of the tongue. The mandible represents a kind of fulcrum for the tongue between the cranial base and the hyoid bone (Figure 3.14).

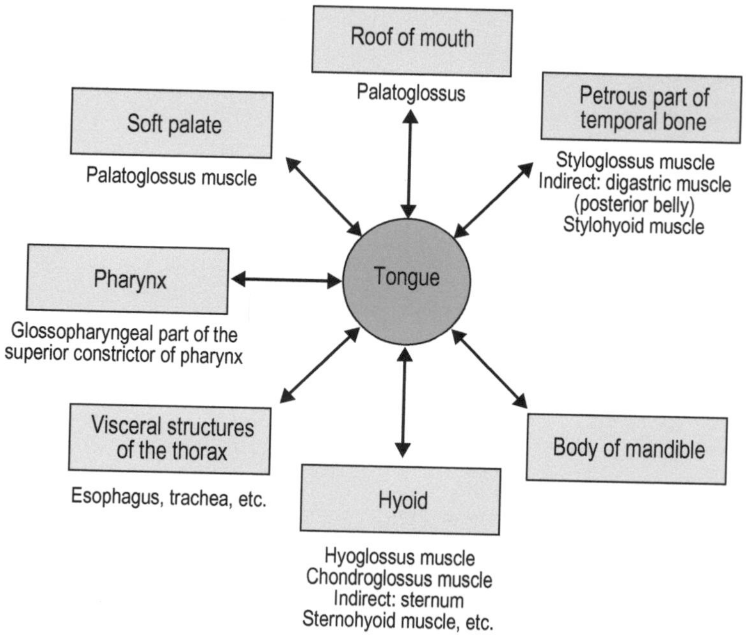

Figure 3.14
The anatomical relations of the tongue

The muscles of the tongue

The tongue consists of extrinsic muscles that are attached to bony structures and of intrinsic muscles that are contained exclusively within the tongue (Figure 3.13). The extrinsic muscles move the tongue as a whole, the intrinsic muscles change its shape. The hypoglossal nerve (CN XII) innervates all the muscles apart from the palatoglossal (glossopharyngeal nerve, CN IX).

> **NOTE** In the case of peripheral deficit of the hypoglossal nerve, the protruded tongue tends to be directed to the paralyzed side because of the preponderance of the muscles on the healthy side.
> The hypoglossal nerve (CN XII) can be impaired in, for instance, dysfunction of the occipital bone and the upper cervical vertebrae. (The ventral fibers of C1 and C2 temporarily attach themselves to the hypoglossal nerve and subsequently form the superior root of the ansa cervicalis.)

Extrinsic muscles

- The genioglossus arises from the mental spine on the inner surface of the body of the mandible and spreads out into the tongue in a fan-like form (CN XII). This is the most important muscle for the positioning and for the resting position of the tongue in the oral cavity, and for drawing the tongue forward. It also moves the tongue upward.
- The hyoglossus: from the body and the greater horn of the hyoid into the sides of the tongue (CN XII).
- The chondroglossus: from the lesser horn of the hyoid into the sides of the tongue (CN XII).
- The styloglossus: from the styloid process into the sides of the tongue (CN XII).
- The palatoglossus: from the palatine aponeurosis into the sides of the tongue (CN IX).
- The myloglossus (inconstant) runs from the posterior end of the mylohyoid line to the root of the tongue.

Intrinsic muscles

- Superior longitudinal.
- Inferior longitudinal.
- Transverse muscle of the tongue.
- Vertical muscle of the tongue.

The nerves of the tongue

The tongue is richly innervated (Figures 3.15 and 3.16).

Motor innervation

- Glossopharyngeal nerve (CN IX): palatoglossus muscle.
- Hypoglossal nerve (CN XII): intrinsic muscles of the tongue, genioglossus, hyoglossus, chondroglossus, and styloglossus muscles.

Sensory innervation

- Lingual nerve from the mandibular nerve (CN V_3): anterior two-thirds of the lingual mucosa.
- Glossopharyngeal nerve (CN IX): posterior third of the lingual mucosa.
- Vagus nerve (CN X): the area around the valleculae (Table 3.1).

Special sense innervation (taste)

- Facial nerve (CN VII), chorda tympani: anterior two-thirds of the lingual mucosa.
- Glossopharyngeal nerve (CN IX): posterior third of the lingual mucosa.

Table 3.1 Sensory and special sense innervation of the tongue

Innervation	Anterior two-thirds of tongue	Posterior third of tongue
Sensory	CN V_3	CN IX, (CN X in region of valleculae)
Special sense (taste)	CN VII	CN IX, (CN X at root of tongue)

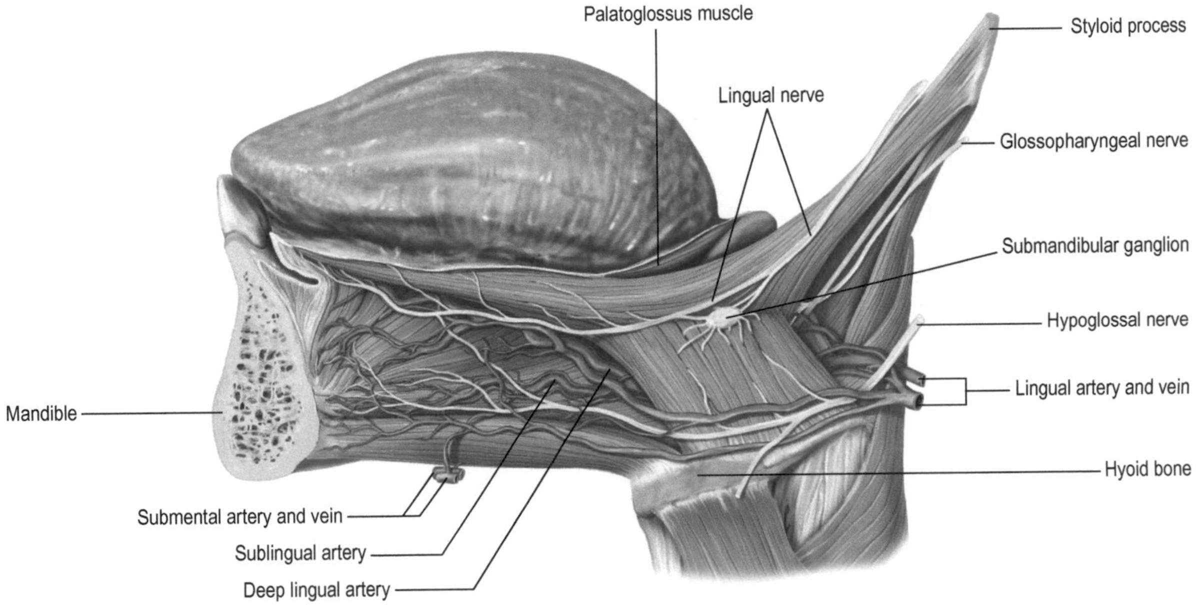

Figure 3.15
Hypoglossal nerve. (From: Schünke, M., Schulte, E., Schumacher, U. [2015] *Prometheus LernAtlas der Anatomie. Kopf, Hals und Neuroanatomie*. Illustrations by M. Voll and K. Wesker, 4th ed. Stuttgart: Thieme)

- Vagus nerve (CN X): scattered taste cells at the root of the tongue (Table 3.1).

Vessels Lingual artery arising from the external carotid artery.

Buccinator muscle

- Origin: outer surface of the alveolar processes of the maxilla and mandible in the region of the three molars and the buccinator crest.
- Insertion: angle of the mouth, intermingles in the modiolus with fibers of the orbicularis oris, in the skin of the upper and lower lip.
- In contrast to other muscles involved in facial expression the buccinator has its own fascia, the buccopharyngeal fascia, and is attached to the superior constrictors of pharynx by the pterygomandibular raphe (Volume 2, section 4.2.2).
- Function: shapes the contour of the cheeks, presses the cheeks against the teeth, presses food out of the lateral oral vestibule into the oral cavity; is involved in blowing and whistling and is particularly important to sucking in neonates; supports laughing and weeping.

Hyoid bone

This horseshoe-shaped bone has a transverse course and is located at the bend where the floor of the mouth meets the angle of the neck at the level of the third cervical vertebra. The hyoid is connected to other bones only by muscles, ligaments, and fasciae: mandible, temporal bone, sternum, clavicle, scapula, vertebral column.[22] The position of the hyoid is an expression of the structures fixed to it. Consequently, any imbalance and change of tension in the aforesaid structures and also in the viscera can alter the hyoid's position.

The hyoid protects the larynx and the pharynx and exhibits a certain freedom of movement, which is important both for the act of swallowing and for the movement of the tongue and cervical spine. Via the

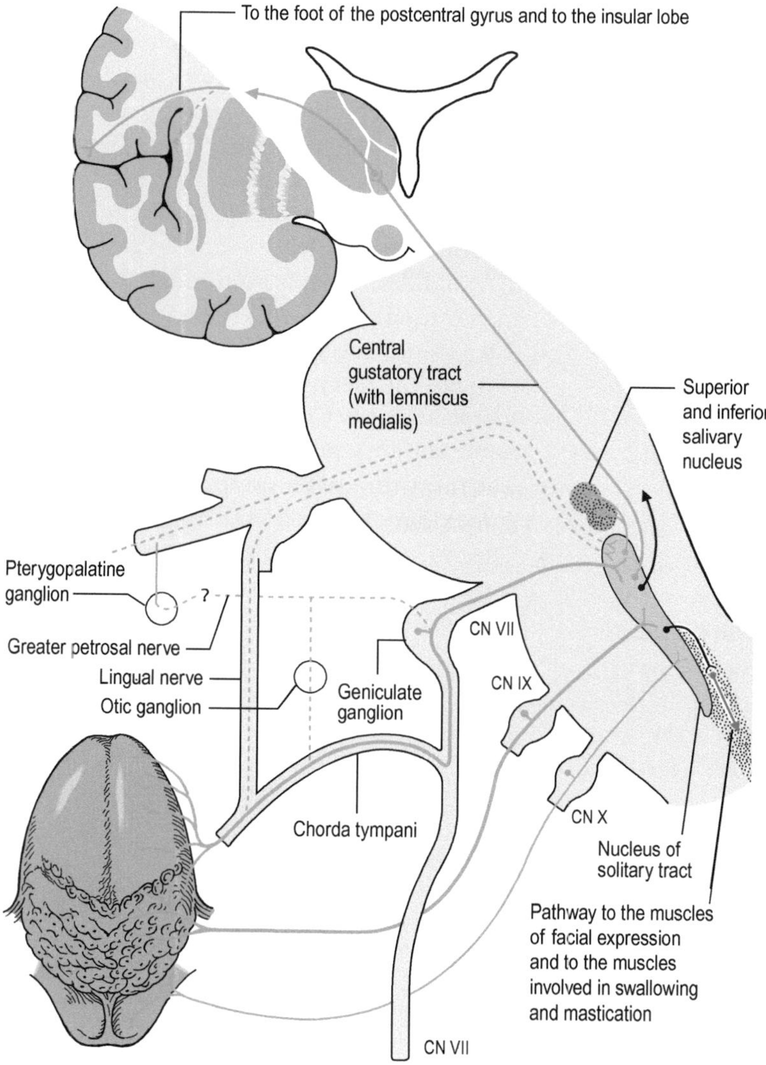

Figure 3.16
Gustatory innervation of the tongue. (From: Bähr, M., Frotscher, M. [2014] *Neurologisch-topische Diagnostik*, 10th ed. Stuttgart: Thieme)

suprahyoid and infrahyoid muscles, the hyoid also acts as a fulcrum for the movement of the mandible. Although the suprahyoid muscles are located in the neck, they belong to the muscles of the head and are innervated by cranial nerves. The infrahyoid muscles, on the other hand, are a continuation of the anterior wall of the torso and are innervated by cervical nerves. During swallowing the hyoid is moved upward and forward, while the infrahyoid muscles and the thyroid cartilage move downward (see also section 2.1.7 and Figures 2.56, 2.62):

- **Suprahyoid muscles**
  - Geniohyoid.
  - Mylohyoid.
  - Digastric.
  - Stylohyoid.
  - Hyoglossus.
  - Chondroglossus.
- **Infrahyoid muscles**
  - Sternohyoid.
  - Thyrohyoid.
  - Omohyoid.

- **Muscles located behind the hyoid**
  - Middle constrictor of pharynx.
  - Stylohyoid.
  - Digastric.
- **Ligamentous connections**
  - Stylohyoid ligament.
  - Lateral thyrohyoid.
  - Medial thyrohyoid.
  - Thyrohyoid membrane.
- **Fascial connections**
  - Cervical fascia, superficial layer.
  - Cervical fascia, pretracheal layer.
  - Suprahyoid lamina.
  - Pharynx.

3.1.2 The pterygopalatine fossa

The fissure that is the pterygopalatine fossa (Figure 3.17) is part of the infratemporal fossa. It contains the pterygopalatine ganglion. It is bounded:

- Anteriorly: by the rounded eminence of the maxillary tuberosity.
- Posteriorly: by the pterygoid process of the sphenoid bone.

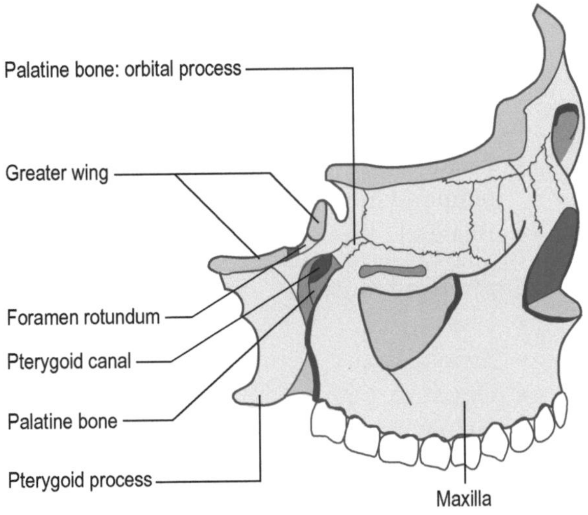

Figure 3.17
The pterygopalatine fossa

- Superiorly: by the under surface of the greater wing and body of the sphenoid bone.
- Medially: by the perpendicular plate of the palatine bone.
- Laterally: by the pterygomaxillary fissure (closed by connective tissue).
- Inferiorly: by the greater palatine canal.

It communicates with:

- The middle cranial fossa through the foramen rotundum (maxillary nerve [CN V_2]).
- The inferior surface of the cranial base through the pterygoid canal/Vidian canal (nerve and artery of pterygoid canal, running to the auditory tube).
- The infratemporal fossa through the pterygomaxillary fissure (maxillary artery).
- The oral cavity through the greater palatine canal (greater palatine nerve and descending palatine artery).
- The nasal cavity through the sphenopalatine foramen (nasal branches from CN V_2 and the sphenopalatine artery).
- The orbit through the inferior orbital fissure (infraorbital nerve, zygomatic nerve).

3.1.3 The pterygopalatine ganglion

Approximately 4 mm in diameter, the parasympathetic pterygopalatine ganglion (Figure 3.18) is one of the important "little things" in cranial osteopathy. This ganglion is linked superiorly to the maxillary nerve via two (ganglionic) branches and is suspended in the pterygopalatine fossa like an "overhead traffic light" (Volume 2, section 7.6).

It contains the perikarya of the postganglionic parasympathetic nerve fibers for the lacrimal gland and the small glands in the mucous membranes of the nose and palate. The preganglionic fibers run from the nerve of the pterygoid canal into the ganglion. The nerve of the pterygoid canal is formed from:

- The parasympathetic preganglionic greater petrosal nerve that issues from the intermedius nerve (CN VII), and

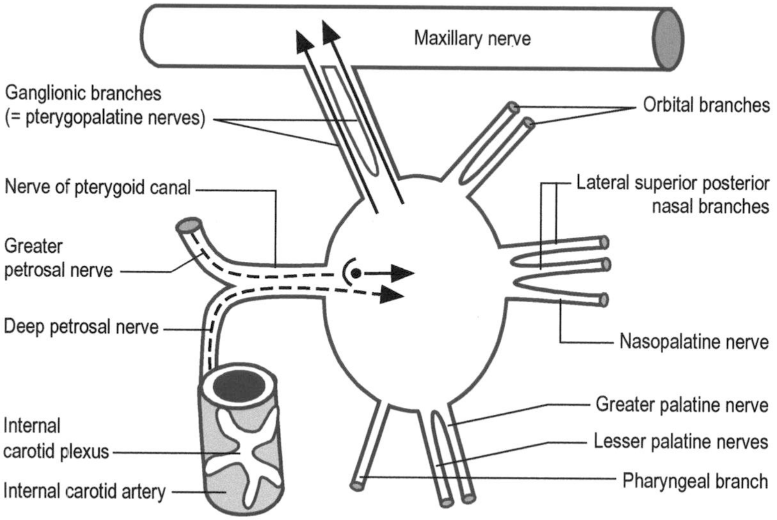

Figure 3.18
The pterygopalatine ganglion

- The sympathetic deep petrosal nerve, which receives its postganglionic fibers from the internal carotid plexus; these in turn derive from the superior cervical ganglion.

Parasympathetic and sympathetic nerve fibers emerge from the ganglion, as well as sensory elements from the maxillary nerve which, just like the sympathetic fibers, either pass through the ganglion without establishing synapses or else bypass it.

- The orbital branches enter the orbit through the inferior orbital fissure and continue into the mucous membrane of the posterior ethmoidal cells and the sphenoidal sinus.
- The lateral posterior superior nasal nerves (5–10 fine branches) pass through the sphenopalatine foramen to the superior and middle nasal conchae and to the mucous membrane of the posterior ethmoidal cells.
- The medial posterior superior nasal nerves also pass through the sphenopalatine foramen into the nasal cavity to supply the mucous membrane of the upper part of the nasal septum, traveling, as the nasopalatine nerve, through the incisive fossa to supply the mucous membrane of the anterior part of the palate and the gingiva behind the upper incisors.
- The greater palatine nerve descends through the greater palatine canal to supply the mucous membrane of the hard palate. In addition, immediately before it traverses the greater palatine foramen, it gives off branches that supply the mucous membrane of the inferior nasal concha and the inferior and middle nasal meatus.
- The lesser palatine nerves pass through canals of the same name to innervate the mucous membrane of the soft palate and the palatine tonsils.
- The pharyngeal branch runs posteriorly and medially to supply the mucous membrane of the nasopharynx.

3.1.4 The pharynx

The pharynx (Figure 3.19) is a musculomembranous tube, some 12–15 cm in length and with openings into the nasal and oral cavities. It communicates laterally with the middle ear, and contributes to both the respiratory and the digestive tracts. It can be subdivided into a nasal, an oral, and a laryngeal part. However, the limits of these subdivisions are not rigidly defined.

The pharynx is suspended on the cranial base. Below, it is continuous with the esophagus at about

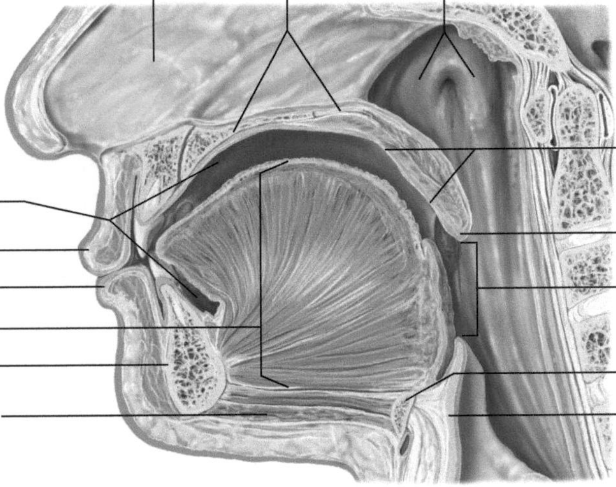

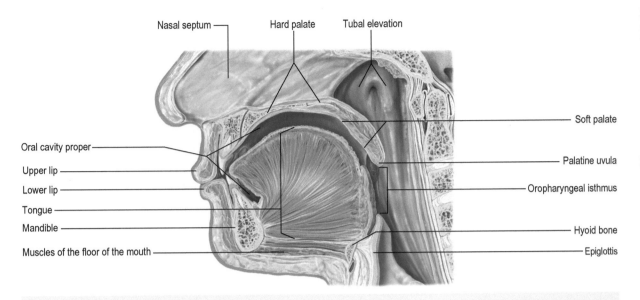

Figure 3.19
The pharynx: sagittal section, medial view. (From: Schünke, M., Schulte, E., Schumacher, U. [2015] *Prometheus LernAtlas der Anatomie. Kopf, Hals und Neuroanatomie*. Illustrations by M. Voll and K. Wesker, 4th ed. Stuttgart: Thieme)

the level of the sixth cervical vertebra. Posteriorly, the pharyngeal wall lies against the cervical spine and the paravertebral muscles. Anteriorly, it opens into the respiratory and digestive tracts.

Openings

- Choanae: the paired openings between the nasopharynx and the nasal cavity.
- Pharyngeal opening of the auditory tube laterally in the nasopharynx.
- Oropharyngeal isthmus: the opening of the oropharynx into the oral cavity.
- Mouth of the esophagus: the opening of the larynopharynx into the esophagus.
- Inlet of the larynx: the opening of the laryngopharynx into the larynx.

The nasopharynx

The nasal part of the pharynx is located at the level of the nasal cavity. It is bounded:

- Superiorly: by the roof of the pharynx at the floor of the sphenoidal sinus where the pharyngeal tonsils are located.
- Posteriorly: by the continuous downward slope of the posterior wall and the anterior arch of the atlas. At the back of the pharynx there is a collection of lymphoid tissue, known as the lateral pharyngeal bands.
- Anteriorly: by the opening into the choanae.
- Laterally: the opening of the auditory tube, approximately 1–1.5 cm behind the inferior nasal meatus; the lymphoid tissue present in the opening of the auditory tube is known as the tubal tonsils. The opening of the tube is surrounded by the tubal elevation.
- Inferiorly: by the soft palate.

Pharyngobasilar fascia

The wall at the roof of the pharynx contains no muscle fibers and is formed by the pharyngobasilar fascia (Figure 3.20), by which it is attached to the cranial base.

The pharyngobasilar fascia originates at the upper margin of the superior constrictor muscle of the pharynx as a fusion of muscle fascia. Posteriorly,

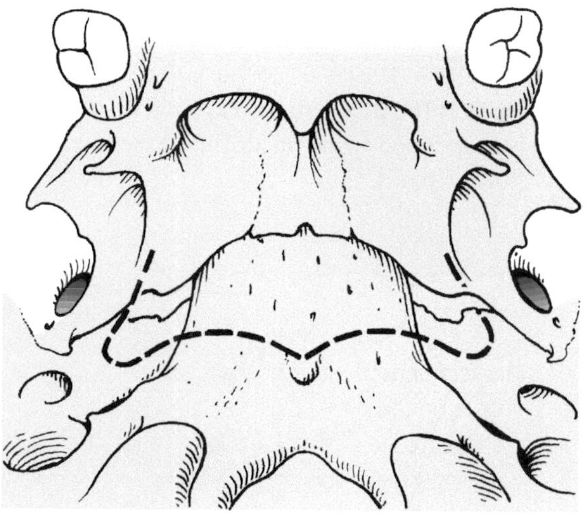

Figure 3.20
Attachment of the pharyngobasilar fascia. (From: Dauber, W. [2008] *Feneis' Bild-Lexikon der Anatomie*, 10th ed. Stuttgart: Thieme)

the pharyngeal raphe runs between the right and left pharyngeal muscles and runs to the inferior end of the pharyngeal wall, providing attachment for the constrictor muscle of the pharynx.

Attachment from posterior to anterior

- Pharyngeal tubercle of the occipital bone.
- Bilaterally over the basilar portion of the occipital bone.
- Petrous part of the temporal bone up to the carotid canal.
- Sweeps round ventrally.
- Passes medially to the tubal cartilage.
- Medial to the medial pterygoid process of the sphenoid bone.
- Attaches to the lateral border of the choanae.
- Follows the pterygomandibular raphe.
- Mylohyoid line of the mandible.

The oropharynx

The oral part of the pharynx, in which the respiratory and digestive tracts cross, opens anteriorly into the oral cavity and is located approximately on a level with the second cervical vertebra. It is bounded:

- Anteriorly: by the oropharyngeal isthmus; this consists of the root of the tongue, the soft palate with the uvula and the anterior (palatoglossal) and posterior (palatopharyngeal) palatal arches, and the muscles of the same name.
- Inferiorly: approximately on a level with the epiglottis.

The laryngopharynx

The laryngeal part of the pharynx opens below into the esophagus and is on a level approximately with the third to sixth cervical vertebrae. It is bounded:

- Superiorly: by the epiglottis.
- Anteriorly: by the inlet of the larynx and the larynx itself.
- Inferiorly: by the cricoid cartilage.

The transitional zone from the laryngopharynx to the inlet of the larynx is bounded above by the epiglottis and laterally and below by the aryepiglottic folds. A mucosal recess, termed the piriform fossa, serves as a swallowing channel in which a large part of the bolus travels from the root of the tongue to the esophageal opening.

In neonates the nasopharynx is still relatively low and the laryngopharynx has barely developed. Neonates are able to feed without closing the epiglottis because the larynx is still in a very high position.

Structure of the pharyngeal wall

The wall of the pharynx is composed of mucous membrane, submucosal connective tissue, glands, lymphoid tissue, muscle, and the adventitia. The mucous membrane does not possess a muscular layer. While the epithelium of the nasopharynx is columnar and ciliated and is interspersed with goblet cells, the other parts of the pharynx are covered with non-keratinized stratified squamous epithelium. In the upper part of the pharynx where muscle fibers are absent, the submucosal connective tissue thickens to become the pharyngobasilar fascia (see above). The submucosal layer is separated from the pharyngeal muscles by elastic connective tissue. The nasopharynx contains seromucous glands, whereas the other parts of the pharynx possess only mucous glands. The adventitia is connected to the spinal column by loose connective tissue and this enables the pharynx to glide in relation to the spinal column.

Muscles

See Figures 3.21 and 3.22.

The constrictor muscles of the pharynx

- Fiber pattern The constrictor muscles of the pharynx are annular, being open anteriorly. Posteriorly at the pharyngeal wall, ascending, horizontal, and descending fiber patterns are mingled. All the constrictor muscles of the pharynx have their attachment at the **pharyngeal raphe**. The pharynx is suspended from the cranial base by this fibrous band.

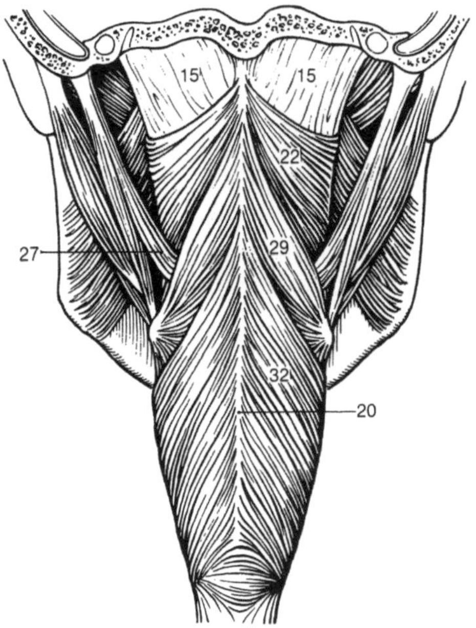

Figure 3.21
The muscles of the pharynx, posterior view.
15 Pharyngobasilar fascia. **20** Pharyngeal raphe. **22** Superior constrictor muscle of the pharynx. **27** Stylopharyngeus muscle. **29** Middle constrictor muscle of the pharynx. **32** Inferior constrictor muscle of the pharynx. (From: Dauber, W. [2008] *Feneis's Bild-Lexikon der Anatomie*, 10th ed. Stuttgart: Thieme)

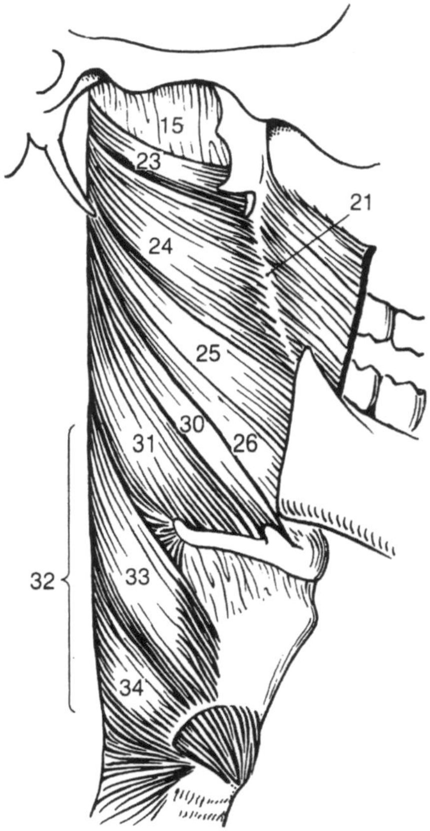

Figure 3.22
The muscles of the pharynx, lateral view. **15** Pharyngobasilar fascia. **21** Pterygomandibular raphe. **23–26** Superior constrictor muscle of the pharynx. **23** Pterygopharyngeal part. **24** Buccopharyngeal part. **25** Mylopharyngeal part. **26** Glossopharyngeal part. **30–31** Middle constrictor muscle of the pharynx. **30** Chondropharyngeal part. **31** Ceratopharyngeal part. **32** Inferior constrictor muscle of the pharynx. **33** Thyropharyngeal part. **34** Cricopharyngeal part. (From: Dauber, W. [2008] *Feneis's Bild-Lexikon der Anatomie*, 10th ed. Stuttgart: Thieme)

- Function To constrict the pharynx; in some cases, because of their muscle fiber pattern, they may also elevate or lower the pharynx.
- Innervation: The constrictor muscles of the pharynx are innervated by the **pharyngeal plexus** – in the upper pharynx more by the glossopharyngeal nerve (CN IX), and in the lower pharynx more by the vagus nerve (CN X).
- Muscles:
  - Superior constrictor muscle of the pharynx (four parts), origin:
    - Pterygopharyngeal part: the medial pterygoid plate and the pterygoid hamulus of the sphenoid.
    - Buccopharyngeal part: pterygomandibular raphe.
    - Mylopharyngeal part: the posterior end of the mylohyoid line.
    - Glossopharyngeal part: intrinsic muscles of the tongue.
  - Middle constrictor muscle of the pharynx, origin:
    - Chondropharyngeal part: lesser horn of the hyoid bone.
    - Ceratopharyngeal part: greater horn of the hyoid bone.
  - Inferior constrictor muscle of the pharynx, origin:
    - Thyropharyngeal part: oblique line of the lamina of the thyroid cartilage.
    - Cricopharyngeal part: cricoid cartilage.

The elevator muscles of the pharynx The elevator muscles of the pharynx run from above (cranial base, palatine aponeurosis, auditory tube) down to the pharyngeal wall:

- Stylopharyngeus
  - Origin: styloid process of the temporal bone.
  - Insertion: passes through the annular muscle layer between the superior and middle constrictor muscles of the pharynx, to the pharyngeal wall, thyroid cartilage, and epiglottis.
  - Function: to elevate and widen the pharynx.
  - Innervation: glossopharyngeal nerve (CN IX) and vagus nerve (CN X).
- **Palatopharyngeus**
  - Origin: palatine aponeurosis and pterygoid hamulus of the sphenoid.
  - Insertion: lateral wall of the pharynx, thyroid cartilage.
  - Function: the most powerful elevator muscle of the pharynx; to narrow the oropharyngeal isthmus, lower the soft palate, basis of the posterior pharyngeal arch; according to Magoun, it also assists in the opening of the auditory tube.[37]
  - Innervation: pharyngeal plexus (glossopharyngeal nerve [CN IX] and vagus nerve [CN X]).
- **Salpingopharyngeus**
  - Origin: posterior medial part of the lip of the auditory tube cartilage; in some cases, the longitudinal muscles of the wall of the pharynx.
  - Insertion: lateral wall of the pharynx.
  - Function: to elevate the pharynx, and prevent downward slippage of the levator veli palatini.
  - Innervation: pharyngeal plexus (glossopharyngeal nerve [CN IX]).

The muscles of the soft palate and palatal arches

- **Tensor veli palatini**
  - Origin: the spine of the sphenoid on the under-surface of the greater wing, the scaphoid fossa at the pterygoid process, and the anterior lateral wall of the auditory tube.
  - Insertion: after turning round the pterygoid hamulus, it inserts into the palatine aponeurosis.
  - Function: to tense the soft palate (elevation to the level of the hamulus), widen the auditory tube, and seal off the nasopharynx during the acts of swallowing and speaking.

- Innervation: branch of the mandibular nerve (CN V_3).
- **Levator veli palatini**
  - Origin: inferior surface of the petrous part of the temporal bone, anterior to the carotid canal, cartilaginous inferior surface of the auditory tube.
  - Insertion: palatine aponeurosis.
  - Function: to tense and elevate the soft palate, widen the auditory tube, and seal off the nasopharynx during the acts of swallowing and speaking.
  - Innervation: pharyngeal plexus (glossopharyngeal nerve [CN IX] and vagus nerve [CN X], in some cases fibers from the facial nerve [CN VII]).
- **Musculus uvulae**
  - Origin: palatine aponeurosis.
  - Insertion: connective tissue at the tip of the uvula.
  - Innervation: pharyngeal plexus (vagus nerve [CN X]).
  - Function: to shorten and thicken the uvula, and seal off the nasopharynx.
- **Palatoglossus**
  - Origin: palatine aponeurosis.
  - Insertion: transverse muscle of the tongue.
  - Function: to elevate the root of the tongue, lower the soft palate, narrow the oropharyngeal isthmus; basis of the anterior palatopharyngeal arch.
  - Innervation:
    - Glossopharyngeal nerve (CN IX).
    - Palatopharyngeal muscle.
    - See The elevator muscles of the pharynx (above).

The nerves of the pharynx

The glossopharyngeal nerve (CN IX), the vagus nerve (CN X), and the sympathetic trunk together form the pharyngeal plexus in the wall of the pharynx. This plexus sends motor fibers to muscles, and sensory and secretory fibers to the mucosa.

Motor innervation See the sections on the respective muscles (above). The upper pharynx tends to be supplied by branches of the glossopharyngeal nerve (CN IX), and the lower pharynx by branches of the vagus nerve (CN X).

Sensory innervation

- **Maxillary nerve (CN V_2)**: roof of the pharynx and area around the opening of the auditory tube.
- **Glossopharyngeal nerve (CN IX)**: root of tongue, lower nasopharynx, palatine tonsils, oropharynx.
- **Vagus nerve (CN X)**: the laryngopharynx and sometimes the oropharynx.

Vessels

Arterial supply

- **Ascending pharyngeal artery** (from the external carotid artery): most important artery, it ascends lateral to the wall of the pharynx as far as the cranial base.
- **Ascending palatine artery** (from the facial artery): wall of the pharynx.
- **Superior laryngeal artery** (from the superior thyroid artery).
- **Sphenopalatine artery** (from the maxillary artery): wall of the pharynx.
- **Inferior thyroid artery** (from the subclavian artery): inferior region of the pharynx.

Venous supply

- The **pharyngeal veins** form a venous network (pharyngeal plexus) around the muscles of the pharynx. Close to the inlet to the esophagus the veins form a kind of cushion that lends the mucous membrane a degree of elasticity, confers protection against pressure forces, and may constrict the lumen in certain circumstances.
- The pharyngeal veins flow into the **internal jugular vein**. They additionally communicate with the pterygoid venous plexus and the meningeal veins.

- The superior laryngeal vein, superior thyroid vein, and the lingual vein are located on a level with the larynx.

Lymphatic supply

Retropharyngeal lymph nodes and deep cervical lymph nodes.

The act of swallowing

Oral phase Contraction of the muscles at the floor of the mouth produces cranial and anterior movement of the hyoid bone, causing the tongue to be squeezed against the bony palate. The tongue (hyoglossus and styloglossus muscles) propels the bolus backward into the pharynx (see also section 3.2.2). This part of the act of swallowing is under voluntary control.

- Raising the larynx and bending round the epiglottis across the inlet of the trachea. While the thyrohyoid muscle draws the larynx toward the hyoid bone, the pre-epiglottic adipose body presses the epiglottis onto the inlet of the larynx, thus closing it.
- The soft palate closes the nasopharynx. Through contraction of the levator and tensor veli palatini muscles, the soft palate is elevated and brought into a horizontal position. By contraction, the superior constrictor muscle of the pharynx also forms Passavant's ridge; in that form it approximates itself to the soft palate. This has the effect of closing the nasopharynx.

Pharyngeal phase During the act of swallowing there is serial contraction of the constrictor muscles of the pharynx downward from superior to inferior. This phase is an involuntary reflex sequence which involves several cranial and spinal nerves.

Esophageal phase During the esophageal phase the food is propelled into the stomach in a peristaltic wave. This is accompanied by the reflex opening of the upper esophageal sphincter, the passage of the food along the esophagus, primary peristalsis (continuation of the initiated act of swallowing), and secondary peristalsis (regulation by mechanical stimuli and the enteric nervous system).

The swallowing reflex Once the bolus comes into contact with the wall of the pharynx, the further act of swallowing takes place involuntarily. The swallowing center is located in the medulla oblongata above the respiratory center. Afferent fibers run in the glossopharyngeal and vagus nerves to the swallowing center. In addition to the named nerves, efferent fibers also run in the trigeminal nerve (muscles of the floor of the mouth), the hypoglossal nerve (muscles of the tongue), and the cervical nerves (infrahyoid muscles). In early childhood the act of swallowing occurs as a purely reflex process and is intimately linked to the suckling process.

> **NOTE** During the act of swallowing the tongue delivers a flexion impulse to the SBS (sphenobasilar synchondrosis). During sucking, too, the tongue exerts pressure on the anterior part of the roof of the mouth and thus stimulates the SBS.

Waldeyer's lymphoid (tonsillar) ring

Waldeyer's lymphoid (tonsillar) ring (Figure 3.23) is located at the points where the oral and nasal cavities open into the pharynx. Its principal function is to identify pathogens which have penetrated into the pharynx and, where appropriate, to activate the immune defense mechanism. The ring consists of the palatine tonsils, the pharyngeal tonsils, the lingual tonsils, the tubal tonsils and, in addition, the lateral pharyngeal bands, and also lymphoepithelial organs with no specific name. These organs consist of primary and especially secondary follicles containing abundant B-lymphocytes and plasma cells.

The palatine tonsils, paired Each tonsil is placed in the tonsillar fossa between the palatoglossal and palatopharyngeal arches. The tonsil is extremely variable in size. When inflamed, especially in childhood, it may become enlarged to such

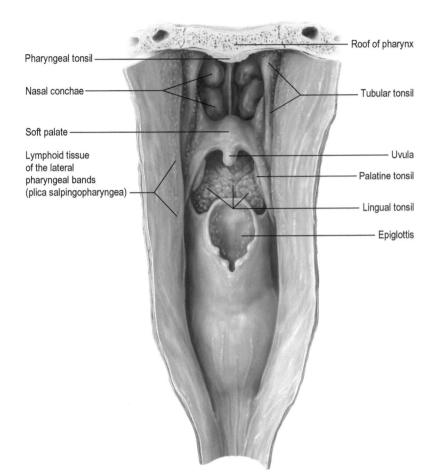

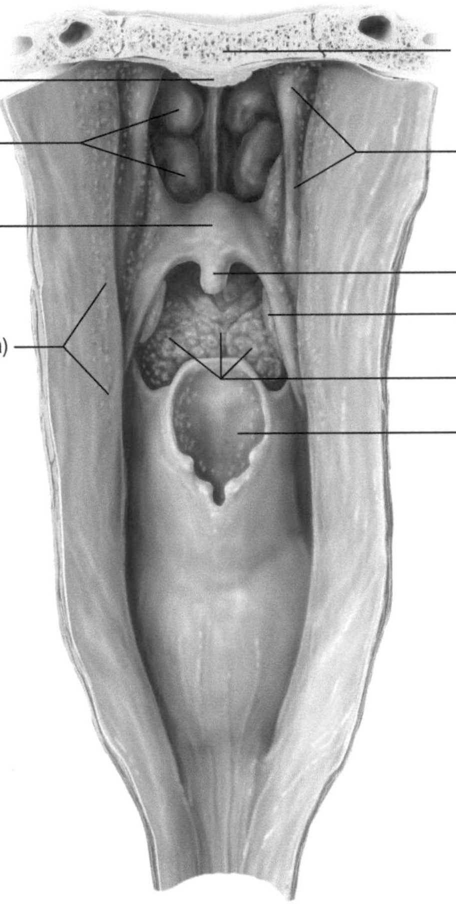

Figure 3.23
Waldeyer's lymphoid (tonsillar) ring. (From: Schünke, M., Schulte, E., Schumacher, U. [2015] *Prometheus LernAtlas der Anatomie. Kopf, Hals und Neuroanatomie.* Illustrations by M. Voll and K. Wesker, 4th ed. Stuttgart: Thieme)

an extent that swallowing is impaired. It is situated on the superior constrictor muscle of the pharynx, from which it is separated by connective tissue. The surface of the tonsil consists of some 10 to 20 crypts (epithelial pockets) which lead into the tonsillar fossulae (apertures of the crypts). Each tonsil is supplied by the facial, maxillary, and ascending pharyngeal arteries. Regionally, it is drained, inter alia, to the jugulodigastric lymph node. This is located beneath the angle of the mandible, at the intersection of the internal jugular vein and the digastric muscle. It is a clinically important finding that this lymph node becomes swollen when the palatine tonsils are inflamed. The palatine tonsils receive sensory innervation from the glossopharyngeal nerve.

The lingual tonsil, non-paired This is located at the root of the tongue and presents as a collection of lymphoid follicles. Following extraction of the palatine tonsils, the lingual tonsil may exhibit marked compensatory enlargement and produce symptoms similar to those associated with the palatine tonsils.

The pharyngeal tonsil, non-paired This is located at the roof of the pharynx, behind the choanae. In childhood the pharyngeal tonsil can grow to such a size that nasal breathing is hampered. This may lead to mouth breathing, with development of a high palate, increased susceptibility to infection due to bypassing the nasal filter, and sleep disturbances with resultant disturbed concentration (sections 2.6.2 and 3.2.4).

The tubal tonsils, paired The tubal tonsils are located around the opening of the auditory tube, on a level with the inferior nasal meatus (Figure 3.24).

Lateral pharyngeal bands, paired Formed from scattered lymphoid tissue on the salpingopharyngeal fold (Figures 3.23 and 3.24).

3.1.5 The larynx

The larynx consists of portions of cartilage, muscles, and strands of fiber (see Figure 3.25). It separates the esophagus from the trachea and serves in the protection of the airways (closing the rima glottidis and the epiglottis), phonation, and also to support abdominal muscular pressure.

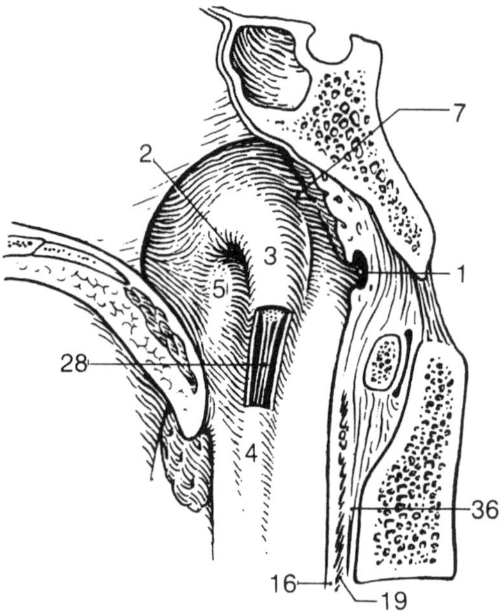

Figure 3.24
The opening of the auditory tube. **1** Pharyngeal bursa. **2** Pharyngeal opening of the auditory tube. **3** Tubal elevation. **4** Salpingopharyngeal fold. **5** Torus levatorius. **7** Pharyngeal recess. **16** Submucosal layer. **19** Muscular tunic of the pharynx. **28** Salpingopharyngeus muscle. **36** Retropharyngeal space. (From: Dauber, W. [2008] *Feneis's Bild-Lexikon der Anatomie*, 10th ed. Stuttgart: Thieme)

Three levels
- Supraglottis: from the laryngeal inlet to the space between the vestibular folds.
- Glottis: from the rima vestibuli to the rima glottidis proper.
- Subglottis: caudal to the rima glottidis to the inferior margin of the cricoid cartilage.

Cartilage framework
Suspended cranially from the hyoid bone:
- Cricoid cartilage.
- Thyroid cartilage.
- Epiglottic cartilage.
- Arytenoid cartilages.

Laryngeal joints
- **Cricothyroid joint** Hinge joint to regulate the length and tension of the vocal folds. The inferior horn of the thyroid cartilage and dorsal lateral surface of the cricoid cartilage form the articular surfaces.
- **Cricoarytenoid joint** Rotating-gliding-hinge joint (cricothyroid muscle), enables phonation by regulating the width of the rima glottidis. The cricoid cartilages move mostly cranially, to allow the arytenoid cartilages room dorsally and thus ensure frictionless movement of the vocal folds. The joint cavity of the arytenoid cartilages and the articular surfaces of the cricoid cartilage form the joint surfaces.

Muscles
- Extrinsic laryngeal: cricothyroid muscle, general pre-tensing of the vocal folds.
- Intrinsic laryngeal: posterior cricoarytenoid (opener of the glottis), lateral cricoarytenoid, transverse arytenoid, oblique arytenoid, thyroarytenoid, vocalis (fine control of tension of the vocal folds), etc.
- These serve to regulate the tension of the vocal folds and to open the rima glottidis.
- The suprahyoid and infrahyoid muscles move the larynx as a whole.

Ligaments Cricothyroid ligament, vocal ligament, lateral thyrohyoid ligament, middle thyrohyoid ligament, thyrohyoid membrane.

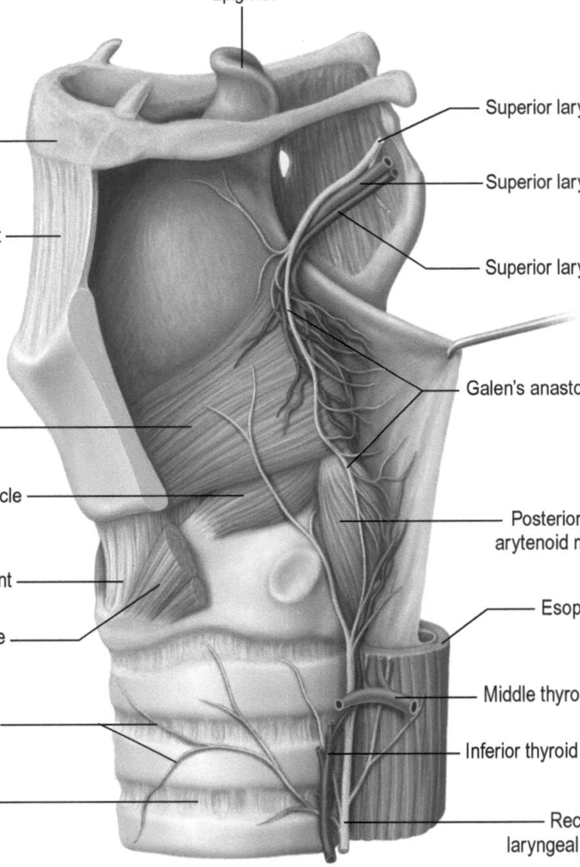

Figure 3.25
The larynx. (From: Schünke, M., Schulte, E., Schumacher, U. [2015] *Prometheus LernAtlas der Anatomie. Kopf, Hals und Neuroanatomie*. Illustrations by M. Voll and K. Wesker, 4th ed. Stuttgart: Thieme)

Fascial attachments

- Cervical fascia, superficial layer.
- Cervical fascia, pretracheal layer.

Innervation Motor and sensory via branches of the vagus nerve:

- Superior laryngeal nerve (CN X): cricothyroid muscle, sensory the mucosa above the rima glottidis
- Recurrent laryngeal nerve (CN X): intrinsic laryngeal muscles, sensory the mucosa below the rima glottidis.

Vessels

- Superior laryngeal artery (from the superior thyroid artery), superior laryngeal vein.
- Inferior laryngeal artery (from the inferior thyroid artery), inferior laryngeal vein.
- Superficial and deep lateral cervical lymph nodes (sides of the neck).
- Anterior cervical lymph nodes (front of the neck).
- Trunk of the jugular vein.

3.2 The causes of dysfunction in orofacial, pharyngeal, and laryngeal structures

Because of the manifold functions of the orofacial system, many and various factors can interact to cause dysfunctions in the mouth and face, and also in the pharynx and larynx. These include sequences of movement and coordination, the muscular balance between all the structures concerned with swallowing (hyoid, mandible, teeth, cervical spine, the muscles of the cheeks, lips, and tongue, nerves, blood vessels, etc.). For the differential diagnosis of pathological processes in the facial area, see also Volume 2, Chapter 4.

FURTHER INFORMATION

Disturbances in early childhood

Through stimulation of the lips and tongue, the infant receives important impulses for the development of the nervous system, speech, and personality. Innate reflexes form the basis for learned and practiced complex motor skills.
If the tone of certain muscles is disturbed, reflexes are unable to develop properly, with the result that complex motor skills also cannot subsequently be learned as they should be. If the chewing, sucking, or swallowing reflex is disturbed, complex masticatory patterns, articulation, voluntary sucking, and swallowing will later be limited and may be executed with diminished coordination.
For example, differentiated TMJ movement skills are necessary for the second babbling phase of language development at age 6 months. Abnormal structural development of the teeth or jaw leads in particular to disturbed articulation (apical, lingual, palatal, and uvular sounds).
Kinesthetic development is co-determined by early childhood experiences involving the oral region, for example during breastfeeding.
Somatopsychic interactions may occur in a wide range of ways. Limitation of masticatory function may also be reflected in personality development, for example in the form of a diminished determination to see things through to completion (or to "grit your teeth and get on with it").

Structural factors All the cranial bones may be involved in orofacial structure dysfunction and may require treatment in such cases.

Dysfunction of the SBS (sphenobasilar synchondrosis) or temporal bone (perinatally or postnatally) may lead to disturbances in the oral cavity, via ligamentous, fascial, and vascular connections, but also because of the influence of the cranial base on the growth of the middle and lower thirds of the face.[22]

Special attention should therefore be focused on the mandible and the maxillary complex. A narrow maxillary complex may in some cases restrict the space available for the tongue, which is then displaced forward. The young child may then develop into a mouth breather with additional follow-on symptoms (e.g., problems with sleep and concentration, etc.).[7]

For Magoun,[24:213] diet is an especially important factor in the development of problems involving the jaws, oral cavity, or pharynx.

3.2.1 Potential dysfunctions of the orofacial system, with particular reference to swallowing disorders

- **Osseous dysfunctions:** maxilla, palatine bone, mandible/TMJ, temporal bone, hyoid, cervical spine.
- **Cartilage dysfunctions:** cricoid cartilage, thyroid cartilage, epiglottic cartilage, arytenoid cartilage, epiglottis.
- **Muscular dysfunctions:** masticatory muscles (e.g., medial pterygoid), suprahyoid, infrahyoid and retrohyoid, pharyngeal and elevator muscles of the pharynx, muscles of the tongue, muscles of the soft palate, esophageal muscles, diaphragm.
- **Body posture:** in dysphagia, the head can sometimes poke forward as a postural adaptation secondary to painful swallowing disorders.[29]
- **Ligamentous dysfunctions:** frenulum of tongue, stylohyoid ligament.
- **Fascial disturbances** (see also muscular dysfunctions): the fasciae of head and neck are functionally closely connected and clinically significant in CMD and TMJ pain, and also in pain associated with chewing and swallowing, tension headache, nuchal and shoulder pain, tinnitus, dizziness, visual disturbances, sinusitis, pharyngitis, and laryngitis. Special attention should be given to the palatine

aponeurosis (as the attachment of many muscles), the pterygomandibular raphe, and the buccopharyngeal fascia (see section 2.6.4 and Volume 2, section 4.2.2).

- **Disturbances of the nerves:** swallowing center in the medulla oblongata, trigeminal nerve (CN V), facial nerve (CN VII), glossopharyngeal nerve (CN IX), vagus nerve (CN X), hypoglossal nerve (CN XII), cervical nerves C1–C3.
- **Autonomic nervous system disturbances**
  - Parasympathetic: vagus nerve (CN X), esophageal branches of the recurrent laryngeal nerve, esophageal plexus.
  - Sympathetic: stellate ganglion, thoracic aortic plexus, esophageal plexus.
- **Disturbance of the oral microbiome:** involved in the origin of intervertebral disk prolapse,[1,14] cardiovascular disease (arteriosclerosis), and diabetes[38] and dental health.
- **Disturbances of the enteric nervous system**
  - Autonomic nervous system.
  - Intramural nervous system: myenteric plexus (Auerbach's plexus), submucosal plexus (Meissner's plexus).
- **Vascular dysfunctions:** temporal artery, ascending pharyngeal artery, superior and inferior thyroid arteries, lingual artery, esophageal branches of the thoracic aorta, inferior phrenic artery, left gastric artery, pharyngeal plexus, inferior thyroid veins, azygos vein, hemiazygos vein, esophageal plexus.
- **Fascial dysfunctions:** superficial layer, pretracheal layer, and prevertebral layer of the cervical fascia, retropharyngeal space, interpterygoid fascia, palatine fascia, pharyngeal fascia, pharyngobasilar fascia.
- **Emotions, stress:** psychological and physical overload, situations of chronic emotional stress and conflict.
- **Conditions in which swallowing disorders occur:** esophageal disorders, space-occupying lesions, mechanical influences, neurological conditions, orthopedic conditions, medical conditions, rheumatologic conditions, endocrine disturbances, "swallowing the wrong way," psychological disturbances.

3.2.2 Potential dysfunctions of the tongue

- Obstruction of nasal breathing leads to downward displacement of the tongue to allow increased mouth breathing. This results in narrowing of the maxillary arch.
- Enlargement of the lingual tonsils and, sometimes, of the pharyngeal tonsils (adenoids) may displace the tongue forward.
- A shortened frenulum will fix the tongue in a lowered position.
- Dysfunction of the cervical spine, especially hyperlordosis, may cause a functional disturbance of the tongue.
- Muscular dysfunctions: hypertonicity of the styloglossus and palatoglossus muscles or a distal bite will cause the tongue to be drawn backward. Hypertonicity of the posterior fibers of the genioglossus muscle or a mesial bite causes the tongue to be drawn forward. A change in tongue position will in turn impair dental and jaw growth.
- A disturbance of the glossopharyngeal nerve (CN IX) and hypoglossal nerve (CN XII; in paresis, deviation of the tongue to the affected side) or a flexion dysfunction of the SBS lead to dysfunction of the styloglossus, palatoglossus, and other muscles of the tongue, with subsequent swallowing disorders.
- Frymann states the following: a **vertical strain dysfunction of the SBS** increases fascial tension in the cervical region, with restriction of the hyoid bone and hence of the tongue; in superior vertical strain dysfunction, there is flexion of the sphenoid and ER of the maxilla, with resultant maxillary widening and shortening. In addition, extension of the occipital bone produces IR of the temporal bone and mandible, causing the mandible to be moved posteriorly. As a result the tongue is displaced forward. In inferior

vertical strain dysfunction there is narrowing of the maxilla and widening of the tongue, possibly causing the latter to push against the teeth. Conversely, the tongue exerts an effect on the SBS. During the act of swallowing the tongue delivers a flexion impulse to the SBS.

- In **parafunctions** such as squeezing of the tongue impressions of the teeth are visible on the tongue.
- When the **tip of the tongue is squeezed** against the teeth the result is an overjet.
- **Glossoptosis** is a special condition that is associated with strong pressure exerted by the root of the tongue against the cervical spine. Pressure on the glottis and blockage of the nasopharyngeal space lead to mouth breathing.
- Common causes of **burning tongue** are mechanical stresses from rubbing the tongue on the edges of the teeth or dentures or from habits such as sucking and squeezing.

Consequences of an incorrect or fixed tongue position

- **Posterior position of the tongue**
  - Swallowing disorder with impulse delivered to the cranium in the direction of the exhalation phase of primary respiratory movement (PRM) (Figure 3.26).
  - The mandible is drawn backward.
  - Disturbance of articulation and auditory tube function, and of pharyngeal drainage.
- **Anterior position of the tongue**
  - Swallowing disorder with impulse delivered to the cranium in the direction of the inhalation phase of PRM (Figure 3.27).
  - The mandible is drawn forward.
  - Disturbance of articulation.
  - Crooked teeth (especially front teeth) with subsequent jaw disturbance.
  - The tongue may sometimes protrude between the teeth and lips.

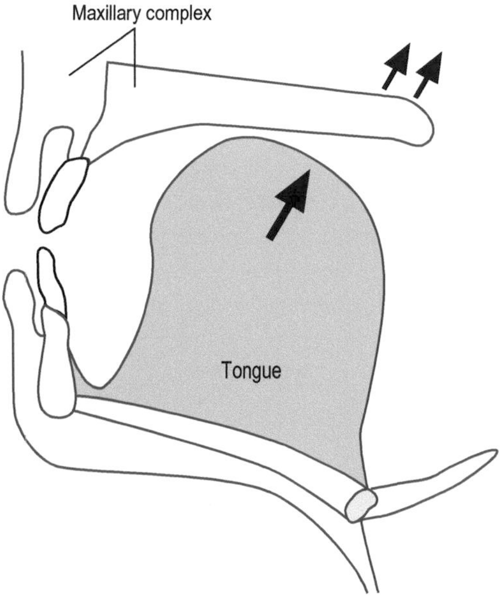

Figure 3.26
Incorrect tongue position and swallowing disturbance: backward displacement of the tongue (modified from Amigues[4])

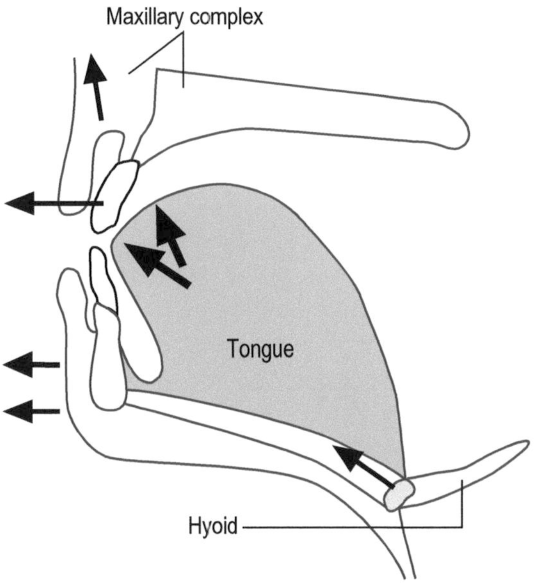

Figure 3.27
Incorrect tongue position and swallowing disturbance: forward displacement of the tongue (modified from Amigues[4])

  - During the act of swallowing the orbicularis oris muscle is unable to contract in order to resist the pressure exerted by the tongue.
  - Atonic lips.
  - According to Knapp,[16] a fixed anterior position of the tongue exerts traction on the hyoid bone via the hyoglossus and genioglossus muscles. This tension is transmitted to the temporal bone (digastric muscle, posterior belly) and the cervico-occipital junction.
- **Possible symptoms**
  - Nasal breathing disturbed when patient is supine.
  - Common ENT symptoms.
  - Impaired chewing and swallowing.
  - Speech disturbances.
  - Delayed neuromotor development.
  - Emotional instability.
  - Dental problems, malocclusion, and TMJ disturbances.

3.2.3 Potential dysfunctions involving the teeth/periodontal ligament

The maxilla, the mandible, and the palatine bone (the incisive, intermaxillary, transverse palatine, and median palatine sutures) are in direct contact with the teeth. Dental dysfunction and pain may occur as a result of incorrect diet (e.g., extreme overload due to gum-chewing), TMJ problems, dental treatments, nasal diseases, positional anomalies of the tongue, trauma, and faulty tension of the masticatory muscles (temporal, masseter, digastric). Dental braces affect the entire viscerocranium, and traumatic injury, postural misalignment, and scoliosis can cause an ascending or descending dysfunction.

Dental alignment is treated for both medical (transmission of forces) and aesthetic reasons.

Causes of dental misalignment

Genetics (cleft palate, pressure from crooked molars), body posture, facial development, diet, jaw shape, dental alignment, breathing (mouth breathing, displaced nasal breathing, etc.), swallowing pattern (infantile swallowing), tongue position and function, lip function, cheek function, occlusion, parafunctions/habits, CMD.

Oral parafunctions/habits can cause (inter alia) hypersensitivity of the neck of the teeth, dental damage (dental wear, cracked teeth, chipped teeth, loosening of teeth, fracture of the edge of the teeth), and, more rarely, periodontal disease.

Orthodontic correction with dental braces can restrict craniofacial function, leading to manually measurable restrictions of motion in remote large joints.[37]

Sequelae of **traumatic injury** to the tooth-bearing bones can in their turn cause disturbances of the eyes, nose, ears, and pharynx. An ascending dysfunction (e.g., postural misalignment, scoliosis) can cause malocclusion which in turn produces descending compensation.

Malocclusion, e.g., early contact, can cause bruxism, tension of the masticatory muscles, periodontal pocket formation, headache, and tinnitus. A malocclusion can manifest itself when the dorsum of the tongue touches the roof of the mouth during swallowing and squeezing.

According to Travell,[44:236,219,273] toothache can be caused by pain radiating from the temporal, masseter (superficial part), and digastric (anterior belly) muscles. Dental pain can radiate to the entire region innervated by the trigeminal nerve; dental, TMJ, or nuchal pain can exacerbate each other or facilitate the trigeminal nucleus (see also section 2.6.6).

Gingiva (gums) and oral mucosa

Burning tongue syndrome, oral dysesthesia, pulpitis/gangrene, gingivitis, periodontitis, a crack in the dental crown, and periodontal ligament pain can cause painful conditions.[7] Osteomyelitis in the head and nape of the neck, vascular disorders, high blood pressure, menstruation, menopause, and changes in air pressure in-flight can also cause pain in the dental region.[10,54]

Burning mouth syndrome or burning tongue (glossodynia)[39] can be caused by Sjögren's syndrome or by systemic disease, e.g., chronic iron deficiency anemia. However, it could also be of psychological origin, especially when no trophic changes are detectable or if no systemic disease has been diagnosed. Nonspecific psychogenic factors (depression, stress) are then the cause. It predominantly affects older women with dentures. The symptoms do not correspond to the regions supplied by specific nerves.

Muscles (buccinator, posterior digastric, mylohyoid) can also cause radiated pain in the gingiva.

Causes of dysfunctions in the pterygopalatine ganglion

These are produced by blows or falls, dysfunctions of the frontal bone, of the zygomatic bone, of the maxilla, of the SBS, of the temporal bone, of the ethmoid bone, or of the upper cervical spine (see also section 3.1.3).

3.2.4 Potential dysfunctions of the pharynx

See under orofacial dysfunctions (section 3.2.1); only a few more myofascial dysfunctions are addressed here.

Muscular dysfunctions of the pharynx

- Muscular dysfunctions of the pharynx can occur from **hypertonicity of muscle chains** (e.g., anterior). In unilateral hypertrophy of the thyrohoid, stylohyoid, and sternocleidomastoid muscles, the slight rotation of the cranium and vertical manubrium of sternum can exert pressure on the pharynx.[50]
- **Superior constrictor of pharynx** (four parts) The function of this muscle may be disturbed in dysfunctions involving the sphenoid, occipital, and palatine bones and as a result of abnormal tension in the cervical fascia. On the other hand, according to Magoun, by drawing the mandible forward, this muscle can induce upper pharyngeal inflammation and lymph stasis.[24:214]
- **Middle constrictor of pharynx** The motion of the hyoid bone may be restricted by this muscle.
- **Inferior constrictor of pharynx** Motion restriction of the thyroid and cricoid cartilage may impair vocal fold function.
- **Constrictor muscles of the pharynx** Through the attachment of the pharyngeal raphe at the cranial base, a flexion dysfunction of the SBS may increase the tension in the fibers of the constrictor muscles of the pharynx. A torsion or sidebending–rotation dysfunction may cause deviation of the pharyngeal raphe and other fascial structures. The consequence may be reduced lymphatic drainage and swelling of the tubal mucosa with resultant auditory problems.
- **Tensor veli palatini** If the pterygoid processes are unequally positioned, the result may be asymmetric tension in the right and left tensor veli palatini muscles. According to Magoun,[24:215] this may cause increased tension in the pharynx, associated with problems when swallowing or, in singers, with difficulty in reaching high-pitched sounds.
- **Levator veli palatini** Asymmetric dysfunctions of the temporal bones (petrous parts) may contribute to asymmetric tension in the left and right levator veli palatini muscles.

Fascial dysfunctions of the pharynx

The **pterygomandibular raphe** requires special mention here. For dysfunctions of this and other fasciae see sections 3.2.1 and 2.6.4.

3.2.5 Potential dysfunctions in laryngeal disorders

These generally present with symptoms such as hoarseness, vocal problems, ventral neck pain, and a globus sensation (functional dysphonia). The neuromuscular elements generally predominate in laryngeal disorders.

- **Osseous dysfunctions**
  - Hyoid (in functional dysphonia, this is cranially displaced during articulation:[17,23] cervical spine,[26] TMJ,[30,31,40] viscerocranium,[26] vertical position or reduced

mobility of the manubrium of sternum,[50] thoracic structures).
  - Posture of head (e.g., anterior displacement or unilateral rotation) or craniocervical posture,[26] body posture.[9,17]
- **Cartilaginous dysfunctions:** larynx (cranially displaced during articulation in functional dysphonia[19,23,36,47]), thyroid cartilage, cricoid cartilage, epiglottic cartilage, arytenoid cartilages, epiglottis, laryngeal joints.
- **Muscular dysfunctions:** neuromuscular elements are especially important in laryngeal dysfunctions.
  - Clearly visible high nuchal tension.[3]
  - Supraglottal contraction with ensuing compression of the vestibular folds.[28]
  - Hypertonicity of the extrinsic and intrinsic laryngeal muscles, parapharyngeal and suprahyoid muscles,[19] cricothyroid[17] (or with surgery or radiotherapy to the thyroid gland). In functional dysphonia with anteroposterior supraglottal compression, the tone of the thyrohyoid muscle has usually been found to be high.[5]
  - Hypertonicity of muscle chains, e.g., anterior with cranial larynx, shortened stylohyoid and sternocleidomastoid muscles and weak deep flexors,[36] relationship between high tone of the geniohyoid, sternocleidomastoid, and cricothyroid, and posterior weight displacement, cranial hyoid, and anterior position of the head.[17]
  - Masticatory muscles[31] (e.g., medial pterygoid), suprahyoid, infrahyoid, and retrohyoid, pharyngeal, elevator muscles of the pharynx, muscles of the tongue, muscles of the soft palate, esophageal muscles, diaphragm.
- **Ligamentous dysfunctions:** cricothyroid ligament, vocal ligament, lateral thyrohyoid ligament, medial thyrohyoid ligament, thyrohyoid membrane.
- **Fascial disturbances** (see also muscular dysfunctions): fasciae of neck and head in relation to posture of the head; superficial and pretracheal layers of the cervical fascia.
- **Disturbances of the nerves:** superior laryngeal nerve (CN X), and recurrent laryngeal nerve (CN X).
- **Disturbances of the autonomic nervous system:** sympathetic: stellate ganglion, thoracic aortic plexus, esophageal plexus.
- **Disturbances of the enteric nervous system**
  - Autonomic nervous system.
  - Intramural nervous system: myenteric plexus (Auerbach's plexus), submucous plexus (Meissner's plexus).
- **Vascular dysfunctions:** superior thyroid artery/vein, inferior thyroid artery/vein, superficial and deep lateral cervical lymph nodes, anterior cervical lymph nodes, trunk of the jugular vein.
- **Emotions:** stress,[19] tendency to upper respiratory tract infections.[13,19]
- **Other aspects:** gastroesophageal reflux, vocal strain.[3]

3.3 Diagnostic investigations for orofacial, pharyngeal, and laryngeal structures

3.3.1 History-taking

- The following symptoms can occur in **orofacial dysfunction**: incomplete lip closure; mouth breathing; increased salivary production; disturbances of sucking, of chewing, of swallowing, of the salivary glands and of the mucosa, of articulation, of the lacrimal glands; special sense deficits and sensory deficits of the tongue and restricted mobility of the tongue; non-physiological resting position of the tongue; forward displacement of the tongue when speaking; disturbed muscle balance in the region of the mouth, face, and neck; and also pain or paresis in the oropharyngeal region. Also consider dental disorders; dental misalignment; diseases and disturbances of the upper respiratory tract, including Waldeyer's tonsillar ring (enlarged tonsils).

- **Sequelae** include disturbed development of chewing, biting, and swallowing, and of articulation ("slurred" enunciation). Tongue protrusion against the teeth in swallowing can predispose to misalignment of teeth and jaws.
- **Clinical signs of the pterygopalatine ganglion:** e.g., dry or irritated nasal, nasopharyngeal, and palatal mucosa, disturbances of lacrimal secretion, asthma, etc.
- **Larynx:** changes can occur in the voice, mainly hoarseness, vocal problems, and also ventral neck pain and globus sensation (functional dysphonia): also, laryngeal crepitation, cough, breathing problems, dysphagia, etc. Symptoms can be precisely localized (in which case mostly unilateral), infrahyoid in the form of cramping sensations, or can manifest as a diffuse sensation of pressure throughout the neck.
- Regarding **etiology**, also consider trauma to the larynx and its environs (nape of neck, respiratory and digestive tracts) and diseases of the respiratory and digestive tracts, gastroesophageal reflux, CMD, and juvenile rheumatoid arthritis.
- **Also enquire about** inflammations, surgery, hearing problems, vocal strain (occupational, nicotine, and alcohol abuse), parafunctions, stress.

3.3.2 Inspection

Assess the symmetry, position, and shape of the oral cavity, the shape of the tongue, the condition of the teeth, dental alignment, mucosal changes, and also the size, color, and coating of the tonsils.

Also evaluate the symmetry, position, shape, and mobility of the mandible, hyoid, larynx, shoulder, cervical spine, cranium, and manubrium of sternum, and also the shape or contours of the associated muscles, e.g., nuchal, hyoid, and extrinsic laryngeal.

If dysfunction is present you can perceive asymmetries and abnormal positions and movement patterns of the structures mentioned:

- Mouth breathing with incompetent, shortened upper lip, incomplete lip closure, and associated increased tone of the mentalis (dimple and crease formation below the lower lip).
- Pouched cheeks, unilateral or bilateral? Indicates tension in the buccinator (leads to narrowness of the maxilla with risk of crossbite).
- Hypertrophy of the muscles of mastication?
- Cranial translation or rotation?
- Shoulder elevation?
- Asymmetry and altered contour of the nuchal muscles, of the sternocleidomastoid, semispinalis, and/or trapezius?
- Hyoid and/or larynx elevated?
- Unilateral or bilateral hypertrophy of the thyrohyoid and stylohyoid muscles?
- Manubrium of sternum in vertical position?
- Dyskinesia evaluation: see section 2.10.
- Evaluation of the oral microbiome: UV illumination to evaluate *Propionibacterium acnes*; gingival bleeding can indicate a dysfunctional oral microbiome.

3.3.3 Larynx questionnaire

- **RBH-Index:** a subjective rating scale for auditory assessment of voice quality (roughness [R], breathiness [B], hoarseness [H]), e.g., by speech and language pathologists or speech therapists.
- **Voice Handicap Index (VHI):** for the patient's own subjective assessment of a vocal impairment.

3.3.4 General test

General tests for the orofacial and pharygolaryngeal region are described below. Test affected structures specifically: e.g., the periodontium, tongue, floor of the mouth, hyoid, pharynx, larynx, and also the muscles of facial expression, masticatory muscles, nuchal muscles, suprahyoid and infrahyoid muscles, extrinsic and intrinsic laryngeal muscles, and the nerves and blood vessels involved. These are listed under the treatment techniques in section 3.4.

Palpation and listening tests

Do these in the region of the oropharynx and the ventral region of the neck, taking account of regional structures. These include:

- Oral cavity.
- Pharynx.
- Hyoid, larynx, in particular thyroid cartilage and cricoid cartilage.
- Muscles of facial expression, suprahyoid, infrahyoid, extrinsic and intrinsic laryngeal muscles.
- Cervical spine, in particular nuchal muscles and upper cervical region.
- Sternum.
- Nerves (CN V, CN VII, CN IX, CN X, CN XII, pterygopalatine ganglion, otic ganglion) and blood vessels (e.g., external carotid artery, facial artery, maxillary artery, greater palatine artery, superior and inferior thyroid arteries), tonsils.

Perform listening and elasticity tests and muscular palpation, taking account of tenderness to pressure, allodynia, active trigger points, asymmetry, etc.

The cervical spine, hyoid, and larynx during the act of swallowing

Patient: Seated.

Practitioner: Take up a position beside the patient.

Hand position: Place one hand on the neck muscles. With your other hand span the hyoid and/or the larynx (Figure 3.28).

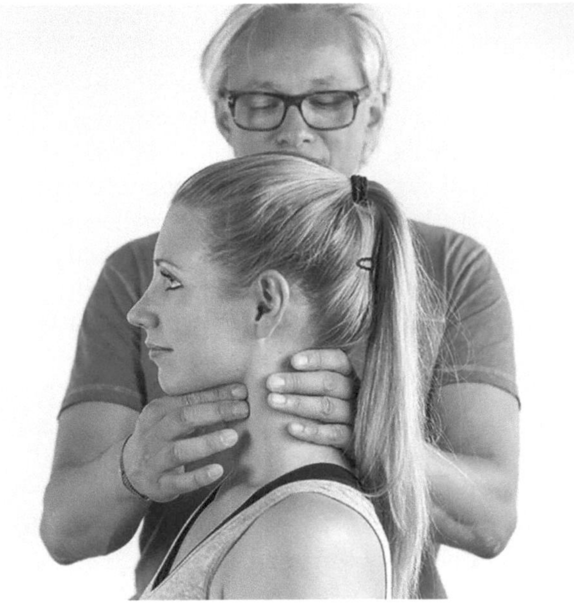

Figure 3.28 Testing the relationship between the cervical spine, hyoid, and larynx while swallowing

Method:

- Ask the patient to swallow.
- During swallowing, there should normally be no or only minimal activity in the cervical spine and no head movement (e.g., minimal rotation or translation) or lifting of the shoulders. There should be minimal activity of the lips during swallowing. A rapid craniocaudal movement at the hyoid should be detected.
- In a swallowing impairment there is prolonged activity of laryngeal movement and also of the submental muscles. This finding seems to act as compensation for weak pharyngeal musculature, by keeping the larynx closed and raised for longer in order to enable swallowing without aspiration.[52]
- Diminished anterior-vertical laryngeal movement is also associated with disordered opening of the upper esophageal sphincter.[27]

The cervical spine, cranium, hyoid, and larynx while speaking and/or singing

Patient: Seated.

Practitioner: Take up a position beside the patient.

Hand position: Place one hand on the neck muscles. With the other hand span the hyoid and/or the larynx (Figure 3.29).

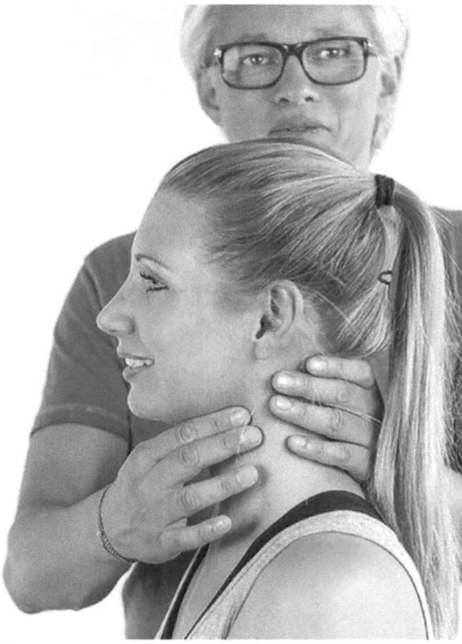

Figure 3.29 Testing the relationship between the cervical spine, cranium, hyoid, and larynx while speaking and/or singing

Method:

- Ask the patient to speak and sing.
- During this, evaluate pain or vocal impairments.
- Examine the movement of the hyoid and larynx during speaking and/or singing.
- Normally, during speaking and singing, there should be little or no activity in the cervical spine and no head movement (e.g., head rotation).
- Also note shoulder elevations or restricted movement of the sternum.

Swallowing and the tongue:

- Using cheek retractors, keep the patient's mouth open.
- Ask the patient to swallow.
- Observe the activity of the tongue during the swallowing process.
- The test is positive if the tongue presses against the teeth (visceral swallowing pattern), additional muscular activity is visible in the nuchal region, or bubbles of saliva are produced.

Swallowing and lips:

- With your index finger and thumb, take hold of the patient's lips, press them together, and hold firmly, while instructing the patient to swallow.
- The test is positive if the patient is unable to swallow while the lips are held firmly in this way.
- This is a physiological finding in early childhood but later it provides a pointer to a functional developmental disturbance of the tongue.

Alternative method: With your thumb and index finger, pull the patient's lower lip forward and hold it firmly in that position while the patient swallows.

Testing the hyoid, thyroid/cricoid cartilage, and other laryngeal cartilage: passive and active

Hand position: With the index finger and thumb of the relevant hand, span the structure or the relational structure under investigation, e.g., for the hyoid and thyroid cartilage (Figure 3.30):

- With the index finger and thumb of the cranial hand span the hyoid.
- With the index finger and thumb of the caudal hand span the thyroid cartilage.

Method:

- Passively test (passive sensing of tension patterns) and then actively test laterality, rotation, sidebending, tilting, craniocaudal and anteroposterior mobility.
- You can test the structures individually and in relation to one another, in particular the hyoid (cranial traction) in relation to the thyroid cartilage, and also other laryngeal cartilages in relation to one another.

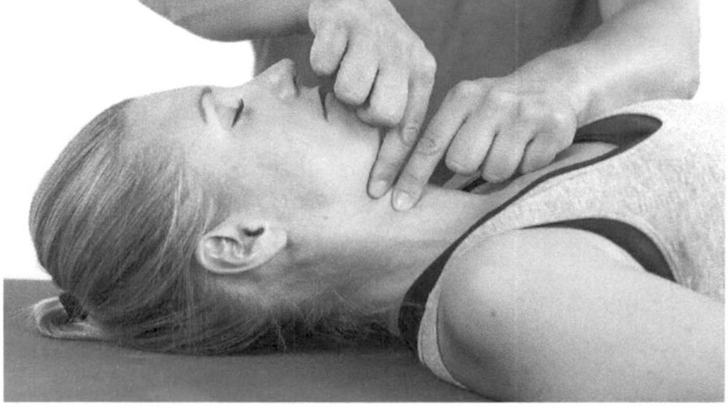

Figure 3.30 Testing the hyoid, thyroid/cricoid cartilage, and other laryngeal cartilages: passive and active

Chapman reflex points

Chapman points are neurolymphatic reflex points in tissue which are the expression of viscerosomatic reflexes. Local obstruction of lymphatic drainage occurs deep in the tissues of the reflex zone affected, presumably mediated by the sympathetic nervous system.

The points are palpated deep in the skin and subcutaneous tissues and, in particular, in the deep fascial layer or in the periosteum (Figure 3.31). Positive points are tender to pressure and tense to the touch, similar to a blister, with or without granular connective-tissue hardening.

Chapman reflex points of the tongue

- Anterior: on the second costal cartilage, 2 cm lateral to the sternum.
- Posterior: above and midway between the spinous process and the transverse process of the axis.

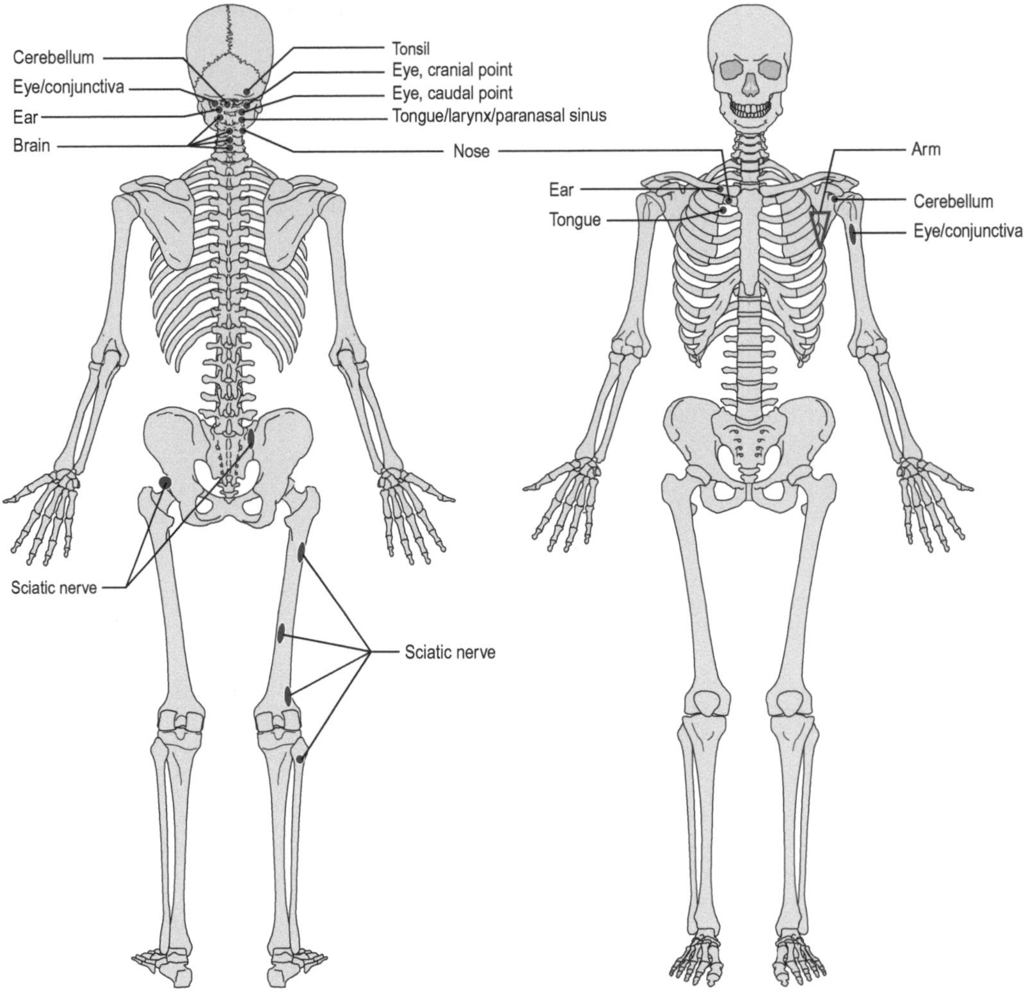

Figure 3.31
Chapman reflex points

Chapman reflex points of the pharynx

- **Pharyngitis**
  - Anterior: on the first rib, 2 cm medial to the point of intersection with the clavicle.
  - Posterior: midway between the spinous process and transverse process of the axis.
- **Tonsillitis**
  - Anterior: first intercostal space, next to sternum.
  - Posterior: midway between the spinous process and transverse process of the atlas.
- **Laryngitis**
  - Anterior: superiorly, on the second rib, 5–6 cm lateral to sternum.
  - Posterior: midway between the spinous process and transverse process of the axis.

3.4 Treatment of the orofacial structures

In treatment, it is necessary to distinguish between peripheral and central sensitization (section 2.6.6).

Tip for practitioners

Treatment method for the orofacial structures
According to Magoun,[24] all the cranial structures should be restored to normal.

- The treatment should focus on the following aspects
  - Normal facial development.
  - Normal acts of swallowing (with no involvement of the mentalis muscle).
  - Nasal breathing.
  - Normal position of tongue and lips.
  - Assisting neutral occlusion and straight teeth.
  - Resolving dysfunctional nuchal tension associated with swallowing.
  - Reducing or resolving dysfunctional patterns involved.
  - Cranial base and the atlanto-occipital joint.
  - Viscerocranium intraosseous and interosseous, in particular maxilla, incisive suture, palatine bone, vomer.
  - Masticatory muscles.
  - Temporal bone, mandible, and the TMJ, including ligaments.
  - Periodontal ligament.
  - Muscles of the floor of the mouth, further hyoid muscles, as well as the hyoid bone and tongue.[22]
  - Cervical spine, especially the upper part, nuchal muscles, and craniocervical fasciae.[22]
  - The following cranial nerves: mandibular (CN V_3), maxillary (CN V_2), greater palatine (CN V_2), facial (CN VII), glossopharyngeal (CN IX), vagus (CN X), hypoglossal (CN XII), otic ganglion (CN IX), submandibular ganglion (CN VII; Volume 2, Chapter 7).
  - External carotid artery/maxillary artery (section 2.8.5).
  - Greater palatine artery (maxillary artery; section 3.4.9).
  - Venous structures, e.g., pterygoid venous plexus (Volume 2, section 2.5.4).
  - Lymphatic drainage of the oral cavity, deep lymphatic pharyngeal drainage.
  - Dietary counseling.[24:213]
  - Microbiome.

Tip for practitioners

Treatment methods for pharyngeal structures, e.g., in sore throat
When treating sore throat, it is important first to find out whether it is a group A beta-hemolytic streptococcal infection or diphtheria (a notifiable disease in Germany and many other countries worldwide). Antibiotics are indicated for these diseases because of the risk of dangerous complications.

Therapy is directed primarily at stimulating the immune system, at removing toxic waste products, and at improving venous drainage. In this context, too, treatment must of course be preceded by a global examination:

- Palatine bone, maxilla, SBS.
- If appropriate, lateral pterygoid muscle (pharyngeal pain) and digastric muscle (swallowing disorder).[44:249,276]
- Craniocervical fasciae.
- Cervicothoracic diaphragm, superior costal articulations, sternoclavicular and acromioclavicular joints, sternum (thymus), release of scalene muscles, etc.[22]
- Muscles of the floor of the mouth, tongue, further hyoidal muscles, and also hyoid bone.[2,22]
- Upper cervical vertebrae and the atlanto-occipital joint (superior cervical ganglion) and pre-ganglionic on a level with the seventh cervical vertebra to second thoracic vertebra and first rib.
- 11th and 12th ribs and thoracic vertebrae (adrenals).
- **Local drainage of the tonsils (section 3.4.13) and auditory tube technique (Volume 2, section 6.4.2).**
- **Lymph techniques**
    - Release of diaphragmatic tension (= primary lymphatic pump).
    - Lymphatic pump technique for the feet.
    - CV-4 technique.
    - Recoil technique for the upper thoracic region and the upper cervicothoracic junction.
    - Osteopathic drainage of the palatine and tubular tonsils.
    - Drainage of the retropharyngeal lymph nodes and of the deep cervical lymph nodes.
- Cranial nerves: mandibular nerve (CN V_3), maxillary nerve (CN V_2), facial nerve (CN VII), glossopharyngeal nerve (CN IX), vagus nerve (CN X), hypoglossal nerve (CN XII; Volume 2, Chapter 7).
- Arteries: external carotid, external carotid/maxillary, external carotid/facial, superior thyroid.
- Harmonization and stimulation of immune defense organs: spleen, liver, thymus, and appendix.
- Resolution of psychosocial stress factors.
- Regulation of diet: cutting down on or avoiding dairy products, cutting down on refined sugar, bread, farinaceous foods, and fried foods. More fruit and vegetables instead.
- **Self-help techniques**
    - Drainage of the palatine tonsils.
    - "Roaring lion."

Tip for practitioners

Methods for the treatment of laryngeal structures, e.g., in functional dysphonia:

- Viscerocranium: intraosseous and interosseous.
- Craniomandibular.
- Hyoid.
- Larynx[1,2]
    - Thyroid cartilage, cricoid cartilage[2] and other laryngeal cartilages, arytenoid cartilage.
    - Thyrohyoid muscle, thyrohyoid membrane: see technique for the thyroid cartilage (section 3.4.7).
    - Cricothyroid muscle, intrinsic laryngeal muscles: see technique for the thyroid cartilage (section 3.4.7).
    - Cricothyroid ligament, thyrohyoid membrane, vocal ligament, lateral thyrohyoid ligament, median thyrohyoid ligament: see technique for the thyroid cartilage (section 3.4.7).
    - Mobilization of the larynx.[2]
    - Circumlaryngeal technique.
- Muscle chains: anterior, posterior, lateral, spiral.
- Suprahyoid muscles.[2]
- Cervical spine, especially upper cervical region, nuchal muscles, and craniocervical fasciae.[2]
- Muscles of facial expression and fasciae.
- Craniosternosacral axis, especially the manubrium of sternum.

- Superior thoracic aperture (thoracic inlet), thoracic structures, including sternocleidomastoid, trapezius muscles.[2]
- Respiratory regulation.
- Head/body posture.[2]
- Superior laryngeal nerve, recurrent laryngeal nerve, glossopharyngeal nerve (CN IX).
- Superior thyroid artery/vein, inferior thyroid artery/vein.
- Lymphatic drainage of the neck: see Volume 2, section 5.1.5.
- Self-help exercises to relax the nuchal, neck, and scapular muscles.[2]
- If appropriate, resting the voice.
- Relaxation exercises, stress reduction, if appropriate psychological support.
- Further: interdisciplinary cooperation, e.g., speech therapy, voice therapy, medical support, in some circumstances surgical intervention.

References and notes

[1] Treatment of laryngeal structures seems to be especially indicated for functional dysphonia.[6,13,15,21,25,33,34,35,47,48,49]

[2] Osteopathic treatment combined with voice therapy improved many variables in occupational dysphonia[25] (see "Further Information").

FURTHER INFORMATION A study of the interdisciplinary treatment of occupational dysphonia by osteopathic manipulative therapy and voice therapy showed a statistically significant improvement in many variables.[25] The following treatment setting was chosen:

- General techniques for the occipital bone, the nape of the neck, and the cervicothoracic junction: fascial general nuchal normalization, strain/counterstrain for the cervical spine and for the suprahyoid muscles, facilitated positional release techniques for the sternocleidomastoid.
- Laryngeal techniques: laryngeal mobilization through stretching of the cricothyroid space, mobilization of the hyoid in the direction of the thyroid cartilage, mobilization of the hyoid during swallowing, lateral mobilization of the hyoid, fascial relaxation of suprahyoid muscles, facilitated positional release techniques for the cervical joints and specifically for the region C0/C1.
- Self-help techniques: post-isometric relaxation for the trapezius, levator scapulae, active relaxation of the nuchal fasciae, relaxation of the suprahyoid muscles.

3.4.1 Treating the periodontal ligament

Testing the periodontal ligament

Since the dental root is connected to the alveolar bone via the periodontal ligaments, the fibrous joint (syndesmosis or gomphosis) between tooth and bone can also be affected by abnormal tension, just like any other articulation.

Practitioner: Take up a position beside the patient's head.

Hand position: Place your index and middle fingers on the occlusal surface of the teeth (Figure 3.32).

Method: Treat the tooth that appears to move in the direction of your fingers or generally appears to move more than the other teeth.

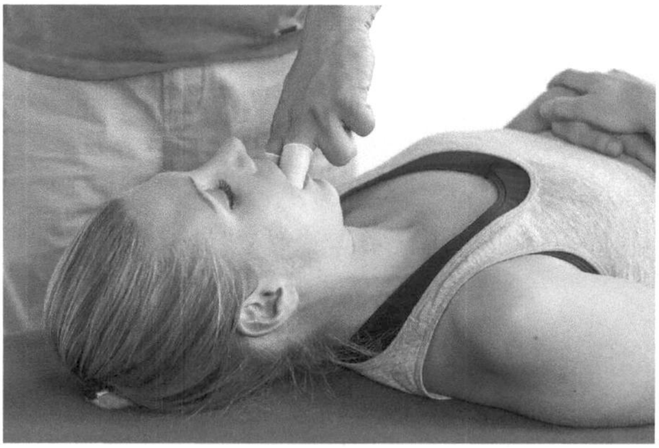

Figure 3.32 Testing the periodontal ligament

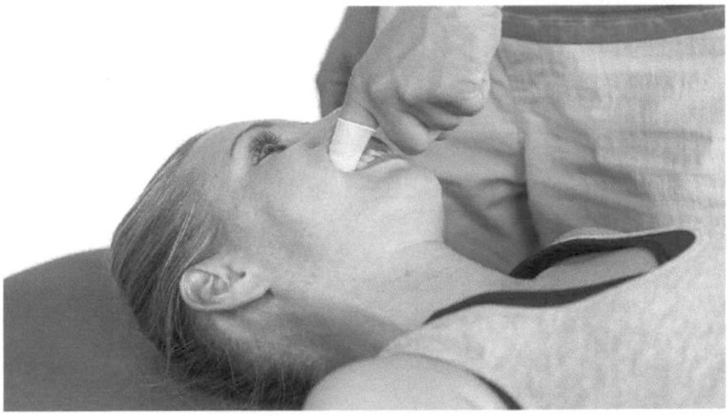

Figure 3.33 Alternative method of testing the periodontal ligament

Alternative test: Place one finger against the buccal surface of the row of teeth and ask the patient to chatter his/her teeth (Figure 3.33). Treat the tooth that presses outward against your finger.

Treatment of the teeth

Practitioner: Take up a position beside the patient's head.

Hand position: Take hold of the affected tooth between your thumb and index finger (Figure 3.34).

Method: Follow the intrinsic movements of the tooth. Perform an "unwinding" of the tooth in its periodontal ligament. Then establish the PBLT in the periodontal ligament.

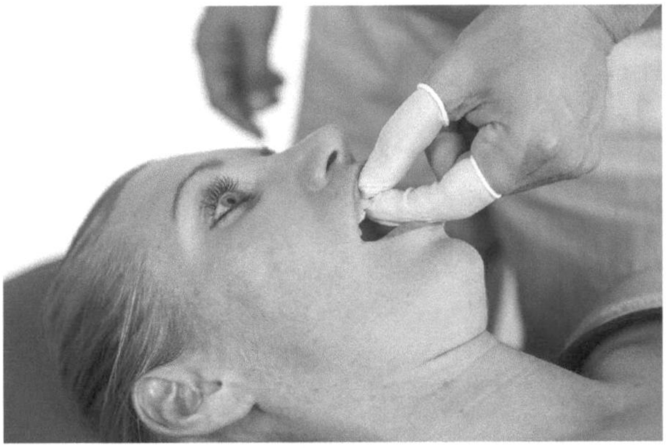

Figure 3.34 Treatment of the teeth

Alternative treatment:

With your thumb and index finger, test each tooth in internal rotation and external rotation, and then treat using the exaggeration principle (indirect technique).

3.4.2 Disorders which are sequelae of dental trauma

Causes: Condition following traumatic injury and subsequent dental and/or orthodontic surgery.

Sequelae: Intraosseous lesions in the maxilla and/or mandible, devitalized teeth, further systemic symptoms possible as sequelae of accident.

Treatment methodology: Supporting dental treatments:

- Affected teeth and related intraosseous lesion.
- Temporomandibular joint.
- Fascial structures of the oral system and also of the viscerocranium.
- Bony cranial structures.
- Craniosacral rhythms.
- Cervical spine, especially atlas and axis.
- Hyoid.
- Shock centers: e.g., lungs, diaphragm, celiac ganglion.
- If appropriate, treatment of further relational structures, depending on case history and diagnostic investigations.
- Psycho-emotional integration,[232] e.g., bifocal integration.
- If appropriate, referral for psychotherapy or hypnotherapy.

3.4.3 Treatment of the tongue

Stretching the frenulum

Method: Place your index finger on the underside of the patient's tongue and stretch the frenulum laterally (Figure 3.35).

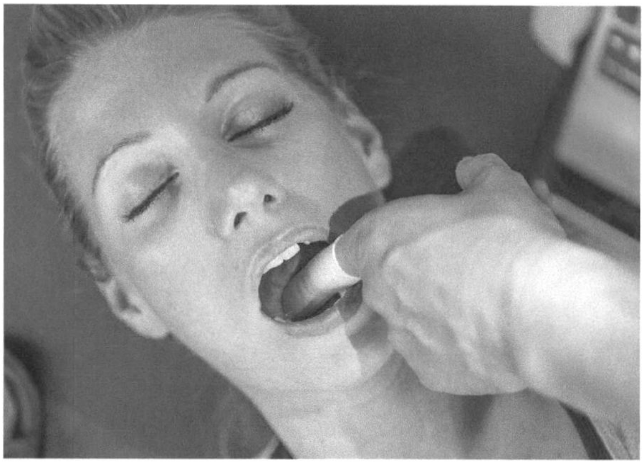

Figure 3.35 Stretching the frenulum

"Unwinding" the tongue

Practitioner: Take up a position beside the patient's head.

Hand position: Take hold of the patient's tongue between your thumb, index finger, and middle finger (Figure 3.36).

Method:
With your fingers, follow all the movements of the tongue ("unwinding") until you sense that release of the tongue has occurred.

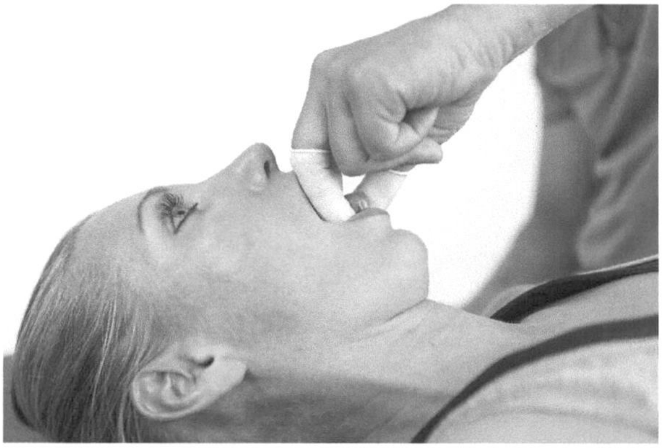

Figure 3.36 "Unwinding" the tongue

General loosening of tension in the tongue

Practitioner: Take up a position beside the supine or seated patient.

Hand position: Take hold of the patient's tongue between your thumb, index finger, and middle finger (Figure 3.36).

Method:

- Ask the patient to swallow while you fix the tongue in place with a handkerchief.
- During this, the patient maintains his/her head in the position of maximal tongue tension, e.g., in sidebending or rotation, etc.
- Repeat this procedure three times. Then perform a gentle "unwinding" of the tongue.
- The patient can also practice this at home as a self-help technique.

Drainage of the tongue

The anterior part of the underside of the tongue is drained toward the tip of the chin; the posterior part posteriorly toward the deep cervical lymph nodes.

3.4.4 Treatment of the floor of the mouth and the omohyoid muscle

Palpation of the floor of the mouth

- Geniohyoid muscle: on intraoral palpation, a band of muscle running from the inferior mental spine of the mandible to the hyoid.
- Mylohyoid muscle: on intra- and extraoral palpation, a sheet of muscle extending from the mylohyoid line of the mandible to the hyoid.
- Digastric muscle: posterior belly: posterior to the angle of the mandible (test for tenderness to pressure during jaw movement).
- Anterior belly: palpate from outside at the floor of the oral cavity.

Technique for the suprahyoid muscles

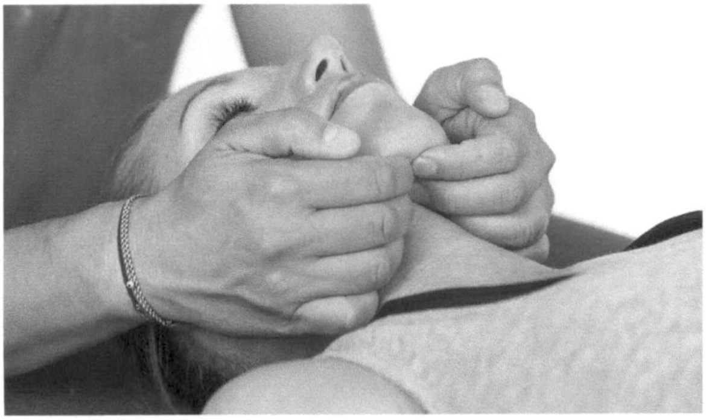

Figure 3.37 Technique for the suprahyoid muscles

Indication: Hypertonicity of the suprahyoid muscles, globus sensation. In the case of a craniomandibular dysfunction the floor of the mouth is often tensed.

Practitioner: Take up a position at the head of the patient.

Hand position: Place the index, middle, and ring fingers of both hands on the midline at the floor of the mouth.

Method: With your index, middle, and ring fingers, apply gentle pressure cranially. While maintaining this pressure, stroke your fingers mediolaterally along the floor of the mouth (Figure 3.37).

Alternative technique I

Practitioner: Take up a position at the head of the patient.

Hand position: Place your hands over both sides of the mandible. From below, place the tips of the fingers of both hands on the muscles of the floor of the mouth.

Method: With your fingers, apply cranial and medial traction (Figure 3.38). Maintain traction until you sense release of tension.

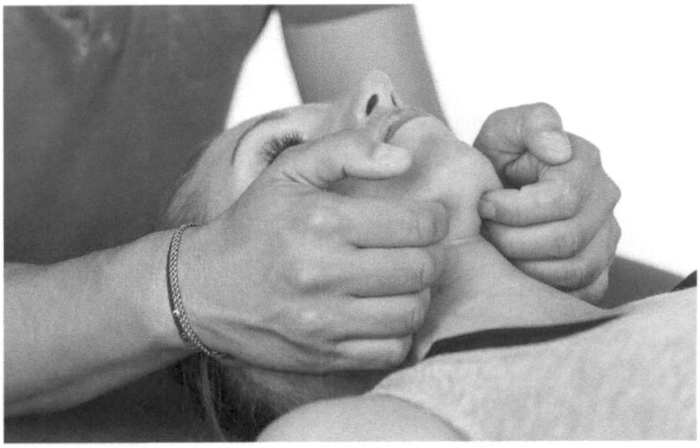

Figure 3.38 Alternative technique I

Alternative technique II, intraoral

Practitioner: Take up a position beside the patient's head.

Hand position: Place the index finger of your cranial hand intraorally on the floor of the mouth. From outside the patient's mouth, position the index finger of your caudal hand on the floor of the mouth, at the same site as the other finger.

Method: With the index finger which is inside the patient's mouth, perform gentle circling movements on the muscles at the floor of the oral cavity, using the index finger outside as a fulcrum (Figure 3.39).

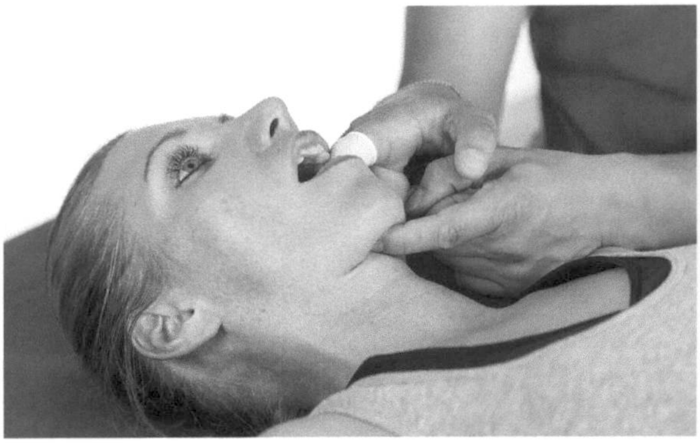

Figure 3.39 Alternative technique II

NOTE Both methods should be comfortable for the patient. Stop the procedure if the patient experiences discomfort.

Technique for the omohyoid muscle

Indication: Dysfunctions of the thoracic spine, of the scapula, and the shoulder girdle; venous drainage disturbances of the cranium and ensuing headaches, compression of the common carotid artery.

Practitioner: Take up a position beside the patient's head.

Hand position: Place the thumb of one hand at the posterior attachment of the muscle to the scapula. Place your other hand on the underside of the mandible (Figure 3.40).

Method:

- The posterior inferior attachment of the omohyoid muscle cannot be treated directly.
- With your thumb, first push the trapezius in a posterior direction.
- Your thumb is now positioned along the course of the omohyoid muscle.

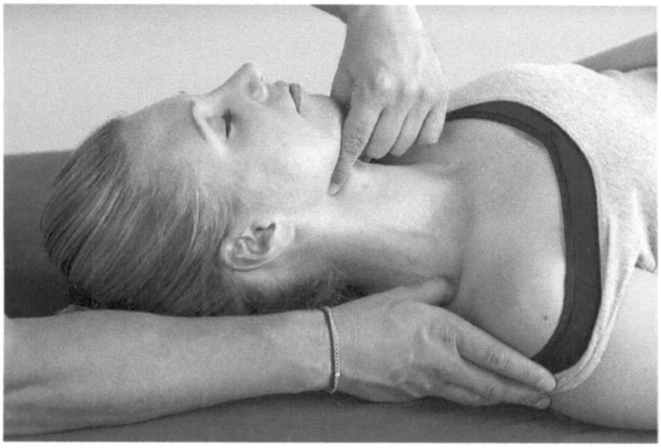

Figure 3.40 Technique for the omohyoid muscle

- By gentle contraction against resistance from the practitioner, the muscles covering the posterior margin of this muscle can reduce the pressure on the jugular vein.

3.4.5 Treatment of the hyoid bone

Indication: Hypertonicity of the suprahyoid and infrahyoid muscles, swallowing disorders, hoarseness, disturbances of phonation and articulation, disturbances of tongue movement; thyroid dysfunctions; dysfunctions of the occiput, cervical spine, and thoracic spine; cranial venous drainage disturbances causing headache; compression of the common carotid artery.

Practitioner: Take up a position beside the patient, on a level with the hyoid.

Hand position:

- With one hand, span the hyoid between index finger and thumb.
- Place the other hand either at the back of the cervical spine or on the relevant structure to test specific anatomical relations. For instance, for the relationship between the hyoid and the thyroid cartilage, span the thyroid cartilage with index finger and thumb (Figure 3.42).

Method:

- **Passive test** Evaluation of the position and passive tensile stress on the hyoid.
- **Active test** Active testing of laterality, rotation, sidebending, tilting, craniocaudal, and anteroposterior mobility of the hyoid.
- **Indirect technique**
  - Then move the hyoid to its limit in the direction of ease.
  - Once the tissues soften, seek the new limit of motion.
  - Repeat this process until no further tissue softening can be detected.
  - Then return the hyoid bone to the neutral position.

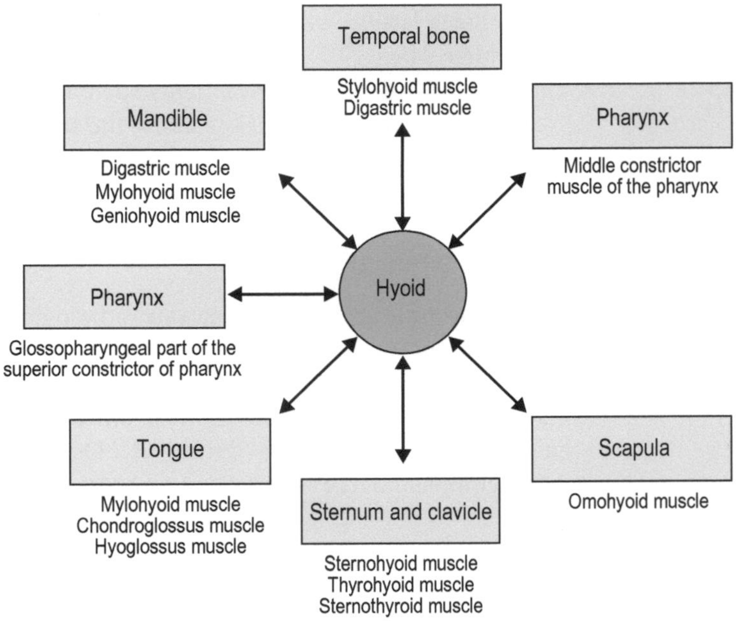

Figure 3.41 Interactions between the hyoid bone and its muscular/musculofascial relations

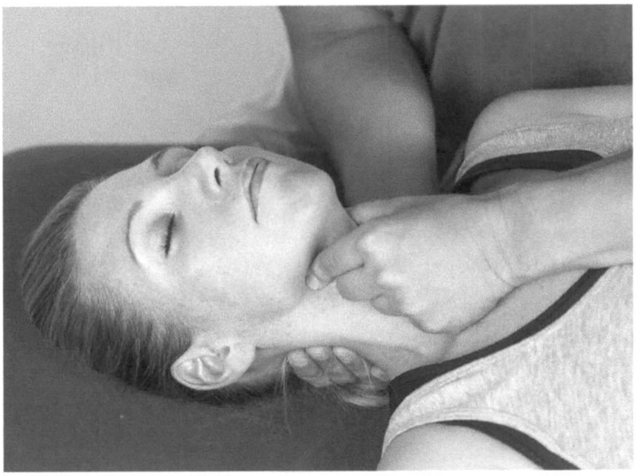

Figure 3.42 Technique for the hyoid bone

- **Direct technique**
  - Move the hyoid bone in the direction of the restriction of motion.
  - Remove the hand supporting the cervical spine. Use it to fix the cranium laterally on the side of the restriction of motion.
  - Finally, place one hand on and the other hand under the patient's neck and perform tissue release on the fasciae of the neck as for the diaphragm. In this, the uppermost hand applies a very gentle posterior pressure and follows the motions of unwinding of the tissues.
- **Specific treatment** of the anatomical relations of the hyoid bone (Figure 3.41), with palpation of the relevant structure with the other hand
  - Temporal bone: traction cranioposteriorly (Figure 3.43): digastric (posterior belly), stylohyoid muscle.
  - Mandible (Figure 3.44):
    - Traction cranially, anteriorly, and medially: digastric (anterior belly), geniohyoid muscle.
    - Cranioanterior traction into the inner margin of the mandible: mylohyoid muscle.
  - Tongue: traction cranially tongue direction (Figure 3.45): hyoglossus, chondroglossus.
  - Pharynx: posterior traction (Figure 3.46): middle constrictor of pharynx.
  - Thyroid cartilage: traction caudally in the direction of the thyroid cartilage (Figure 3.47): thyrohyoid muscle.

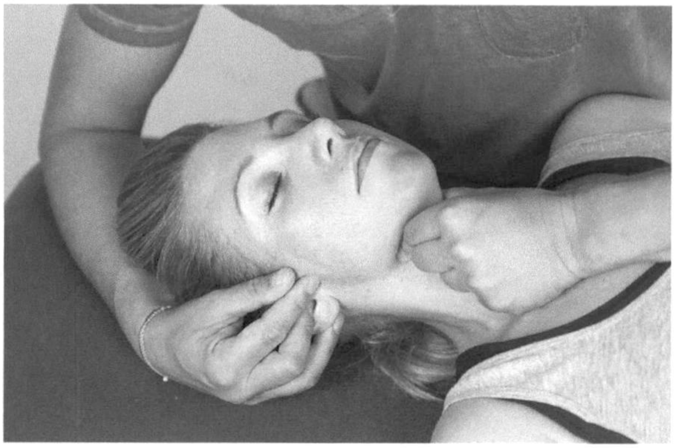

Figure 3.43 Specific treatment for the hyoid bone–temporal bone

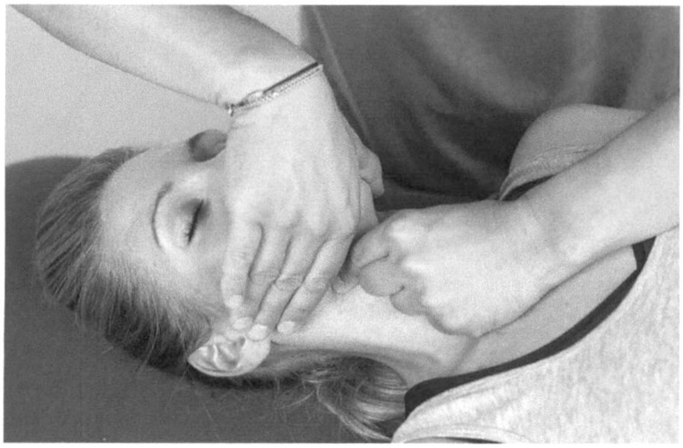

Figure 3.44 Specific treatment for the hyoid–mandible

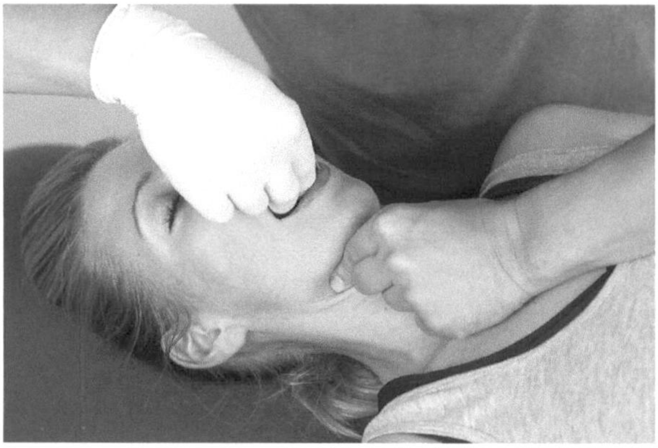

Figure 3.45 Specific treatment for the hyoid–tongue

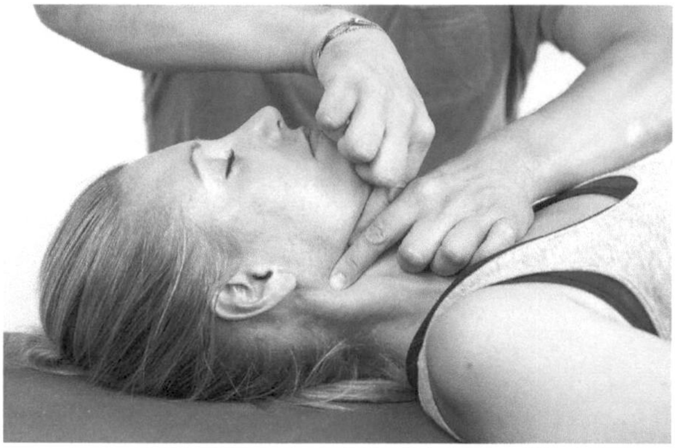

Figure 3.46 Specific treatment for the hyoid–pharynx

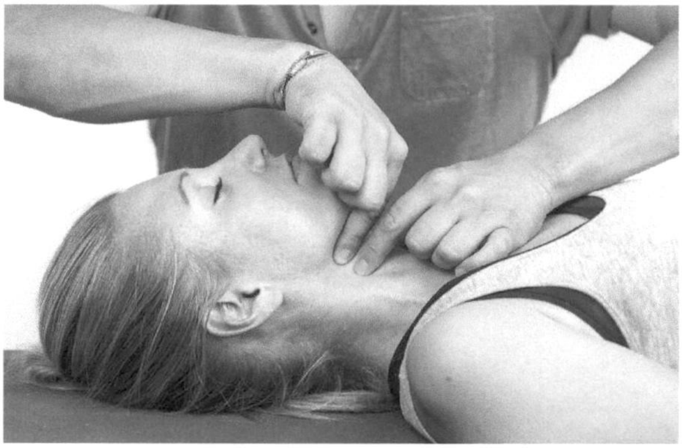

Figure 3.47 Specific treatment for the hyoid–thyroid cartilage

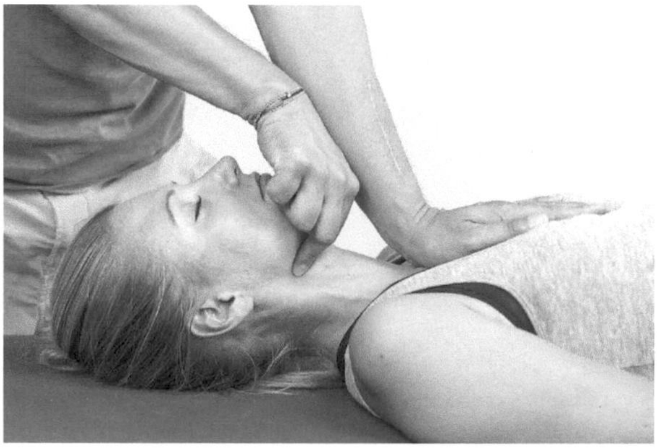

Figure 3.48 Specific treatment for the hyoid–sternum

    - Sternum: traction caudally in the direction of the sternum (Figure 3.48): sternohyoid muscle.
    - Scapula: traction posteriorly and inferiorly, in the direction of the scapula (Figure 3.49): omohyoid muscle.
    - Cervical fascia, superficial layer and pretracheal layer (Figure 3.50).
- Effect: on the hyoid bone (Figure 3.41) and its muscles, ligaments, and fasciae, the first to seventh cervical vertebrae, the swallowing process and phonation, the thyroid gland and psychological effect.

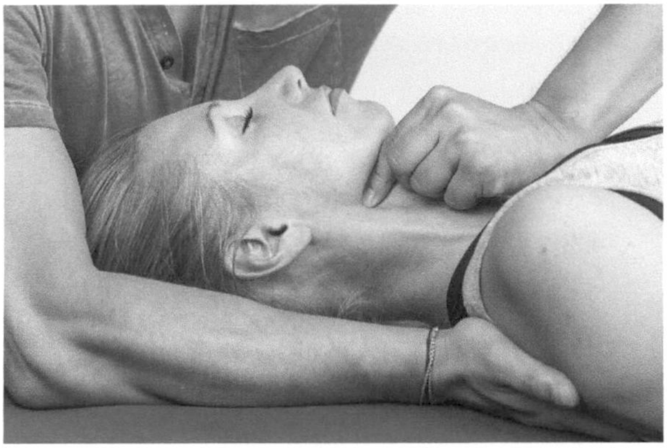

Figure 3.49 Specific treatment for the hyoid–scapula

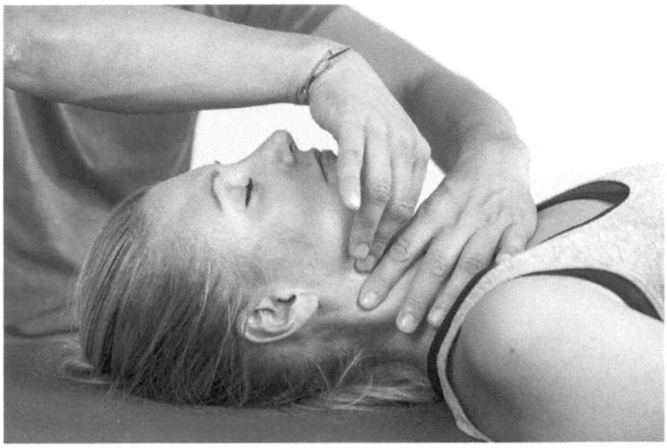

Figure 3.50 Specific treatment for the hyoid–superficial layer and pretracheal layer of the cervical fascia

Alternative technique

Another option for releasing restrictions of the hyoid bone is to fix it inferiorly while asking the patient to initiate swallowing.

The cervical spine and the act of swallowing

Practitioner: Take up a position beside the patient.

Hand position: Place one hand on the neck muscles. With your other hand take the hyoid between the thumb and index finger. (This treatment can also be given when the patient is supine.)

Method: Establish a kind of PBT between the cervical spine and the hyoid (Figure 3.28).

NOTE This component may also be integrated into the technique for the hyoid described above.

It is of course essential to conduct further tests of the postural pattern and to implement all techniques required to eliminate dysfunctions involving the cervical spine.

3.4.6 Technique for the pharynx

Hand position:

- With the cranial hand span the nape of the neck.
- Caudal hand
    - Superior constrictor of pharynx: the caudal hand spans both sides of the angle of the mandible.
    - Middle constrictor of pharynx: the caudal hand spans both sides of the hyoid.
    - Inferior constrictor of pharynx: the caudal hand spans both sides of the thyroid cartilage.

Test:

- Passive test: evaluating the position and passive traction tensions directed posteriorly on mandible, hyoid, and thyroid cartilage.

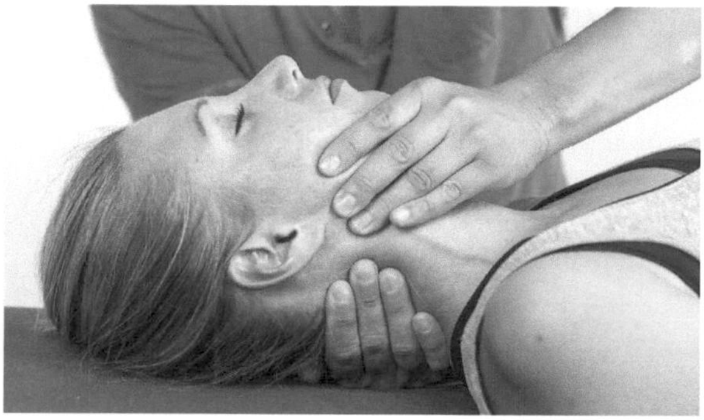

Figure 3.51 Technique for the pharynx, superior constrictor muscle of the pharynx

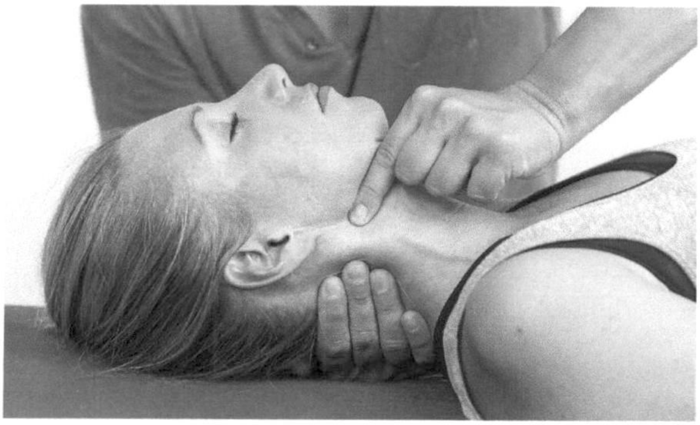

Figure 3.52 Technique for the pharynx, middle constrictor muscle of the pharynx

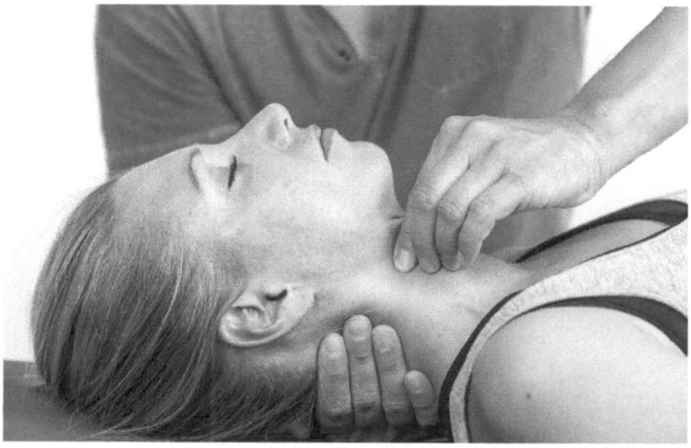

Figure 3.53 Technique for the pharynx, inferior constrictor muscle of the pharynx

- Active test: perform traction directed anteriorly on each of the following: the mandible, hyoid, and thyroid cartilage.

Method:

- Superior constrictor of pharynx: traction directed anteriorly on the mandible (Figure 3.51).
- Middle constrictor of pharynx: traction directed anteriorly on the hyoid (Figure 3.52).
- Inferior constrictor of pharynx: traction directed anteriorly on the thyroid cartilage (Figure 3.53).
- The specific method can be performed as described in the treatment of the hyoid (section 3.4.5).

Thyrohyoid and cricothyroid muscles

See technique for the thyroid cartilage (section 3.4.7).

3.4.7 General laryngeal mobilization

Hand position: With one hand span the nape of the neck, and with the other span the laryngeal structures.

Method: Mobilize the laryngeal structures in their entirety (cartilages: thyroid, cricoid, arytenoid, and epiglottic and associated muscles, ligaments, and fasciae) laterally, in rotation, sidebending, tilting, craniocaudally, and anteroposteriorly (Figure 3.54).

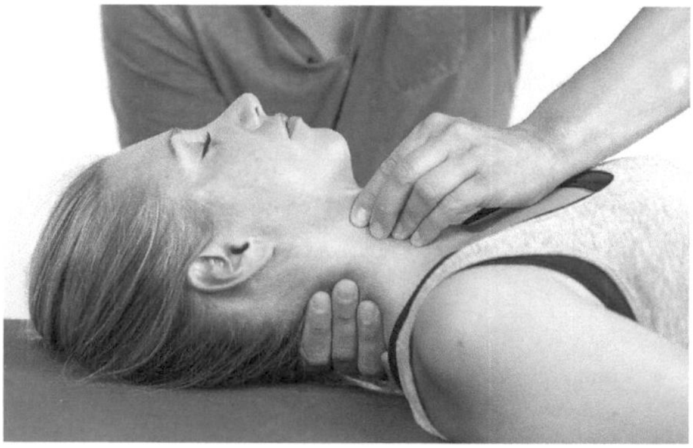

Figure 3.54 General mobilization of the larynx

Technique for the thyroid cartilage

Indication: Laryngeal swallowing disturbance, voice production difficulties, hoarseness; for the crico-thyroid muscle: speech problems, problems with the production of high tones.

Test:

- Passive test: evaluating the position and passive tensile stresses on the thyroid cartilage.
- Active test: active testing of laterality, rotation, sidebending, tilting, craniocaudal and antero-posterior mobility of the thyroid cartilage.

Method:

- **Thyroid cartilage—hyoid**
  - With the thumb and index finger of the cranial hand span the hyoid, with the thumb and index finger of the caudal hand span the thyroid cartilage (Figure 3.55).
  - Exert traction on the hyoid superiorly and/or on the thyroid cartilage inferiorly to regulate the tension of the thyrohyoid muscle and the thyrohyoid membrane.
- **Thyroid cartilage—sternum**
  - With the thumb and index finger of the cranial hand span the thyroid cartilage, place the caudal hand on the manubrium of sternum (Figure 3.56).
  - Exert traction on the thyroid cartilage superiorly to regulate tension in the sternothyroid muscle (swallowing disturbance, reduced volume of sound in speech and singing).
  - You can also carry out a release laterally on the belly of the sternothyroid muscle between the greater horn of the hyoid and the oblique line of the thyroid cartilage.
- **Thyroid cartilage—cricoid cartilage**
  - With the thumb and index finger of the cranial hand, span the thyroid cartilage; with the thumb and index finger of the caudal hand, span the cricoid cartilage (Figure 3.57).
  - Exert traction on the thyroid cartilage superiorly to regulate tension in the cricothyroid muscle (problems with vocal fold tension or voice frequency).
  - You can also palpate the cricothyroid muscles lateral to the cricothyroid ligament and carry out a release.
  - Exert traction on the thyroid cartilage anteriorly to regulate tension in the vocalis muscle (laryngeal swallowing disturbance, problems with voice production).
- **Inferior constrictor of pharynx**
  - With the thumb and index finger of the cranial hand span the thyroid cartilage, with the caudal hand span the nape of the neck (Figure 3.58).
  - Exert traction on the thyroid cartilage anteriorly to regulate tension in the inferior constrictor of pharynx.

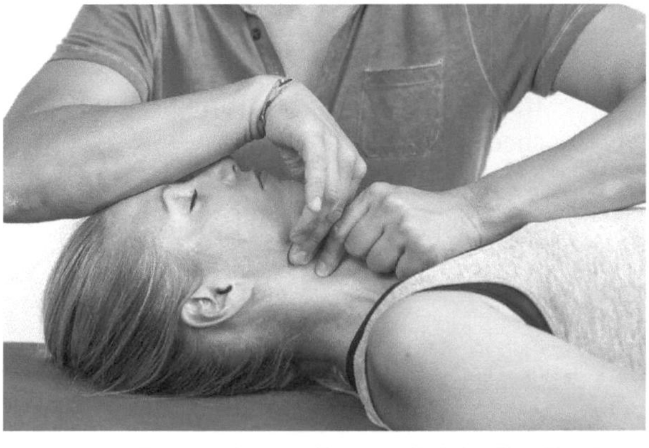

Figure 3.55 Technique for the thyroid cartilage. Thyroid cartilage–hyoid

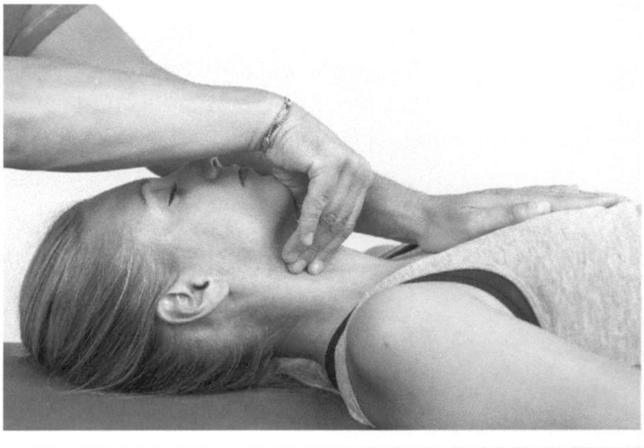

Figure 3.56 Technique for the thyroid cartilage. Thyroid cartilage–sternum

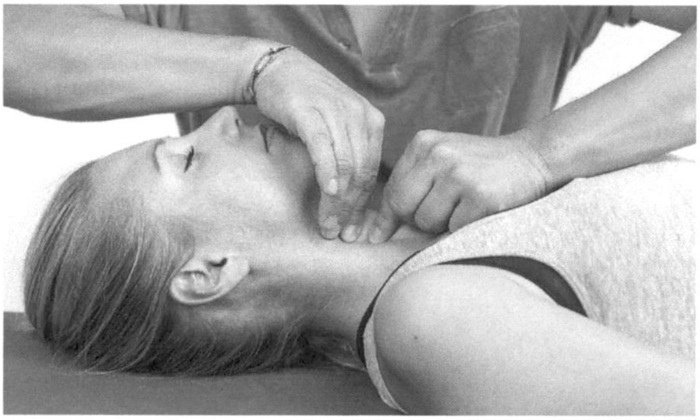

Figure 3.57 Technique for the thyroid cartilage. Thyroid cartilage–cricoid cartilage

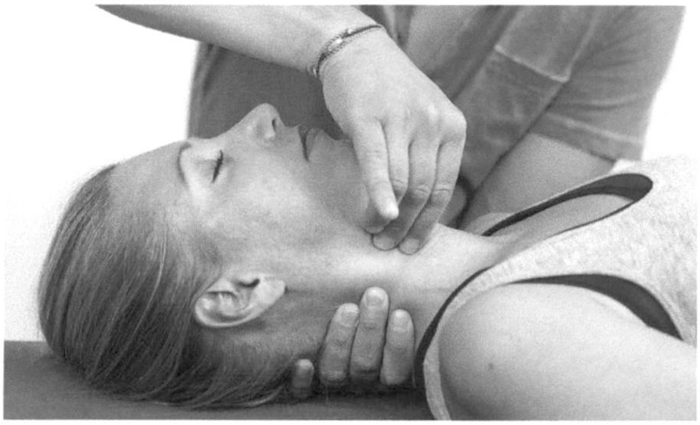

Figure 3.58 Technique for the thyroid cartilage. Inferior constrictor muscle of the pharynx

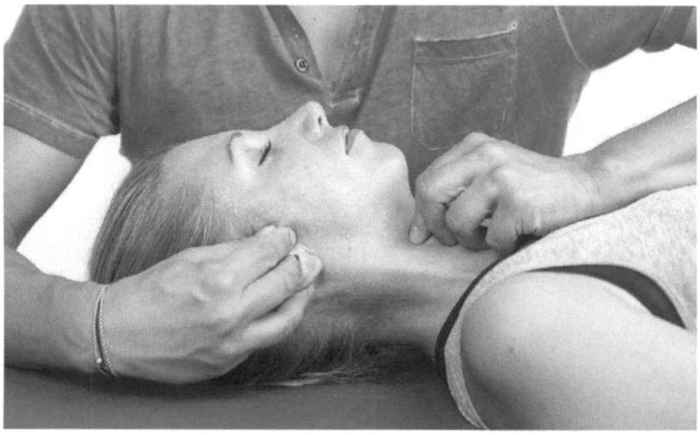

Figure 3.59 Technique for the thyroid cartilage. Thyroid cartilage–temporal bone

- **Thyroid cartilage—temporal bone**
  - Use the five-finger technique on the temporal bone with the cranial hand (contralaterally); with the thumb and index finger of the caudal hand span the thyroid cartilage (Figure 3.59).
  - Exert traction on the thyroid cartilage caudally to release tension in the stylopharyngeus ligament (cranially displaced thyroid cartilage).

Circumlaryngeal technique, modified

Indication: Cranial larynx, hypertonicity and firmness of the hyoid-laryngeal muscles.[6,13,21,34,35,47]

Hand position: Place the thumb, index, and if appropriate middle finger on the affected laryngeal structures (Figure 3.60).

Method:

- Exert a gentle pressure on various sites of the larynx while following the myofascial inductions.
- Depending on what you sense on palpation, you can establish a PBT or DBT at various laryngeal structures.
- For this, start superficially and with slight pressure.
- Then, if necessary and the patient tolerates it, exert a deeper pressure.

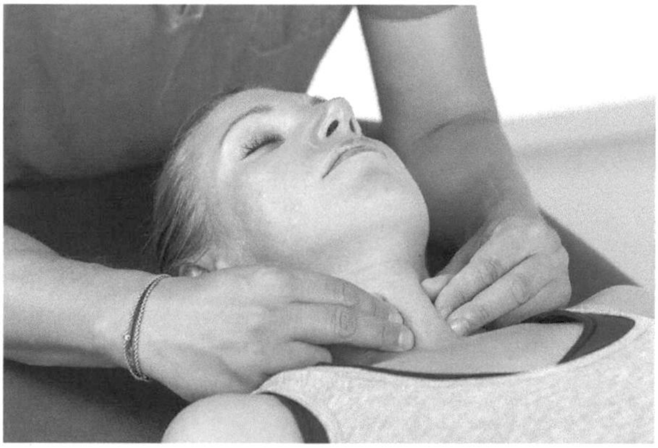

Figure 3.60 Circumlaryngeal technique, modified

- While the technique is being carried out, the patient hums or vocalizes sounds; during this, the patient and practitioner register any change in voice quality. An improvement in voice quality and/or reduction in pain and in laryngeal cranial displacement indicates a normalization of the tension.
- Finally, carry out a general laryngeal mobilization.
- An improvement in symptoms should be achieved in the first session.

Test and technique for the sternum (e.g., anterior dysfunction of the manubrium of sternum)

Hand position: Place one hand on the sternum, with the ball of the hand in the region of the manubrium and the fingers aligned caudally on the body of the sternum (Figure 3.61).

Test: This tests the posteriority and anteriority of the manubrium in relation to the body of sternum. A restriction of movement posteriorly can be eliminated by a direct technique or mobilization in the region of the manubrium.

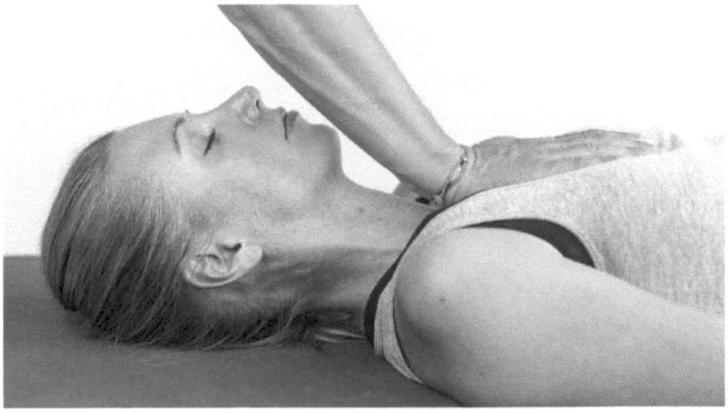

Figure 3.61 Test and technique for the sternum (e.g., anterior dysfunction of the manubrium of sternum)

3.4.8 Techniques for the cranial nerves

- **Technique for the infraorbital nerve and branches of the maxillary nerve (CN V_2):** in sensory disturbances of the lips, palate (and also in the region of the roof of the pharynx and of the auditory tube); see Volume 2, section 7.5.2.
- **Technique for the greater palatine nerve**; see Volume 2, section 7.5.2.
- **Technique for the facial nerve (CN VII):** special sense disturbances in the anterior two-thirds of the mucosa of the tongue: see testing the mobility of the facial nerve and technique for the facial nerve (Volume 2, section 7.6.2).
- **Glossopharyngeal nerve (CN IX):** for sensory and special sense disturbances in the posterior third of the mucosa of the tongue, motor disturbance of the palatoglossus muscle (problems with sensory and motor function of the lower nasopharyngeal and oropharyngeal space); see Volume 2, section 7.8.2.
- **Technique for the superior laryngeal nerve (CN X):** for sensory disturbances in the mucosa above the rima glottidis, disturbances of the cricothyroid muscle (speech problems, problems with producing high pitch sounds); see Volume 2, section 7.9.2.
- **Technique for the recurrent laryngeal nerve (CN X):** in restricted mobility of the nerve, trapping is a strong possibility (differential diagnosis: bronchial carcinoma, etc.): hoarseness (differential diagnosis: bronchial carcinoma, aortic aneurysm), sensory disturbances in the region of the mucosa below the rima glottidis, thyroid problems; see Volume 2, section 7.9.2.
- **Technique for the vagus nerve (CN X):** in sensory and special sense disturbances in the root of tongue (motor and sensory disturbances of the laryngopharynx and sometimes of the oropharynx); see Volume 2, section 7.9.2.
- **Technique for the hypoglossal nerve (CN XII):** in disturbances of the motor function of the tongue; see Volume 2, section 7.11.2.
- **Technique for the otic ganglion:** in parotid gland dysfunction; see Volume 2, section 7.8.2.
- **Technique for the submandibular ganglion:** in dysfunction of the submandibular gland and the sublingual gland; see Volume 2, section 7.6.2.

Technique for the pterygopalatine ganglion: in disturbances of the mucosa of the nose, palate, and pharynx, of the soft palate, and of the lacrimal gland; see Volume 2, section 7.6.2.

3.4.9 Treatment of the arteries, veins, and lymph vessels

Technique for the greater palatine artery

Patient: Supine.

Practitioner: Take up a position at the head of the patient.

Hand position:

- Place the tip of the middle finger of one hand at the level of or above the hyoid on the external carotid artery.
- Place the tip of the middle finger of the other hand within the mouth at the greater palatine foramen and palpate the pulse of the artery (Figure 3.62).

Method:

- Bend the head contralaterally to the side and rotate it.
- With the middle finger on the external carotid artery exert caudal traction.
- With the middle finger on the greater palatine artery carry out local tissue release.
- Maintain the local tissue release in the region of the greater palatine artery and the caudal traction in the region of the external carotid artery until you sense a normalization of glide and improvement of pulsation.

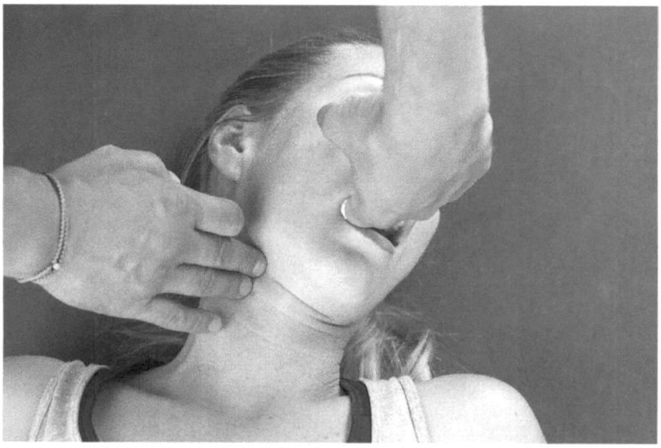

Figure 3.62 Technique for the greater palatine artery

Technique for the common carotid artery/external carotid artery

See section 2.8.5.

Technique for the external carotid artery/facial artery, external carotid artery/maxillary artery

This treats the site where the facial artery and maxillary artery branch off from the external carotid artery.

Aim: To improve the arterial supply to the pharynx.

Patient: Turn the head contralaterally to the side of treatment.

Practitioner: Take up a position at the patient's head.

Hand position:

- **Facial artery** With the cranial hand span the mandible. Place the thumb or another finger on the facial artery (Figure 3.63).

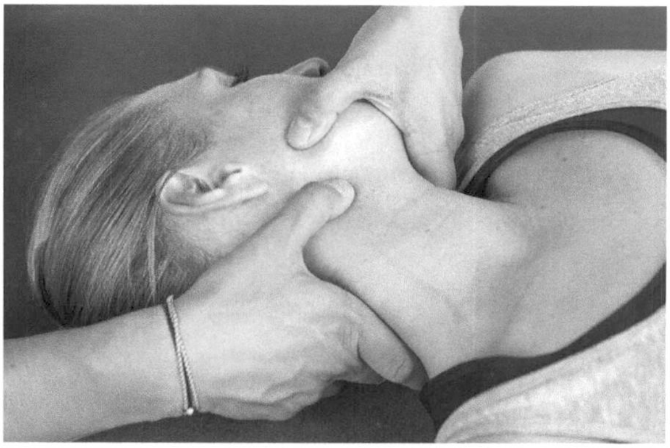

Figure 3.63 Technique for the external carotid artery/facial artery

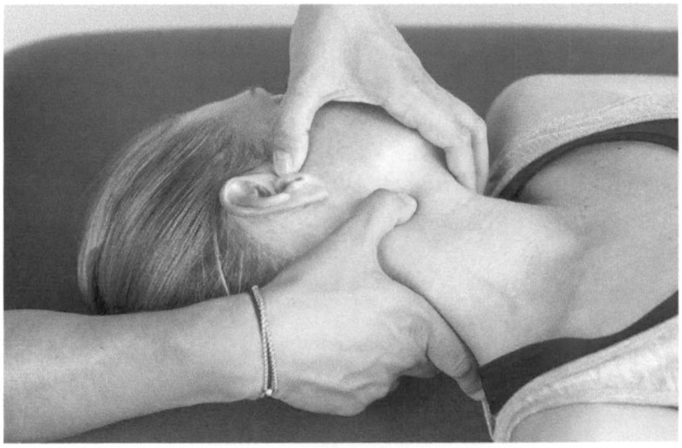

Figure 3.64 Technique for the external carotid artery/maxillary artery

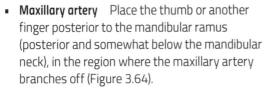

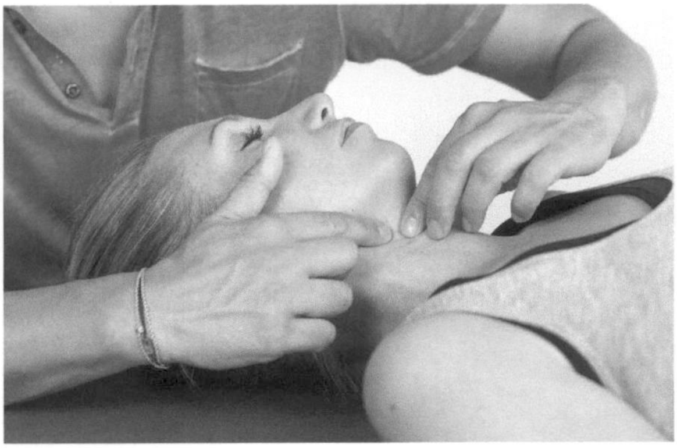

Figure 3.65 Technique for the superior thyroid artery

- **Maxillary artery** Place the thumb or another finger posterior to the mandibular ramus (posterior and somewhat below the mandibular neck), in the region where the maxillary artery branches off (Figure 3.64).
- With the caudal hand span the occipital bone. Place the thumb directly below the angle of the mandible.

Method:

- The thumbs apply a gentle pressure onto the tissues, each moving simultaneously toward the other and away from each other again.
- With the fingers cautiously exert a gentle longitudinal traction.
- Maintain this extremely slight tension until you sense a softening and inherent motion of the surrounding tissues.
- Then apply a gentle pressure on the tissues. During the expanding expression of tissue elasticity and the gentle yielding of pressure follow all the tissue dynamics which have been sensed.

Technique for the superior thyroid artery

Hand position:

- Place the index and/or middle finger of one hand medial to the sternocleidomastoid, laterally and slightly cranially to the thyroid cartilage at the external carotid artery.
- With the other index and/or middle finger palpate the origin of the superior thyroid artery at the level of the space between the hyoid and the thyroid cartilage. (Although the artery continues caudally along the side of the thyroid cartilage, in this case palpate only at the level of the space between the hyoid and the thyroid cartilage.)

Method:

- First evaluate the pulsation by comparison with the other side. A diminished pulsation is a positive finding.
- Bend the head contralaterally to the side. To test for glide, first use your index fingers to exert a divergent longitudinal traction onto the vessel. Then test the glide of the superior thyroid artery caudally.
- For treatment, fix the external carotid artery and with the other hand exert caudally directed traction at the superior thyroid artery (Figure 3.65), while following tissue relaxations or the micromovements.
- Maintain the tension until you can palpate a normalization of glide.
- Then apply a gentle pressure on the tissues. During the expanding expression of tissue

elasticity and the gentle yielding of pressure, follow all the tissue dynamics which have been sensed.

Technique for the inferior thyroid artery/vein

Hand position (Figure 3.66):

- Place the index and/or middle finger of one hand on the subclavian artery lateral to the sternocleidomastoid muscle and posterior to the clavicle.
- Place your index and/or middle finger on the inferior portion of the thyroid gland.

Method:

- First, evaluate the pulsation by comparison with the other side. A diminished pulsation is a positive finding.
- Bend and rotate the head contralaterally to the side.
- Fix the subclavian artery, and with the other hand exert a mediocranial traction at the inferior thyroid artery.
- Evaluate the elasticity or glide by comparison with the other side.
- In the case of dysfunction, fix the subclavian artery and exert mediocranial traction on the inferior thyroid artery. Then continue as with the superior thyroid artery (see above).

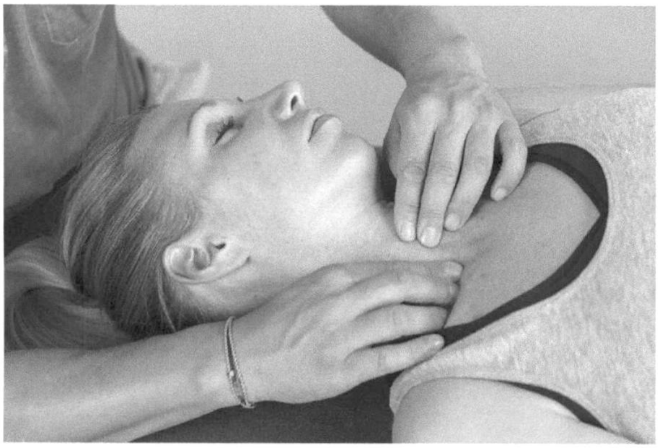

Figure 3.66 Technique for the inferior thyroid artery

3.4.10 Treatment of venous structures

Technique for the pterygoid venous plexus

See Volume 2, section 2.5.4.

Deep venolymphatic pharyngeal drainage

Indication: To improve the venolymphatic drainage of the oral and pharyngeal cavity, the nose, and the brain.

Practitioner: Take up a position at the head of the patient.

Hand position: Place one hand, from the side, under the neck. Place the other hand on the roof of the skull.

Method:

- Alternately compress and decompress the nape of the neck.
- During this, carry out the compression with constantly changing combinations of sidebending and rotation of the nape of the neck (Figure 3.67).
- Carry out these alternating movements in the region of the nape of the neck about 5–10 times.

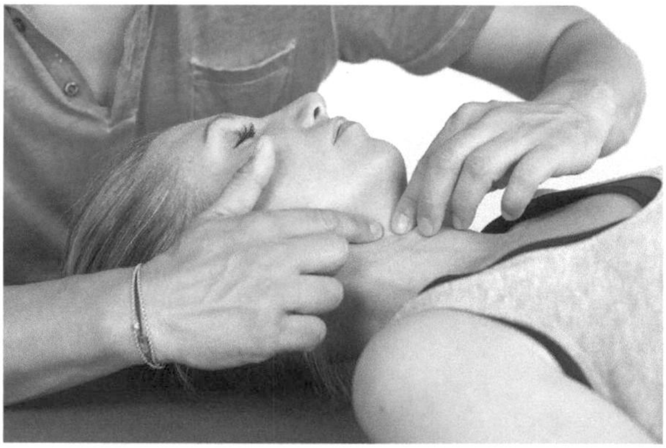

Figure 3.67 Deep venolymphatic pharyngeal drainage

Lymphatic drainage of the oral cavity

The back of the oral cavity can be drained off posteriorly to the deep cervical lymph nodes and the front to the submental and cervical lymph nodes.

3.4.11 Further procedures for chronic inflammation of the tonsils and also of the oral cavity, pharynx, and larynx

- Strengthening the physical barriers (oral/intestinal).
- Gentle regular exercise.
- Interval fasting (16:8 method) and dietary regulation (e.g., cutting down on high-sugar foods).
- Regulating sleep/wake behavior.

3.4.12 Procedures in the case of a dysfunctional microbiome of the oral cavity

Indications: E.g., burden of *Porphyromonas gingivalis, Streptococcus mutans, Clostridium difficile, Propionibacterium acnes.*

Therapeutic procedures: Professional dental cleaning at a dental practice, regular tooth brushing and cleaning of the interdental spaces, cleaning the tongue, oral probiotics,[42,51,53] a low-sugar diet, if relevant smoking cessation, if relevant treating mouth breathing, and if relevant stress reduction; if *Propionibacterium acnes* is present, also, in some circumstances, mouth rinse (1 minute each time after brushing the teeth in the evening, then spitting out) with hydrogen peroxide solution (0.1–0.5%) for 3 months and taking purified lactoferrin (200 mg) for 3 months.

3.4.13 Self-help techniques, exercise programs

If there are problems with the mouth and jaws, daily exercise programs are generally necessary for therapeutic success; these must be tailored to the individual. For children and adolescents in particular these comprise breathing (Volume 2, section 2.5.12), tongue, swallowing, and lip exercises.

Drainage of the palatine tonsils

Use your own index finger to demonstrate to the patient how to reach the palatine tonsils, which are located bilaterally behind the palatoglossal arch.

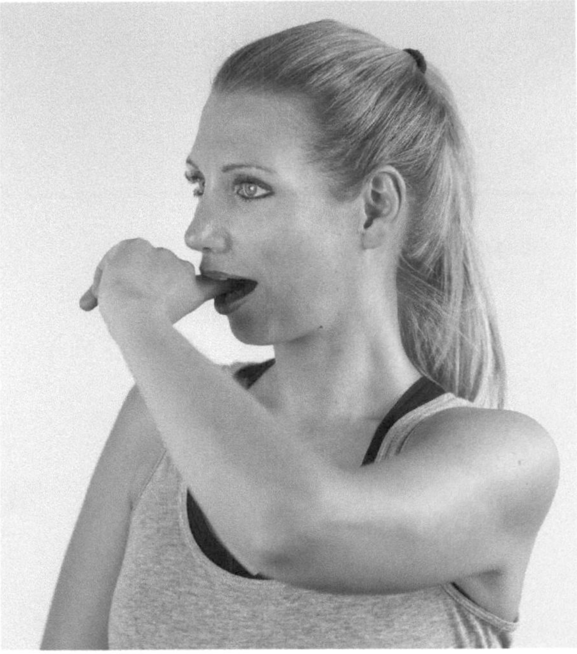

Figure 3.68 Drainage of the palatine tonsils

The patient may then finger-massage and drain the palatine tonsils once daily (Figure 3.68).

The "roaring lion"

This exercise represents another way to improve the milieu in the pharynx, including the tongue and tonsils. It also has a positive effect in people with halitosis.

Method: (instruct the patient as follows)

- Squat on your heels, with your hands on your knees, arms straight, and fingers spread.
- Shift your bodyweight on to your knees.
- Push your stomach and chest forward. Stretch your back so that it is in slight extension. Relax your shoulders.
- Open your mouth wide and stick your tongue out as far as possible toward your chin. You may also adopt a cross-eyed look.
- Start to breathe in; then, while breathing out, roar like a lion.

- Over a period of about 3 weeks perform this exercise at least once a day for 1–2 minutes.

Tongue training:
Each exercise builds upon the other. Therefore, it is usually helpful to do the tongue exercises in the order set out below. You should not work on the exercises for longer than 2–5 minutes daily. Several of the exercises below can be done daily. Do the tongue training for about 4 months.

- **Ideal resting position for the tongue** (Figure 3.69)
  - A piece of wafer can be stuck to the site immediately behind the top incisors, or you can find the site where the tip of the tongue is positioned by saying the consonant "n."
  - Then place the whole of the body of the tongue in a relaxed manner against the palate.
  - Keep the lips and cheeks relaxed during the exercise.
  - Gently close the lips.
  - Keep the side teeth slightly open.
  - Duration: about 1 minute.
- **Tongue clicking** (supports the tongue position at the palate and coordination)
  - Start with the tip of the tongue at the ideal resting position, the body of the tongue lying flat on the palate.
  - Click loudly and powerfully.
  - During this process, the mandible should barely move.
  - Duration: approximately 1 minute, until you can place the tongue well against the palate.
  - Alternatively, you can place a piece of wafer in the middle of the palate, so that it sticks there. Using the tip of the tongue, click until the wafer has disappeared.
- **Stretching the tongue after sucking it against the palate** (trains coordination, mobility, and strength; Figure 3.70)
  - Suck the tongue against the palate and simultaneously stretch the tongue.
  - Keep the muscles of the chin, lips, and cheeks relaxed during the exercise.

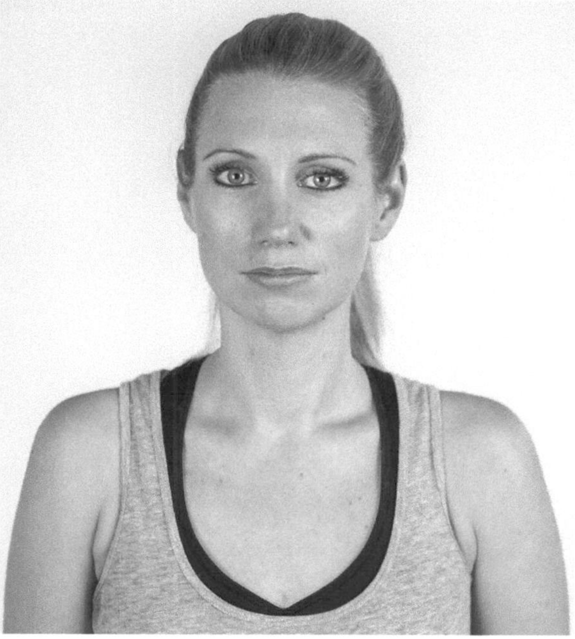

Figure 3.69 Tongue training. Ideal resting position of the tongue

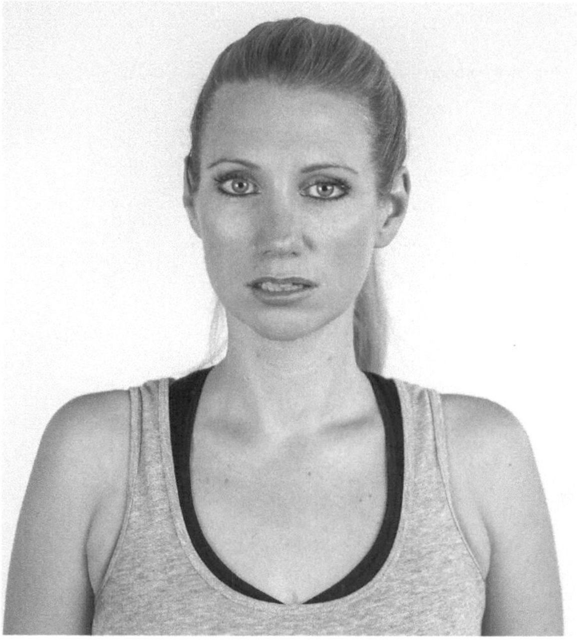

Figure 3.70 Tongue training. Stretching the tongue which has been sucked against the palate

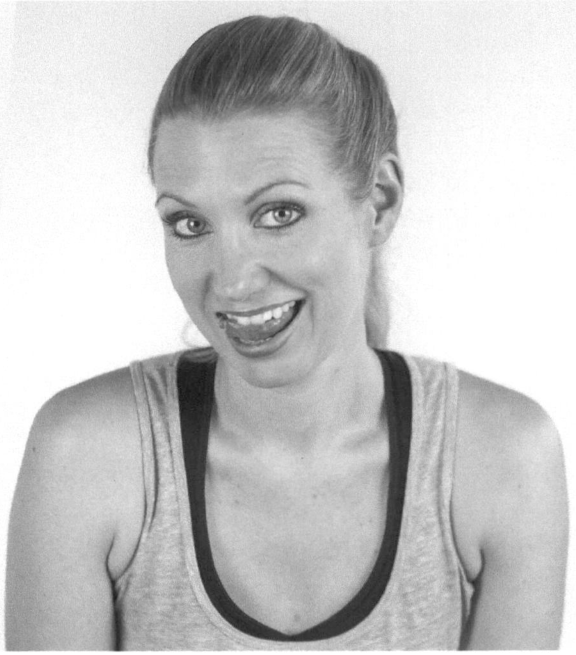

Figure 3.71 Tongue training. Counting the teeth

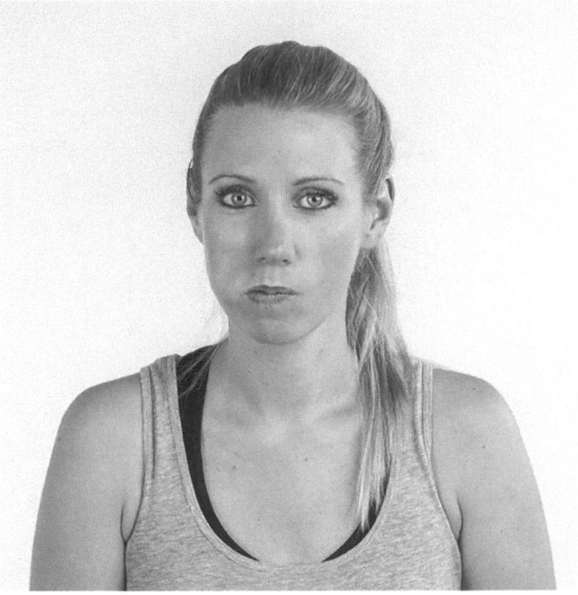

Figure 3.72 Tongue training. Pressing the tongue against the cheek

  - ▸ Duration: hold the position of the tongue for about 1 minute.
  - ▸ Do this exercise for about 1 month.
- **Counting teeth** (trains mobility and coordination; Figure 3.71): touch each individual tooth with the tongue.
- **Place the tongue laterally on the lower lip** (trains coordination, especially of the genioglossus). Repeat the exercise about 5–10 times.
- **Press the tongue against the cheek** (trains coordination, especially of the styloglossus; Figure 3.72). Press the tongue about 5–10 times against the cheek from inside.

The following exercises are used to prepare for the swallowing exercises.

- **Straight tongue** (trains the tongue muscles, especially the superior and inferior longitudinal muscles; Figure 3.73)
  - ◆ The exercise begins and ends in the ideal resting position.
  - ◆ You should do this exercise in front of a mirror.

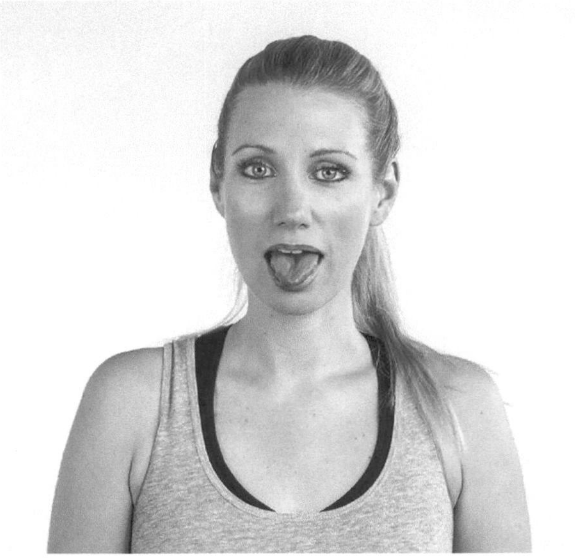

Figure 3.73
Tongue training. Straight tongue

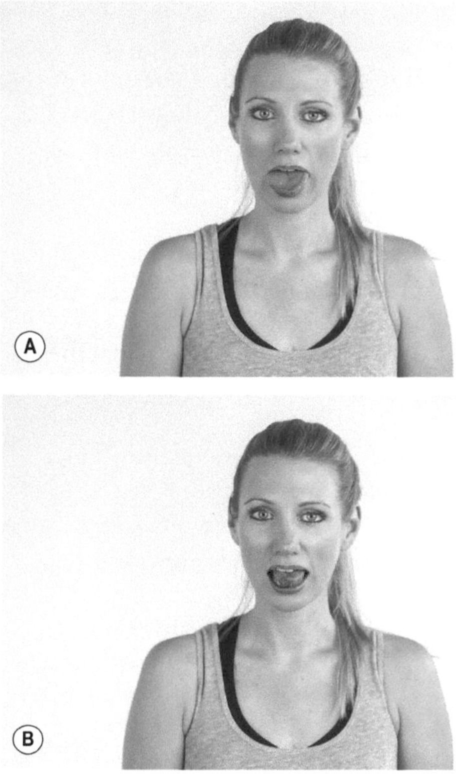

Figure 3.74
Tongue training: **A** wide and **B** narrow tongue

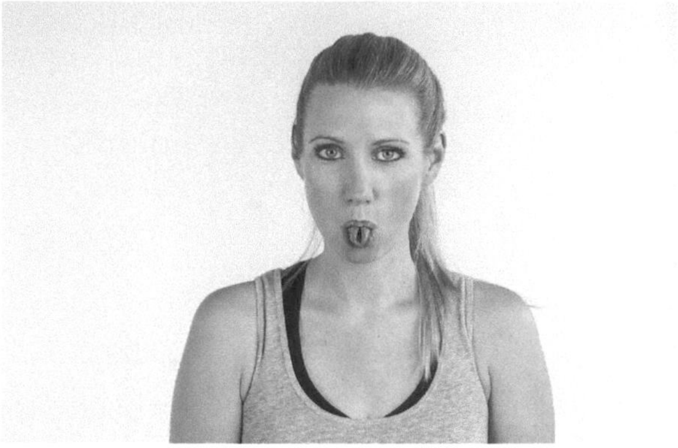

Figure 3.75
Tongue training. Rolling tip of tongue inward

- Open the mouth as wide as possible and stick out the tongue like a plank, keeping the tongue as straight as possible.
- Do not touch either the teeth or the floor of the mouth with your tongue.
- If you can no longer maintain the position or your tongue starts to quiver return the tongue to its ideal resting position.
- Practice the exercise for about a month.

The following exercises are to be done together for about 1 month:

- **Wide and narrow tongue** (trains the intrinsic and extrinsic tongue muscles; Figure 3.74)
  - Starting position as in the previous exercise.
  - Narrow and then widen the outstretched tongue.
  - Initially, the exercise can be done without stretching the tongue out completely. However, this should be achieved with increasing practice.
  - Hold these positions for at least 2 seconds each time and repeat about 10 times.
  - Alternatively, a tongue depressor can be placed on the tongue. At first the tongue is relaxed, and then the tip of the tongue is placed on the narrow edge of the depressor. Then the depressor is moved forward and backward. The tongue touches the depressor at the front, so that the tongue narrows. If the tongue is placed down on the depressor it widens.
- **Rolling the tip of the tongue inward** (serves to prepare for swallowing, especially with the aid of the vertical muscle; Figure 3.75). Roll the tip of the tongue inward about 5–10 times.
- **Tongue backward and downward** (serves to prepare for swallowing, especially with the aid of the hypoglossus; Figure 3.76). Move the tongue forward and backward about 5–10 times.

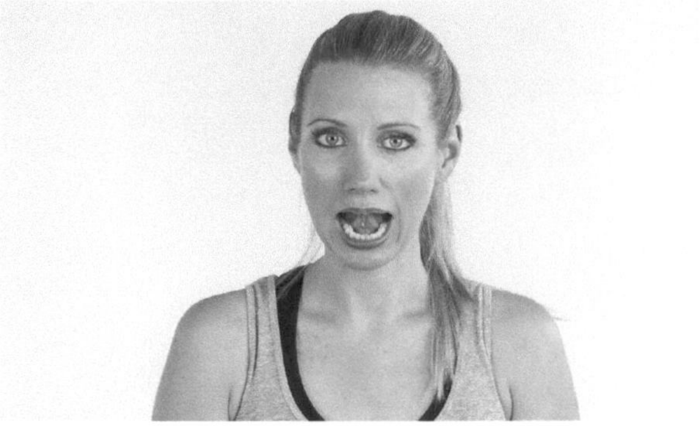

Figure 3.76
Tongue training. Tongue backward and downward

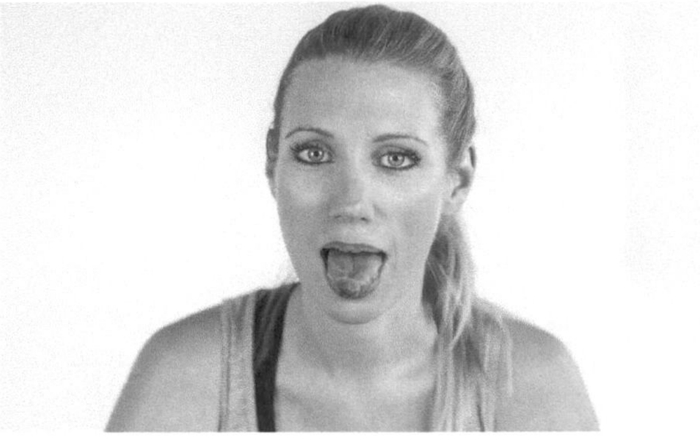

Figure 3.77
Tongue training. Tongue exercise with rubber ring

- **Tongue exercise with rubber ring** (Figure 3.77) A rubber ring is pulled onto the tongue and the tongue must narrow at the front in order to brush the ring off.

Swallowing exercises

The swallowing exercises are not started until the tongue exercises can be successfully done. Swallowing chiefly involves cranial nerves IX and XII. The precondition for normal swallowing is good muscle balance of the orofacial muscles and good mobility of the hyoid and the tongue. It is also important to be able to move the head free from the movement of the shoulders (body exercises can be offered for this). The tongue's points of contact in swallowing correspond with those for articulation. When doing the exercises, take care to keep the muscles of facial expression and the cervical muscles relaxed during swallowing. Do the exercises for about 3 months.

- **Correct swallowing** (learning to observe extraoral signs during swallowing in front of the mirror)
  - For these exercises place the tongue in the ideal resting position at the beginning and end of every exercise.
  - During the exercises take care that there is no sign of movement in the muscles of the cheeks, chin, and lips.
  - Quite often during the exercises, contact is made with the teeth. However, the side teeth ought only to come into contact for a brief moment during swallowing.
  - Do the exercises for about 1 month.
- **Pulling the mouth sideways in both directions while swallowing** (learning to observe intraoral signs during swallowing; Figure 3.78)
  - With the index and middle fingers, gently pull the corners of the mouth sideways in both directions.
  - Place the tongue in the ideal resting position at the beginning and end of each exercise.

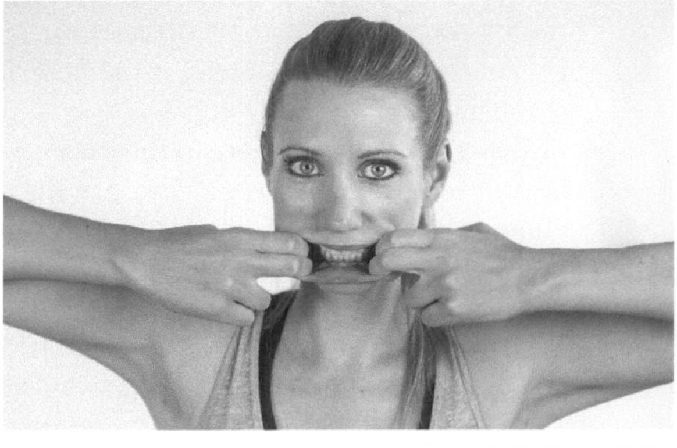

Figure 3.78
Swallowing exercises. Pulling the mouth sideways in both directions while swallowing

- ◆ The patient swallows. The fingers should not be able to detect any tension in the cheeks during swallowing.
- ◆ Also, the teeth should not be compressed and no bubbles of saliva should be forced forward through the teeth.
- ◆ Do the exercises for about 1 month.

The last two exercises are done together.

- **Swallowing and drinking**
  - ◆ The patient can start this exercise when the two previous ones can be correctly done.
  - ◆ During drinking and swallowing the muscles of the cheeks, chin, and lips should not move.
  - ◆ Do not compress the tongue.
  - ◆ The tongue should form a correct seal against the palate.
  - ◆ Do for about 1 month.
- **Smiling and swallowing** (Figure 3.79)
  - ◆ Place a drinking straw with a diameter of 3 mm on the tip of the tongue and use the tongue to press the straw into the middle of the palate.
  - ◆ During this exercise, the tongue should not press against the teeth.
  - ◆ Smile as you swallow.

Lip exercises, exercises for the orbicularis oris muscle

Lip exercises can be done at any time when incomplete lip closure (lip incompetence) is present. Otherwise you can perform the lip exercises after the swallowing exercises, in order to help the mouth close during the swallowing process:

- **Face Former/lip trainer** (Figure 3.80)
  - ◆ These training devices are particularly useful for lip incompetence, decompensated lip closure, and mouth breathing. This can become necessary at any time during therapy.
  - ◆ Place the trainer behind the lips and in front of the teeth.
  - ◆ Encircle the trainer with the lips.
  - ◆ Establish an angle of about 90 degrees between chin and neck.
  - ◆ Place the tongue in the ideal resting position.
  - ◆ During the exercises the mentalis muscle must not tighten.
  - ◆ Pull the Face Former or other lip trainer forward for 6 seconds, while the lips tighten in order to keep it in the mouth. Over another 6 seconds release the traction again.
  - ◆ Repeat this 20 times.

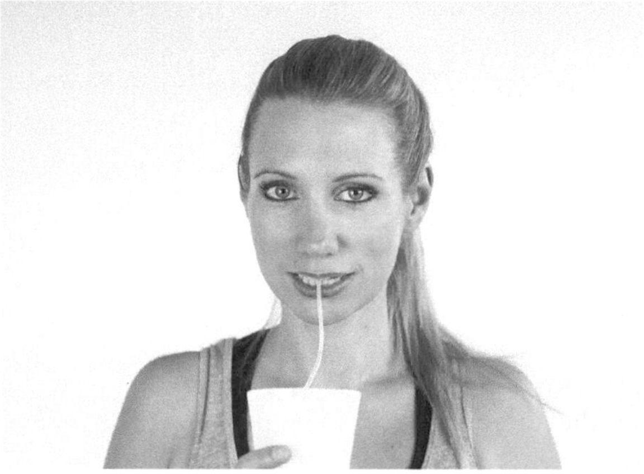

Figure 3.79
Swallowing exercises. Smiling while swallowing

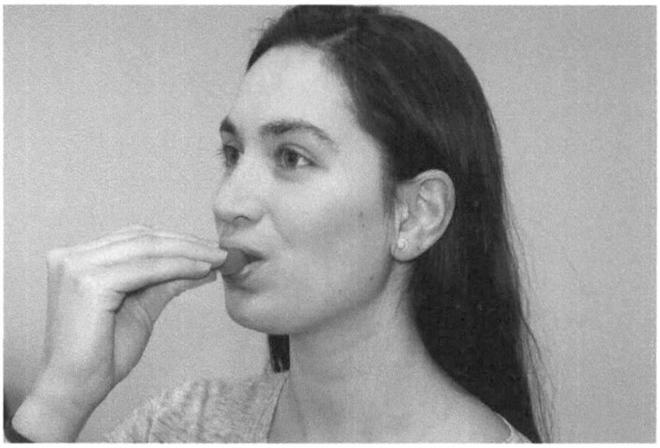

Figure 3.80
Lip exercises. Face Former/lip trainer. (Beate Siemers, Hamburg)

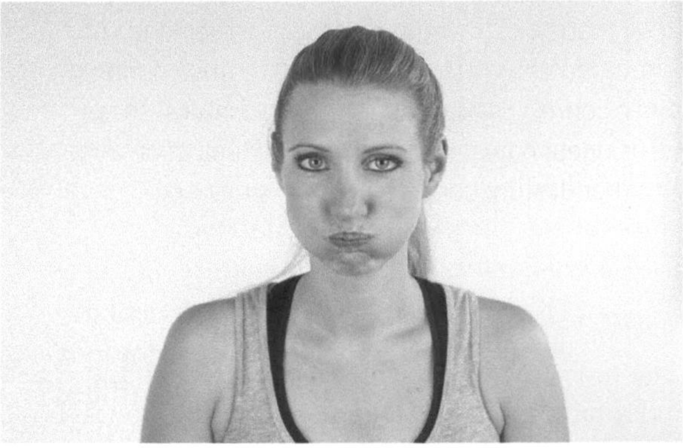

Figure 3.81
Lip exercises. Puffing out the cheeks

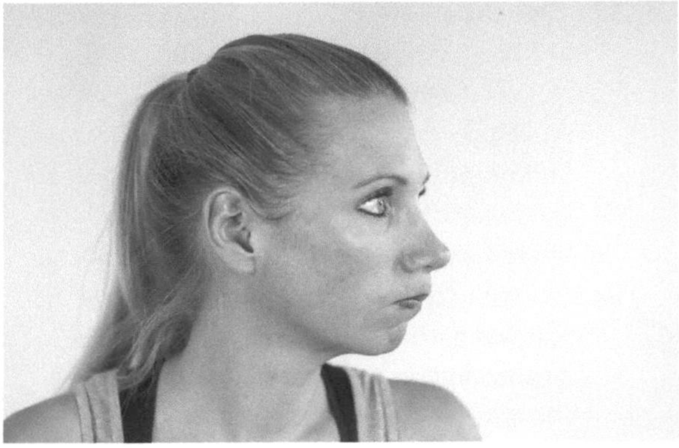

Figure 3.82
Lip exercises. Upper lip exercises with chew bone

- Later you can also pull the trainer upward/downward or swallow at the same time during the exercise.

One of the modes of action of the Face Former is to create negative pressure in the mouth and is intended to treat complex etiologies, e.g., craniocervical dysfunction syndromes.[8]

- **Lip popping**
  - This exercise can be done once the exercises with the lip trainer have been mastered.
  - At the start and end of every lip popping, place the tongue in the ideal resting position.
  - The lip popping must be as loud as possible.
  - Ask the patient first to press the lips together and then push them apart as forcefully as possible.
  - Do for about 1 month.
- **Puffing out the cheeks** (stretching the orofacial muscles, especially the mentalis)
  - Close the mouth and puff out the cheeks (Figure 3.81).
  - During this exercise, ensure that you inhale and exhale calmly through the nose (into the abdomen).
  - Continue with the last two exercises for about 1 month.
- **Sucking on a sucking device** (training lip closure, activating the orofacial muscles, stimulating cranial nerve VII and many other cranial nerves, improving ventilation of the auditory tube, normalizing salivary flow)
  - Suck on the device with as much noise and lip activity as possible.
  - Keep the muscles of the front and back of the neck relaxed.
  - Initially, do this exercise for about 30 seconds. Over about 1 week increase to about 2 minutes.
  - **Note** This exercise can be made more complicated by sucking up water through a straw (diameter: 1 mm or 0.5 mm) drawn through a hole in the device.
- **Upper lip exercise with chew tool** (especially in the case of incompetent upper lip, short upper lip, short frenulum)
  - You can tie a chew tool to a length of dental floss and place it behind the upper lip (Figure 3.82).

Chewing exercises

See section 2.9.4.

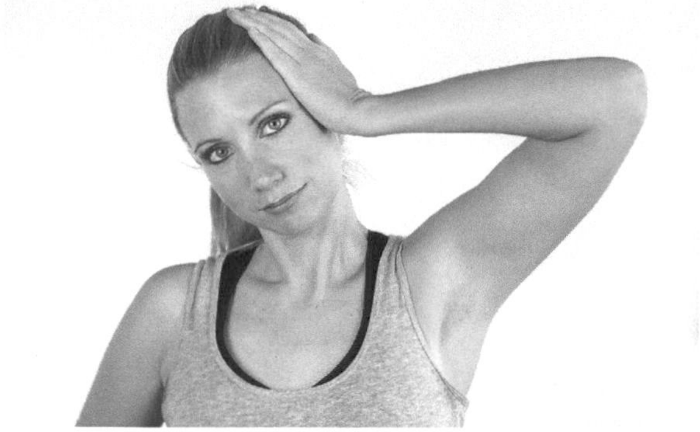

Figure 3.83
Post-isometric relaxation of the trapezius

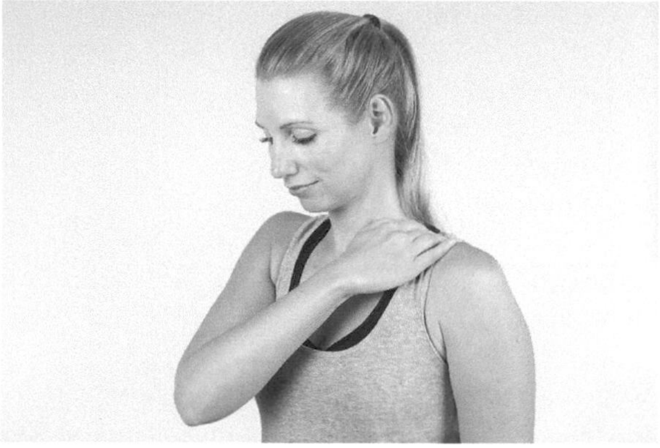

Figure 3.84
Post-isometric relaxation of the levator scapulae

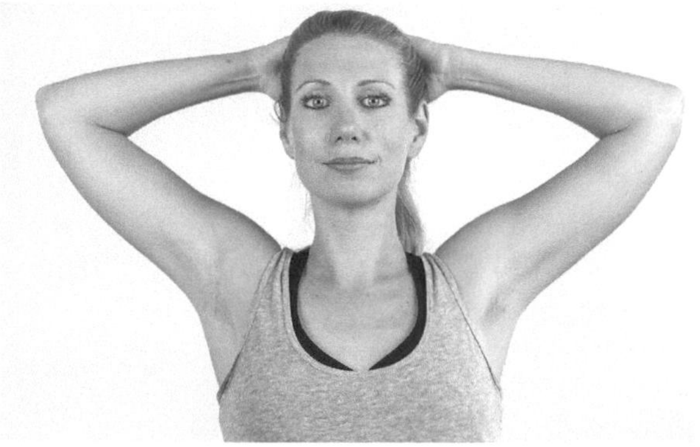

Figure 3.85
Active relaxation of the nuchal fasciae

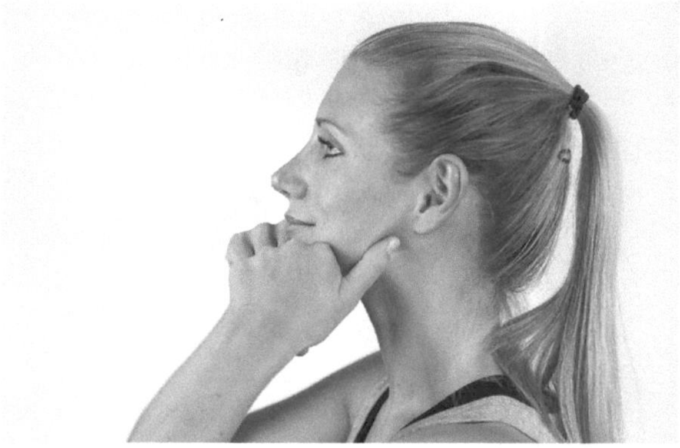

Figure 3.86
Relaxation of the suprahyoid muscles

Myofascial relaxation

- **Post-isometric relaxation of the trapezius** (Figure 3.83). The patient positions the hand contralaterally at the side of the head. The head is stretched sideways until the first sensation of stretch. From here resist the pressure isometrically for 8 seconds and then again seek out the limit of motion. Repeat 3 times.
- **Post-isometric relaxation for the levator scapulae** (Figure 3.84). Place the hands on the head and move the head obliquely backward. For further procedure see above.
- **Active relaxation of the nuchal fasciae** (Figure 3.85). Press the tender point of the trapezius muscle with the flat of the hand, while the patient actively bends and stretches the head several times.
- **Relaxation of the suprahyoid muscles** (Figure 3.86). Position the thumb on the angle of the jaw and move it slowly toward the tip of the chin.

3.5 References

1 Albert, H. B., Lambert, P. and Rollason, J. (2013) 'Does nuclear tissue infected with bacteria following disc herniations lead to Modic changes in the adjacent vertebrae?' *Eur. Spine J.* 22, 690–696.

2 Allain, A. (1992) 'Le complexe musculo-aponevrotique sous-hyoidien et la circulation veineuse de retour cranien à propos de 10 études échotomographiques.' Dijon: Mémoire.

3 Altman, K. W., Atkinson, C. and Lazarus, C. (2005) 'Current and emerging concepts in muscle tension dysphonia: a 30-month review.' *J. Voice. 19*, 2, 261–267.

4 Amigues, J. P. (1992) *L'A.T.M. Une articulation entre l'osteopathe et le dentiste.* Aix en Provence: Verlaque, p. 142.

5 Angsuwarangsee, T. and Morrison, M. (2002) 'Extrinsic laryngeal muscular tension in patients with voice disorders.' *J. Voice. 16*, 3, 333–343.

6 Aronson, A. (1990) *Clinical Voice Disorders: An Interdisciplinary Approach*, 3rd Ed. New York, NY: Thieme Stratton.

7 Bahnemann, F. (Ed.) (1993) *Der Bionator in der Kieferorthopädie. Grundlagen und Praxis.* Heidelberg: Haug, pp. 28, 30–44.

8 Berndsen, K. and Berndsen, S. (2007) 'Myofunktionelle Behandlungen und ihr Einfluss auf die sprachliche Artikulation.' In: Schöler, H. and Welling, A. (Ed.) *Handbuch Sonderpädgagogik der Sprache*, Vol. 1. Göttingen: Hogrefe, pp. 866–888.

9 Cardoso, R., Lumini-Oliveira, J. and Meneses, R. F. (2017) 'Associations between posture, voice, and dysphonia: a systematic review.' *J. Voice.* doi: 10.1016/j.jvoice.2017.08.030.

10 Catlin, F. I. (1963) 'Differential diagnosis of facial pains.' *JAMA. 186*, 4, 291–295.

11 Drenckhahn, D. (Ed.) and Zenker, W. (1985) *Benninghoff, Anatomie*, Vol. 1, 15th Ed. München: Urban and Schwarzenberg.

12 Feneis, H. (1988) *Anatomisches Bildwörterbuch*, 6th Ed. Stuttgart: Thieme.

13 Greene, M. and Mathieson, L. (1991) *The Voice and its Disorders.* London, UK: Whurr Publishers.

14 Javanshir, N., Salehpour, F., Aghazadeh, J. et al. (2017) 'The distribution of infection with *Propionibacterium acnes* is equal in patients with cervical and lumbar disc herniation.' *Eur. Spine J. 26*, 3135–3140.

15 Khoddami, S. M., Nakhostin Ansari, N., Izadi, F. et al. (2013) 'The assessment methods of laryngeal muscle activity in muscle tension dysphonia: a review.' *ScientificWorldJournal.* doi: 10.1155/2013/507397.

16 Knapp, C. (1985) 'Succion du pouce et charnière cervico-occipitale.' *Annales de Médécine Ostéopathique. 1*, 1.

17 Kooijman, P. G., de Jong, F. I., Oudes, M. J. et al. (2005) 'Muscular tension and body posture in relation to voice handicap and voice quality in teachers with persistent voice complaints.' *Folia. Phoniatr. Logop. 57*, 3, 134–147.

18 Larsen, C. (2007) *Die zwölf Grade der Freiheit.* Petersberg: Via Nova.

19 Lee, E. K. and Son, Y. I. (2005) 'Muscle tension dysphonia in children: voice characteristics and outcome of voice therapy.' *Int. J. Pediatr. Otorhinolaryngol. 69*, 7, 911–917.

20 Leonhardt, H., Tillmann, B., Töndury, G. and Zilles, K. (Ed.) (1987) *Rauber/Kopsch: Anatomie des Menschen, Vol. 1. Nervensystem.* Stuttgart: Thieme.

21 Lieberman, J. (1998) 'Principles and techniques of manual therapy: application in the management of dysphonia.' In: Harris, T., Harris, S., Rubin, J. and Howard, D. (Ed.) *Voice Clinic Hand Book.* London, UK: Whurr Publishers, pp. 91–138.

22 Liem, T. (2018) *Kraniosakrale Osteopathie. Ein praktisches Lehrbuch*, 7th Ed. Stuttgart: Thieme.

23 Lowell, S. Y., Kelley, R. T., Colton, R. H., et al. (2012) 'Position of the hyoid and larynx in people with muscle tension dysphonia.' *Laryngoscope. 122*, 2, 370–377.

24 Magoun, H. I. (1976) *Osteopathy in the Cranial Field*, 3rd Ed. Kirksville, MO: Journal Printing Company.

25 Marszalek, S., Niebudek-Bogusz, E., Woznicka, E. et al. (2012) 'Assessment of the influence of osteopathic myofascial techniques on normalization of the vocal tract functions in patients with occupational dysphonia.' *Int. J. Occup. Med. Environ. Health. 25*, 3, 225–235.

26 Miller, N. A., Gregory, J. S., Semple, S. I. et al. (2012) 'Relationships between vocal structures, the airway and craniocervical posture investigated using magnetic resonance imaging.' *J. Voice. 26*, 1, 102–109.

27 Müller, F., Walther, E. and Herzog, J. (2014) *Praktische Neurorehabilitation. Behandlungskonzepte nach Schädigung des Nervensystems.* Stuttgart: Kohlhammer.

28 Ogawa, M., Yoshida, M., Watanabe, K. et al. (2005) 'Association between laryngeal findings and vocal qualities in muscle tension dysphonia with supraglottic contraction.' *Nihon. Jibiinkoka. Gakkai. Kaiho. 108*, 7, 734–741.

29 Olmos, S. R. (2016) 'Comorbidities of chronic facial pain and obstructive sleep apnea.' *Curr. Opin. Pulm. Med. 22*, 570–575.

30 Pereira, T. C., Brasolotto, A. G., Conti, P. C. et al. (2009) 'Temporomandibular disorders, voice and oral quality of life in women.' *J. Appl. Oral Sci. 17,* Suppl., 50–56.

31 Piron, A. and Roch, J. B. (2010) 'Temporomandibular dysfunction and dysphonia (TMD).' *Rev. Laryngol. Otol. Rhinol. (Bord). 131,* 1, 31–34.

32 Pothmann, R. (Ed.) (1996) *Systematik der Schmerzakupunktur.* Stuttgart: Hippokrates.

33 Roy, N. (2008) 'Assessment and treatment of musculoskeletal tension in hyperfunctional voice disorders.' *Int. J. Speech Lang. Pathol. 10,* 4, 195–209.

34 Roy, N. and Leeper, H. A. (1993) 'Effects of the manual laryngeal musculoskeletal tension reduction technique as a treatment for functional voice disorders: perceptual and acoustic measures.' *J. Voice. 7,* 242–249.

35 Roy, N., Bless, D. M., Heisey, D. et al. (1997) 'Manual circumlaryngeal therapy for functional dysphonia: an evaluation of short- and long-term treatment outcomes.' *J. Voice. 11,* 321–331.

36 Rubin, J. S., Blake, E. and Mathieson, L. (2007) 'Musculoskeletal patterns in patients with voice disorders.' *J. Voice. 21,* 4, 477–484.

37 Seider, R. (1999) 'Der Einfluss von kraniosakraler Therapie auf den Bewegungsumfang entfernt liegender großer Gelenke, bei Zustand nach kieferorthopädischer Zahnstellungskorrektur mittels Zahnspange.' Diplomarbeit. Hamm.

38 Seymour, G. J., Ford, P. J., Cullinan, M. P. et al. (2017) 'Relationship between periodontal infections and systemic disease.' *Clin. Microbiol. Infect. 13,* Suppl. 4, 3–10.

39 Siccoli, M. M., Bassetti, C. L. and Sándor, P. S. (2006) 'Facial pain: clinical differential diagnosis.' *Lancet. Neurol. 5,* 3, 257–267.

40 Silva, A. M., Morisso, M. F. and Cielo, C. A. (2007) 'Relationship between the severity of temporomandibular disorder and voice.' *Pro. Fono. 19,* 3, 279–288.

41 Stecco, C. (2016) *Atlas des menschlichen Fasziensystems.* München: Elsevier.

42 Teanpaisan, R., Piwat, S. and Dahlén, G. (2011) 'Inhibitory effect of oral *Lactobacillus* against oral pathogens.' *Lett. Appl. Microbiol. 53,* 4, 452–459.

43 Tillmann, B. (1997) *Farbatlas der Anatomie. Zahnmedizin—Humanmedizin.* Stuttgart: Thieme.

44 Travell, J. G. and Simons, D. G. (1983) *Myofascial Pain and Dysfunction,* Vol. 1. Baltimore: Williams and Wilkins.

45 von Treuenfels, H. (2012) 'Kindesentwicklung, Kieferanomalien und Kieferorthopädie.' In: Liem, T., Schleupen, A., Altmeyer, P. and Zweedijk, R. (Ed.) *Osteopathische Behandlung von Kindern,* 2nd Ed. Stuttgart: Haug.

46 Upledger, J. E. (1987) *Craniosacral Therapy II. Beyond the Dura.* Seattle: Eastland Press, p. 1.

47 Van Houtte, E., Van Lierde, K. and Claeys, S. (2011) 'Pathophysiology and treatment of muscle tension dysphonia: a review of the current knowledge.' *J. Voice. 25,* 202–207.

48 Van Lierde, K. M., De Bodt, M., Dhaeseleer, E. et al. (2008) 'The treatment of muscle tension dysphonia: a comparison of two treatment techniques by means of an objective multiparameter approach.' *J. Voice. 24,* 3, 294–301.

49 Van Lierde, K. M., De Bodt, M., Dhaeseleer, E. et al. (2010) 'The treatment of muscle tension dysphonia: a comparison of two treatment techniques by means of an objective multiparameter approach.' *J. Voice. 24,* 3, 294–301.

50 Voith, C. and Piekartz, H. (2017) 'Neuromuskuläre Untersuchung und Behandlung bei funktioneller Dysphonie.' *Manuelle Therapie. 21,* 214–220.

51 Vuotto, C., Longo, F. and Donelli, G. (2014) 'Probiotics to counteract biofilm-associated infections: promising and conflicting data.' *Int. J. Oral Sci. 6,* 189–194.

52 Warnecke, T. and Dziewas, R. (2013) *Neurogene Dysphagien: Diagnostik und Therapie.* Stuttgart: Kohlhammer.

53 Wu, C. C., Lin, C. T. and Wu, C. Y. (2015) 'Inhibitory effect of *Lactobacillus salivarius* on *Streptococcus mutans* biofilm formation.' *Mol. Oral Microbiol. 30,* 1, 16–26.

54 Zakrzewska, J. M. (2013) 'Differential diagnosis of facial pain and guidelines for management.' *Br. J. Anaesth. 111,* 1, 95–104.

4.1	Morphology of the occipital bone according to Rohen	260
4.2	Location, causes, and clinical presentation of osteopathic dysfunctions of the occipital bone	261
4.2.1	Osseous dysfunctions	261
4.2.2	Muscular dysfunctions	262
4.2.3	Ligamentous dysfunctions	263
4.2.4	Fascial dysfunctions	263
4.2.5	Dysfunctions of intracranial and extracranial dural membranes	263
4.2.6	Disturbances of nerves, parts of the brain, and CSF spaces	263
4.2.7	Vascular disturbances	263
4.3	Diagnosis of the occipital bone	264
4.3.1	History-taking	264
4.3.2	Inspection	264
4.3.3	Palpation of the position of the atlanto-occipital joint	264
4.3.4	Palpation of the position of the occipital bone	264
4.3.5	Palpation of PRM rhythm	264
4.3.6	Motion testing	266
4.4	Treatment of the occipital bone	266
4.4.1	Atlanto-occipital joint	266
4.4.2	Intraosseous dysfunctions	270
4.4.3	Fluid/electrodynamic techniques	272
4.5	References	275

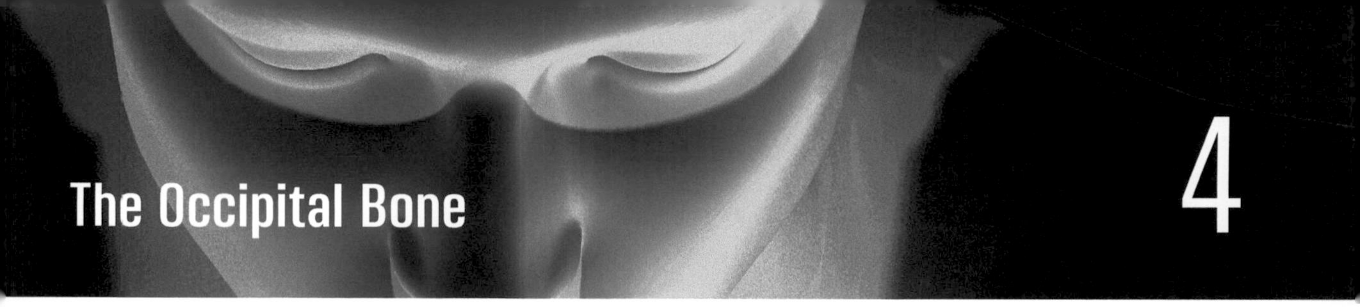

4 The Occipital Bone

The occipital bone, forming, as it does, part of the base of the skull, is an important bone of the cranial region. This is reflected in its many muscular, ligamentous, and fascial relations with connections to the vertebral column, scapula, clavicle, sternum, and visceral compartment. At the same time it serves as the point of attachment for all the intracranial dural folds. The sagittal nuchal ligament connects the deep and superficial cervical fasciae and is important for rotation movements of the cervical spine.

As well as venous outflow and the inflow of the vertebral and posterior meningeal arteries, the many neural structures at the occipital bone manifest its interaction with functional structures and systems; for example, the tongue (CN XII), pharynx (CN IX), digestive system (CN X), sensory innervation of the cranium, innervation of the masticatory muscles (CN V), the sternocleidomastoid, the trapezius (CN XI), and the sympathetic innervation of the face (superior cervical ganglion).

The suboccipital muscles, which attach to the occipital bone, serve as useful instruments of measurement on account of their significant proprioceptive innervation, and are important in connection with the organs of sight and balance.

Another aspect which is clinically important in childhood is to consider the ossification of the bone. The anterior intraoccipital synchondrosis, which runs directly through the condyles, only ossifies between the fifth and eighth years of life. Consequently, falls and asymmetric forces can contribute to the development of scolioses.

4.1 Morphology of the occipital bone according to Rohen[13]

The sphenoid and occipital bone are closely connected in the cranial base. Together they exhibit all the formal elements of a vertebra. In this metamorphosis of the vertebrae into the cranial base, however, the order in which the formal elements of vertebrae are arranged to become the cranial bones is reversed. The anterior vertebral body finds its counterpart in the occipital bone, while the vertebral processes find their counterpart in the processes of the body of the sphenoid.

Rohen sees the basilar bone (occipital bone and sphenoid) as representing not simply the vertebra but the vertebral column of the skull—expressing, so to speak, the formal elements of all the vertebrae and thus the vertebral column as a whole, and integrating them in one ideal form. So a complete reversal takes place at the craniocervical transition zone: anterior and posterior are exchanged and a new space is created.

For Rohen, the substantia spongiosa system of the extremities, which ossifies intracartilaginously from the inside and is related to the physical substance and blood vessel system (and is adapted to the static stresses caused by the trajectories), metamorphoses into the viscerocranium. The compact substance, meanwhile, which ossifies periosteally from the outside, gives shape to the long bones, and is closely connected to the locomotor system via numerous muscle attachments, he sees as metamorphosing into the roof of the cranium. Seen in this light the base of the skull represents the connection between the roof of the skull, with its cosmic orientation, and the terrestrially oriented viscerocranium.

Via the sensory nerves, located particularly at the base of the skull, the external world impinges on the brain; in return, individuality communicates itself to the external world by means of language and facial expression. This reciprocal or counter-sensory flow takes place primarily at the cranial base.

4.2 Location, causes, and clinical presentation of osteopathic dysfunctions of the occipital bone

4.2.1 Osseous dysfunctions

- **Lambdoid suture**
  - The squamous interdigitated suture prevents overlapping of the bones, but can be compressed by a fall or blow.
- **Occipitomastoid suture and the condylo-squamoso-mastoid pivot point (CSMP)**
  - Causes:
    - Bilateral compression: fall or blow to the occipital squama.
    - Unilateral compression: fall or blow to the side of the occipital squama or mastoid process. This forces the squama in an anterior direction, the basilar part of the occipital bone inferiorly and the temporal bones into internal rotation. The concave mastoid border of the occipital bone is forced anteriorly and superiorly, wedging it into the convex posterior edge of the mastoid process of the temporal bone, which moves posteriorly and medially.
    - Whiplash injuries and direct thrust techniques to the back of the head can also result in compression of this suture.
  - Compression at this suture leads to opposite motion of the temporal bone relative to the occipital bone. In other words, the occiput moves into flexion and the temporal bone into internal rotation.
  - Clinical presentation/hypothetical pathology:
    - Abnormal tensions of the tentorium cerebelli.
    - Venous congestion of the sigmoid sinus.
    - Disturbances in the fluctuation of the cerebrospinal fluid (CSF) with possible disturbance to the cranial nerve nuclei at the fourth ventricle.
    - Disturbances to the cerebellum, medulla oblongata, or other centers of the brain, and of the vagus nerve (nausea, vomiting, etc.).
  - Sequelae Dysfunction of the SBS and a change in the frequency and amplitude of PRM rhythm, impairing homeostasis of the body as a whole.
- **Petro-occipital fissure (petro-occipital synchondrosis; this fissure is also known as the petrobasilar suture)** The lateral margins of the base of the occipital bone form a ridge, which articulates with a groove on the lower posterior portion of the petrous part of the temporal bone. This construction enables a turning and sliding motion.
  - **Causes** In association with the occipital bone: usually as a result of trauma, e.g., tooth extraction with mouth opened wide.
  - **Clinical presentation/hypothetical pathology** Disturbance at the jugular foramen (Figure 4.1) and foramen lacerum and the nerves and blood vessels that pass through these (Figure 4.2).
- **Petrojugular suture** The jugular process of the occipital bone articulates with the jugular articular surface of the petrous part of the temporal bone. This location can be seen as

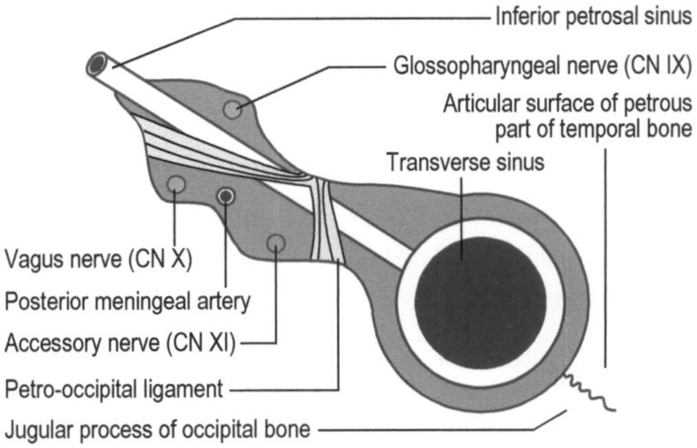

Figure 4.1
Jugular foramen

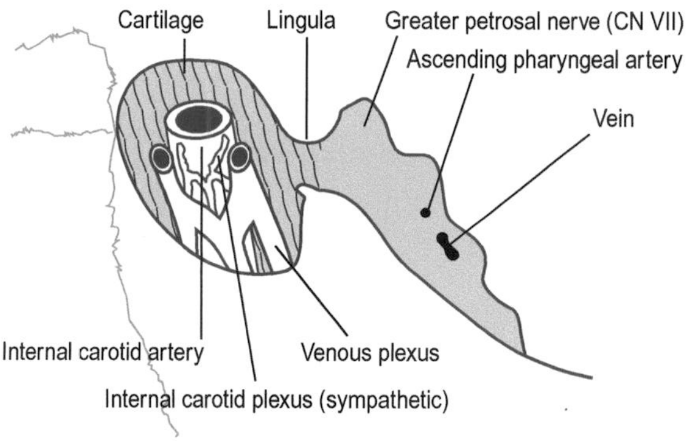

Figure 4.2
Foramen lacerum

a pivot point for the dynamics of the occiput and the temporal bone.
  - Causes and clinical presentation: see petro-occipital fissure (petro-occipital synchondrosis) (above).
- **Atlanto-occipital joint** The many neural, vascular, muscular, and fascial associations and attachments mean that this region is responsible for a large number of symptoms.
  - Causes: birth trauma, falls, and blows. Secondary lesions can result from dysfunctions of the SBS or sacrum, hypertonicity of the nuchal muscles, abnormal fascial tensions, psychological tension and stress, abnormal asymmetric stress, poor working position, etc.
  - Clinical presentation/hypothetical pathology:
    - Upper cervical syndrome, pain in the nuchal area.
    - Headache and other functional disturbances affecting the brain (obstruction of venous drainage of the jugular vein).
    - Stenosis of the vertebral artery with disturbance of the sympathetic fibers of the inferior cervical ganglion.
    - Disturbances of the salivary glands and eyes (superior cervical ganglion).
    - Cranial nerve symptoms (disturbance of the vagus, glossopharyngeal nerve, accessory nerve, and hypoglossal nerve).
    - Disturbance of fine motor function and motor skills (decussation of pyramids).
    - Dysfunction of the medulla oblongata.
    - Spinal scoliosis.
    - Disturbance of the pituitary, thyroid, and parathyroid.
    - Possible dull pain in the lower half of the body (irritation of fibers of the spinal cord).
    - Abnormal dural tensions, sometimes accompanied by compression of the SBS or sacrolumbar transition zone, etc.

4.2.2 Muscular dysfunctions

The tonus of all nuchal muscles can impair the mobility of the occiput and thus the SBS.

- **Sternocleidomastoid** Clinical presentation/hypothetical pathology
  - Hypertonicity: motion restriction of the occipitomastoid suture, migraine, or hemicranial headache.
  - Cranial nerve XI runs through the jugular foramen, which can be impaired by hypertonicity of the sternocleidomastoid or trapezius. This in turn can lead to further increase in tonus of these two muscles via CN XI.
- **Trapezius** Clinical presentation/hypothetical pathology
  - Headache affecting the back of the head, pain and stiffness of the shoulder, aggravation of pain in the masticatory muscles.
  - Bilateral hypertonicity: flexion dysfunction of the SBS.
- **Semispinalis capitis** Clinical presentation/hypothetical pathology
  - Headache affecting the back of the head; temporal headache.
  - Bilateral hypertonicity: flexion dysfunction of the SBS.

- Unilateral hypertonicity: torsion dysfunction of the SBS.
- Hypertonicity of the splenius capitis muscle can lead to pain at the nape of the neck, and headache affecting the back of the head, and the parietal region.

- **Longus capitis and rectus capitis anterior** Clinical presentation/hypothetical pathology
  - Bilateral hypertonicity: extension dysfunction of the SBS.
  - Unilateral hypertonicity: torsion dysfunction of the SBS.
- **Rectus capitis lateralis** Clinical presentation/hypothetical pathology
  - Venous reflux to the inside of the cranium and disturbances of CN IX, CN X, and CN XI.
  - Unilateral hypertonicity: torsion dysfunction of the SBS.
- **Rectus capitis posterior major and minor** Clinical presentation/hypothetical pathology
  - Headache affecting the back of the head.
  - Bilateral hypertonicity: flexion dysfunction of the SBS.
  - Unilateral hypertonicity: torsion of the SBS.
  - In the case of muscle atrophy: possible slight compression of spinal cord due to connective tissue link between the rectus capitis posterior minor and the posterior part of the dura mater.[5]
- **Obliquus capitis superior** Clinical presentation/hypothetical pathology
  - Headache affecting the back of the head.
  - Bilateral hypertonicity: flexion dysfunction of the SBS.
  - Unilateral hypertonicity: sidebending/rotation dysfunction of the SBS.
- **Superior pharyngeal constrictor** Clinical presentation/hypothetical pathology
  - Pain and dysfunction of the floor of the mouth and pharynx.
  - In the case of hypertonicity: via the pharyngeal raphe, flexion and extension dysfunctions of the SBS.

4.2.3 Ligamentous dysfunctions

- Abnormal tension of the **nuchal ligaments** can impair the mobility of the occipital bone.
- **Posterior atlanto-occipital membrane** The vertebral artery and suboccipital nerve pierce this membrane. Tensions in the membrane can therefore impair their function.
- Other ligaments in the region of the occipital bone may also be involved in any dysfunctions: the anterior atlanto-occipital membrane, anterior longitudinal ligament, apical ligament of the dens, alar ligaments, tectorial membrane, and posterior longitudinal ligament.

4.2.4 Fascial dysfunctions

- **Investing layer of cervical fascia:** extending to the superior nuchal line.
- **Prevertebral layer of cervical fascia:** extending from its attachment to the pharyngeal tubercle to the occipitomastoid suture.
- **Pharynx:** at the pharyngeal tubercle.

4.2.5 Dysfunctions of intracranial and extracranial dural membranes

See section 6.3.1.

4.2.6 Disturbances of nerves, parts of the brain, and CSF spaces

See sections 6.3.2 and 6.3.3.

4.2.7 Vascular disturbances

- **Occipital artery** Causes: dural tensions in the occipital groove, medial to the mastoid notch.
- **Jugular vein** (responsible for drainage of about 95% of the venous blood that leaves the head)
  - Causes: abnormal dural tension at the jugular foramen, dysfunction of the occipital and temporal bones, occipitomastoid and petrojugular sutures, and petro-occipital fissure (petrobasilar suture; petro-occipital synchondrosis).

The jugular foramen is like a broad suture between the occiput and temporal bone and so liable to be impaired when there is any dysfunction of these two bones.

- Clinical presentation/hypothetical pathology: venous congestion within the cranium → headache, memory disturbances, and impairment of brain function.

4.3 Diagnosis of the occipital bone

4.3.1 History-taking

See clinical presentation of dysfunctions in section 4.2.

4.3.2 Inspection

- Occipital squama bent: occiput in flexion.
- Occipital squama flattened: occiput in extension.

4.3.3 Palpation of the position of the atlanto-occipital joint

Patient: Supine.

Practitioner: Take up a position at the head of the patient.

Hand position:

- Place your hands underneath the patient's head, to each side of the occiput.

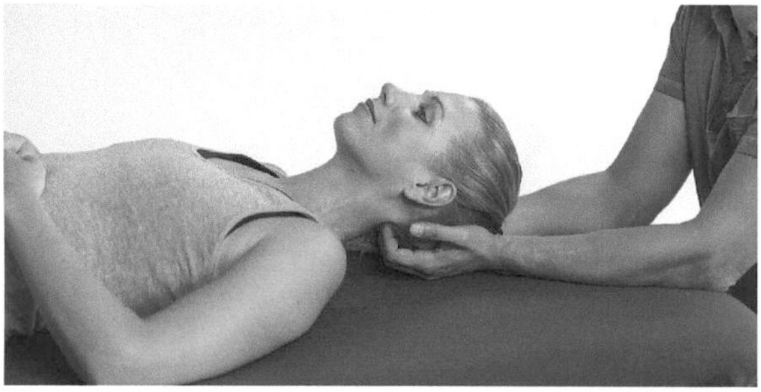

Figure 4.3 Palpation of the position of the atlanto-occipital joint

- Place the index and middle fingers as close as possible to the occipital condyles (Figure 4.3).

Method:

- Compare the two sides.
- The side that is lying farther anterior and inferior than the other may be the side where the compression is present, if any.

4.3.4 Palpation of the position of the occipital bone

- Supraoccipital part: inferior (ER) or superior (IR)?
- The angle of the squama and condyles: reduced or enlarged?
- External occipital protuberance: whether or not laterally displaced?
- Condylar part: compressed anteroposteriorly or mediolaterally?
- Lambda: depressed, e.g., in the case of primary traumatic injury due to force, or elevated?
- Occipitomastoid suture: depressed or elevated?
- Flexibility of the occipital bone: pliant or hard?

4.3.5 Palpation of PRM rhythm

Tip for practitioners

Biomechanical, inhalation phase

The occipital bone turns about a transverse axis, which runs through both condylo-squamoso-mastoid pivot points (CSMP), above the foramen magnum:

- The basilar part and foramen magnum move superiorly and anteriorly.
- The articulations with the atlas move anteriorly.
- The inferior lateral parts of the occipital squama move inferiorly and anteriorly.
- Lambda and the cranial part of the occipital squama move posteriorly and inferiorly.
- The peripheral, lateral parts of the occipital bone at asterion move inferiorly and laterally.
- The mastoid border moves anteriorly.

Developmental dynamic, inhalation phase

- The occipital squama moves centrifugally (outward motion).
- The convexity of the squama decreases; i.e., it flattens.

If a motion restriction is discovered on palpation, the practitioner may induce motion in the direction of restricted motion. This will emphasize the restriction and make it clearer to identify. The practitioner is then better able to sense which structure is the origin of the motion restriction:

- Intraosseous tension.
- Sutural/osseous restriction relative to adjoining bones.
- Dural restriction.
- Fascial or ligamentous restriction.
- Muscular restriction.
- Vascular effect.
- Neuronal activity.

Practitioner: Take up a position at the head of the patient.

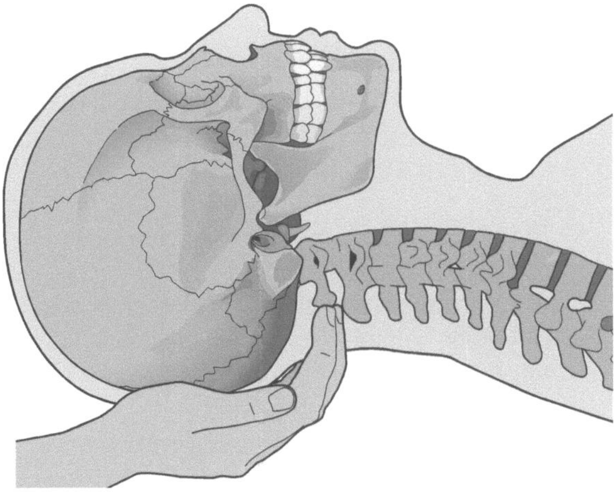

Figure 4.4 Palpation of PRM rhythm of the occipital bone

Hand position:

- Place your hands under the patient's head, one each side, so that the occiput is cradled in your hands.
- Place your index and middle finger as close as possible to the occipital condyles (Figure 4.4).

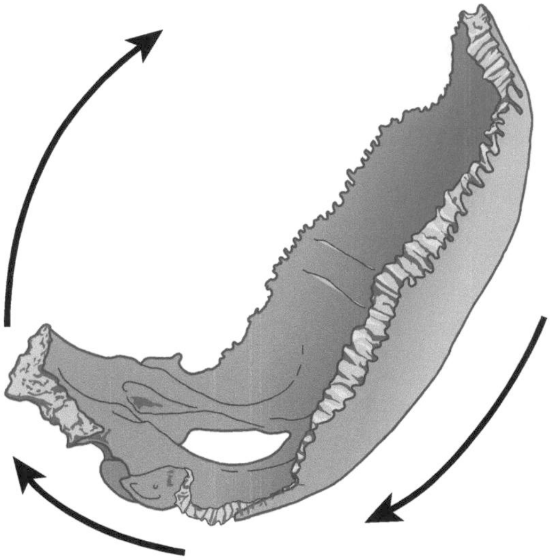

Figure 4.5 PRM inhalation phase: biomechanical

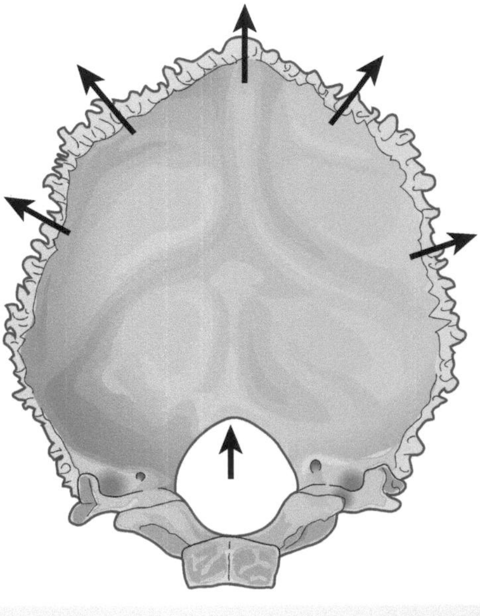

Figure 4.6 PRM inhalation phase: developmental dynamic

Biomechanical approach: inhalation phase of PRM, normal finding (Figure 4.5)

- The joint articulations with the atlas move anteriorly.
- The inferior lateral parts of the occipital squama move inferiorly and anteriorly.
- Lambda and the cranial part of the occipital squama move posteriorly and inferiorly.
- The peripheral, lateral parts of the occipital bone at the asterion move inferiorly and laterally in an external rotation motion. (The mastoid border [of the occipital with the temporal bone] moves anteriorly. The basilar part of the occipital bone moves superiorly and anteriorly.)

Exhalation phase of the PRM, normal finding

- The joint articulations with the atlas move posteriorly.
- The inferior lateral parts of the occipital squama move superiorly and posteriorly.
- Lambda and the cranial part of the occipital squama move anteriorly and superiorly.
- The peripheral, lateral parts of the occiput at asterion move superiorly and medially in an internal rotation motion. (The mastoid border [of the occipital with the temporal bone] moves posteriorly. The basilar part moves inferiorly and posteriorly.)

Developmental dynamic approach: inhalation phase of PRM, normal finding (Figure 4.6)

- The occipital squama moves centrifugally (outward motion).
- The convexity of the squama is reduced: the squama flattens.

Exhalation phase of PRM, normal finding

- The occipital squama moves centripetally (inward motion).
- The convexity of the squama increases.
- Compare the amplitude, strength, ease, and symmetry of the motions of the occiput.

4.3.6 Motion testing

Hand position: See palpation of PRM rhythm, section 4.3.5 above.

Method: Apply slight cephalad traction to the occiput to test the mobility of the atlanto-occipital joint.

- Restrictions or compression may be unilateral or bilateral.
- Compare the amplitude and ease of motion of the occiput, or the amount of force required to produce motion.

4.4 Treatment of the occipital bone

4.4.1 Atlanto-occipital joint

Indication: Primary or secondary dysfunctions presenting with: upper cervical syndrome, pain at nape of neck, headache, obstruction of venous drainage of the jugular vein, stenosis of the vertebral artery with disturbance of the sympathetic fibers of the inferior cervical ganglion, disturbances of the salivary glands and eyes, cranial nerve symptoms, disturbance of fine motor function and motor skills, dysfunction of the medulla oblongata, scoliosis, endocrine disturbances, dull pain in the lower half of the body, abnormal dural tensions, sometimes accompanied by compression of the SBS or sacrolumbar transition zone, etc.

Bilateral release of the atlanto-occipital joint and decompression of the occipital condylar region

Practitioner: Take up a position at the head of the patient.

Hand position:

- Place both hands underneath the occiput with the palms facing anterior.
- The patient's head should at this stage be resting in the palms of your hands.
- Bend your fingers upward at a right angle so that they are pointing directly anterior.

- Place your fingers immediately by the inferior palpable border of the occiput, very close to the arch of the atlas. (During the course of the treatment, when the nuchal muscles relax, your fingers will rest on the posterior arch of the atlas.)

Method:

- Do not apply any additional pressure with your fingers. The weight of the skull alone, with your fingers acting as a lever, is used to release the nuchal muscles (Figures 4.7 and 4.8).
- Readjust your fingers into the upright position as often as necessary if the release of the nuchal muscles causes them to shift to an oblique angle.

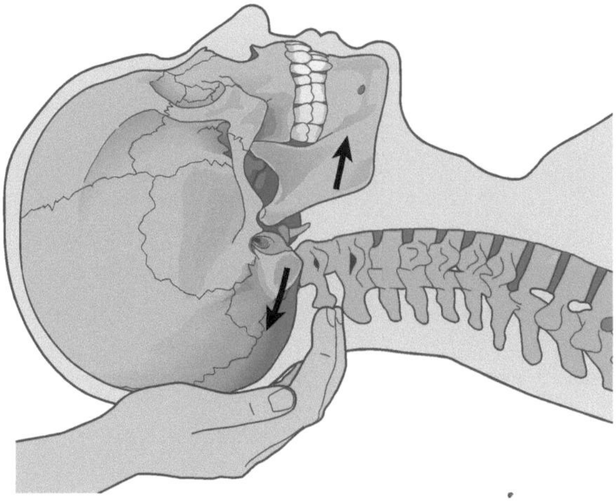

Figure 4.7 Bilateral release of the atlanto-occipital joint and decompression of the occipital condylar region

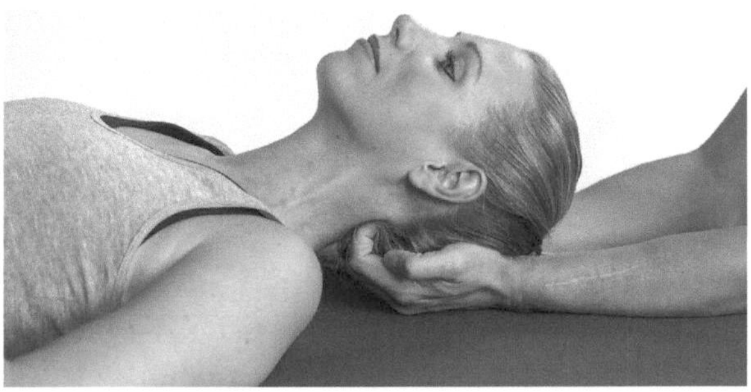

Figure 4.8 Bilateral release of the atlanto-occipital joint and decompression of the occipital condylar region

- As the nuchal muscles relax it will gradually become possible to feel the bony arch of the atlas.
- At the end of treatment the skull will no longer be resting on your palms but will be supported at the atlas by your fingers alone.
- After releasing the nuchal muscles you can also go on to release the occipital condyles from the atlas. To do this, hold the arch of the atlas in place with your middle fingers alone, using the ring fingers and little fingers to draw the occipital bone gently cephalad.
- Then decompress the occipital condyles transversally. Continue to point your fingers toward the foramen magnum at a 45° angle corresponding to the arrangement of the occipital condyles. Draw your elbows together so that your fingers move outward at the occipital condyles. Continue until you sense a softening and inherent motion of the tissues.

Contraindications:

- Fracture of the dens axis, e.g., as a result of whiplash injury.
- Risk of intracranial bleeding, in acute aneurysm or cerebrovascular accident.
- Fracture of the cranial base.

Bilateral release of the atlanto-occipital joint

Practitioner: Take up a position at the head of the patient.

Hand position:

- Grasp the arch of the atlas with the thumb and index finger (or middle finger) of one hand.
- Hold the occiput with the other hand, placing your thumb and little finger on the lateral parts of the occipital bone.
- Place your index and middle finger next to inion, on the superior nuchal line.

Method:

- Begin by palpating the motion of the occiput in extension and flexion (phases of PRM).
- Then hold the atlas firmly in position (Figures 4.9 and 4.10).

- As you do so, go with the occiput in the direction of greater ease (indirect technique). Establish a position of the occiput (in terms of flexion or extension, sidebending, and rotation) that achieves the best possible balance of ligamentous and membranous tensions in the joint (PBLT and PBMT).
- This position will enable the ligamentous/membranous tensions to normalize.
- Now you should also draw the occiput gently cephalad, to disengage the joint.
- Allow all further unwinding of the tissue, without slackening the gentle cephalad traction to the occipital bone and all the time maintaining the PBLT and PBMT.

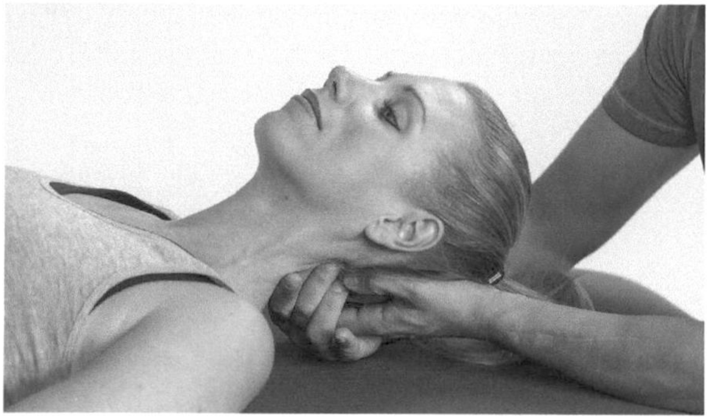

Figure 4.9 Bilateral release of the atlanto-occipital joint

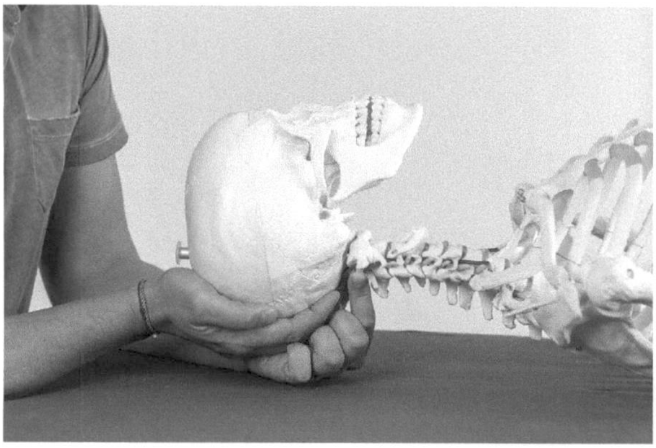

Figure 4.10 Bilateral release of the atlanto-occipital joint (shown on model)

- Maintain the PBT of the atlanto-occipital joint until you sense that the unwinding of the tissues is complete and that a release of the motion restriction has occurred.

Sutherland's technique

Practitioner: Take up a position at the head of the patient.

Hand position:

- Place the tip of your middle finger on the posterior tubercle of the atlas (Figure 4.11).
- Place your other hand on the frontal bone with your fingers pointing caudad.

Method:

- Hold the atlas anterior and prevent it from moving posterior.
- Ask the patient to make a slight nod of the head.
- The anteriorly directed pressure of your finger on the atlas prevents bending anywhere other than at the atlanto-occipital joint, involving the rest of the cervical spine.
- The nodding movement releases the occipital condyles from the atlas. At the same time there is an increase in tension of the atlanto-occipital ligaments.
- Induce a PBLT (and PBMT). The point of balanced tension (PBT) is the position in which the tension in the ligaments (dural membranes) between the occiput and the atlas is as balanced as possible.

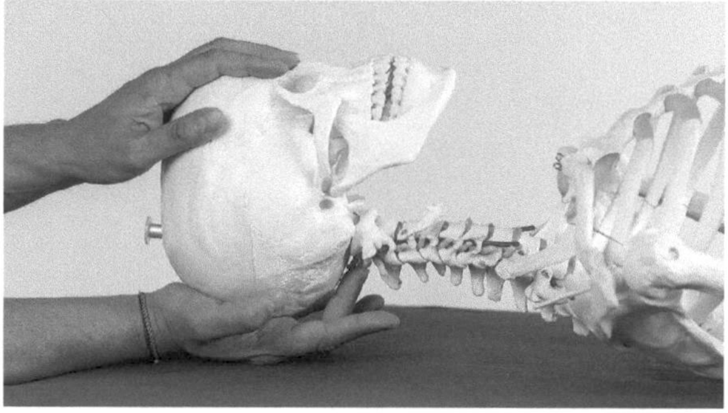

Figure 4.11 Sutherland's technique

- Maintain the PBT until the ligamentous/membranous tension is normalized.
- Breathing assistance: ask the patient to hold their breath at the end of an in- or out-breath for as long as possible. The moment just before the patient has to breathe out, or draw the next involuntary breath, is when release of the motion restriction usually occurs.

Tip for practitioners

As strictly defined, Sutherland's technique is only concerned with the ligamentous tension of the atlanto-occipital joint. However, in view of the fact that the dura mater spinalis is attached at the foramen magnum and C2 and that there is also some attachment at C1, a PBMT should also be induced.

Unilateral release of the atlanto-occipital joint

If the above technique fails to release a condyle, it can be treated individually.

Patient: Supine, with head slightly turned toward the side of the restricted condyle.

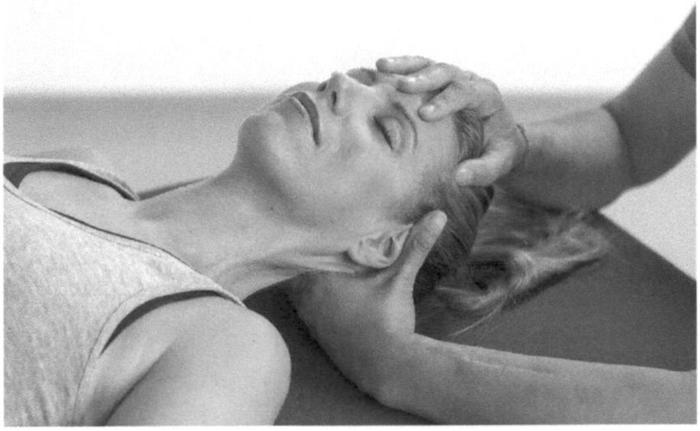

Figure 4.12 Unilateral release of the atlanto-occipital joint

Practitioner: Take up a position at the head of the patient.

Hand position:

- Place the hand that is on the same side as the restricted condyle under the atlas. Your hand is supported on the little finger, the side of which rests on the table (Figure 4.12).
- Align the basal joint of your index finger so that it provides the main contact with the articular surface of the atlas that is restricted. Place the thumb to the side of the patient's head, but do not exert any pressure.
- Place the other hand on the patient's forehead.

Method:

- The patient's head should not be in contact with the table. Support it entirely on the hand that is underneath the atlas.
- Apply gentle posterior pressure with the hand on the frontal bone, from the contralateral side to the restricted joint, in the direction of that joint (Figure 4.12).
- Maintain this pressure until the occiput moves posterior on the articular surfaces of the atlas, so that the restricted joint opens.

Unilateral release of the atlanto-occipital joint using the V-spread technique to direct energy

Place the finger that is to direct the energy on the frontal tuber (Figure 4.13; V-spread technique[11]).

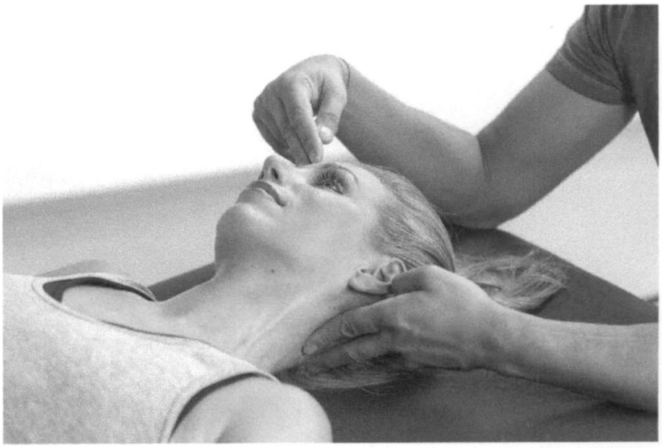

Figure 4.13
Unilateral release of the atlanto-occipital joint using the V-spread technique. The sending finger is seen on the frontal tuber

4.4.2 Intraosseous dysfunctions

Cranial base-occiput-foramen magnum technique in young children

Practitioner: Take up a position at the head of the patient.

Hand position:

- Place the index and middle fingers of one hand on the occipital squama and between the atlas and occiput. The thumb should be placed a little higher on the occipital squama.
- Place the other hand on the frontal bone with the index finger lying along the metopic suture (Figure 4.14).

Method:

- Anterior–posterior decompression of the SBS and anterior intraoccipital synchondrosis between the lateral and basilar parts of the occipital bone: apply traction in an anterior direction with the hand on the frontal bone.
- Posterior–anterior decompression of the posterior intraoccipital synchondrosis between the squama and the lateral parts of the occipital bone (and to the anterior intraoccipital synchondrosis): apply traction in a posterior direction to the occipital squama, using the index and middle fingers.
- Lateral decompression of the lateral parts of the occipital bone: spread the index and middle fingers, focusing your attention toward the lateral parts of the occipital bone.
- Rotation of the occipital squama: rotate the occipital squama against the restriction, using the thumb that is placed on the squama (direct technique).
- Establish the PBMT.
- In addition the other hand, which is placed on the frontal bone, can be used to direct a fluctuation wave in the direction of the restriction.

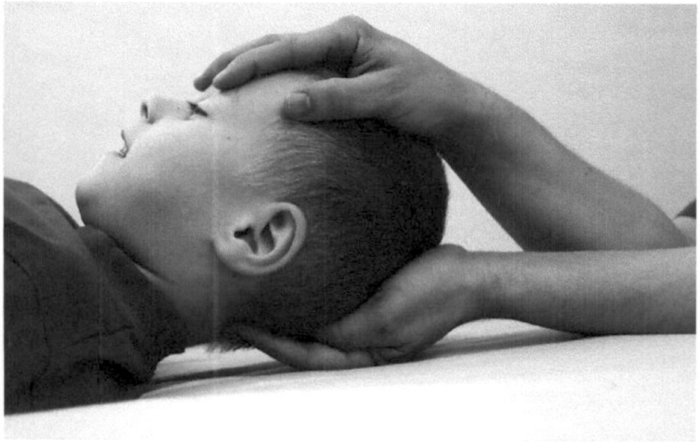

Figure 4.14 Cranial base-occiput-foramen magnum technique in young children. (Liem, T., Schleupen, A., Altmeyer, P., Zweedijk, R. (eds) (2012) *Osteopathische Behandlung von Kindern*, 2nd edn. Stuttgart: Haug. Photographer: Thomas Möller, Ludwigsburg)

Platybasia technique

Practitioner: Take up a position at the head of the patient.

Hand position:

- Place your thumbs on the greater wings of the sphenoid.
- Your index fingers should be positioned on the temporal bones anterior to the occipitomastoid suture.
- Position your middle, ring, and little fingers on the occiput (Figure 4.15).

Method:

- Anterior–posterior decompression of the SBS: with your thumbs on the greater wings of the sphenoid, apply traction in an anterior direction.

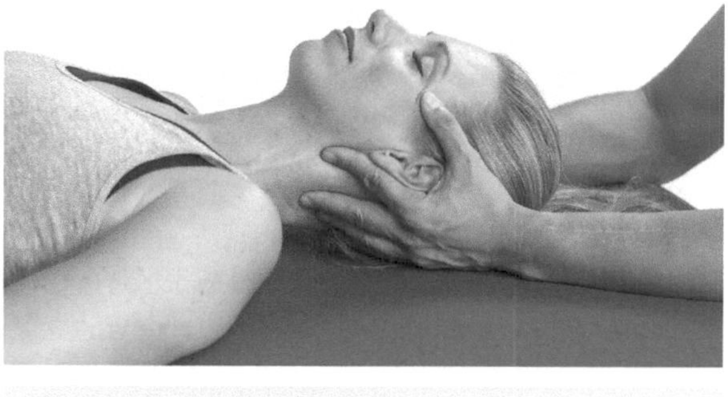

Figure 4.15 Platybasia technique

- Decompression of the occipitomastoid suture: separate your index and middle fingers.
- Posterior–anterior decompression: apply traction to the occiput in a posterior direction with your middle, ring, and little fingers, so as to decompress the squama from the lateral parts of the occipital bone, the lateral parts from the basilar parts, and the basilar parts of the occipital bone from the sphenoid.
- Establish the PBMT and PBFT.

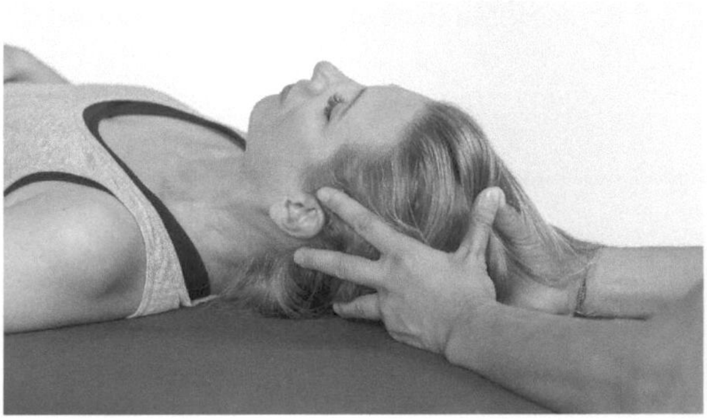

Figure 4.16 Occipital squama technique

Occipital squama technique

Practitioner: Take up a position at the head of the patient.

Hand position:

- Place your hands symmetrically on each side of the patient's head.
- Position your little fingers bilaterally on the interparietal occiput.
- Position your ring fingers mainly on the supraocciput, posterior to the lambdoid suture.
- Position your middle fingers anterior to the lambdoid suture.
- Let your index fingers rest lightly on the parietal bones, without exerting any pressure.
- Your thumbs should be touching each other above the vertex, but not in contact with the patient's head (Figure 4.16).

Method:

- Decompress the lambdoid suture by spreading the middle and ring fingers.
- Harmonize intraosseous tensions with your little finger and ring finger.
- **Testing the occipital squama** Test the motion of the squama in rotation, flexion, extension, and sidebending. Encourage the particular motion that you are testing, by means of impulses from your little finger and ring finger, and compare the amplitude, ease, and symmetry of this motion.

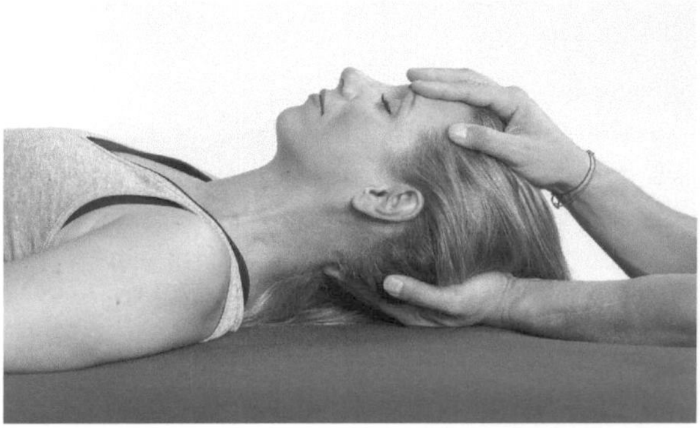

Figure 4.17 Alternative hand position: fronto-occipital palpation

- **Treating the occipital squama**
  - Using your little finger and ring finger, guide the squama in the direction of the motion restriction and wait for the release of the tissue (direct technique).
  - Alternatively, guide the squama in the direction of ease (indirect technique).
  - Establish the PBMT and PBFT.

Alternative hand position: fronto-occipital palpation

- Place your upper hand on the frontal bone, with the fingers pointing caudad.
- Position your middle finger on the metopic suture above nasion.

- Your ring and index fingers should rest laterally beside it, above the arch of the eyebrows.
- Place your thumb and little finger on the frontal bone near the coronal suture.
- Place your other hand under the patient's head, so that the occipital squama rests on the palm (Figure 4.17).

4.4.3 Fluid/electrodynamic techniques

Compression of the fourth ventricle (CV-4)

Explanation of effect from the biomechanical viewpoint Compression (Figure 4.18) applied to the lateral parts of the occiput reduces the accommodation of the occipital squama to the changes in pressure of the intracranial fluid.[7] This produces a rise in intracranial pressure, leading to an increase in the motion and exchange of fluid.[8:51] As a result, the CSF flows not only through the larger openings but also penetrates right into the smallest reaches of its distribution, to the sheaths of nerves and blood vessels, the fasciae, and the extracellular and intracellular fluid. The overall effect is an improved supply to the cells, an improved motion of the lymph and a regeneration of the tissue, as well as the stimulation of the cranial nerve centers in the region of the fourth ventricle. The biodynamic, bioelectric, and biochemical qualities of the CSF mean that all the body's exchange processes are stimulated.[1,8:51,9:112f.] The CV-4 technique tends to work in a centripetal direction.

Effect and indication:

- Normalization of PRM rhythm.
- Reduces tonicity of the sympathetic nervous system, with positive effects on stress symptoms, anxiety states, and insomnia.[9:112f.,12:54]
- Reduces tonicity of the entire connective tissue system. It is therefore indicated in acute and chronic muscular disturbances, degenerative joint disorders, and period pains.
- Lowers fever by up to 2°C within 30–60 min.[12:54]
- Raises core body temperature on compression of the occipital squama.[10]

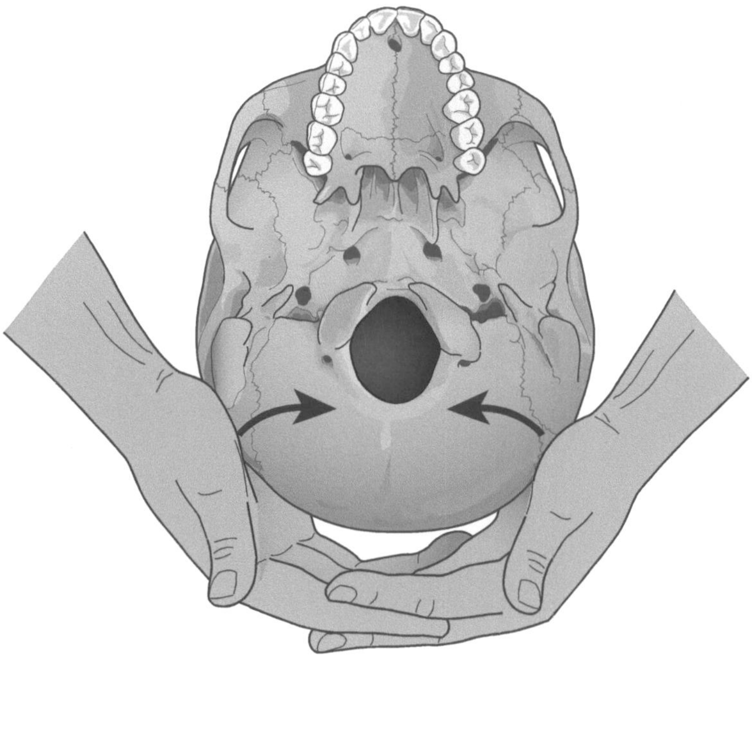

Figure 4.18
CV-4 technique. The arrows indicate the direction of extension/internal rotation

- In hypertension.
- In tachycardia.[2]
- In edema due to venous congestion.[9:114]
- In inflammation and infections.[9:114]
- Promotes ossification.[8:56]
- In cases of depression.
- In cases of headache due to disturbances of venous drainage.[9:114]
- In neuroendocrine disturbances.[8:56]
- In cases of thyroid hyperactivity.
- Epilepsy (care must be taken not to trigger a seizure).
- Promotes uterine contraction and so aids the birth process and induction of labor.
- Arthritic disorders.[12:54,9:114]
- Can release secondary, slight dysfunctions of the spinal column.[11:204]
- Lymphatic pump effect.[9:110]
- This technique can reveal primary dysfunctions elsewhere in the body so that they can be recognized.[8:56]
- Sutherland describes it as a universal technique: 'When you do not know what else to do, compress the fourth ventricle.'[11:37] The CV-4 can also be used to counteract the negative effects of another technique.
- Lowers blood sugar.[9:112f.]

Contraindications:

- Where there is a risk of cerebral bleeding, e.g., in acute cerebrovascular accident or aneurysm, or malignant hypertension (on account of the increase in intracranial pressure).
- Fractures of the base of the skull, head injuries, especially fractures of the occipital bone.
- Pregnancy from the seventh month onward, as there is a risk of inducing labor. (However, V. Frymann is of the view that the effect of CV-4 on the birth is homeostatic only.[3,4])
- In much-weakened elderly patients, as they may lack the strength to come back out of the exhalation phase/emptying phase. It is better to induce a still point in the inhalation phase in such patients.

Practitioner: Take up a position at the head of the patient.

Hand position:

- Place your slightly cupped hands one inside the other, and place the tips of your thumbs together in the form of a letter V (Figure 4.20).
- Position the tips of your thumbs roughly at the spinous process of the patient's second or third cervical vertebra, pointing distally.
- The ball of your thumbs should lie medially on the occipital squama (Figure 4.19).

> **CAUTION** Do not position the ball of your thumbs over the occipitomastoid suture. According to Magoun, this could predispose to fracture.

Method:

- Direct your attention throughout the procedure to the fluid in the fourth ventricle.
- During the exhalation phase, follow the narrowing motion of the occipital squama with the ball of the thumbs.
- In the inhalation phase, hold the ball of the thumbs so as to prevent the external rotation or broadening of the occipital squama. This is achieved, according to Magoun, by contraction of the flexor digitorum profundi muscles alone.[9:111]

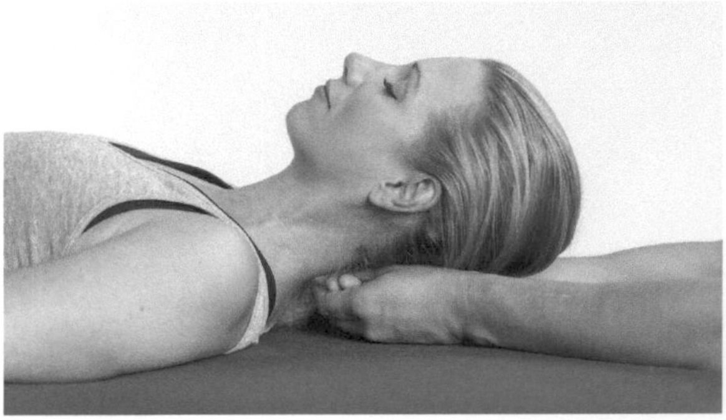

Figure 4.19 CV-4 technique (side view)

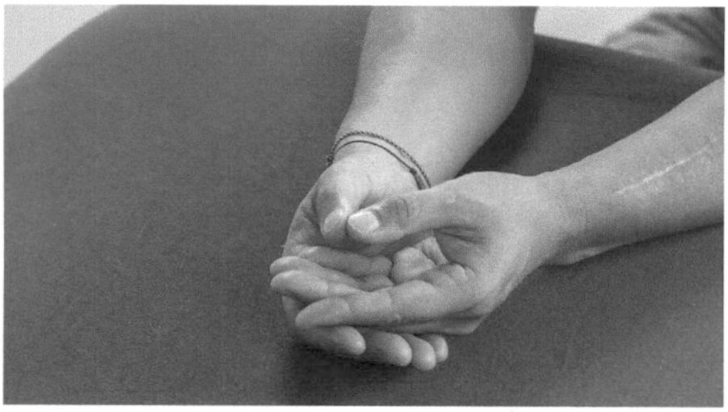

Figure 4.20 CV-4 technique: hand position

- In the next exhalation phase, follow the occipital bone further into internal rotation with your hands, and resist it once more as it tries to broaden in the following inhalation phase.
- During the exhalation phase, follow the narrowing motion of the occipital squama with the ball of the thumbs.
- After a few cycles, the pressure against your thumbs in the inhalation phase will be felt to reduce. This means that the flexion/extension motion has stopped: the still point has been reached.
- Keep your hands on the occiput during the still point, following any minor motion of the nuchal muscles if this occurs. This motion is a kind of unwinding and release of the fasciae, muscles, and bones.
- The still point may last anywhere from a few seconds to several minutes.
- The signs of a successfully induced still point are: deeper breathing; slight sweat formation on the forehead; reduction in muscle tonus; patient falling asleep.
- End of the still point: the practitioner will sense a strong, even pressure on each side of the occiput, in the direction of external rotation. Follow this motion passively, noting the quality of the rhythm.
- Once you have assessed the quality of the craniosacral rhythm, you will be able to decide whether it is necessary to induce a further still point.

Tip for practitioners

The CV-4 can also be induced from any other point on the cranium or the sacrum. The procedure is essentially the same: follow the exhalation phase and offer resistance to the inhalation phase.

Expansion of the fourth ventricle (EV-4 technique)

Effect, indication, and contraindications:
See under CV-4 technique, above. The EV-4 works in a centrifugal direction. Performance of a CV-4 or EV-4 is decided by the inherent forces.

Practitioner: Take up a position at the head of the patient.

Hand position:

- Let the patient's occiput rest on the palms of your hands.
- Your fingertips should meet in the middle. Direct the fingertips anteriorly (Figure 4.21).

Method:

- During the inhalation phase, go with the occipital squama into external rotation.

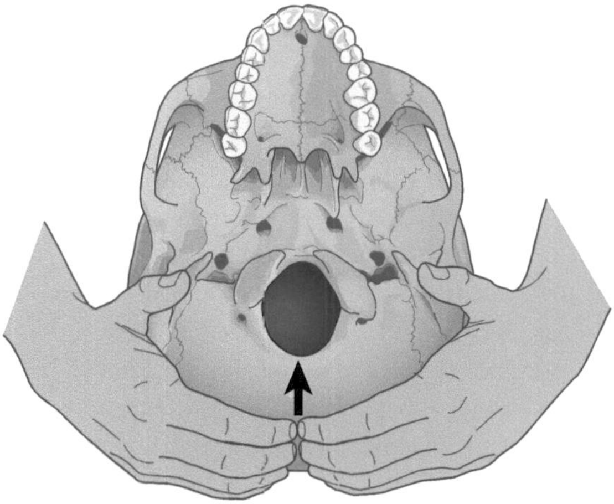

Figure 4.21 Expansion of the fourth ventricle (EV-4)

- In the exhalation phase, resist the extension and internal rotation of the occipital squama by applying gentle pressure with your fingertips in an anterior direction at the midline of the occiput.
- In the next inhalation phase, go with the occipital squama further into external rotation.
- Continue as for CV-4.

Vitalist approach It is the body itself that sets the healing processes in motion through the medium of mechanisms such as spontaneous local or system-wide still points, e.g., as a CV-4 or EV-4. The practitioner can encourage these processes by synchronization with the inherent homeodynamic forces and rhythmic patterns. This method demands no meeting of tissue resistance and no confrontation with it. Nor does it require the exercising of resistance in a phase of primary respiration.

4.5 References

1 Bolet, P. (1993) *La compression du 4ème ventricule modifie-t-elle le profil ionique chez le patient.* St Etienne: Mémoire.

2 Courty, F. (1998) *Compression du IVème ventricule et rythme cardiaque.* Marseille: Mémoire.

3 Frymann, V. M. (1976) 'Learning difficulties of children viewed in the light of the osteopathic concept.' *J. Am. Osteopath. Assoc.*, p. 76.

4 Frymann, V. M. (1966) 'Relation of disturbances of craniosacral mechanisms to the symptomatology of the newborn: study of 1250 infants.' *J. Am. Osteopath. Assoc.*, p. 65.

5 Hack, G. D., Koritzer, R. T., Robinson, W. L. et al. (1995) 'Anatomic relation between the rectus capitis posterior minor muscle and the dura mater.' *Spine. 20*, 2484–2486.

6 Kasack, A. (1998) 'Die osteopathische Behandlung für Kinder mit Down-Syndrom mit Schwerpunkt auf dem Os occipitale.' Master's thesis. Bonn.

7 Liem, T. (2018) *Kraniosakrale Osteopathie. Ein praktisches Lehrbuch*, 7th Ed. Stuttgart: Thieme.

8 Lippincott, H. A. (1948) 'Compression of the bulb.' *J. Osteopath. Cranial Assoc.*, Meridian, Cranial Academy.

9 Magoun, H. I. (1976) *Osteopathy in the Cranial Field*, 3rd Ed. Kirksville: Journal Printing Company.

10 Puylaert, M. (1988) 'Der Einfluss der Kompression der Squama occipitalis auf die Erhöhung der Körpertemperatur.' Master's thesis. Munich.

11 Sutherland, W. G. (1991) *Teachings in the Science of Osteopathy.* Fort Worth: Sutherland Cranial Teaching Foundation.

12 Upledger, J. E. and Vredevoogd, J. D. (2016) *Lehrbuch der CranioSacralen Therapie I*, 7th Ed. Stuttgart: Haug.

13 Rohen, J. W. (2002) *Morphologie des menschlichen Organismus*, 2nd Ed. Stuttgart: Verlag Freies Geistesleben, pp. 362–365.

5.1 Morphology of the sphenoid according to Rohen 278

5.2 Location, causes, and clinical presentation of osteopathic dysfunctions of the sphenoid 278
5.2.1 Osseous dysfunctions 278
5.2.2 Muscular dysfunctions 280
5.2.3 Ligamentous dysfunctions 280
5.2.4 Fascial dysfunctions 280
5.2.5 Dysfunction of intracranial and extracranial dural membranes 281
5.2.6 Disturbances to nerves, parts of the brain, and CSF spaces 281
5.2.7 Vascular disturbances 281
5.2.8 Endocrine disturbances 281

5.3 Diagnosis of the sphenoid 281
5.3.1 History-taking 281
5.3.2 Inspection 281
5.3.3 Palpation of position 282
5.3.4 Palpation of the PRM rhythm 282
5.3.5 Motion testing 283

5.4 Treatment of the sphenoid 283
5.4.1 Intraosseous dysfunctions 283
5.4.2 Fluid/electrodynamic techniques 285
5.4.3 Dural techniques 286
5.4.4 Sutural dysfunctions 287

5.5 References 287

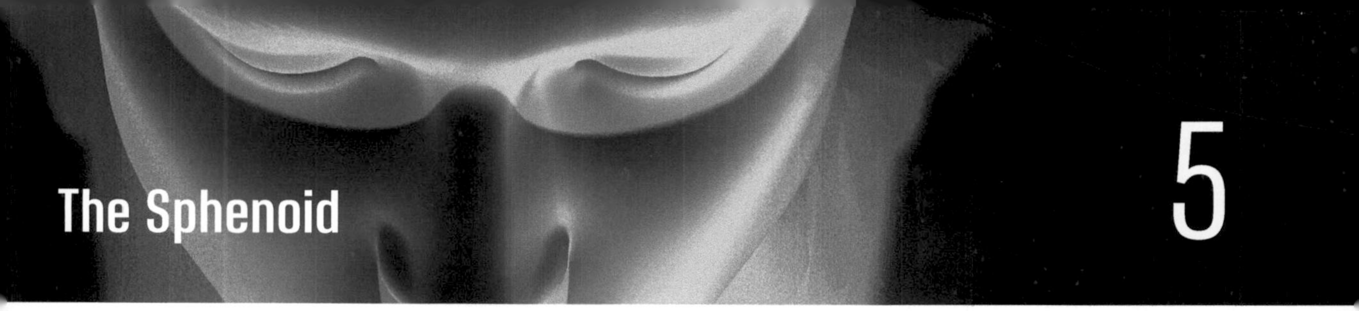

5 The Sphenoid

The unpaired sphenoid is the central bone of the cranial base. It is also described as being the supporting structure of the base of the skull.[4]

The posterior parts of the sphenoid adapt to the growth of the neurocranium, so that its periods of growth are largely complete by the age of 10. However, the anterior parts (greater wing and pterygoid process) also form part of the viscerocranium and adapt to the growth of this part of the skull. Therefore, further marked periods of growth are also found during adolescence, and postnatal growth in this area is greater overall than in the posterior region.

The sphenoid's many points of passage for nerves and blood vessels make it a means of transmission between the brain, orbits, oronasal space, face, and soft tissue regions of the neck.[6] According to Sutherland, many dysfunctions affecting the face are connected with the sphenoid.[1,10]

On account of its relations, the sphenoid is involved in many functional systems, e.g., sight, breathing, digestion, and endocrine functions. For example, there are myofascial connections with the masticatory system, visual apparatus, palate, and pharynx. There are also ligamentous connections to the mandible and irregular ones to the ear.

Neural connections exist between the sphenoid and functions of the pituitary, Broca's speech area, the taste center—the gustatory cortex, the third ventricle, the temporal lobe, and the hypothalamus. There is also a connection with the visual functions of cranial nerves II, III, IV, and VI, the sensitivity of the face, dural innervation (CN V_2, CN V_3), and with the innervation of the parotid glands (lesser petrosal nerve [CN IX]) and autonomic innervation of the oronasal space (pterygopalatine ganglion, internal carotid plexus, pterygoid canal). Vascular connections with the internal carotid artery, middle meningeal artery, ophthalmic artery, and venous drainage via the cavernous sinus are also important.

5.1 Morphology of the sphenoid according to Rohen[8]

The seven posterior vertebral processes, which in the vertebra reflect the three dimensions of space, find their counterpart in the processes of the body of the sphenoid: lateral to the body of the sphenoid are the greater wings, superiorly the lesser wings, inferiorly the pterygoid processes, and anteriorly the sphenoidal rostrum.

For Stone, the sphenoid is the positive pole of the coccyx.[9]

5.2 Location, causes, and clinical presentation of osteopathic dysfunctions of the sphenoid

5.2.1 Osseous dysfunctions

The orbits

The mobility of the orbits may be disturbed, and restriction of the fine mobility and position of the sphenoid may impair the muscles and nerves of the eye and the optic nerve.

Clinical presentation: visual disturbances.

Sutures

- **Sphenosquamous suture and sphenosquamous pivot point (SSP)**
  - Causes: primary trauma as a result of a fall or blow to the cheek or mastoid process of the temporal bone on the same side. Secondary lesions can result from dysfunctions of the sphenoid or viscerocranium or hypertonicity of the temporalis muscle (in psychological stress or temporomandibular syndrome).

- Clinical presentation:
  * At the vertical portion of the suture: middle meningeal artery → migraine.
  * At the horizontal portion of the suture: greater and lesser petrosal nerves. From the greater petrosal nerve to the pterygopalatine ganglion: disturbance of the lacrimal gland, dry or irritated mucosa of the nose, nasopharynx, and palate, allergic rhinitis (see also pterygopalatine fossa, section 3.1.2). Lesser petrosal nerve: disturbance of the parotid gland.
  * Functional disturbance of neighboring parts of the brain.
- Sequelae: dysfunction of the SBS and a change in the frequency and amplitude of the PRM rhythm, impairing homeostasis of the body as a whole.

- **Sphenopetrosal synchondrosis:** see also sphenopetrosal ligament in section 5.2.3 below. This lies in the region of the suture. Widens to form the foramen lacerum (Figure 4.2).
- **Sphenoparietal suture, sphenofrontal suture**
  - Clinical presentation/hypothetical pathology: the mobility of the SBS can be restricted by force to the sutures.
- **Sphenozygomatic suture**
  - Causes: a fall or blow to the cheek, or SBS dysfunctions.
  - Clinical presentation/hypothetical pathology:
    * The zygomatic bone is an important integration point for influences arriving from the occipital bone, sphenoid, and viscerocranium. Traumatic injuries can impair this important integrative function.
    * Maxillary sinusitis, disturbance of the orbits.
- **Sphenoethmoidal suture** Clinical presentation/hypothetical pathology: dysfunctions of the SBS, sphenoid, and ethmoid bones can disturb the transmission of motion from the spine of the sphenoid to the ethmoid bone, and the drainage of the nasal cavities.
- **Sphenovomerine suture, sphenopalatine suture** The tips of the pterygoid processes of the sphenoid move within grooves on the back of the small palatine bones. The pterygoid processes converge anteriorly and separate posteriorly, so that, in the inhalation phase, the sphenoid spreads the palatine bones apart and moves them into external rotation. According to Sutherland this slight pendulum motion between the tips of the pterygoid processes of the sphenoid and these grooves on the palatines is particularly important for the effective transmission of motion to the palatine and maxillary bones, and also for its function as a "speed reducer." This mechanism is frequently disturbed, for example in SBS dysfunctions or in traumatic injuries to the face.
  - Causes: extreme or sustained opening of the mouth or tooth extraction.
  - Clinical presentation/hypothetical pathology: disturbance of motion transmission to the maxillary complex, motion restriction of the maxillary complex, disturbance of the pterygopalatine ganglion or maxillary nerve, venous congestion of the pterygoid plexus.

Intraosseous dysfunctions

- **Between presphenoid and post-sphenoid**
  - The pre- and post-sphenoid fuse in about the eighth month in utero.
  - According to observations made by Sutherland, prenatal disturbances in the linking of pre- and post-sphenoid in the early stages of development of the cranial base could be expressed in the development of a slanted shape of the orbits, a characteristic typical of Down syndrome.[3]
- **Between the complex of the body of sphenoid and lesser wings, and the complexes of the greater wing and pterygoid process**
  - At birth, the sphenoid consists of three parts: in the middle, the body with its two lesser wings, to each side, the greater

wings with their respective pterygoid process. Ossification of the sphenoid bone is complete around the seventh month of life.
  - Disturbances between the complex of the body and lesser wings and that of the greater wings and pterygoid processes can lead to disturbances in the development of the orbits, and visual disturbances (CN II, CN III, CN IV, CN VI). The function of CN V_1 can also be affected, as can that of the adjacent cavernous sinus.
- Causes: primary trauma as a result of direct force to the sphenoid during birth or traumatic injury in infancy; secondary lesion caused by dysfunction of the sacrum.
- Sequelae: reduced pliancy of the bone, SBS dysfunction, development of scolioses, disturbances of the foramen lacerum and jugular foramen, and impairment of the function of all structures involved.

5.2.2 Muscular dysfunctions

- **Masticatory muscles**
  - The muscles to mention here are the temporalis, lateral pterygoid, and medial pterygoid.
  - Clinical presentation/hypothetical pathology: dental malocclusion; grinding of teeth, temporomandibular joint pain, headache, pain in the upper jaw, central region of the face, floor of the mouth, or ear.
- **Muscles of the eye**
  - Superior rectus, inferior rectus, medial rectus, lateral rectus, and superior oblique.
  - Dysfunction of the sphenoid, of the rest of the orbits, or of innervation produces changes in tension of these muscles resulting in visual disturbances.
- **Tensor veli palatini** Affects the auditory tube and soft palate.
- **Palatopharyngeus** (longitudinal muscle of pharynx) **and superior pharyngeal constrictor** (constrictor muscle of pharynx) Clinical presentation/hypothetical pathology: disturbances in swallowing.

5.2.3 Ligamentous dysfunctions

- **Petrosphenoidal ligament** (Gruber's ligament) at the petrosphenoidal suture (fissure)
  - Causes: dysfunction of the petrous part of the temporal bone, tooth extractions, and ossification of the ligament.
  - Clinical presentation/hypothetical pathology: abducent nerve (CN VI) symptoms, eye disturbances, squinting when tired in small children, etc.

FURTHER INFORMATION Magoun states that tooth extraction from the upper jaw can lead to ipsilateral dysfunction of the petrosphenoidal ligament. Tooth extraction from the lower jaw can lead to dysfunction of the ligament on the opposite side. Cranial nerves III, IV, and VI (supplying the eye muscles) run along the side of the body of the sphenoid, close to this ligament. CN VI in particular is vulnerable to tensions from the tentorium and from the ligament, because of the fibrous link between this and the petrosphenoidal ligament, and because it runs in an osteofibrous canal formed by the ligament and the temporal bone.

- **Sphenomandibular ligament** Excessive strain of the sphenomandibular ligament can occur unilaterally as a result of dental surgery.[7:296]

5.2.4 Fascial dysfunctions

- **Interpterygoid aponeurosis** At the spine of the sphenoid and anterior border of the foramen ovale and foramen spinosum.
- **Pterygo-temporo-mandibular aponeurosis** From the lateral pterygoid plate to the foramen ovale.
- **Palatine aponeurosis** At the medial pterygoid plate.
- **Orbital fascia** The fascial structures of the orbit.

- **Investing layer of cervical fascia** Over the muscular and ligamentous attachment to the styloid process.
- **Visceral compartment and pharynx** At the medial pterygoid plate and foramen lacerum.
  - Causes: dysfunctions may be caused by hypertonous muscular tension, dysfunctions of the locomotor system and internal organs (e.g., esophagus, stomach, lung).
  - Sequelae: motion restrictions of the SBS, dysfunctions of involved structures.

5.2.5 Dysfunction of intracranial and extracranial dural membranes

See section 6.3.1.

5.2.6 Disturbances to nerves, parts of the brain, and CSF spaces

See also sections 6.3.2 and 6.3.3.

- **Greater and lesser petrosal nerves:** in each case, in the groove for the nerve of that name
  - Causes: abnormal dural tension in groove; the greater petrosal nerve runs along its groove to the foramen lacerum, an opening in the sphenopetrosal synchondrosis. Vertical strain in particular can impair this nerve (a parasympathetic branch of the intermediate nerve).
  - Clinical presentation/hypothetical pathology:
    - Greater petrosal nerve: dysfunction of the lacrimatory and nasal glands and of the palate.
    - Lesser petrosal nerve: dysfunction of the parotid gland.
- **Cingulate gyrus** Clinical presentation/hypothetical pathology: depression, disturbances of concentration, etc.

5.2.7 Vascular disturbances

- **Internal carotid artery**
  - Causes: abnormal dural tension in the carotid canal, foramen lacerum, and cavernous sinus, and alteration in the position of the sphenoid (especially in torsion and sidebending dysfunctions of the SBS).
  - Clinical presentation/hypothetical pathology: disturbance of the sympathetic nervous system brought about by impingement of the internal carotid plexus, disturbance of the voluntary control of the muscular system (the frontal lobe center that controls this is supplied by the middle cerebral artery, a terminal branch of the internal carotid artery).
- **Middle meningeal artery**
  - Causes: compression of the sphenosquamous suture and the sphenosquamous pivot point (SSP), abnormal tension of the dura mater in the middle cranial fossa.
  - Clinical presentation/hypothetical pathology: migraine and raised intracranial pressure.

5.2.8 Endocrine disturbances

Hormonal control is centered in the pituitary, which is located in the sella turcica of the sphenoid. Any alteration in the fine mobility of the sphenoid, abnormal dural tension of the diaphragma sellae, and tensions in the lateral walls of the cavernous sinus impair the function of the pituitary.

NOTE The opening in the diaphragma sellae is thought to enlarge during the inhalation phase of PRM for the stalk of the pituitary, and to become smaller again during the exhalation phase.

5.3 Diagnosis of the sphenoid

5.3.1 History-taking

See clinical presentation (section 5.2).

5.3.2 Inspection

See dysfunctions of the SBS (section 6.3) and reference 5.

5.3.3 Palpation of position

- Greater wing: lowered (ER) or raised (IR).
- Temporal fossa: shallow (ER) or deep (IR).

Sutherland's cranial vault hold

This hold (Figure 5.1) is often used for the diagnosis and treatment of the sphenoid and SBS.

Patient: Supine.

Practitioner: Take up a position at the head of the patient.

Hand position:

- Place your hands on each side of the patient's head.
- Position your index fingers at the level of the greater wings, behind the lateral corners of the eyes.
- Position your middle fingers on the temporal bones, in front of the ears.
- Position your ring fingers on the temporal bones, behind the ears.
- Position your little fingers on each side of the occiput.
- Place your thumbs on top of the patient's head, if possible in contact with each other to act as a "fulcrum" or fixed point.

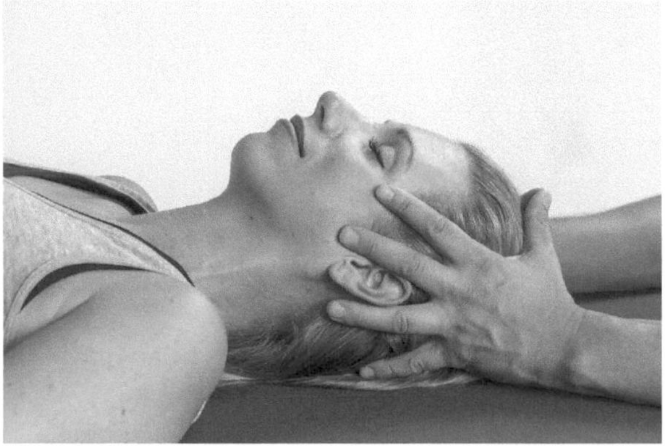

Figure 5.1 Cranial vault hold

5.3.4 Palpation of the PRM rhythm

Tip for practitioners

Biomechanical approach, inhalation phase

- The sphenoid moves about a transverse axis in front of the sella turcica, running through the two SSPs.
- The posterior part of the body of the sphenoid rises and the anterior part dips down.
- The sella turcica shifts in a superior and anterior direction.
- The pterygoid processes move posteriorly and outward.
- The greater wings perform an external rotation, and move outward, forward, and downward.
- The lesser wings glide anteriorly, downward, and outward.
- The zygomatic border moves in an anterior, inferior, and lateral direction.

Developmental dynamic, inhalation phase

- The sphenoid moves anteriorly, the posterior part rises and the anterior part dips down.
- The greater wings move laterally.

If palpation detects a motion restriction, the practitioner can deliver an impulse in the restricted direction of motion. This makes the restriction more evident, and enables you better to sense which structure is the origin of the motion restriction.

Biomechanical approach: inhalation phase of PRM, normal finding (Figure 5.2)

- The greater wings move outward, anterior, and inferior.

Exhalation phase of PRM, normal finding

- The greater wings move inward, posterior, and superior.

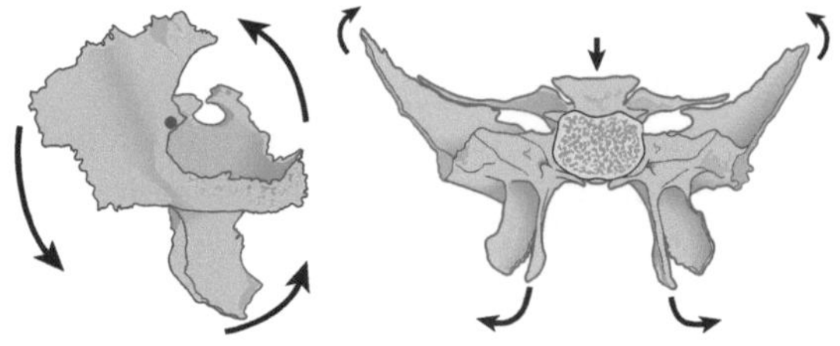

Figure 5.2
Inhalation phase of PRM, biomechanical

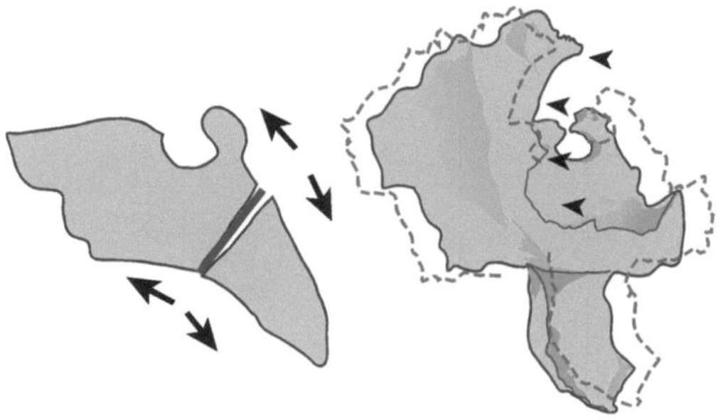

Figure 5.3
Inhalation phase of PRM, developmental dynamic

Developmental dynamic approach: inhalation phase of PR, normal finding (Figure 5.3)

- The sphenoid moves anteriorly, the posterior part rises and the anterior part dips down.
- The greater wings move laterally.

Exhalation phase of PRM, normal finding

- The sphenoid moves posteriorly, the posterior part dips down and the anterior part rises.
- The greater wings move medially. Compare the amplitude, strength, ease, and symmetry of the motions of the sphenoid.

5.3.5 Motion testing

Hand position: Cranial vault hold (section 5.3.3).

Method: Compare the amplitude and ease of the motions of the sphenoid, or the strength needed to induce motion.

5.4 Treatment of the sphenoid

5.4.1 Intraosseous dysfunctions

Indication Molding: in cases of functional impairment due to disturbances of prenatal development of the sphenoid, birth trauma or traumatic injury during infancy, or secondary to dysfunctions of the sacrum, such as: reduced pliability of the bone, SBS dysfunctions, scolioses, disturbances of the foramen lacerum, and of the jugular foramen.

Technique to release tensions between the pre- and post-sphenoid

NOTE This technique is particularly indicated in newborns and small children.

Patient: Supine.

Practitioner: Take up a position at the head of the patient.

Hand position: Cranial vault hold (Figure 5.4).

Method:

- Begin by sensing the tissue tension between the pre- and post-sphenoid.

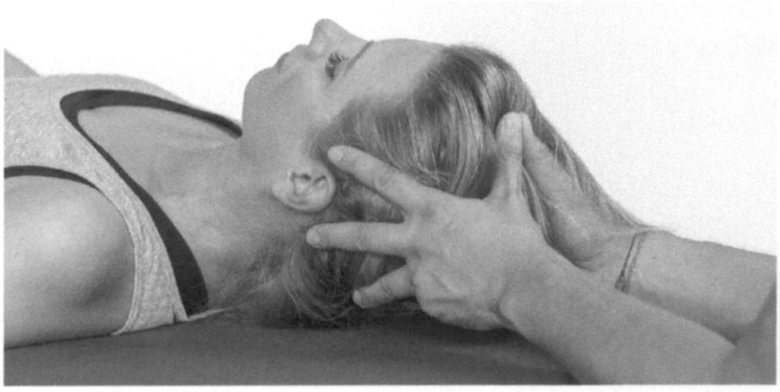

Figure 5.4 Technique to release tensions between the pre- and post-sphenoid

- Move both parts of the bone in the direction of their motion restriction.
- Establish the PBMT and PBFT between the pre- and post-sphenoid.
- Maintain this position until you sense a release of tension between the pre- and post-sphenoid.

Cant hook technique for disengagement of the complex of the body of sphenoid and lesser wings from the complex of the greater wings and pterygoid process, right

NOTE Before carrying out this technique, the sphenofrontal suture must be free to move.

Patient: Supine.

Practitioner: Take up a position beside the patient's head, on the side opposite the dysfunction.

Hand position:

- Place the little finger of your left hand intraorally, positioning it on the side of the right pterygoid process. To locate this position, pass your little finger back along the side of the alveolar part of the maxilla as far as you can, until the front of your finger pad rests on the pterygoid process.
- Place the index finger of your left hand laterally on the greater wing.

Freeing the sphenofrontal suture

Method:

- Right hand: grasp the two sides of the frontal bone by its lateral surface (zygomatic process) with your thumb and index finger.
- If possible, the end of your left thumb (the distal phalanx) should rest on the left greater wing.
- With your left hand, hold the sphenoid firmly in position (Figure 5.5).
- Keep your right thumb immobile, and also your left thumb which is resting on the side opposite the dysfunction. Your right thumb is acting as the pivot around which the movement is organized.
- During the inhalation phase, begin to apply traction to the frontal bone in a superior and very slightly anterior direction with your middle finger (disengagement of the frontal bone from the greater wing).
- Without reducing the gentle disengagement, permit all motions and unwinding of the frontal bone.
- At each release of the tissues, seek the next limit of motion of the frontal bone in the superior direction on the side of the dysfunction.
- Allow yourself to be guided by the fluctuations of the PRM until you achieve the PBMT between the frontal bone and the greater wing. The PBMT is the position in which the dural membrane tension between the frontal bone and the greater wing is as balanced as possible.
- Maintain the PBMT until a correction of the abnormal membranous tension has been achieved and the inherent homeostatic forces (PRM rhythm, etc.) have brought the correction into effect.
- When this has happened, begin again during the inhalation phase to apply traction in an anterior direction to the frontal bone, with your middle finger (disengagement of the frontal bone from the lesser wing).
- Continue according to the method for the greater wing (see below).

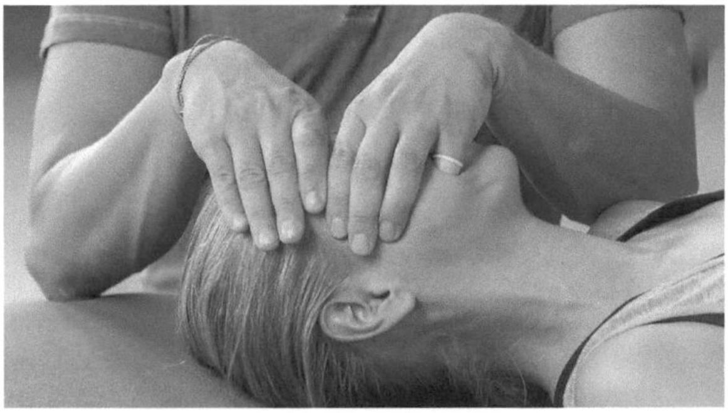

Figure 5.5 Freeing the sphenofrontal suture

To disengage the complex of the body of the sphenoid and lesser wings from the complex of the greater wings and pterygoid process

Method:

- Now place the fingers of your right hand on the right superior orbital margin of the frontal bone, level with the lesser wing.
- Release your left thumb from the left greater wing.
- Use your right hand to sense the motion of the lesser wing (Figure 5.6).
- At the same time, use your left hand (which is in contact with the greater wing and pterygoid process) to sense the motion of the greater wing–pterygoid process complex.
- If you sense dysfunctional tensions, guide the two parts of the bone in the direction of motion restriction (direct technique).
- Permit minute unwinding motions of the tissue, but do not relax the gentle pressure in the direction of the restriction.
- Establish the PBMT between the complex of the body of the sphenoid and lesser wings, and the complex of the greater wings and pterygoid process.
- Maintain this position until you sense a release between the two parts of the bone.

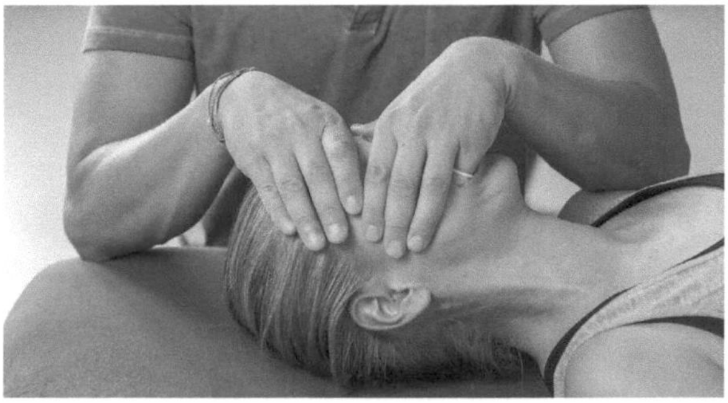

Figure 5.6 Release of the complex of the body of the sphenoid and lesser wings from the complex of the greater wings and pterygoid process

5.4.2 Fluid/electrodynamic techniques

Tip for practitioners

The CV-3 is the method of choice for:

- Restrictions in the third ventricle.
- Asymmetries in the rhythmic rolling and unrolling of the cerebral hemispheres.
- Dysfunctions of the hypothalamus, pituitary, and epiphysis.
- Dysfunction of the lamina terminalis.

Compression of the third ventricle (CV-3)

Indication and effect: Similar to those for the CV-4 (section 4.4.3).

Practitioner: Take up a position at the head of the patient.

Hand position:

- Place your index and/or middle finger on the greater wings.
- Your thumbs should rest on the coronal suture (Figure 5.7).

Method:

- Begin by sensing and differentiating the movement or restriction at the base (the hypothalamus and pituitary stalk), the top (epiphysis), and the anterior borders of the third ventricle.
- During the exhalation phase, go with the greater wings in a superior, posterior, and medial direction.
- During the inhalation phase, resist external rotation of the greater wings by means of gentle pressure in a superoposterior direction and bilaterally in the medial direction.
- In the next exhalation phase, follow the greater wings further into internal rotation with your hands.
- Focus your attention constantly on the intracranial fluid in the third ventricle at the level of the

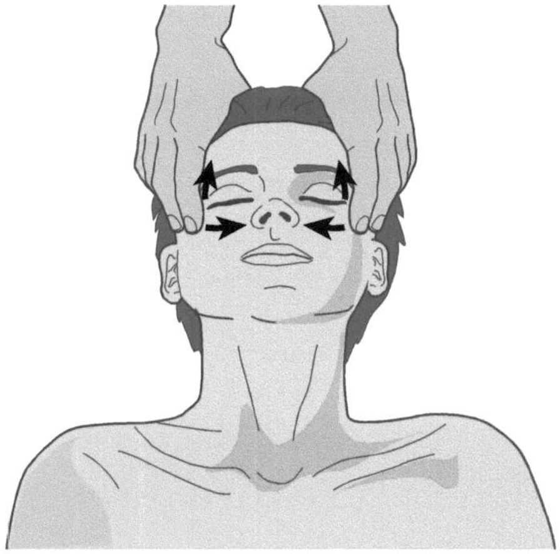

Figure 5.7 Compression of the third ventricle (CV-3)

restriction and on the lamina terminalis, which represents the anterior boundary of the third ventricle; it is a fulcrum point for the central nervous system (CNS), or for the rhythmic rolling and unrolling of the cerebral hemispheres.
- After a few cycles, the pressure against your fingers in the inhalation phase reduces. The flexion/extension motion has come to a standstill: the still point has been reached.
- When the tensions have subsided and you sense a strong, even pressure in the direction of external rotation, follow this impulse.
- Evaluate the qualities of the craniosacral rhythm and the motion of the cerebral hemispheres; having done so you can decide whether you should induce another still point.

Vitalist approach: See EV-4 technique (section 4.3.3).

5.4.3 Dural techniques

Modified anterior dural girdle technique according to Jim Jealous

Part of the anterior dural girdle (a term derived from embryology) forms a dural fold along the posterior margin of the lesser wing, running to the parietal bone, posterior to the coronal suture (Figures 5.7 and 5.8).

Indication: Dysfunction of the temporomandibular joint (TMJ), migraine, abnormal dural tension.

Palpation of the cranial dural sac and the anterior dural fold

Practitioner: Take up a position at the head of the patient.

Hand position: Sutherland's cranial vault hold, with the difference that your thumbs are placed on the patient's head, aligned along the anterior dural girdle, directly behind the coronal suture (Figure 5.8).

Method:
- Begin by sensing the entire dural sac and dural folds: sense the tension and PRM rhythm.
- Then sense the PRM rhythm of the anterior dural girdle.
- Compare the tension, the amplitude, strength, ease, and symmetry of motion of the anterior dural girdle.

Jealous states that the practitioner should sense the reaction of the anterior dural girdle to the "Breath of Life" and wait for the appearance of a lateral fluctuation.

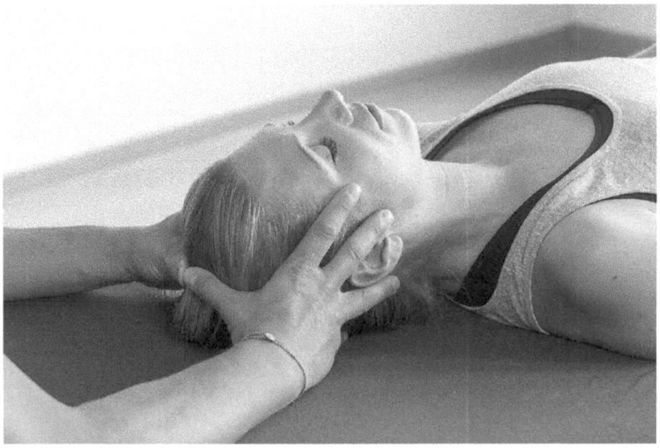

Figure 5.8 Palpation of the cranial dural sac and the anterior dural fold

Anterior girdle and tentorium

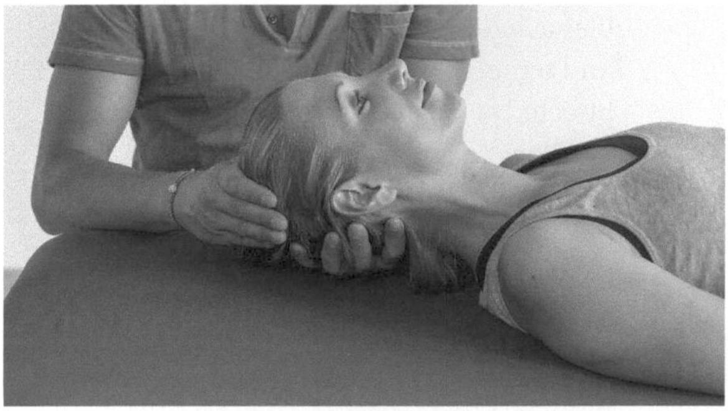

Figure 5.9 Anterior dural girdle and tentorium

Practitioner: Take up a position beside the head of the patient.

Hand position:

Superior transverse attachment of the tentorium

- Hold the occiput with one hand so that the superior transverse attachment of the tentorium (approximately along the course of the superior nuchal line) lies in the palm of your hand.
- Place your other hand immediately behind the coronal suture, holding the anterior dural girdle. Place your thumb on one side and the other fingers on the other, in the hollow often found posterior to the coronal suture.

Inferior transverse attachment of the tentorium

- The hand position is the same except that the palm of the hand on the occiput now lies on the inferior transverse attachment of the tentorium (slightly lower than the superior attachment).

Method: Establish the PBMT and PBFT (Figure 5.9).

5.4.4 Sutural dysfunctions

- Sphenosquamous suture: see temporal bone, section 9.4.8.
- Sphenopetrosal synchondrosis (petrosphenoidal fissure/suture): see temporal bone, section 9.4.8.
- Sphenoparietal suture: see parietal bone, section 11.4.6.
- Sphenofrontal suture: see frontal bone, section 10.4.5.
- Sphenozygomatic suture: see zygomatic bone, section 14.4.3.
- Sphenoethmoidal suture: see ethmoid bone, section 7.2.1.
- Sphenovomerine suture: see vomer, section 8.2.5.
- Sphenopalatine suture: see palatine bone, section 13.3.2.

5.5 References

1 Eser-Bindl, U. (2002) 'Os sphenoidale und os ethmoidale—Entwicklung, Verknöcherung und Frage nach der Möglichkeit einer Mobilität.' Master's thesis. Munich: COE.

2 Hack, G. D., Koritzer, R. T., Robinson, W. L. et al. (1995) 'Anatomic relation between the rectus capitis posterior minor muscle and the dura mater.' *Spine. 20*, 2484–2486.

3 Kasack, A. (1998) 'Die osteopathische Behandlung für Kinder mit Down-Syndrom mit Schwerpunkt auf dem Os occipitale.' Master's thesis. Bonn.

4 Kuta, A. J. and Laine, F. J. (1993) 'Imaging the sphenoid bone and basiocciput: anatomic considerations.' *Semin. Ultrasound. CT MRI. 14*, 3, 146–159.

5 Liem, T. (2018) *Kraniosakrale Osteopathie. Ein praktisches Lehrbuch*, 7th Ed. Stuttgart: Thieme.

6 Lustrin, E. S., Robertson, R. L. and Tilak, S. (1993) 'Normal anatomy of the skull base.' *Neuroimag. Clin. North. Am. 4*, 3, 465–478.

7 Magoun, H. I. (1976) *Osteopathy in the Cranial Field*, 3rd Ed. Kirksville: Journal Printing Company.

8 Rohen, J. W. (2002) *Morphologie des menschlichen Organismus*, 2nd Ed. Stuttgart: Verlag Freies Geistesleben, pp. 362–365.

9 Stone, R. (1994) *Polaritätstherapie*, 2nd Ed. Hugendubel, p. 204.

10 Sutherland, W. G. (1944) 'The cranial bowl.' *J. Am. Osteopath. Assoc. 1944*, 348–353.

6.1 Rohen's concept of the metamorphosis of vertebrae into the cranial base 290

6.2 Significance of the SBS 290

6.3 Location, causes, and clinical presentation of osteopathic dysfunctions of the SBS 291
6.3.1 Dysfunctions of intracranial and extracranial dural membranes 293
6.3.2 Disturbances to nerves and parts of the brain 294
6.3.3 Disturbances in CSF spaces 296
6.3.4 Vascular disturbances 296

6.4 Diagnosis and treatment of the SBS 296
6.4.1 Flexion and extension 297
6.4.2 Right and left torsion 297
6.4.3 Right and left lateroflexion-rotation 298
6.4.4 Superior and inferior vertical strain 299
6.4.5 Right and left lateral strain 299
6.4.6 Compression of the SBS 300

6.5 References 301

6 The Spheno-Occipital Synchondrosis/Synostosis (Sphenobasilar Synchondrosis) (SBS)

The cranial base, with the spheno-occipital synchondrosis (SBS) that lies within it, represents a kind of fulcrum in the development of the skull. Its rate of growth, together with that of the brainstem, is comparatively slow; the enlargement of the frontal and temporal lobes of the cerebrum and the cerebellum, on the other hand, leads to strong growth of the anterior, middle, and posterior cranial fossa.

In childhood, the SBS has an importance as a mobile fulcrum. Beyond the 13th to 17th years of life, the SBS is ossified and possesses only a certain intraosseous elasticity. This could indicate a function as a "punctum fixum," a fixed point. The role of the SBS in relation to osteopathic dysfunctions and disorders is unclear, owing to the inadequate quality of the available study results.

Primary dysfunctions in the region of the SBS are assumed to originate probably in the prenatal, perinatal, or postnatal period or early childhood: birth trauma, falls onto the head or sacrum, head injury, severe dural tension, restrictions of a number of cranial bones, etc. It is also possible for tensions at the cranial base to emerge secondary to musculoskeletal issues (such as hypertonic tensions of the nuchal muscles) and visceral dysfunctions. The extent to which dysfunctions at the cranial base and SBS affect the other cranial bones, cranial mobility, and the craniosacral system, and possible consequences affecting connected structures (such as nerves and regions of the brain, intra- and extracranial dural membranes, vessels, and the endocrine system), is purely speculative.

6.1 Rohen's concept of the metamorphosis of vertebrae into the cranial base

The evolutionary developments associated with upright gait mean that the cranial base lies at a different angle in humans compared to mammals in general, and the viscerocranium therefore lies more beneath the roof of the skull.[20]

The idea that the bones of the cranium were metamorphosed vertebrae dates back to an insight by the German poet and polymath Goethe in 1790; an idea later taken up by the researcher and philosopher Oken.

An account of individual elements such as that given by Mees[19] does not greatly assist the understanding of the structures. The functional dynamics of the tissue are more important.

6.2 Significance of the SBS

A review examining histological and radiological studies on the ossification of the SBS was published by Schalkhaußer in 2010.[12,17] According to this study, the SBS begins to ossify from around the sixth (13th or 16th) year of life.[6,14,16,17] Ossification is complete between the 13th and 17th years of life.[14,16,17]

This finding was also in essence confirmed by a study by Bassed et al.,[1] in which 666 individuals aged between 15 and 25 underwent a routine full body CT scan. The authors showed that fusion begins as early as the age of 15 and is complete by the 17th year of life. Fusion starts superiorly and progresses in an inferior direction. Scar formation could be demonstrated on the side of the fusion until the 25th year of life.[1]

Regarding the mobility of the spheno-occipital joint, the state of research is not clear. Osteopathic studies have been carried out on this subject, but using very different study designs. Many of these studies are of an early date, which partly explains why few standards were observed. The reporting of these studies was also inadequate.[11]

It is unlikely that the ossified SBS in adults evidences any articular movement or mobility, a situation that Magoun had indeed assumed to be so.[15] However, there are many indications that there is mobility in the sutures of the roof of the skull.[12]

The main decisive factors in the stability of the SBS region are its thickness (one of the strongest regions of the skull) and the thin surrounding layer of cortical bone (compacta). From adolescence onward the cranial base should no longer be seen as a beam of bony, compact structure, but rather as a more or less continuously pneumatized region that can extend from the ethmoid to the basilar part of the occipital bone.[4]

According to Latkowski, the multi-walled structure of the paranasal sinuses, the elastic qualities of the bony paranasal sinus system, and their air content give them an energy-absorbing, force-absorbing, or dampening function against the effect of traumatic force,[8] dissipating the incoming force. Although purely angular movements in the sense of flexion/extension of the SBS seem unlikely, Eser-Bindl believes that mobility, in the sense of the elasticity and pliability of a global cranial base that is more or less strongly pneumatized, can be considered.[4]

It remains unclear how far and to what extent trabecular structures in the SBS region confer elasticity in this region. But even if this region does turn out to have a certain intraosseous elasticity in adulthood, it seems more likely that the cranial base, as a central location in the midline of the cranium and attachment for numerous fascial structures, must have a significance in later years as a stable fulcrum/fixed point, in no way comparable with the mobility of the synchondrosis in childhood.

Cook[3] assumes that it is, rather, the region between the body and greater wing of the sphenoid that is examined in an investigation of the cranial base. To him, it is this that seems to be mobile, because of the sphenoidal sinus and orbital fissures. However, this appears to be just as speculative as other assumptions previously mentioned.

What role does the SBS then play in adults, in osteopathic palpation? In all events, the SBS of an adult will display more resistance in its reaction to rhythmic phenomena than the SBS of a four-year-old. This chronological element should therefore be taken into account in palpation.

A further question relates to what it is that we sense when we try to palpate the region of the SBS. Although this matter does not form part of the present chapter, we can point to certain parameters here, such as resonance, instability, and sensitivity and other subjective means of approach.[9] Para-ideological influences are another possibility (see, for example, reference 10 on this subject). Most studies of the palpation of cranial patterns in the SBS region show a high risk of bias, which means that study results are generally open to question.[11]

Until studies of high methodological quality and reliable results are performed, it will not be possible to make any definitive statements of general relevance about palpation and the role of the SBS, for example regarding dysfunctions and disorders. It is also unclear how far radiological or other technical or imaging methods correlate with palpation findings. Here, too, the quality of the studies available so far tends to be low, which reduces their reliability.

Another question that needs to be discussed is whether the traditional descriptions of the SBS are still adequate, or whether the understanding of them needs to be rendered in more appropriate models.[12]

6.3 Location, causes, and clinical presentation of osteopathic dysfunctions of the SBS

Table 6.1 is based on the experience of osteopaths and accounts they have provided. The extent of their clinical relevance is as yet unclear.

Table 6.1 Dysfunctions of the SBS[12]

Dysfunction	Axes	Causes	Clinical presentation	Severity
Flexion	2 transverse axes	• Compensatory, e.g., visceral disturbance • Rarely traumatic (birth: pressure from the mother's pubic bone on the occiput) • Adrenal or thyroid hyperactivity; hydrocephalus	• Headache • Endocrine disturbances • Far-sightedness • Sinusitis, rhinitis • Masked allergy • Weakness in lumbar spine and sacrum • Extroversion	1
Extension	2 transverse axes	• Compensatory, e.g., visceral disturbance • Rarely, prenatal or perinatal trauma • Pituitary disturbance • Microencephaly	• Severe migraine • Asthma and sinusitis • Near-sightedness • Moodiness • Loner behavior	1–2
Torsion	1 longitudinal axis	• Compensatory in disturbances of the myofascial-skeletal system, viscera, etc. • Rarely primary trauma	• Severe migraine • Pain syndrome • Scoliosis • Endocrine disturbance • Visual disturbances • Sinusitis, allergy • Dyslexia • Sense of inner conflict • Disturbances of balance	2
Lateral flexion-rotation	2 vertical, 1 longitudinal axis	• Compensatory in disturbances of the myofascial-skeletal system, viscera, etc. • Rarely primary trauma	Also: • Dental malocclusion and TMJ syndrome • Hypermobility of the upper cervical spine • Mild psychological disturbances	2–3

Continued

Table 6.1 Dysfunctions of the SBS[12] *Continued*

Dysfunction	Axes	Causes	Clinical presentation	Severity
Vertical strain	2 transverse axes	• Primary trauma • Superior vertical strain: force from above onto the basilar part, or from behind onto the occiput • Inferior vertical strain: force from above onto the base of the sphenoid or from in front onto the frontal bone • Fall onto the pelvis or heels • Visceral disturbances	• Endocrine disturbances • Dental malocclusion • TMJ syndrome • Visual disturbances • Headache and migraine • Depression • Schizoid states • Inferior vertical strain: sinusitis, allergy • Superior vertical strain: disturbances of hearing	3
Lateral strain	2 vertical axes	• Primary trauma • Lateral force onto the greater wing or occiput, unilateral force from anterior onto the frontal bone or from behind onto the occiput • Prenatal or perinatal • Membranous • Trauma to the temporal bone or occiput • Orthodontic / orthopedic procedures to the jaw	• Visual disturbances • Severe migraine and headache • Endocrine disturbances • Disturbances of balance • Learning disturbances • Severe psychological disturbances	4
Compression		• Compression of: L5–S1, atlanto-occipital joint • Membranous, sutural • Prenatal or perinatal • Emotional stress	Also: • Severe metabolic disturbance • Neuropsychiatric problems • Disturbances; depression • Suicidal tendency, autism, etc.	5

6.3.1 Dysfunctions of intracranial and extracranial dural membranes

Falx cerebri, tentorium cerebelli, falx cerebelli, spinal dura mater

- Causes
  - A torsion dysfunction may lead to a kind of twisting distortion of the falx cerebri on account of its attachments to the frontal bone anteriorly and the occipital bone posteriorly. Anteriorly, the falx is shifted away from the raised greater wing, and posteriorly it moves closer to the side of this greater wing, that is, closer to the side of the lowered occiput. The tentorium cerebelli moves caudad on the side where

the occipt is lowered and cephalad on the opposite side. The spinal dura mater moves caudad on the side where the occiput is lowered.
  - A sidebending/rotation dysfunction causes the falx cerebri to incline toward the convex side, i.e., the side of the dysfunction. The tentorium also inclines toward the side of the convexity. The spinal dura mater moves caudad on the side where the occiput is lowered.
- Clinical presentation/hypothetical pathology: disturbance of venous drainage and drainage of the choroid plexus, and the cranial nerves where they run along and are sheathed in the dura.
- Radiating/referred pain: see Volume 2, section 5.1.3 and reference 12.

6.3.2 Disturbances to nerves and parts of the brain

All the cranial nerves are susceptible, with the following symptoms and sequelae:

Olfactory nerve (CN I)

- Causes: at the level of the lesser wing of the sphenoid; mainly due to dysfunction of the ethmoid bone.
- Clinical presentation: disturbance of sense of smell.

Optic nerve (CN II)

- Causes: abnormal dural tension in the optic canal or alteration in the position of the body of the sphenoid.
- Clinical presentation: disturbance of vision.

Motor nerves of the eye, e.g., oculomotor (CN III), trochlear (CN IV), abducent (CN VI) nerves

- Causes: abnormal tension in the petrosphenoidal ligament (especially CN VI), tentorium, or superior orbital fissure; often found in vertical strain.
- Clinical presentation
  - CN III, motor: lateral deviation of the eyeball, horizontal double vision, divergent strabismus, restriction of the line of sight upward, downward, and medially, ptosis of eyelid.
  - CN III, autonomic: mydriasis, impairment of pupillary reflex, failure of accommodation.
  - CN IV: upward and medial deviation of the eyeball, reduced downward, lateral movement, vertical or oblique double vision, convergent strabismus.
  - CN VI: horizontal double vision, convergent strabismus, medial deviation of the eyeball, restriction of the lateral line of sight, tendency to hold the head turned to one side to compensate for the deficiency.

Trigeminal nerve (CN V)

- Causes: abnormal dural tension of the tentorium cerebelli and the visceral (meningeal) dura of the trigeminal ganglion, alteration in the position of the temporal bone, tensions and stasis in the wall of the cavernous sinus (CN V_1, V_2), abnormal dural tension at the foramen rotundum (CN V_2) or foramen ovale (CN V_3). The foramen ovale lies close to the spine of the sphenoid, which according to Magoun[15:184] is the point of maximum motion of the sphenoid, making it susceptible to dysfunctions.
- Clinical presentation
  - Trigeminal neuralgia.
  - CN V_1: altered sensitivity and pain in the skin of the forehead and upper eyelid, the mucous membrane of the frontal sinus, and the connective tissue membrane, limitation of the corneal reflex, pain in the eye and lacrimation (the trigeminal nerve contains some parasympathetic fibers).
  - CN V_2: disturbances of sensation affecting the center of the face, restriction of the sneezing reflex.

- CN V_3: disturbances of sensation affecting the lower face, disturbance of masticatory muscle function.
- Trigeminal ganglion: all listed symptoms of the trigeminal branches.

Pterygopalatine ganglion

- Causes: force onto the face, or dysfunction of the TMJ with hypertonicity of the medial and lateral pterygoid muscles, can lead to disturbances of the joint between palatine and sphenoid and so potentially affect the pterygopalatine ganglion in the sphenopalatine foramen. The pterygopalatine ganglion can also be affected in SBS dysfunctions.
- Clinical presentation: secretory disturbances of the lacrimal gland and the mucous membranes of the nose and palate (this volume, section 3.2.3).

Facial nerve (CN VII) and intermediate nerve (CN VII)

Pass through the internal acoustic meatus in the facial canal; unite at geniculate ganglion; branching of sensory/special sense fibers in the chorda tympani; main part of nerve through the stylomastoid foramen.

- Causes: dural tensions of the internal acoustic meatus and stylomastoid foramen.
- Clinical presentation
  - Facial nerve (CN VII): disturbance of facial expression.
  - Intermediate nerve (CN VII): disturbance of saliva secretion; taste disturbances of the anterior two-thirds of the tongue, functional disturbance of the lacrimal gland, nasal and palatine glands (via greater petrosal nerve).

Vestibulocochlear nerve (CN VIII)

Through the internal acoustic meatus to the organ of hearing and balance.

- Causes: abnormal dural tension of the internal acoustic meatus, dysfunction of the petrojugular suture.
- Clinical presentation: disturbances of hearing and balance.

Glossopharyngeal nerve (CN IX), vagus nerve (CN X), accessory nerve (CN XI)

At the jugular notch, together with the intrajugular process.

- Causes: dural tensions at the jugular foramen, dysfunction of the occipital and temporal bones, occipitomastoid suture, petrojugular suture, or petro-occipital fissure (petrobasilar suture; petro-occipital synchondrosis).
- Clinical presentation
  - CN IX: disturbances of swallowing (fibers supplying sensation to the pharynx), taste disturbances, dry mouth (parasympathetic fibers serving parotid gland).
  - CN X: functional disturbances of the heart, digestion, pulmonary respiration, speaking, and swallowing.
  - CN XI: torticollis.

Hypoglossal nerve (CN XII)

- Causes: dural tensions of the hypoglossal canal.
- Clinical presentation: restriction of mobility of the tongue, disturbances in sucking.

Basal ganglia

- Causes: disturbance in supply and drainage of the basal ganglia; the basal ganglia are drained through the cavernous sinus and straight sinus, which are directly linked with the sphenoid, occiput, and tentorium.
- Clinical presentation: disturbances of movement and trembling.

Mesencephalon

- Causes: the mesencephalon has to pass through the opening in the tentorium above the SBS, as do all links between the spinal cord and cerebral cortex. Torsions and sidebending dysfunctions can cause disturbance of these structures.

Hypothalamus

- Causes: sidebending/rotation dysfunction of the SBS.
- Clinical presentation: disturbance of temperature regulation, water balance, endocrine system, and emotional disturbances.

Cortical regions

- Clinical presentation/hypothetical pathology: dysfunction of the greater wing of the sphenoid can cause impairment of the sense of taste, of smell, and of hearing. Dysfunction of the lesser wing can affect the speech cortex.

6.3.3 Disturbances in CSF spaces

Cerebral aqueduct and interventricular foramen

- Causes
  - The aqueduct is located between the third and fourth ventricles and can become twisted in the case of torsion, and kinked in that of sidebending of the SBS, resulting in hydrocephalus.
  - The intraventricular foramen between the lateral ventricle and third ventricle can be narrowed in dysfunctions of the SBS.

Fluctuation of CSF in the subarachnoid space

- Causes: particularly in the case of torsion or sidebending-rotation dysfunction of the SBS.

6.3.4 Vascular disturbances

Dural venous sinuses

Sigmoid sinus, superior and inferior petrosal sinus, transverse sinus, cavernous sinus, superior and inferior sagittal sinus, occipital sinus, confluence of sinuses.

- Causes
  - Compression.
  - Abnormal dural tension in the jugular foramen, foramen magnum, tentorium cerebelli, falx cerebri, and falx cerebelli.
  - Motion restriction of the sphenoid and occipital bone.
- Sequelae
  - Sigmoid sinus: congestion affecting the confluence of sinuses and superior petrosal sinus.
  - Superior and inferior petrosal sinuses: congestion affecting the cavernous sinus and basilar venous plexus, the ophthalmic veins, and the veins of the medulla, pons, inferior surface of the cerebellum, and other segments of the brain.
- Clinical presentation/hypothetical pathology
  - Region of the sigmoid sinus → pain behind the ear.
  - Region of the transverse sinus → pain in the temporal region or ipsilateral front of the head or the eye.
  - Confluence of sinuses → pain in the ipsilateral front of the head and in the eye.
  - Region of the superior petrosal sinus → pain in the temporal region.
  - Cavernous sinus → pain in the ipsilateral eye and maxillary region.
  - Region of the superior sagittal sinus and veins running to this area → pain in the frontoparietal region and region of the eye.
  - Venous stasis affecting particular segments of the brain → headache, impairment of relevant brain functions.
  - Venous stasis affecting the eyes → visual disturbances, sensation of pressure.

6.4 Diagnosis and treatment of the SBS

Examination of the SBS region is by passive listening techniques and active motion testing.

SBS dysfunctions may be treated individually, or can be treated simultaneously. When doing so, however, it is important to address the dysfunctions in order of severity. If, for example, palpation has revealed the following SBS dysfunctions— right torsion, left sidebending/rotation, superior vertical strain—the first step in the correction must be to establish the PBMT of the superior vertical strain, then the PBMT of the left sidebending/rotation, and finally the PBMT of the right torsion.

To carry out treatment, **Sutherland's cranial vault hold** should be adopted (section 5.3.3).

Particularly in children, the SBS is fundamentally important where there is delayed or dysfunctional development of orofacial structures. In such cases the SBS is actively mobilized several times.

6.4.1 Flexion and extension

Flexion

The amplitude of flexion motion is greater than that of extension.

Correction

- With your index fingers, guide the greater wings in an inferior and anterior direction (Figure 6.1).
- With your little fingers, guide the lower part of the occipital squama in an inferior and anterior direction.
- Breathing assistance by the patient: at the end of an in-breath, hold the inhalation for as long as possible, while dorsally flexing both feet. Repeat for several breathing cycles.

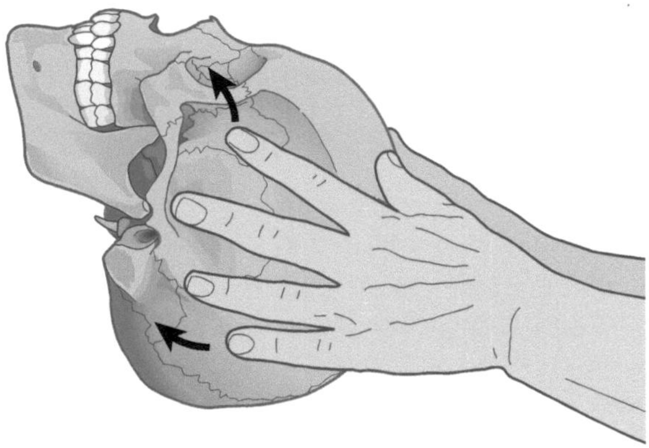

Figure 6.1
Flexion of the SBS

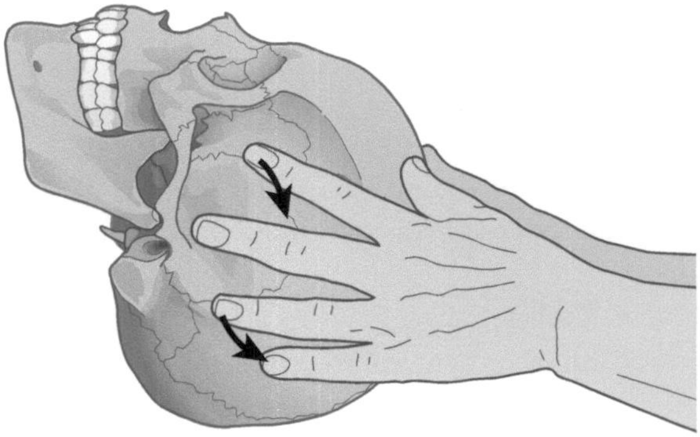

Figure 6.2
Extension of the SBS

Extension

The amplitude of extension motion is greater than that of flexion.

Correction

- With your index fingers, guide the greater wings of the sphenoid in a superior and posterior direction (Figure 6.2).
- With your little fingers, guide the lower part of the occipital squama in a superior and posterior direction.
- Breathing assistance by the patient: at the end of an out-breath, hold the exhalation for as long as possible, while performing plantar flexing of the feet. Repeat for several breathing cycles.

6.4.2 Right and left torsion

Right torsion

The amplitude of induced right torsion is greater than that of induced left torsion.

Correction

- With your right index finger, guide the right greater wing of the sphenoid cephalad (Figure 6.3).
- With your right little finger, guide the right side of the occiput caudad.

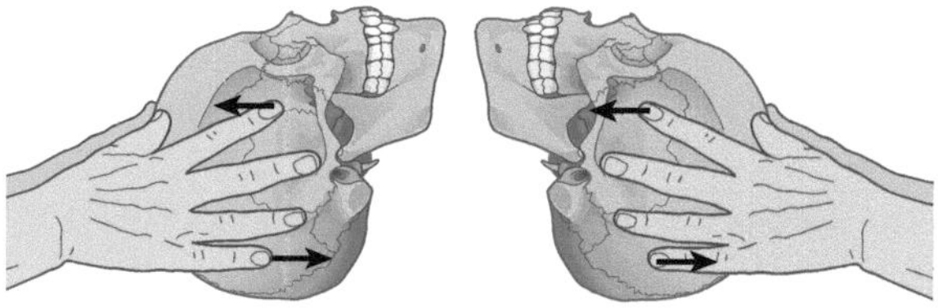

Figure 6.3
Right torsion of the SBS

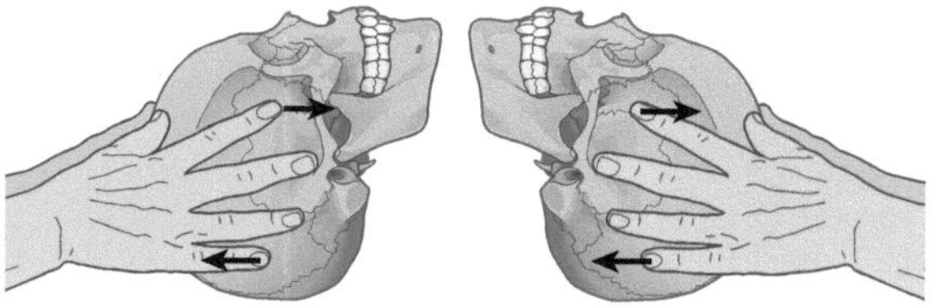

Figure 6.4
Left torsion of the SBS

- With your left index finger, guide the left greater wing caudad.
- With your left little finger, guide the left side of the occiput cephalad.

Left torsion

The amplitude of induced left torsion is greater than that of induced right torsion.

Correction

- With your left index finger, guide the left greater wing of the sphenoid cephalad (Figure 6.4).
- With your left little finger, guide the left side of the occipital bone caudad.
- With your right index finger, guide the right greater wing caudad.
- With your right little finger, guide the right side of the occipital bone cephalad.

6.4.3 Right and left lateroflexion-rotation

Right lateroflexion-rotation

The amplitude of induced right sidebending-rotation is greater than the amplitude of induced left sidebending-rotation.

Correction

- Right hand: move your index finger and little finger apart. Move your right hand caudad (Figure 6.5).
- Left hand: move your index finger and little finger closer together. Move your left hand cephalad.

Left lateroflexion-rotation

The amplitude of induced left sidebending-rotation is greater than the amplitude of induced right sidebending-rotation.

Correction

- Left hand: move your index finger and little finger apart. Move your left hand caudad (Figure 6.6).
- Right hand: move your index finger and little finger closer together. Move your right hand cephalad.

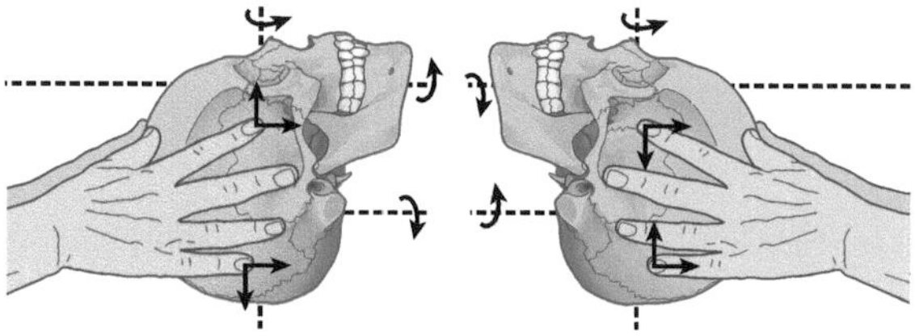

Figure 6.5
Right lateroflexion-rotation

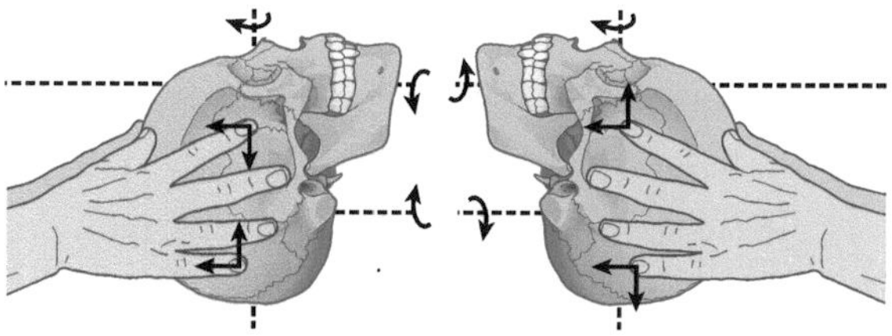

Figure 6.6
Left lateroflexion-rotation

6.4.4 Superior and inferior vertical strain

Superior vertical strain

The amplitude of induced superior vertical strain is greater than that of induced inferior vertical strain.

Correction

- With your index fingers, guide the greater wings in an inferior and anterior direction (flexion) (Figure 6.7).
- With your little fingers, guide the occipital squama in a superior and posterior direction (extension).
- Alternative technique: see dysfunction of the temporal bone in anterior rotation (section 9.4.5).

Inferior vertical strain

The amplitude of induced inferior vertical strain is greater than that of induced superior vertical strain.

Correction

- With your index fingers, guide the greater wings in a superior and posterior direction (extension) (Figure 6.8).
- With your little fingers, guide the occipital squama in an inferior and anterior direction (flexion).
- Alternative technique: see dysfunction of the temporal bone in posterior rotation (section 9.4.5).

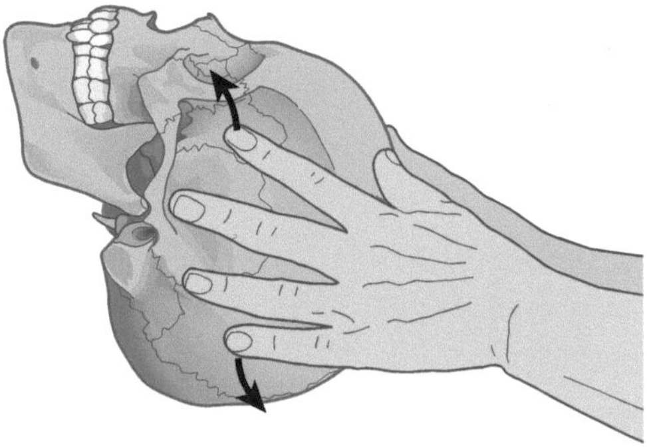

Figure 6.7
Superior vertical strain

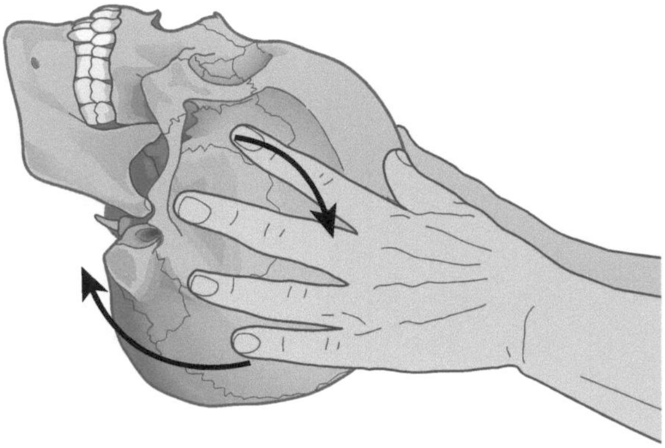

Figure 6.8
Inferior vertical strain

6.4.5 Right and left lateral strain

Right lateral strain

The amplitude of induced right lateral strain is greater than that of induced left lateral strain.

Correction

- With your right index finger, guide the right greater wing of the sphenoid in an anterior direction (Figures 6.9 and 6.10).
- With your right little finger, guide the right side of the occipital bone in an anterior direction.
- With your left index finger, guide the left greater wing in a posterior direction.
- With your left little finger, guide the left side of the occipital bone in a posterior direction.
- When treating the effect of extreme force without dysfunction axes: move your right and left index fingers to the right.[12]

Left lateral strain

The amplitude of induced left lateral strain is greater than that of induced right lateral strain.

Correction

- With your left index finger, guide the left greater wing of the sphenoid in an anterior direction (Figure 6.11).

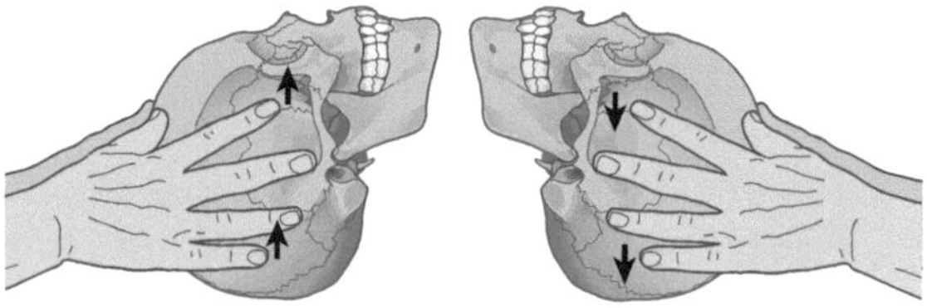

Figure 6.9
Right lateral strain

- With your left little finger, guide the left side of the occipital bone in an anterior direction.
- With your right index finger, guide the right greater wing in a posterior direction.
- With your right little finger, guide the right side of the occipital bone in a posterior direction.
- When treating the effect of extreme force without dysfunction axes: move your left and right index fingers to the left.

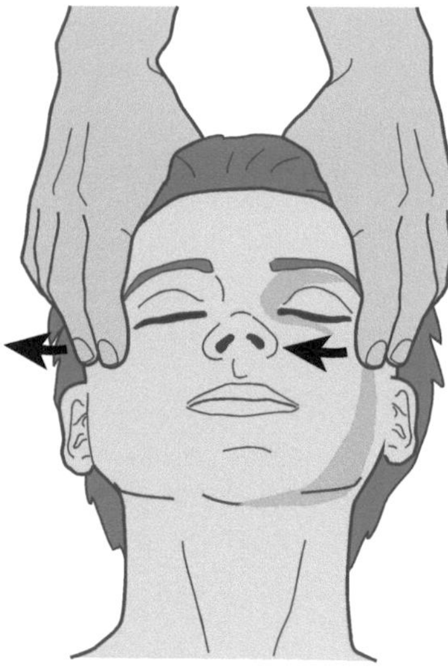

Figure 6.10
Right lateral strain [without axis of dysfunction]

6.4.6 Compression of the SBS

Compression/decompression of the SBS

The sphenoid moves posteriorly, but not anteriorly, i.e., there is no motion away from the occipital bone (Figures 6.12 and 6.13).

Correction

- Compression: begin by moving your index fingers in a posterior direction at the same time as your little fingers move anteriorly.
- Decompression: then move your index fingers anteriorly while at the same time moving your little fingers posteriorly.
- Maintain this traction until the membrane tension is resolved.

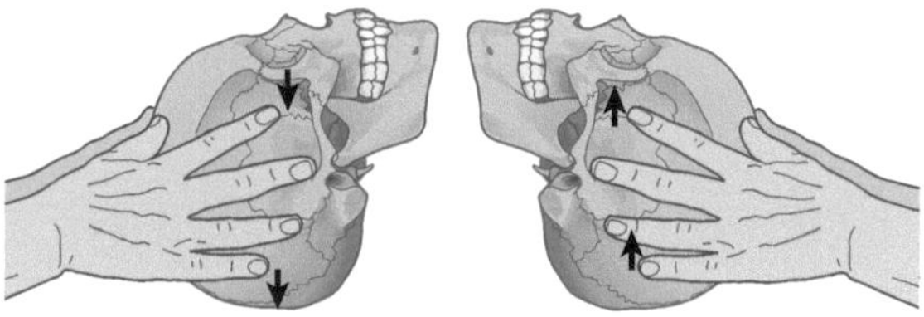

Figure 6.11
Left lateral strain

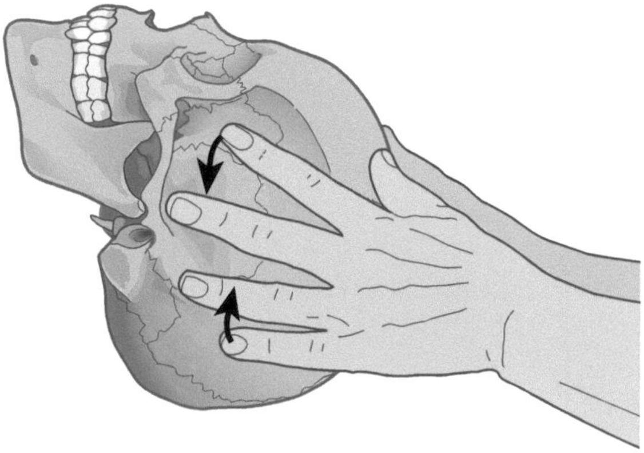

Figure 6.12
Compression of the SBS

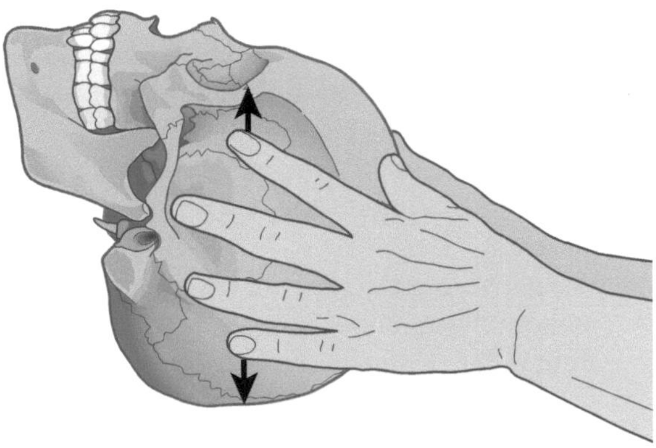

Figure 6.13
Decompression of the SBS

6.5 References

1 Bassed, R. B., Briggs, C. and Drummer, O. H. (2010) 'Analysis of time of closure of the spheno-occipital synchondrosis using computed tomography.' *Forensic Sci. Int. 200*, 161–164.

2 Bolet, P. (1993) *La compression du 4ème ventricule modifie-t-elle le profil ionique chez the patient?* St. Etienne: Mémoire.

3 Cook, A. (2005) 'The mechanics of cranial motion—the sphenobasilar synchondrosis (SBS) revisited.' *J. Bodyw. Mov. Ther. 9*, 177–188.

4 Eser-Bindl, U. (2002) 'Os sphenoidale und Os ethmoidale—Entwicklung, Verknöcherung und Frage nach der Möglichkeit einer Mobilität.' Master's thesis. Munich, COE.

5 Hack, G. D., Koritzer, R. T., Robinson, W. L. et al. (1995) 'Anatomic relation between the rectus capitis posterior minor muscle and the dura mater.' *Spine. 20*, 2484–2486.

6 Ingervall, B. and Thilander, B. (1972) 'The human sphenooccipital synchondrosis. The time of closure appraised macroscopically.' *Acat. Odond. Scand. 30*, 349–356.

7 Kasack, A. (1998) 'Die osteopathische Behandlung für Kinder mit Down-Syndrom mit Schwerpunkt auf dem Os occipitale.' Master's thesis. Bonn.

8 Latkowski, B. (1967) 'Die Rolle der Nasennebenhöhlen bei der Verteilung und Dämpfung einwirkender Gewalten.' *Monatsschr. Ohrenheilkd. Laryngorhinol. 101*, 5, 218–222.

9 Liem, T. (2011) 'Wechselseitige Beziehungsdynamiken und subjektive Ansätze in der Osteopathie.' *Osteopath. Med. 12*, 2, 4–7.

10 Liem, T. (2014) 'Pitfalls and challenges involved in the process of perception and interpretation of palpatory findings.' *Int. J. Osteopath. Med. 17*, 4, 242–249.

11 Liem, T. (2018a) 'Review zur Bedeutung der Schädelbasis in der Osteopathie.' *Osteopath. Med. 19*, 2, 8–15.

12 Liem, T. (2018b) *Kraniosakrale Osteoapthie. Ein praktisches Lehrbuch*, 7th Ed. Stuttgart: Thieme.

13 Lippincott, H. A. (1948) 'Compression of the bulb.' *J. Osteopath. Cranial Assoc.*, Meridian: Cranial Academy.

14 Madeline, L. A. and Elster, A. D. (1995) 'Suture closure in the human chondrocranium. CT assessment.' *Radiolog. 196*, 747–756.

15 Magoun, H. I. (1976) *Osteopathy in the Cranial Field*, 3rd Ed. Kirksville: Journal Printing Company.

16 Okamoto, K., Ito, J., Tokiguchi, S. et al. (1996) 'High resolution CT findings in the development of the sphenooccipital synchondrosis.' *AJNR Am. J. Neuroradiol. 17*, 117–120.

17 Schalkhaußer, A. (2000) *Schließung und Mobilität der Synchondrosis sphenobasilaris*. Munich: COE, pp. 26–27.

18 Upledger, J. E. and Vredevoogd, J. D. (2016) *Lehrbuch der CranioSacralen Therapie I*, 7th Ed. Stuttgart: Haug.

19 Mees, L. C. F. (1981) *Das menschliche Skelett. Form und Metamorphose*. Stuttgart: Verlag Urachhaus.

20 Rohen, J. W. (2002) *Morphologie des menschlichen Organismus*, 2nd Ed. Stuttgart: Verlag Freies Geistesleben, p. 387.

7.1 The morphology of the ethmoid bone according to Rohen 304

7.2 Location, causes, and clinical presentation of osteopathic dysfunctions of the ethmoid bone 304
7.2.1 Osseous dysfunction 304
7.2.2 Dysfunction of the falx cerebri 305
7.2.3 Disturbances of nerves and parts of the brain 305
7.2.4 Vascular disturbances 305

7.3 Diagnosis of the ethmoid bone 305
7.3.1 History-taking 305
7.3.2 Palpation of the PRM rhythm 305
7.3.3 Motion testing 307

7.4 Treatment of the ethmoid bone 307
7.4.1 Intraosseous dysfunctions 307
7.4.2 Flexion dysfunction of the ethmoid bone, indirect technique 309
7.4.3 Extension dysfunction of the ethmoid bone, indirect technique 309
7.4.4 Rotation dysfunction of the frontal bone: in particular, dysfunction in internal rotation 310
7.4.5 Rotation dysfunction of the maxilla 312
7.4.6 The cribriform plate 313
7.4.7 Perpendicular plate 314
7.4.8 The ethmoidal labyrinth (lateral masses) 314
7.4.9 Drainage of the ethmoidal cells 317
7.4.10 Additional techniques for the treatment of the ethmoidal cells 320

7.5 References 320

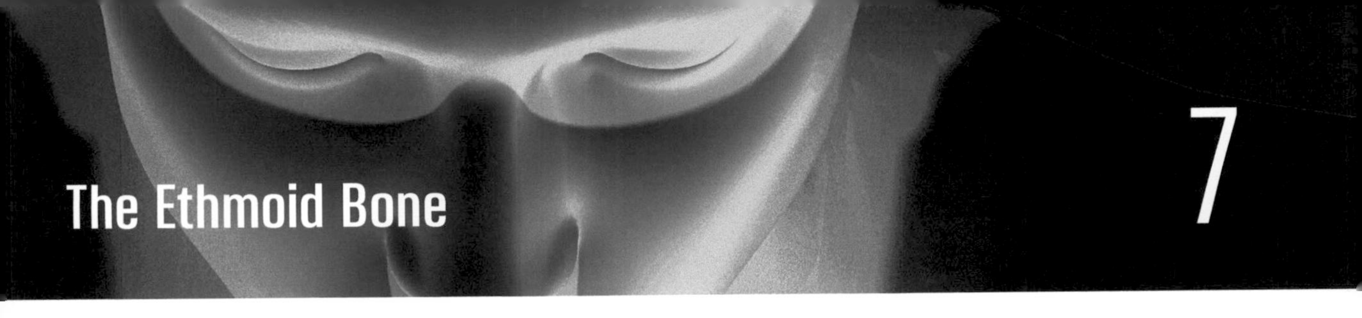

The Ethmoid Bone

7

The unpaired ethmoid contributes to the formation of the cranial base, middle cranial fossa, nasal cavities, and orbits, along with the functions associated with these structures. It is the point of attachment for the anterior falx cerebri and the central site for the embryonic formation of the viscerocranium. Its articulations with the frontal bone, sphenoid, maxilla, etc. make it especially important in dysfunctions in these regions.

The air we breathe in passes through the nasal conchae into the olfactory region and into the respiratory pathways. According to Sutherland, in conditions affecting the paranasal sinuses the frontoethmoidal articulations will be in expansion.[2]

7.1 The morphology of the ethmoid bone according to Rohen[1]

The ethmoid occupies a key position, as important for the adjacent bones of the viscerocranium as the thorax is for the function of the pectoral girdle and upper limbs and for pulmonary respiration. It is the central point for the organization of the viscerocranium. The rhythm of pulmonary breathing may also be able to affect the cerebrospinal fluid system of the brain via the cribriform plate.

7.2 Location, causes, and clinical presentation of osteopathic dysfunctions of the ethmoid bone

Tip for practitioners

Primary dysfunctions

- Intraosseous At birth, the ethmoid consists of the two lateral masses (the ethmoidal labyrinth) and a perpendicular plate. The perpendicular plate fuses with the cribriform plate, uniting with the ethmoidal cells in the second year of life. Developmental disturbances in utero between the pre- and post-sphenoid, or disturbances of ossification between the complex of the body and lesser wings and the complex of the greater wings and pterygoid processes of the sphenoid (ossification around the seventh month of life), can cause tensions transmitted to the intraosseous organization of the ethmoid.
- Primary trauma Birth trauma, falls, blows, or other effects of force in early childhood can also affect the ethmoid bone. In particular, at the sutures, this can lead to unilateral or bilateral posterior displacement of the ethmoid notch. This can result in motion restriction of the ethmoid bone and tensions at the falx cerebri.

Secondary dysfunctions

Dysfunction of the sphenoid (in SBS dysfunctions), frontal bone and maxilla, and the zygomatic bone, or tensions transmitted via the falx cerebri, can cause secondary motion restriction of the ethmoid bone.

7.2.1 Osseous dysfunction

Causes Occurs particularly in dysfunctions of the sphenoid, frontal bone, and maxilla: sphenoethmoidal suture, vomeroethmoidal suture, ethmoidomaxillary suture.

A fall onto the middle of the frontal bone causes flexion or extension dysfunctions of the frontal bone and ethmoid. Unilateral falls onto the frontal bone lead to sidebending-rotation dysfunctions or lateral strain dysfunctions. Sidebending-rotation dysfunctions cause compression of the cranial bones on the side of the concavity.

- **Frontoethmoidal suture:** the region where the cribriform plate of the ethmoid articulates with the ethmoid notch is especially susceptible to dysfunctions.

- **The following locations are also especially susceptible:** ethmoidonasal suture, ethmoidomaxillary suture, palatoethmoidal suture, ethmoidolacrimal suture, ethmoidoseptal suture, ethmoidoconchal suture.

7.2.2 Dysfunction of the falx cerebri

- Causes: occurs in dysfunctions of the ethmoid bone (crista galli), especially in combination with the frontal bone (frontoethmoidal suture).
- Clinical presentation/hypothetical pathology: congestion of the anterior part of the superior sagittal sinus with functional disturbances in the corresponding parts of the brain; pain in the ipsilateral eye.

7.2.3 Disturbances of nerves and parts of the brain

- **Olfactory nerves**
  - Causes: in dysfunctions of the frontal and ethmoid bones, especially in the area where the cribriform plate of the ethmoid articulates with the ethmoidal notch of the frontal bone.
  - Clinical presentation: disturbances of the sense of smell.
- **Anterior and posterior ethmoidal nerves** (both are branches of the nasociliary nerve, branch of the ophthalmic nerve V1)
  - Causes: see olfactory nerves.
  - Clinical presentation: disturbances of sensation and pain in the mucosa and skin of the nose and mucosa of the sphenoidal sinus and posterior ethmoidal cells.

7.2.4 Vascular disturbances

- **Anterior and posterior ethmoidal artery**
  - Causes: see Volume 2, section 2.3.4.
  - Clinical presentation: sinusitis, rhinitis, allergic rhinitis, colds.
- **Anterior ethmoidal artery**: disturbances of the mucosa of the ethmoidal cells and frontal sinus, and disturbances of the nasal cavity.
- **Posterior ethmoidal artery**: disturbances of the mucosa of the ethmoidal cells and of the nasal cavity.

7.3 Diagnosis of the ethmoid bone

7.3.1 History-taking

- Sinusitis, rhinitis, allergic rhinitis, disturbances of the sense of smell, reddened eyes.
- Always take account of previous traumatic injuries.

7.3.2 Palpation of the PRM rhythm

Tip for practitioners

Biomechanical, inhalation phase

- In flexion, the ethmoid bone moves around a transverse axis below the cribriform plate, in the middle of the perpendicular plate.
- The anterior part of the crista galli moves in a superoposterior direction together with the falx cerebri.
- The posterior part of the cribriform plate moves inferior together with the sphenoid.
- The posterior part of the perpendicular plate moves inferior, together with the body of the sphenoid; the anterior part moves superior.
- The inferior part of the anterior surface of the ethmoid moves anterior.
- The posterior part of the ethmoidal cells moves laterally into external rotation controlled by the frontal bone and maxilla, with the effect of opening the nasal cavities.

Developmental dynamic, inhalation phase

- Downward-directed force.

If palpation reveals a restriction, the practitioner may induce motion in the restricted direction. This will emphasize the restriction, making it easier to sense which structure is the origin of the motion restriction.

Palpation of flexion and extension motion (biomechanical)

Testing and treatment of the flexion and extension motion of the ethmoid is done via the frontal bone and nasal bones (Figure 7.1).

Patient: Supine.

Practitioner: Take up a position beside the head of the patient.

Hand position:

- Cranial hand: span the greater wings with your middle or index finger and your thumb.
- Caudal hand: place your middle finger below nasion (the median point of the frontonasal suture) so as to rest on the internasal suture. Place your index finger on glabella (between the arches of the eyebrows).

Inhalation phase of PRM, normal finding (Figure 7.2)

- At glabella (index finger), motion in a posterior (and superior) direction.
- At the internasal suture (middle finger), an anterior motion.

Exhalation phase of PRM, normal finding

- At glabella (index finger), motion in an anterior (and inferior) direction.
- At the internasal suture (middle finger), a posterior motion.

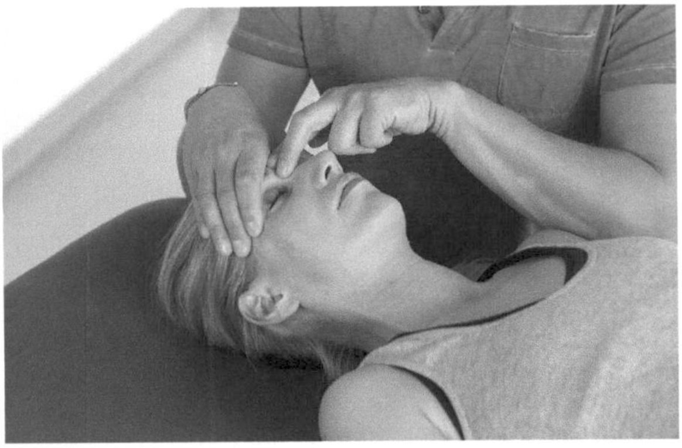

Figure 7.1 Palpation of flexion and extension of the ethmoid bone

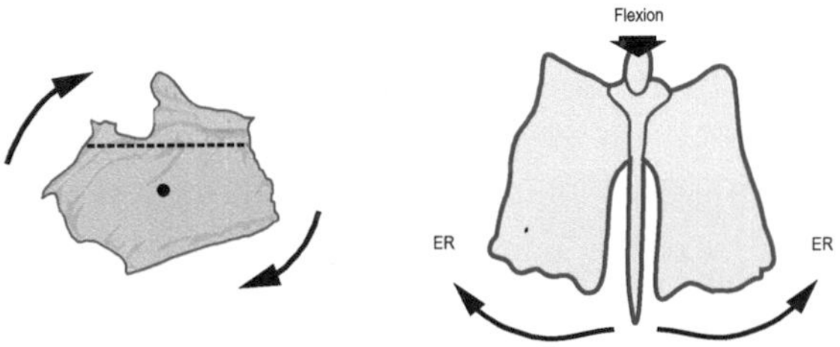

Figure 7.2 PRM inhalation phase/biomechanical

Compare the amplitude, ease, and symmetry of motion of the ethmoidal cells. Other kinds of motion of the ethmoidal cells may arise during the flexion/extension motion: torsion, lateral shear, or sidebending. These provide an indication as to other dysfunctions of the ethmoid bone.

Palpation of the external and internal rotation motion (biomechanical)

The mobility of the ethmoid in external and internal rotation is dependent on that of the frontal bone and maxilla (Figure 7.3). The freedom of motion of the labyrinth (lateral masses) can therefore be reduced by an internal rotation dysfunction of the maxilla. For this reason, the ethmoid should be tested and treated via the frontal bone and maxilla.

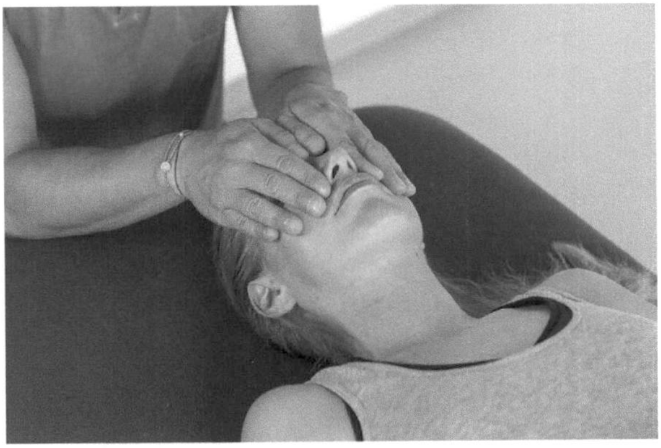

Figure 7.3
Palpation of external and internal rotation of the ethmoid bone

Practitioner: Take up a position at the head of the patient.

Hand position: Place your hands on the frontal bone and maxilla, on either side and pointing caudad.

Method:

- In the inhalation phase, palpate the external rotation motion of the frontal bone and maxilla.
- In the exhalation phase, palpate the internal rotation motion of the frontal bone and maxilla.
- Direct your attention to the ethmoid bone.

Motion testing: This differs from palpation of the PRM rhythm in just one respect: the external and internal rotation of the frontal bone and maxilla is now actively induced (see above).

Palpation of the PRM rhythm (developmental dynamic)

Practitioner and hand position: See palpation of the extension and flexion motion (above).

Method:

Inhalation phase of PRM, normal finding (Figure 7.4)

- Force operating in an anterior and downward direction.

Exhalation phase of PRM, normal finding

- Force operating in a posterior and upward direction.

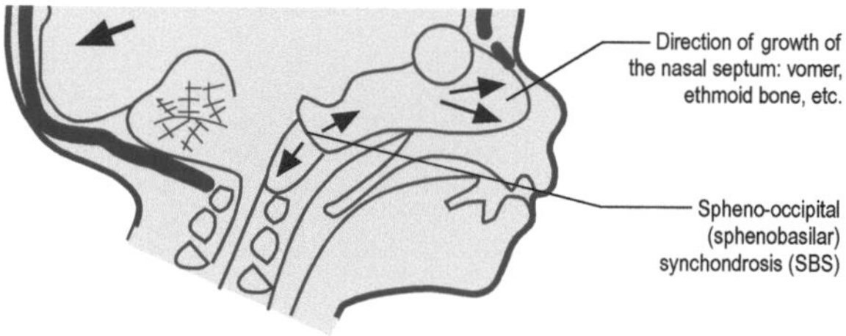

Figure 7.4 PRM inhalation phase/developmental dynamic

7.3.3 Motion testing

Hand position: As above (section 7.3.2).

Method:

During the inhalation phase of PRM

- At the beginning of the inhalation phase, administer a slight impulse to posterior and cephalad motion with the index finger that is on glabella.
- With the middle finger that is on the internasal suture, you will sense a minute anterior motion (flexion of the ethmoid bone) in response to this pressure.

During the exhalation phase of PRM

- At the beginning of the exhalation phase, administer a slight impulse in the posterior direction with the middle finger on the internasal suture.
- With the index finger that is on glabella, you will sense a minute anterior motion (extension of the ethmoid bone) in response to this pressure.

Compare the amplitude and ease of motion or the force needed to bring about motion.

7.4 Treatment of the ethmoid bone

The SBS, frontal bone, and maxilla should also be examined and treated as required.

Indication: Primary and secondary dysfunctions and motion restrictions, and resulting functional disturbances, e.g., sinusitis, rhinitis, allergic rhinitis, disturbances of the sense of smell, reddened eyes.

7.4.1 Intraosseous dysfunctions

It is important for the success of intraosseous techniques to ensure that all the sutural articulations of the ethmoid bone are free to move.

Decompression of the cranial base

Indication: Developmental disturbances in utero, birth trauma, or dysfunctions transmitted to the ethmoid bone due to traumatic injury in early childhood.

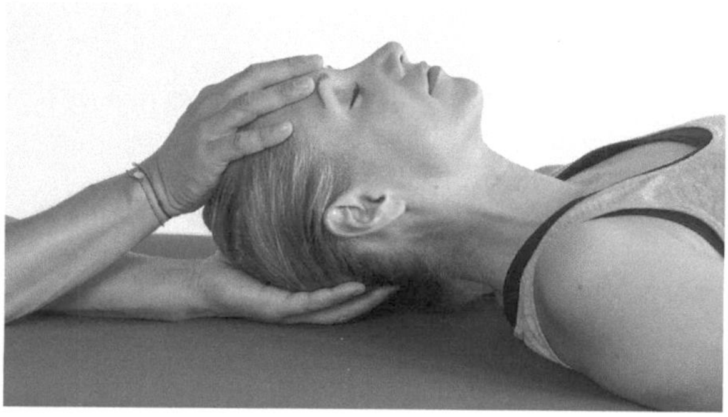

Figure 7.5 Decompression of the cranial base

Practitioner: Take up a position at the head of the patient.

Hand position:
Fronto-occipital cranial hold (Figure 7.5):

- Place your upper hand around the frontal bone, with your fingers pointing caudad.
- Place your lower hand around the occiput, with your fingers pointing caudad.

Method:

- With your upper hand, during the inhalation phase, apply a gentle impulse in the anterior direction to the frontal bone, by pressing your elbow down onto the table.
- Direct your attention as you do this toward the articulations of the ethmoid: anteriorly with the frontal bone and posteriorly with the sphenoid and the SBS. Gently decompress the articulations with the ethmoid bone.
- Establish the PBMT and PBFT.

Intraosseous treatment of the ethmoid

Hand position: See decompression of the cranial base (above).

Method:

- Intraosseous treatment of the ethmoid bone is carried out as follows: with the fingers lying immediately next to the midline, apply gentle compression directed toward the ethmoid bone (i.e., the middle and index fingers on the frontal bone deliver posteriorly directed pressure, and the middle and index fingers on the occipital bone deliver anteriorly directed pressure).
- The compression is only required to establish resonance with the intraosseous tensions of the ethmoid bone.
- At the same time, you can try to copy the former anteriorly directed developmental forces that were expressed in the ethmoid.

NOTE The ethmoidal cells represent the cranial end point of the central midline. You can try to take its relationship to the sphenoid and notochord into account in your palpation.

Ethmoid V-spread technique

Hand position:

- Place your index and middle finger each side of the metopic suture, between nasion and glabella, forming a letter "V" between your two fingers. Place the sending finger at the asterion on the side opposite the dysfunction (Figure 7.6).
- Alternative: position the sending finger at inion and caudally on the midline.

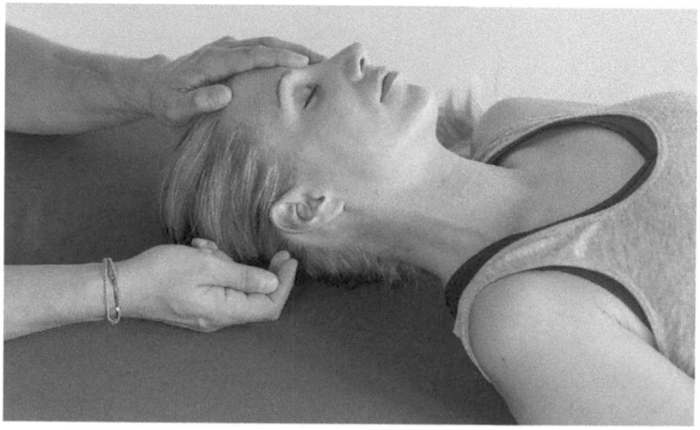

Figure 7.6 Ethmoid V-spread technique

7.4.2 Flexion dysfunction of the ethmoid bone, indirect technique

The motion of the ethmoid bone into extension is reduced.

Practitioner: Take up a position beside the head of the patient.

Hand position:

- Place one hand across the occipital bone, with the squama in the palm of your hand.
- Place the middle finger of your other hand on the glabella, and the index finger below the nasion on the internasal suture (Figure 7.7).

Method:

- Guide the occipital bone into flexion (caudad and anteriorly).
- Go with the ethmoid bone into the direction of the dysfunction, in other words, in the direction of greater motion (of ease). Apply slight pressure on the glabella with your middle finger so as to guide the ethmoid into flexion.
- Establish the PBMT—the position of the ethmoid bone that creates the best possible reciprocal balance of the abnormal intracranial membranous joint tensions—and PBFT.

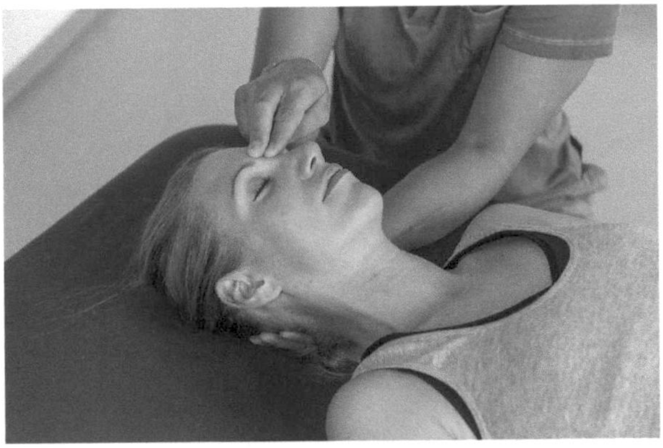

Figure 7.7 Flexion dysfunction of the ethmoid bone, indirect technique

- Maintain the PBT until a correction of the abnormal membranous tension has been achieved and the inherent homeostatic forces (PRM rhythm, etc.) have brought this into effect.
- Breathing assistance: the patient can assist as follows: at the end of an in-breath, hold the inhalation for as long as possible, while performing a plantar flexing of both feet. Repeat for several breathing cycles.
- A fluid impulse may be used to direct energy from the occiput towards the ethmoid bone.

Alternative indirect technique: in harmony with PRM

- During the inhalation phase of PRM, go with the occipital bone into flexion (in a caudad and anterior direction).
- At the same time, administer gentle pressure on the glabella to encourage the flexion motion of the ethmoid bone.
- During the exhalation phase of PRM, just passively follow the motion of the occipital and ethmoid bones.
- In the next PRM inhalation phase, again give an impulse at the occipital and ethmoid bones to encourage motion into flexion, and passively follow the motion during the exhalation phase.
- Continue until you sense a release of the ethmoid.

7.4.3 Extension dysfunction of the ethmoid bone, indirect technique

Hand position: As for flexion dysfunction (Figure 7.7).

Method:

- Guide the occipital bone into extension (in a cranial and posterior direction).
- Go with the ethmoid bone in the direction of the dysfunction, in other words, into the direction of greater motion (direction of ease). To do so, administer gentle pressure with your middle finger to the internasal suture to guide the ethmoid bone into extension.

- Establish the PBMT and PBFT.
- Breathing assistance: the patient can also be asked to assist as follows: at the end of an out-breath, hold the exhalation for as long as possible, while dorsally flexing both feet. Repeat for several breathing cycles.
- A fluid impulse may be used to direct energy from the occiput toward the ethmoid bone.

Alternative indirect technique, in harmony with the PRM rhythm

- During the exhalation phase of PRM, go with the occipital bone into extension (in a cranial and posterior direction).
- At the same time, administer gentle pressure with your middle finger on the internasal suture to encourage the extension motion of the ethmoid bone.
- During the inhalation phase, just passively follow the motion of the occipital and ethmoid bones.
- In the next exhalation phase, again give an impulse at the occipital and ethmoid bones to encourage motion into extension, and passively follow the motion during the inhalation phase.
- Continue until you sense a release of the ethmoid bone.

Vitalist approach See EV-4 technique (section 4.4.3).

7.4.4 Rotation dysfunction of the frontal bone: in particular, dysfunction in internal rotation

Aim: To spread the ethmoid notch of the frontal bone, create freedom of motion of the cribriform plate of the ethmoid, release the surrounding sutures, release the falx cerebri, and improve drainage of the superior and inferior sagittal sinuses.

Indication: Fall or blow to the frontal bone, rhinitis, sinusitis, and functional disturbances to the sense of smell.

Frontal bone spread technique

Practitioner: Take up a position at the head of the patient.

Hand position:

- Hold the outside of the zygomatic processes of the frontal bone with your in-bent ring fingers to provide a firm purchase.
- Support your ring fingers with your little fingers.
- Position your middle and index fingers each side of the midline of the frontal bone.
- Place your thumbs posteriorly, touching or crossing (Figure 7.8).

Method:

- Administer slight pressure in a posterior direction with your index fingers on the midline of the frontal bone.
- At the same time, move your ring fingers in an anterior, lateral, and caudal direction.
- This widens the ethmoidal notch.
- Establish the PBMT and PBFT.
- A fluid impulse may be used to direct energy from the inion.

If this technique is insufficient, a frontal bone lift may be performed.

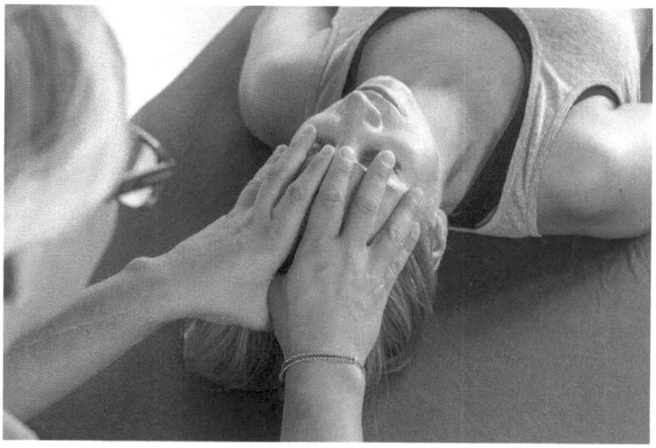

Figure 7.8 Frontal bone spread technique

Frontal bone lift technique

Practitioner and hand position: As for spread technique.

Method:

- During the exhalation phase, begin to administer gentle pressure in a medial direction on the lateral aspects of the frontal bone (Figure 7.9) with your ring fingers, to release the frontal bone from the sphenoid (IR).
- As soon as the frontal bone begins to move anterior, you can relax the medial pressure of your ring fingers. It is very important to do this, as IR of the frontal bone would further narrow the ethmoidal notch.
- Replace this pressure with anterior, slightly cephalad traction. This traction is very gentle and is induced by pressing your elbows slightly down on the table, so that your fingers rise anteriorly. Never let the degree of force rise to the level where the tissue begins to contract in resistance.
- The weight of the cranium is sufficient to keep the occiput, the posterior point of attachment of the falx, in position on the table.

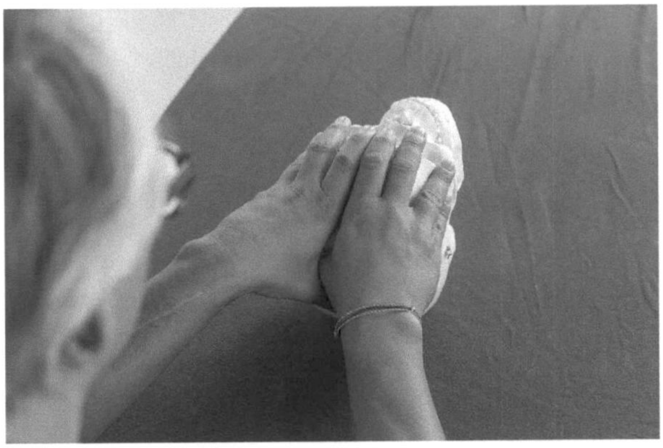

Figure 7.9 Frontal bone lift technique

- At each release of the tissues, seek the new limit of motion of the frontal bone in the anterior direction.
- Permit all motions and tissue unwinding of the frontal bone, without reducing the gentle traction.
- You will be able to sense the various stages of tissue release: first the sutural tensions, then the elastic and collagenous tensions of the falx cerebri (feels like cement or a rubber band or chewing gum). When the falx has been freed of its tension patterns (floating sensation), you can relax the anteriorly directed traction and remove your hands.
- To release the frontoethmoidal suture, focus your attention particularly on this suture.
- A fluid impulse may be used to direct energy from inion.

NOTE—IMPORTANT The degree of tension applied in the lift should be judged by imitating the tension present, and applying about 5 g of extra tension over and above the degree of tension you detect. Never lift your hands suddenly away from the bone while performing the technique.
Always take care to position your hands accurately. Incorrect positioning can cause the technique to be ineffective at best; in the worst case it can exacerbate or give rise to symptoms, especially if your fingers are lying on the sutures.

Tip for practitioners

Another option is to encourage the flexion and extension motion of the frontal bone while administering the gentle anterior traction (in harmony with the PRM rhythm).

7.4.5 Rotation dysfunction of the maxilla

Maxilla lift and spread technique

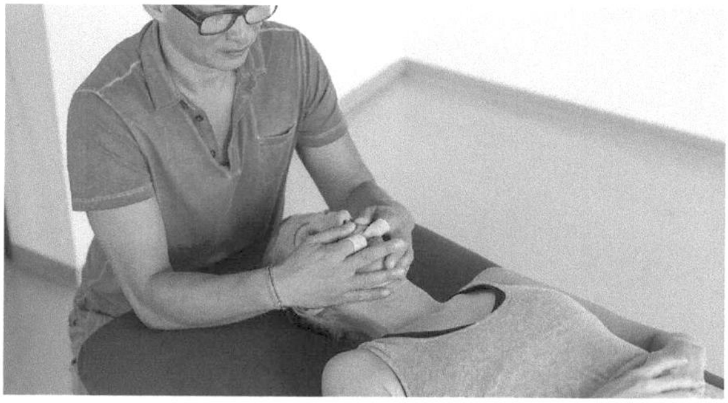

Figure 7.10 Maxilla lift and spread technique

Aim: To release the ethmoidomaxillary, lacrimo-maxillary, and ethmoidolacrimal sutures and create freedom of motion of the perpendicular plate.

Practitioner: Take up a position at the head of the patient.

Hand position:

- Place your hands either side of the patient's head.
- Place your thumbs outside or just above the alveolar processes of the maxillae. Your thumbs should be medially oriented.
- Place your index fingers intraorally on the alveolar processes of the maxillae.
- This means that you are in effect grasping the maxillae between your finger and thumb, from inside and outside (Figure 7.10).

Maxilla lift technique

Method:

- With your thumb and index finger, administer anterior and caudad traction to the two maxillary bones. This frees the maxillae from the ethmoid bone.
- A fluid impulse may be used to direct energy from the opposite lambdoid suture.

NOTE The medial border of the orbital surface of the maxilla is released from the bottom of the ethmoidal cells, the posterior border of the frontal process of the maxilla is freed from the anterior of the ethmoidal labyrinth (lateral masses), and the ethmoidal crest on the medial side of the maxilla released from the middle nasal concha.

Maxilla spread technique

- When you sense a release at the ethmoidomaxillary sutures, you can go on to spread the maxillae away from each other.
- Without reducing the anterior and caudal traction, induce external rotation of the maxillae. Administer posterior pressure on the intermaxillary suture with your thumbs. With your index fingers, guide the alveolar process in a lateral and anterior direction.
- Establish the PBMT and PBFT.
- A fluid impulse may be used to direct energy from the opposite lambdoid suture.

Alternative technique to treat an internal rotation dysfunction of the maxillae

Aim: To release the ethmoidomaxillary suture and create freedom of motion of the perpendicular plate.

Practitioner: Take up a position beside the patient's head.

Hand position:

- Cranial hand: span the greater wings with your thumb and your middle or index finger.
- Caudal hand: place your middle and index fingers intraorally, against the upper teeth on each side (Figure 7.11).

Method:

- During the inhalation phase, deliver a caudad impulse via the greater wings to induce flexion.

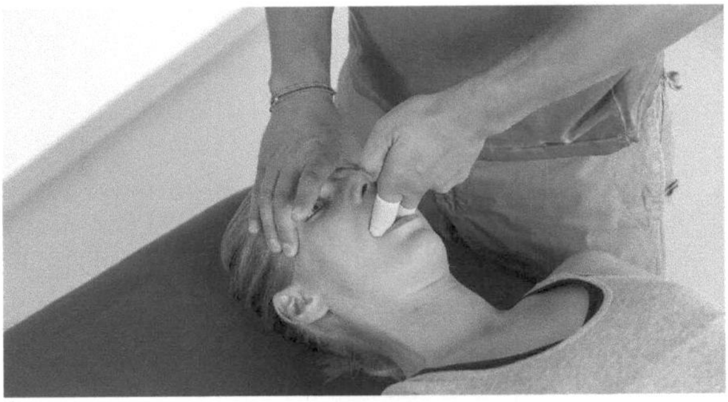

Figure 7.11 Alternative technique to treat an internal rotation dysfunction of the maxillae

- At the same time, spread apart the fingers resting on the upper teeth (external rotation of the maxillae).
- During the exhalation phase, passively follow the motion of the cranial bones.
- Repeat this procedure for several cycles, until the mobility of the perpendicular plate increases.

7.4.6 The cribriform plate

The cribriform plate forms the boundary between the nasal cavity and the anterior cranial cavity. The cribriform plate articulates with the ethmoidal notch of the frontal bone via the frontoethmoidal suture. This is a plane suture.

Technique to treat the cribriform plate

See frontal bone spread and lift (this chapter, section 7.4.4).

Alternative technique to treat the cribriform plate

Practitioner: Take up a position beside the patient's head.

Hand position:

- Cranial hand: span the frontal bone with your thumb and middle finger (and/or index finger) by hooking the thumb and finger around the zygomatic processes of the frontal bone. Place the basal joint of your index finger on glabella.
- Caudal hand: grasp the frontal processes of the maxillae with the middle and index fingers. Place your thumb and ring finger on the anterolateral surfaces of the maxillae.

Method:

- Direct technique (Figure 7.12)
  - Cranial hand: administer gentle posterior and superior pressure with the basal joint of the index finger on glabella, while moving the outer inferior parts of the frontal bone anterior and laterally with your thumb and middle finger (external rotation of the frontal bone). The overall effect is to move the frontal bone into a more shallow-angled position (flexion of the frontal bone).
  - At the same time, induce external rotation of the maxillae with your caudal hand.
  - Also administer inferiorly directed traction to the frontal processes of the maxillae with the index and middle finger of your caudal hand, supporting these fingers with your thumb and ring finger.
- Establish the PBMT and PBFT at the frontal and ethmoid bones.
- Maintain the PBT until a correction of the abnormal membranous tension has been achieved, the inherent homeostatic forces (PRM rhythm, etc.) have put the correction into effect, and you sense a release at the cribriform plate, the ethmoidal notch, and the ethmoidomaxillary sutures, and the motion of the ethmoid and frontal bones has ceased.

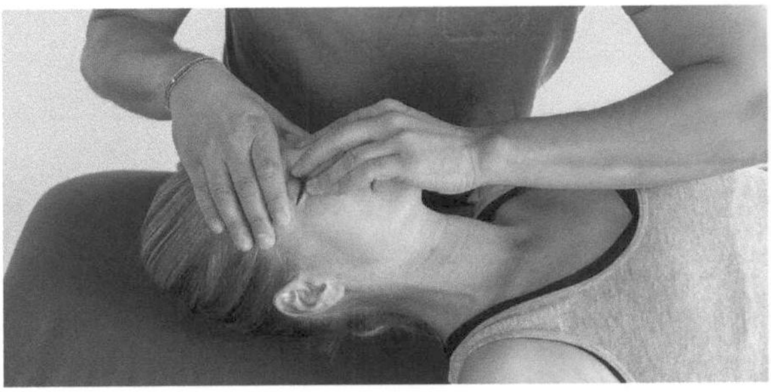

Figure 7.12 Alternative technique to treat the cribriform plate

Unilateral treatment of the cribriform plate, right

Practitioner: Take up a position to the (left) of the patient's head, the opposite side to the dysfunction.

Hand position:

- Cranial hand: span the frontal bone with your thumb and middle finger (and/or index finger), by hooking them around the outside of the zygomatic processes of the frontal bone. Place the basal joint of your index finger on glabella.
- Caudal hand: place your index finger on the (right) frontal process of the maxilla. Position your middle finger on the (right) anterior surface of the maxilla. Position your ring finger on the (right) zygomatic bone.

Method:

- Direct technique (Figure 7.13)
  - ▸ Cranial hand: administer gentle posterior and superior pressure with the basal joint of the index finger on the glabella, while moving the outer inferior parts of the frontal bone anterior and laterally with your thumb and middle finger (external rotation of the frontal bone). The overall effect is to move the frontal bone into a more shallow-angled position (flexion of the frontal bone).
  - ▸ Guide the maxilla into external rotation with the index and middle finger of your caudal hand.
  - ▸ With your ring finger, guide the zygomatic bone into external rotation.
- Establish the PBMT and PBFT at the frontal bone.
- Maintain the PBT until a correction of the abnormal membranous tension has been achieved, the inherent homeostatic forces (PRM rhythm, etc.) have brought the correction into effect, and you sense a release at the cribriform plate, the ethmoidal notch, and the ethmoidomaxillary sutures. Continue until the motion of the frontal bone has ceased.

7.4.7 Perpendicular plate

The perpendicular plate forms the superior part of the nasal septum.

Aim: To create freedom of motion of the perpendicular plate and release the surrounding sutures.
Technique: See under external and internal rotation dysfunction of the ethmoid bone (above).

7.4.8 The ethmoidal labyrinth (lateral masses)

Technique for the ethmoidal labyrinth (lateral masses of the ethmoid bone)

Indication:
Motion restriction of the ethmoidal labyrinth, sinusitis.

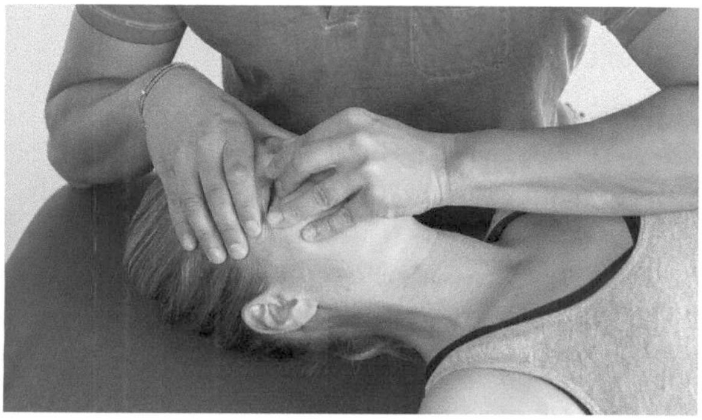

Figure 7.13 Unilateral treatment of the cribriform plate, right

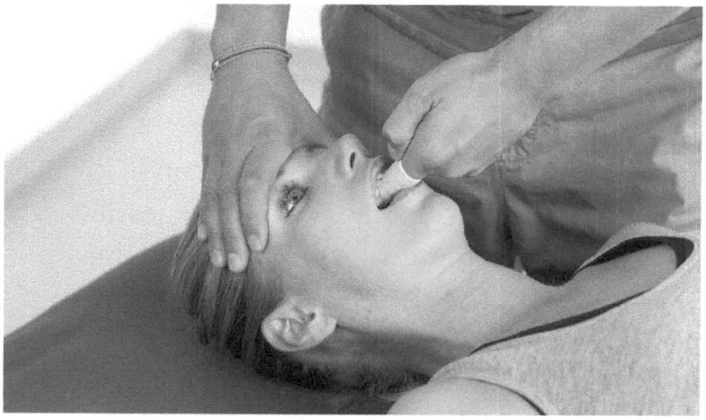

Figure 7.14 Indirect technique for the ethmoidal labyrinth

Indirect technique for the ethmoidal labyrinth

Practitioner: Take up a position beside the patient's head.

Hand position:

- Cranial hand: span the frontal bone with your thumb and middle finger (and/or index finger), by hooking them around the outside of the zygomatic processes of the frontal bone. Place the basal joint of your index finger on the glabella.
- Caudal hand: place your index finger intraorally on the median palatine suture, posterior to the transverse palatine suture (Figure 7.14).

Method:

- Cranial hand: during the exhalation phase, deliver an impulse to the frontal bone to encourage motion into internal rotation and extension. As you do so, gently follow the anterior motion with the basal joint of your index finger on glabella. Meanwhile use your thumb and middle finger to move the outer, inferior parts of the frontal bone posterior and medially (internal rotation of the frontal bone). The overall effect is to move the frontal bone into a more steeply angled position (extension of the frontal bone).
- Caudal hand: at the same time, administer pressure in a superior direction with your index finger. This encourages motion of the ethmoid bone into extension, via the vomer (Figure 7.15). The effect of this is to guide the ethmoidal labyrinth into extension and internal rotation (narrowing of the ethmoidal labyrinth).
- Breathing assistance: you can also ask the patient to hold an exhalation at the end of an out-breath for as long as possible. Repeat for several breathing cycles.
- Establish the PBMT and PBFT at the frontal bone, vomer, and ethmoid bone.
- Maintain the PBT until a correction of the abnormal membranous tension has been achieved, the inherent homeostatic forces (PRM rhythm, etc.) have brought this into effect, and you sense a release of the ethmoidal labyrinth. Continue until the motion of the ethmoidal labyrinth and frontal bone has ceased.

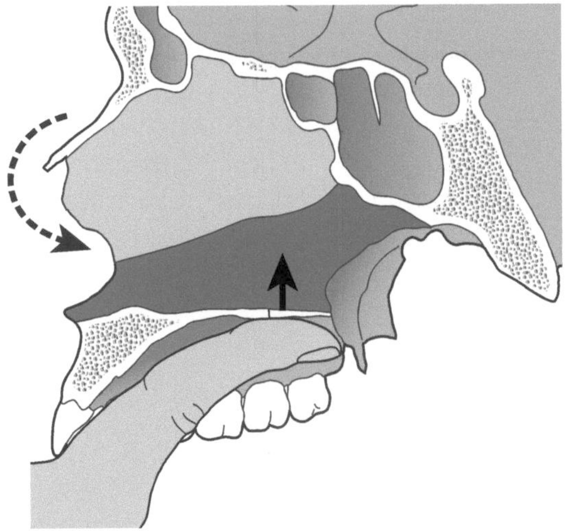

Figure 7.15 Indirect technique for the ethmoidal labyrinth: impulse by index finger to encourage motion of the ethmoid bone into extension

Direct technique for the ethmoidal labyrinth

Hand position:

This differs only very slightly from the position for the indirect technique: the index finger of your caudal hand placed intraorally on the median palatine suture lies anterior to the transverse palatine suture (Figure 7.16).

Method:

- Cranial hand: during the inhalation phase, follow the glabella in a posterior and superior direction with the basal joint of the index finger, while moving the outer inferior parts of the frontal bone anterior and laterally with your thumb and middle finger (external rotation of the frontal bone). The overall effect is to move the frontal bone into a more shallow-angled position (flexion of the frontal bone).

- Caudal hand: at the same time, administer pressure in a superior direction. This encourages motion of the ethmoid bone into flexion, via the vomer (Figure 7.17).
- The effect of this is to guide the ethmoidal labyrinth into flexion and external rotation (spreading of the ethmoidal labyrinth).

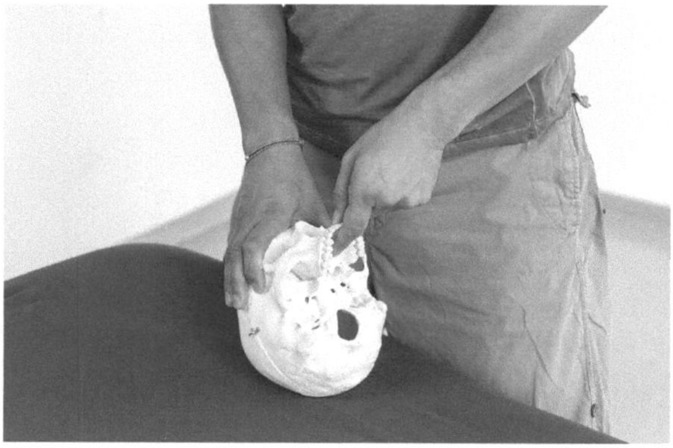

Figure 7.16 Direct technique for the ethmoidal labyrinth

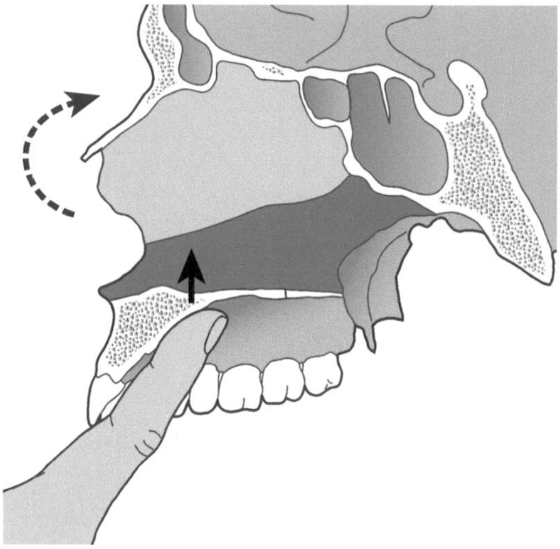

Figure 7.17 Direct technique for the ethmoidal labyrinth: impulse by index finger to encourage motion of the ethmoid bone into flexion

- Breathing assistance: you can also ask the patient to hold an inhalation at the end of an in-breath for as long as possible. Repeat for several breathing cycles.
- Establish the PBMT and PBFT at the frontal bone, vomer, and ethmoid bone.
- Maintain the PBT until a correction of the abnormal membranous tension has been achieved and stabilized by the inherent homeostatic forces (PRM rhythm, etc.), you sense a release of the ethmoidal labyrinth, and the motion of the ethmoidal labyrinth has ceased.

NOTE Always make sure that the amount of force used is not so great as to cause additional tension of the tissue.

Both in the direct and the indirect technique, it is equally possible to deliver the therapeutic impulses simply in harmony with the PRM rhythm.

Unilateral treatment of the ethmoidal labyrinth, right

Practitioner:

Take up a position to the (left) of the patient's head, the side opposite the dysfunction.

Hand position:

- Cranial hand: span the frontal bone with your thumb and middle finger (and/or index finger), by hooking them around the outside of the zygomatic processes of the frontal bone.
- Caudal hand: place your index finger on the frontal process of the (right) maxilla. Place your ring finger intraorally, with the inner edge of the finger on the outside of the alveolar process of the maxilla. Place the thumb, and that of your cranial hand, externally on the zygomatic process of the frontal bone (Figure 7.18).

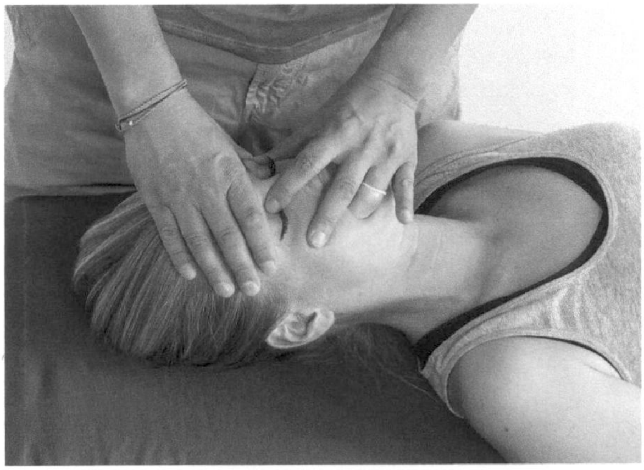

Figure 7.18 Unilateral treatment of the ethmoidal labyrinth,right

Method:

- Stabilize the (right) maxilla with your caudal hand.
- With the index and/or middle finger of your cranial hand, move the frontal bone on the affected side cephalad.
- With your thumbs, stabilize the other (left) side of the frontal bone in its position.
- The effect is to release the frontal bone on the side of the dysfunction from the maxilla, so freeing the ethmoidal labyrinth, which lies between these two bones.
- Establish the PBMT and PBFT.

7.4.9 Drainage of the ethmoidal cells

Ethmoid pump technique

Indication: Sinusitis.

Aim: To drain the ethmoidal cells, to enable secretions to drain away.
This technique is very like the ethmoidal labyrinth release, except that the impulses are always delivered in harmony with the PRM rhythm in the ethmoid pump technique.

Practitioner: Take up a position beside the patient's head.

Hand position:

- Cranial hand: span the frontal bone with your thumb and middle finger (and/or index finger), by hooking them around the outside of the zygomatic processes of the frontal bone. Place the basal joint of your index finger on glabella.
- Caudal hand: place your index finger intraorally on the median palatine suture, anterior to the transverse palatine suture. Position your middle finger intraorally on the median palatine suture, posterior to the transverse palatine suture (Figures 7.19 and 7.20).

Alternative hand position: The index finger only is placed on the median palatine suture, both anterior and posterior to the transverse palatine suture (Figure 7.22; see also Figure 8.1). This method should only be used if you are able to sense and induce the flexion and extension of the vomer using this finger position.

Method:

During the inhalation phase:

- Cranial hand: with the basal joint of the index finger resting on glabella, administer gentle pressure in a posterior and superior direction. As you do this, move the outer, inferior parts of the frontal bone anteriorly and laterally with your thumb and middle finger (external rotation of the frontal bone). The overall effect is to move the frontal bone into a more shallow-angled position (flexion of the frontal bone).

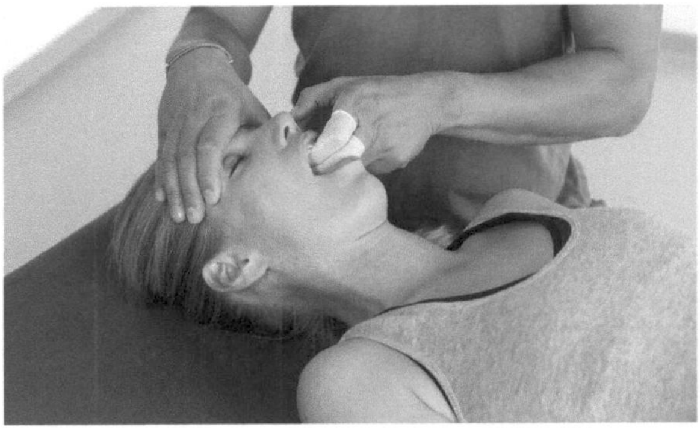

Figure 7.19 Ethmoid pump technique

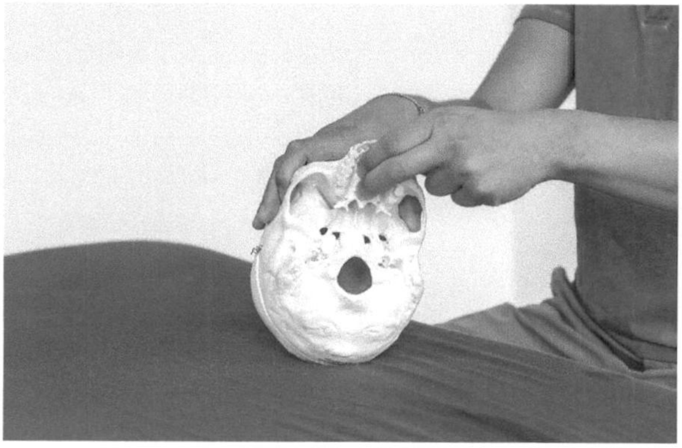

Figure 7.20 Ethmoid pump technique (shown on model)

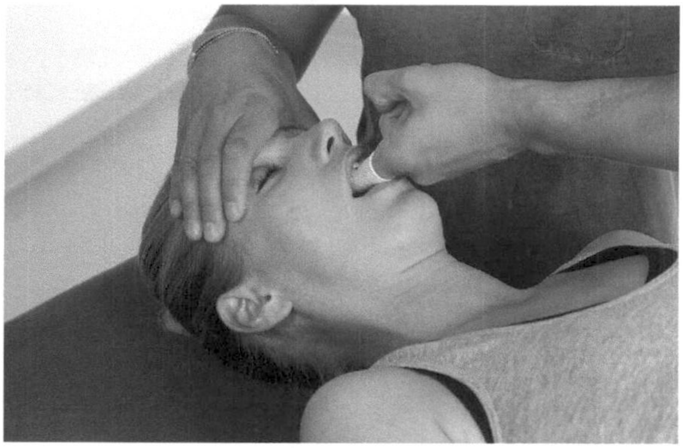

Figure 7.22 Alternative hand position: ethmoid pump technique

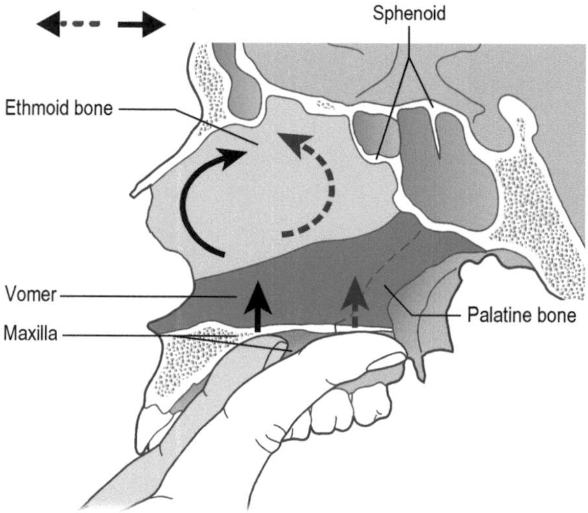

Figure 7.21 Ethmoid pump technique. Continuous arrows: impulse to ethmoid bone during inhalation phase. Dotted arrows: impulse to ethmoid bone during exhalation phase

- Caudal hand: at the same time apply pressure in a superior direction with the index finger of the caudal hand (impulse directed superiorly and anterior to the transverse palatine suture: flexion). This encourages motion of the ethmoid bone into flexion, via the vomer (Figure 7.21, continuous arrows).

During the exhalation phase:

- Cranial hand: with the basal joint of the index finger, gently follow the glabella anterior. As you do this, move the outer, inferior parts of the frontal bone in a posterior and medial direction using your thumb and middle finger (internal rotation of the frontal bone). The overall effect is to move the frontal bone into a more steeply angled position (extension of the frontal bone).
- Caudal hand: at the same time, administer pressure in a superior direction with your middle finger (impulse directed superiorly and posterior to the transverse palatine suture: extension). This encourages motion of the ethmoid bone into extension, via the vomer (Figure 7.21, dotted arrows).
- Repeat for several cycles of the PRM rhythm.

Alternative ethmoid pump technique (opposite physiological motion)

Method:

- With the basal joint of the index finger on glabella, administer gentle pressure in a posterior and superior direction. As you do this, move the outer, inferior parts of the frontal bone in an anterior and lateral direction using your thumb and middle finger (external rotation of the frontal bone). The overall effect is to move the frontal bone into a more shallow-angled position (flexion of the frontal bone).

- At the same time, deliver an impulse in a superior direction with the middle finger of your caudal hand (impulse directed superiorly and posterior to the transverse palatine suture: extension).
- In the next phase of the PRM cycle, gently follow the glabella anteriorly with the basal joint of the index finger. As you do this, move the outer, inferior parts of the frontal bone in a posterior and medial direction using your thumb and middle finger (internal rotation of the frontal bone). The overall effect is to move the frontal bone into a more steeply angled position (extension of the frontal bone).
- At the same time deliver an impulse in a superior direction with the index finger of the caudal hand (impulse directed superiorly and anterior to the transverse palatine suture: flexion).

Unilateral drainage of the ethmoidal cells

Practitioner: Take up a position to the (left) of the patient's head, the side opposite the dysfunction.

Hand position:

- Cranial hand: place the palm of your hand on the frontal bone (right-hand side). Place your thumb on the (left-hand) side of the frontal bone (the side opposite the dysfunction), resting on the side of the bone. Position your index finger on the frontal process of the (right) maxilla. Position your middle finger on the anterior surface of the (right) maxilla. Rest your ring finger and little finger on the (right) zygomatic bone.
- Caudal hand: place your index finger intraorally on the median palatine suture, anterior to the transverse palatine suture. Place your middle finger intraorally on the median palatine suture, posterior to the transverse palatine suture (Figures 7.23 and 7.24).

Alternative hand position: The index finger only is placed on the median palatine suture, both anterior and posterior to the transverse palatine suture (Figure 7.25). This method should only be used if you are able to sense and induce the flexion and extension of the vomer using this finger position.

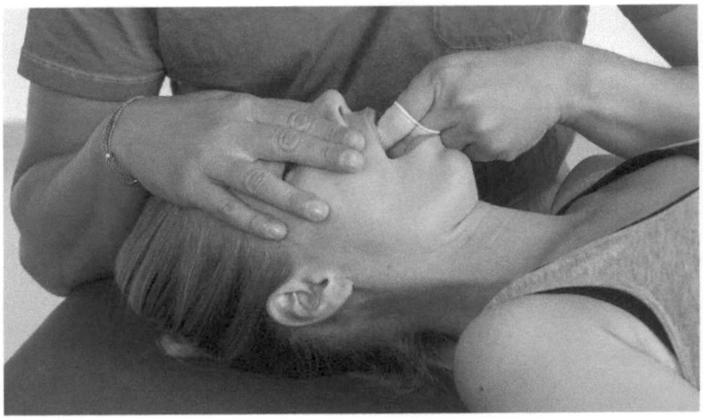

Figure 7.23 Unilateral drainage of the ethmoidal cells

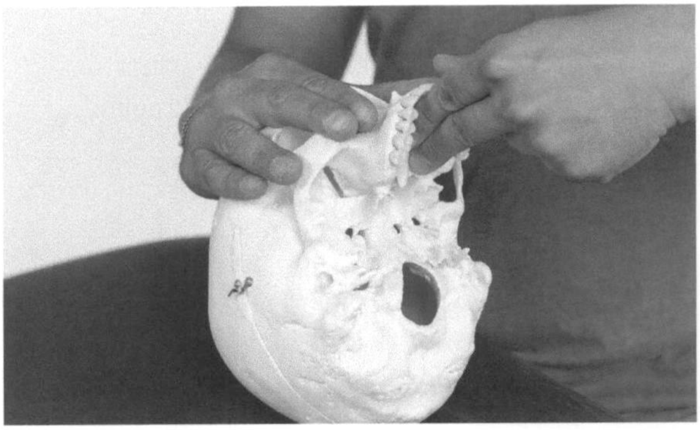

Figure 7.24 Unilateral drainage of the ethmoidal cells (shown on model)

Method:

During the inhalation phase:

- Administer an impulse to the frontal bone, maxilla, and zygomatic bone to encourage motion into external rotation.
- At the same time, administer pressure in a superior direction with the index finger of your caudal hand (impulse directed superiorly and anterior to the transverse palatine suture: flexion). This encourages motion of the ethmoid bone into flexion, via the vomer.

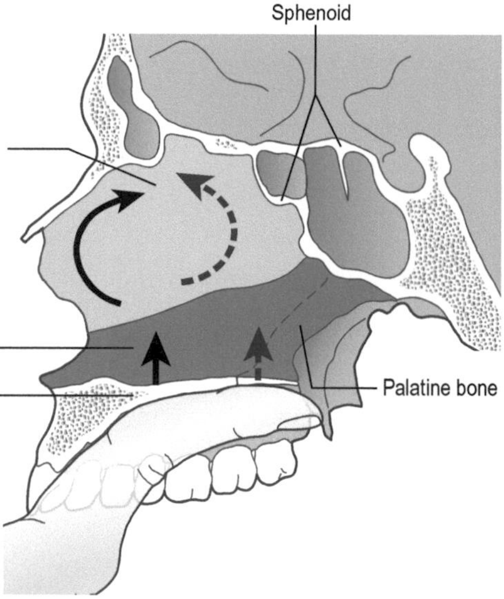

Figure 7.25 Alternative hand position: unilateral drainage of the ethmoidal cells. Continuous arrows: impulse to ethmoid bone during inhalation phase. Dotted arrows: impulse to ethmoid bone during exhalation phase

During the exhalation phase

- Administer an impulse to the frontal bone, maxilla, and zygomatic bone to encourage motion into internal rotation.
- At the same time, administer pressure in a superior direction with the middle finger of the caudal hand (impulse directed superiorly and posterior to the transverse palatine suture: extension). This encourages motion of the ethmoid bone into extension, via the vomer. Repeat for several cycles of the PRM rhythm.

7.4.10 Additional techniques for the treatment of the ethmoidal cells

Zygomatic bone technique

Practitioner: Take up a position at the head of the patient.

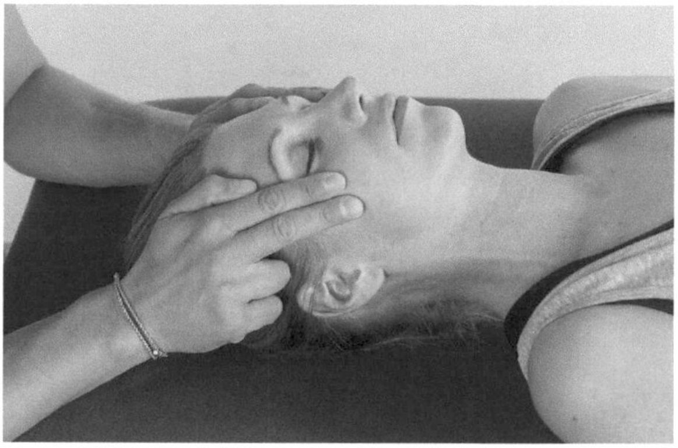

Figure 7.26 Zygomatic bone technique

Hand position: Place the index and middle fingers of both hands on the ipsilateral zygomatic bone (Figure 7.26).

Method:

- Administer gentle medially directed pressure to the zygomatic bones with your fingers. This gentle pressure is transmitted to the maxillae.
- Establish PBMT and PBFT.
- This has an effect on the maxillary sinus, leading to an improvement in breathing.

Frontal bone lift technique

See this volume, section 10.4.4 (frontal bone).

Maxilla lift and spread technique

See this volume, sections 7.4.5 and 12.4.1 (maxillae).

Self-help technique for drainage of the ethmoidal cells
See Volume 2, sections 2.5.8 and 2.5.12.

7.5 References

1 Rohen, J. W. (2002) *Morphologie des menschlichen Organismus*, 2nd Ed. Stuttgart: Verlag Freies Geistesleben, p. 391.

2 Sutherland, W. G. (1944) 'The cranial bowl.' *J. Am. Osteopath. Assoc. 1944*, 348–353.

8.1 Diagnosis of the vomer 322
8.1.1 History-taking 322
8.1.2 Inspection and palpation of the position 322
8.1.3 Palpation of PRM rhythm 322
8.1.4 Motion testing 323
8.1.5 Additional test options 324

8.2 Treatment of the vomer 324
8.2.1 Flexion dysfunction 324
8.2.2 Extension dysfunction 325
8.2.3 Torsion dysfunction, right 326
8.2.4 Lateral shear, e.g., right 326
8.2.5 Sutural dysfunctions 327
8.2.6 Decompression 327
8.2.7 Vomer pump technique 328

8.3 References 329

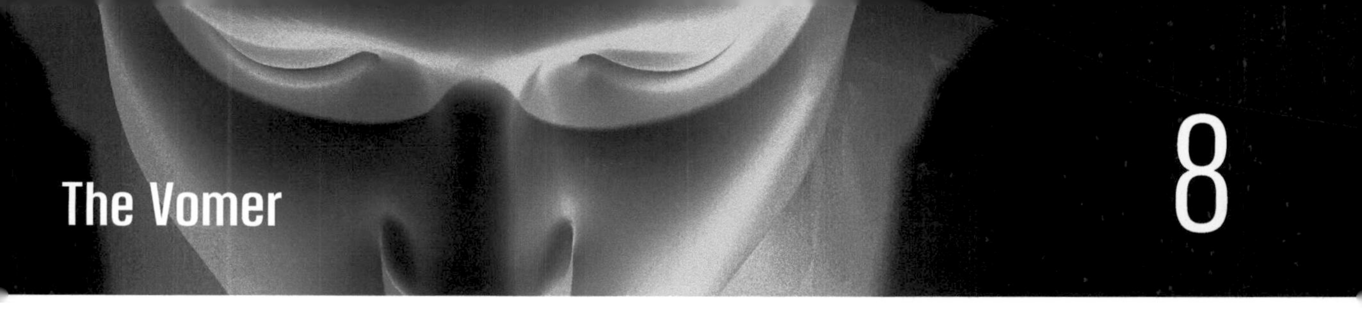

8 The Vomer

The vomer is a four-sided unpaired bone, lying medially, which forms the posterior inferior part of the nasal septum. Since it transmits the antero-inferior growth impulse of the cranial base to the viscerocranium, it has a strong influence on the embryological development of the nasal cavity. According to Magoun, the rhythmic motion of the vomer promotes drainage and circulation in the sphenoidal sinus[2:57] and in the nasal cavity.

8.1 Diagnosis of the vomer

8.1.1 History-taking

- Nasal problems (rhinitis, sinusitis).

8.1.2 Inspection and palpation of the position

- Hard palate: lowered (possibly ER) or elevated (possibly IR).

8.1.3 Palpation of PRM rhythm

Tip for practitioners

Since there is a sutural articulation between the vomer and the hard palate, motion of the vomer can be palpated via a contact with the hard palate.

Biomechanical, inhalation phase

- The vomer moves about a transverse axis in the middle of the vomer.
- The vomer executes a circular motion.
- The vomer descends overall, with the posterior part sinking lower than the anterior part.

Developmental dynamic, inhalation phase

- Forward, downward-directed force.

Practitioner: Take up a position beside the head of the patient.

Hand position:

- Cranial hand: span the greater wings with your thumb and your middle or index finger.
- Caudal hand: place your index finger on the median palatine suture (both anterior and posterior to the transverse palatine suture) (Figures 8.1 and 8.2).

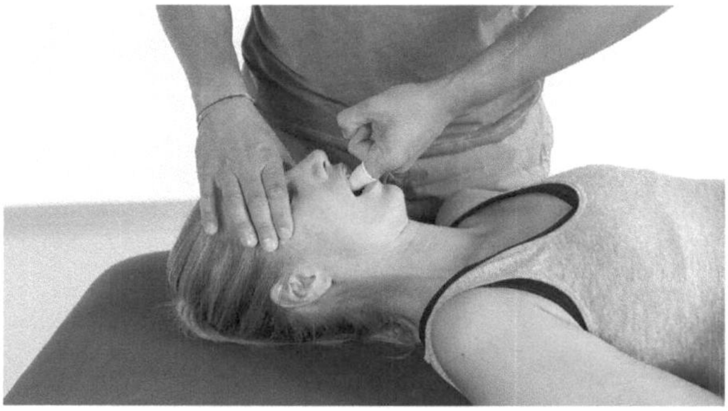

Figure 8.1 Palpation of PRM rhythm of the vomer

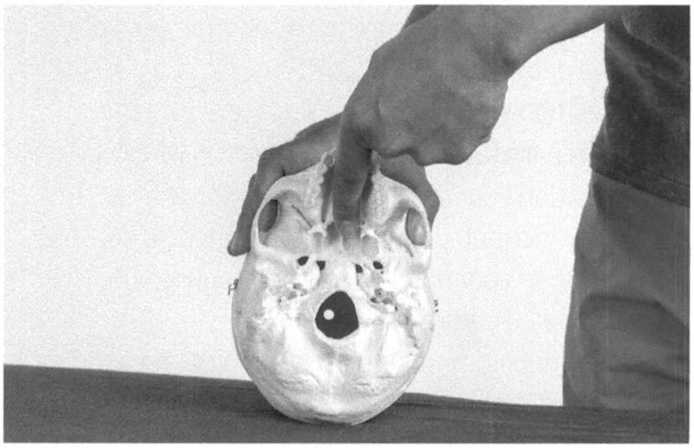

Figure 8.2 Palpation of PRM rhythm of the vomer (shown on model)

Biomechanical approach:

Inhalation phase of PRM, normal finding (Figure 8.3)

- A lowering of the posterior inferior border of the vomer can be palpated posterior to the transverse palatine suture.
- Anterior to the transverse palatine suture there is a cephalad motion of the anterior inferior border of the vomer.

Exhalation phase of PRM, normal finding

- A cephalad motion of the posterior border of the vomer can be palpated posterior to the transverse palatine suture.
- Anterior to the transverse palatine suture there is a lowering of the anterior inferior border of the vomer.

Biodynamic/embryological approach:

Inhalation phase of PRM, normal finding (Figure 8.4)

- Force operating in an anterior and downward direction.

Exhalation phase of PRM, normal finding

- Force operating in a posterior and upward direction.

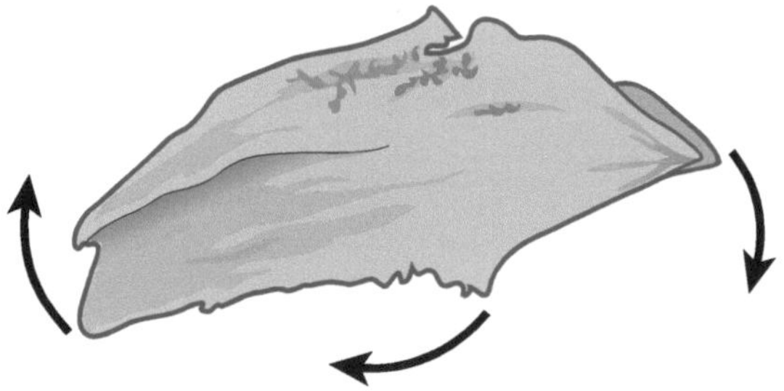

Figure 8.3 Inhalation phase of PRM, biomechanical

Compare the amplitude, strength, and ease of motion of the vomer. Other types of motion of the vomer may occur during the flexion and extension motion: torsion, lateral shear, and sidebending. These provide an indication about further dysfunctions of the vomer.

8.1.4 Motion testing

The only difference between motion testing and palpation of the PRM rhythm is that here the flexion and extension motion of the vomer is actively induced by the practitioner.

Testing of flexion and extension

Hand position: See palpation of PRM rhythm (section 8.1.3).

Method:

During the PRM inhalation phase

- With the thumb and middle finger on the greater wings, administer an impulse in a caudal direction (flexion motion).
- You will sense a reaction to this pressure, via the index finger on the median palatine suture. This reaction is a minute caudad motion behind the transverse palatine suture (flexion motion of the vomer).

During the PRM exhalation phase

- With the thumb and middle finger on the greater wings, administer an impulse in the cranial direction (extension motion).
- You will sense a reaction to this pressure, via the index finger on the median palatine suture.

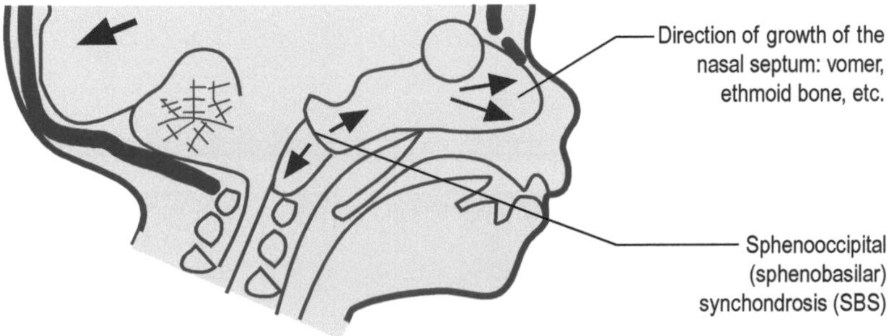

Figure 8.4 PRM inhalation phase/developmental dynamic

This reaction is a minute cephalad motion behind the transverse palatine suture (extension motion of the vomer).

Compare the amplitude and ease of motion, or the amount of force needed to elicit motion.

8.1.5 Additional test options

Testing the motion of the vomer by directly inducing the particular motion

- Testing of **flexion motion**: during the inhalation phase of PRM, move the posterior part of the vomer in a caudal direction and the anterior part cephalad (Figure 8.5A).
- Testing of **extension motion**: during the exhalation phase, move the posterior part of the vomer cephalad and the anterior part caudad (Figure 8.5B).
- Testing of torsion motion: turn the vomer to the right and left while holding the greater wings in a neutral position (Figure 8.5C).
- Testing of lateral shear: shift the vomer to the right and left while holding the greater wings in a neutral position (Figure 8.5D).

Compare the amplitude and ease of motion, and the amount of force needed to elicit motion.

Testing the vomer via the ethmoid bone

- Place your middle finger on the glabella and your index finger below the nasion on the internasal suture.
- Palpate the reaction of the vomer via induction of flexion and extension motion of the ethmoid bone.

8.2 Treatment of the vomer

Indication: Primary and secondary dysfunctions and motion restrictions of the vomer, and resulting nasal problems such as rhinitis, sinusitis, etc.

8.2.1 Flexion dysfunction

Practitioner: Take up a position beside the patient's head.

Hand position:

- Cranial hand: span the greater wings with your thumb and middle or index finger.
- Caudal hand: place your index finger on the median palatine suture (anterior and posterior to the transverse palatine suture).

Method:

Indirect technique (exaggeration technique)

- During the inhalation phase, ease the greater wings in a caudal direction with your thumb and middle finger (flexion motion).
- At the same time, administer a cephalad impulse with the index finger on the median palatine suture, anterior to the transverse palatine suture (flexion motion of the vomer) (Figure 8.6, arrows with continuous lines).
- Hold the sphenoid and vomer in flexion.

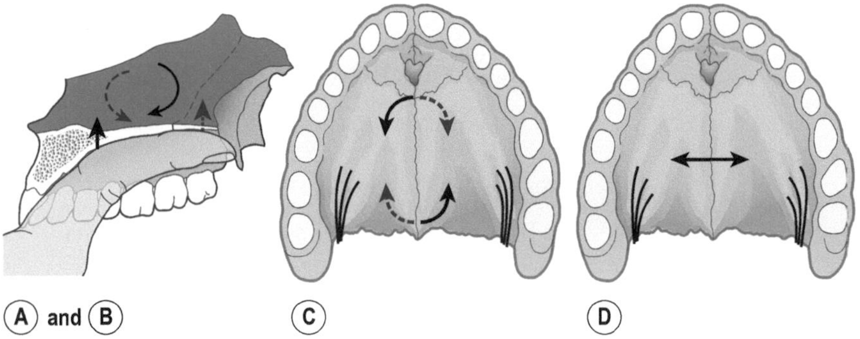

Figure 8.5
Testing of the vomer.
A Testing of flexion motion: continuous line.
B Testing of extension motion: dotted line.
C Testing of torsion motion.
D Testing of lateral shear

- Breathing assistance: ask the patient to hold an inhalation for as long as possible at the end of an in-breath. Repeat for several breathing cycles.
- Establish the PBMT and PBFT.
- A fluid impulse may be used to direct energy from the inion.

Direct technique

- During the exhalation phase, ease the greater wings cephalad with your thumb and middle finger (extension motion).
- At the same time, administer a cephalad impulse with the index finger on the median palatine suture, posterior to the transverse palatine suture (extension motion of the vomer) (Figure 8.6, arrows with dotted lines).
- Hold the sphenoid and vomer in extension.
- Breathing assistance: ask the patient to hold an exhalation for as long as possible at the end of an out-breath. Repeat for several breathing cycles.
- Continue as for indirect technique.

8.2.2 Extension dysfunction

Hand position: See flexion dysfunction (section 8.2.1).

Method:

Indirect technique (exaggeration technique)

- During the exhalation phase, ease the greater wings and vomer into extension and hold them there (Figure 8.7, arrows with continuous lines).
- Breathing assistance: ask the patient to hold an exhalation for as long as possible at the end of an out-breath. Repeat for several breathing cycles.
- Establish the PBMT and PBFT.
- A fluid impulse may be used to direct energy from the inion.

Direct technique

- During the inhalation phase, ease the greater wings and vomer into flexion and hold them there (Figure 8.7, arrows with dotted lines).

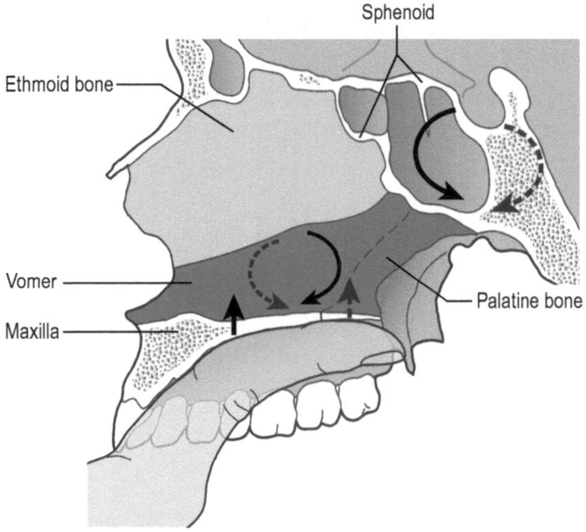

Figure 8.6 Flexion dysfunction of the vomer.

Arrows with continuous lines: indirect technique. Go with the sphenoid into flexion and hold it there. Encourage motion of the vomer into flexion.

Arrows with dotted lines: direct technique. Go with the sphenoid into extension and hold it there. Encourage the motion of the vomer into extension

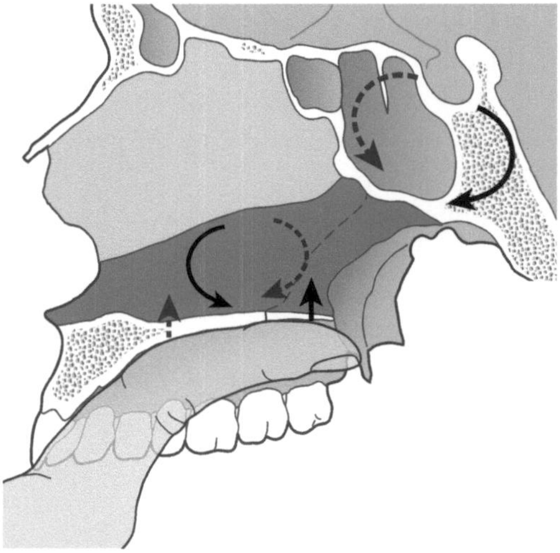

Figure 8.7 Extension dysfunction of the vomer.

Arrows with continuous lines: indirect technique. Go with the sphenoid into extension and hold it there. Encourage the motion of the vomer into extension.

Arrows with dotted lines: direct technique. Go with the sphenoid into flexion and hold it there. Encourage the motion of the vomer into flexion

- Breathing assistance: ask the patient to hold an inhalation at the end of an in-breath for as long as possible. Repeat for several breathing cycles.
- Continue as for indirect technique.

Alternative method to treat flexion or extension dysfunction. Example: flexion dysfunction, indirect technique

- During the inhalation phase, deliver a gentle impulse to encourage motion into flexion.
- During the exhalation phase, passively follow the motion of the vomer.
- In the next inhalation phase, again gently encourage motion into flexion.
- Continue until the restriction is released.

Vitalist approach: See EV-4 technique (section 4.4.3).

8.2.3 Torsion dysfunction, right

Hand position: See flexion dysfunction (section 8.2.1).

Method:

Indirect technique (exaggeration technique)

- Hold the greater wings in a neutral position.
- At the same time, administer an impulse to encourage motion in the direction of ease of the torsion (right) with the index finger on the median palatine suture (Figure 8.8, arrow with continuous line; also Figure 8.5).
- Establish the PBMT and PBFT.
- A fluid impulse may be used to direct energy from the inion.

Direct technique:

- Hold the greater wings in a neutral position.
- At the same time, administer an impulse to encourage motion in the direction of restricted torsion (left) (Figure 8.8, arrow with dotted line; also Figure 8.5) with the index finger on the median palatine suture.
- Continue as for indirect technique.

8.2.4 Lateral shear, e.g., right

Hand position: See Figure 8.9; description, see flexion dysfunction (section 8.2.1).

Method:

Indirect technique (exaggeration technique)

- Hold the greater wings in a neutral position.
- At the same time, administer an impulse in the direction of lateral shear with greater ease of motion (right; see arrow with continuous line in Figure 8.5) with the index finger on the median palatine suture.
- Establish the PBMT and PBFT.
- A fluid impulse may be used to direct energy from the inion.

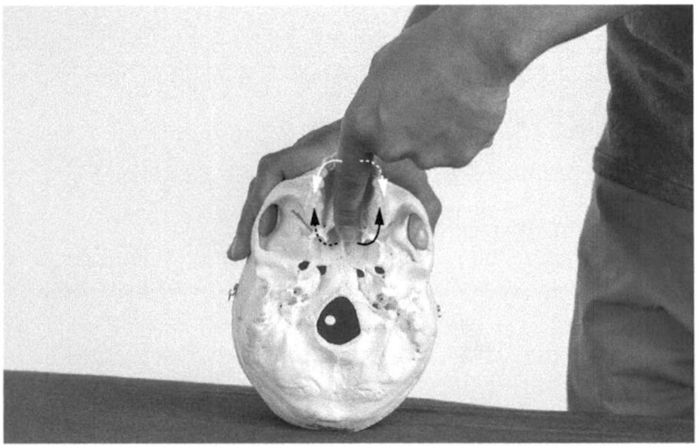

Figure 8.8 Torsion dysfunction of the vomer, right

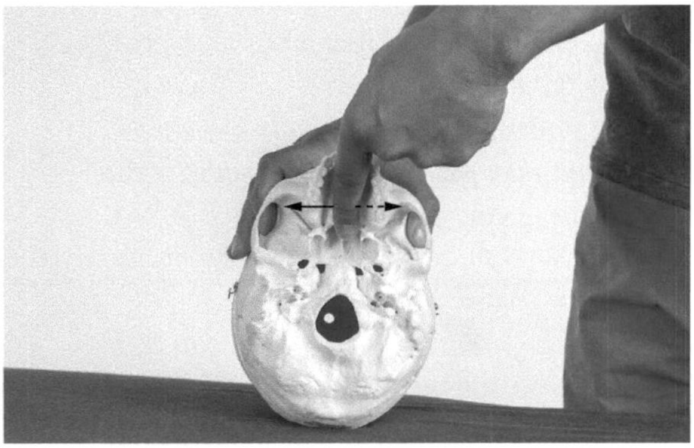

Figure 8.9 Lateral shear of the vomer, right

Direct technique

- Hold the greater wings in a neutral position.
- At the same time, administer an impulse in the direction of restricted lateral shear (left; see arrow with dotted line in Figure 8.5) with the index finger on the median palatine suture.
- Continue as for indirect technique.

8.2.5 Sutural dysfunctions

Sphenovomerine suture

Suture margin: The rostrum of the sphenoid fits between the alae of the vomer.

Suture type: Schindylesis.

Hand position: See flexion dysfunction (section 8.2.1).

Method:

- Indirect technique: with your hands, go with the vomer and sphenoid in the direction of the dysfunction (i.e., the direction of greater ease of motion).
- Establish the PBMT and PBFT between the sphenoid and the vomer.
- Maintain the PBT until a correction of the abnormal tension has been achieved and the inherent homeostatic forces (PRM rhythm, etc.) have brought the correction into effect, and the motion of the vomer and sphenoid has ceased.
- Breathing assistance: ask the patient to hold an inhalation for as long as possible at the end of an in-breath. Repeat for several breathing cycles.
- A fluid impulse may be used to direct energy from the inion.

Vomeromaxillary suture in internal rotation dysfunction of the maxillae

Suture margin: Inferiorly the anterior part of the vomer articulates with the nasal crest of the maxilla.

Suture type: Plane suture.

Aim: To release the vomeromaxillary suture and create freedom of motion of the vomer.

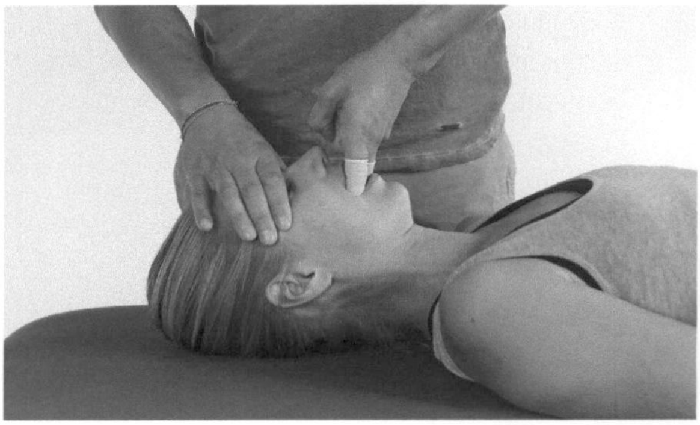

Figure 8.10 Vomeromaxillary suture in internal rotation dysfunction of the maxillae

Practitioner: Take up a position beside the patient's head.

Hand position:

- Cranial hand: span the greater wings with your thumb and middle or index finger.
- Caudal hand: place your middle and index fingers on each side of the maxillae, resting on the teeth.

Method:

- During the inhalation phase, administer an impulse to induce flexion (in a caudal direction) via the greater wings (direct technique).
- At the same time, spread the fingers that are resting on the upper teeth (external rotation of the maxillae; Figure 8.10).
- During the exhalation phase, passively follow the motion of the cranial bones.
- Repeat this procedure for several cycles, until the mobility of the vomer in the vomeromaxillary suture increases.

8.2.6 Decompression

Practitioner: Take up a position beside the patient's head.

Hand position:

- Cranial hand: span the greater wings with your thumb and middle or index finger.

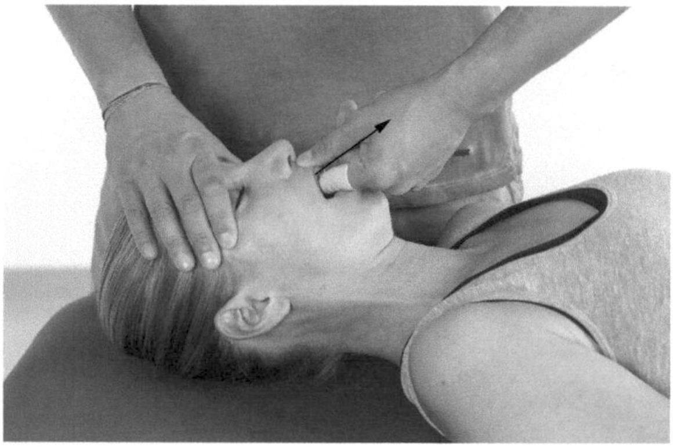

Figure 8.11 Decompression of the vomer

- Caudal hand: position your index finger intraorally, on the median palatine suture (anterior and posterior to the transverse palatine suture). Place your thumb externally below the nose, on the intermaxillary suture.

Method:

- Hold the greater wings in a neutral position.
- At the same time, administer traction in an anterior and inferior direction with the index finger and thumb of your caudal hand, at a roughly 45° angle (Figure 8.11).

8.2.7 Vomer pump technique

Indication: Sinusitis.

Aim: Drainage of the sphenoidal sinus, and to allow secretions to drain away.

Patient: Supine.

Practitioner: Take up a position beside the patient's head.

Hand position:

- Cranial hand: span the greater wings with your thumb and middle and/or index finger.
- Caudal hand: position your index finger intraorally, on the median palatine suture.

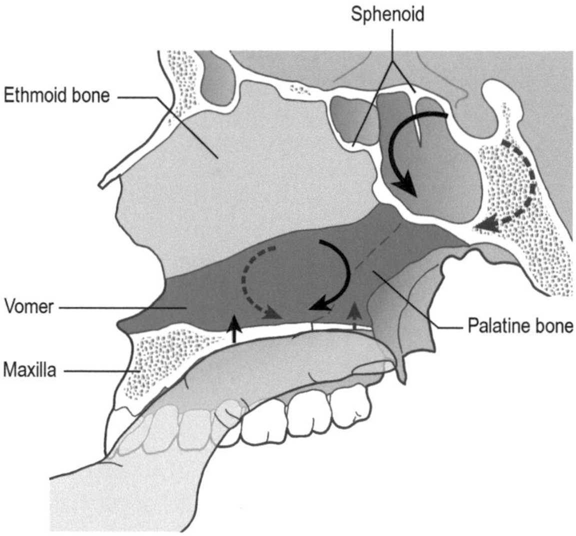

Figure 8.12 Vomer pump technique.

To close the sinus Arrows with dotted lines: during the exhalation phase, impulse to encourage the motion of the vomer into extension and of the sphenoid into extension.

To open the sinus Arrows with continuous lines: during the inhalation phase, impulse to encourage the motion of the vomer into flexion and of the sphenoid into flexion

Method:

To close the sinus

- During the exhalation phase of PRM, administer gentle pressure to the posterior part of the median palatine suture with your index finger (extension of the vomer).
- At the same time, guide the greater wings cephalad, using your thumb and middle finger (extension; Figure 8.12, arrows with dotted lines).

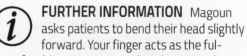

FURTHER INFORMATION Magoun asks patients to bend their head slightly forward. Your finger acts as the fulcrum for this movement, and as the patient's head bends forward, the pressure is transmitted through the posterior part of the vomer to the rostrum of the sphenoid, moving it into extension.[1:172]

- Hold the vomer and sphenoid in extension, and ask the patient to hold an exhalation for as long as possible at the end of an out-breath. Repeat the procedure several times.

To open the sinus

- During the inhalation phase of PRM, administer pressure with your index finger to the anterior part of the median palatine suture (flexion of the vomer).
- At the same time, guide the greater wings caudad using your thumb and middle finger (flexion; Figure 8.12, arrows with continuous lines).
- Hold the vomer and sphenoid in flexion and ask the patient to hold an inhalation for as long as possible at the end of an in-breath. Repeat the procedure several times.

Opposite physiological motion

During the inhalation phase, perform a caudad movement with your middle finger and thumb on the greater wings (flexion motion). At the same time, administer a cephalad impulse to the posterior part of the palatine suture with your index finger (extension motion of the vomer).

During the exhalation phase

- Perform a cephalad movement with your middle finger and thumb on the greater wings (extension motion).
- At the same time, administer a cephalad impulse to the anterior part of the palatine suture with your index finger (flexion motion of the vomer; Figure 8.13, arrows with dotted lines).
- In the next inhalation phase of PRM, again induce opposite physiological motion of the vomer.
- Continue until you sense a relaxation and release of the sphenoid sinuses.

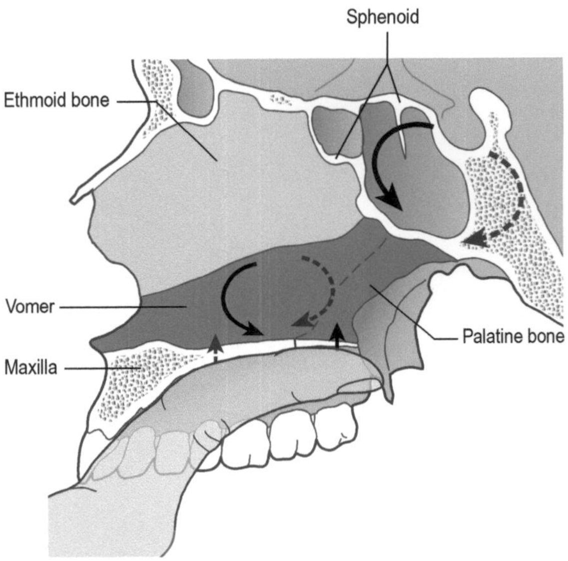

Figure 8.13 Vomer pump technique. Opposite physiological motion.

Arrows with continuous lines: during the inhalation phase, flexion of the sphenoid and encouraging extension of the vomer.

Arrows with dotted lines: during the exhalation phase, extension of the sphenoid and encouraging flexion of the vomer

Finish this technique by resynchronizing the motion of the vomer with that of the sphenoid, in harmony with the PRM rhythm.

During the inhalation phase, go with the sphenoid and the vomer into flexion, and in the exhalation phase, go with both sphenoid and vomer into extension (Figure 8.13, arrows with continuous lines).

8.3 References

1 Magoun, H. I. (1951) *Osteopathy in the Cranial Field*, 3rd Ed. Kirksville: Journal Printing Company.

2 Magoun, H. I. (1976) *Osteopathy in the Cranial Field*, 1st Ed. Kirksville: Journal Printing Company.

9.1 The morphology of the temporal bone according to Rohen 332

9.2 Location, causes, and clinical presentation of osteopathic dysfunctions of the temporal bone 333
9.2.1 Osseous dysfunction (including sutures and other joints) 333
9.2.2 Intraosseous dysfunctions 335
9.2.3 Muscular dysfunction 335
9.2.4 Ligamentous dysfunction 335
9.2.5 Fascial dysfunctions 336
9.2.6 Dysfunction of the tentorium cerebelli 336
9.2.7 Disturbances affecting nerves and parts of the brain 336
9.2.8 Vascular disturbances 338
9.2.9 Disturbances of the endolymphatic ducts 339

9.3 Diagnosis of the temporal bone 339
9.3.1 History-taking 339
9.3.2 Inspection 339
9.3.3 Palpation of position 339
9.3.4 Palpation of PRM rhythm 339
9.3.5 Motion testing 341

9.4 Treatment of the temporal bone 343
9.4.1 Intraosseous dysfunctions 343
9.4.2 Molding 345
9.4.3 Dysfunction in external and internal rotation, unilateral 345
9.4.4 Dysfunction in external and internal rotation, bilateral 348
9.4.5 Dysfunction in anterior and posterior rotation, unilateral 350
9.4.6 Dysfunction in anterior and posterior rotation, bilateral 351
9.4.7 Temporal bone lift technique 352
9.4.8 Sutural dysfunctions 353
9.4.9 Technique for the auditory ossicles 365
9.4.10 Dural techniques 365
9.4.11 Specific testing and technique for the falx cerebri and falx cerebelli 366
9.4.12 Treatment of the tentorium cerebelli 367
9.4.13 Fluid/electrodynamic techniques 368
9.4.14 Auditory tube technique 370

9.5 References 370

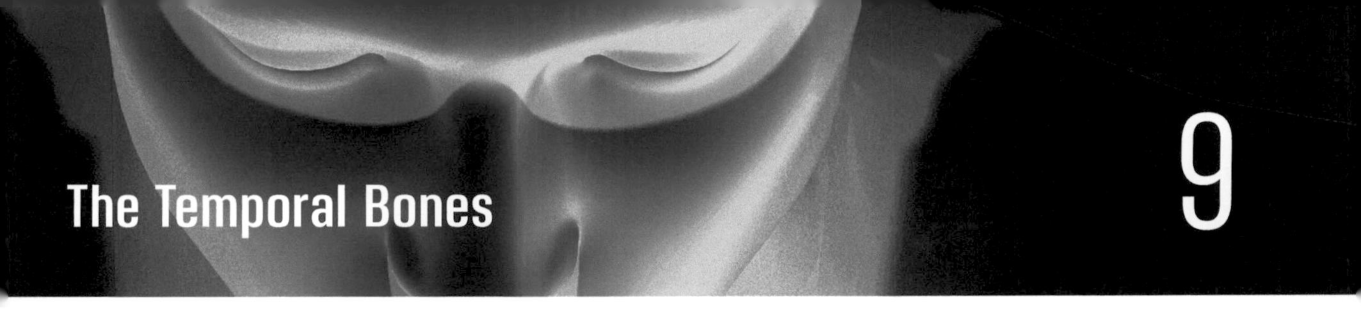

9 The Temporal Bones

The temporal bone consists of three parts (squamous, tympanic, and petrous). At birth, these are still not completely joined.

Seen from the morphological point of view, there are similarities between the paired temporal bones and the bones of the pelvis. Ascending and descending polarities unite in the temporal bone. The squamous part belongs to the calvaria, and spreads upward, fanning out as it does so. It undergoes membranous ossification. The petrous part, whose wedge-like shape thrusts downward, into the cranium, belongs to the cranial base; it ossifies endochondrally. Between the two lies the zygomatic process, aligned horizontally forward.

Muscular connections link with the sternum, clavicle, thoracic spine, hyoid bone, pharynx, palate, masticatory system, eardrum, and middle ear. There are ligamentous connections to the sphenoid, hyoid, mandible, and middle ear. There are fascial connections in the temporal fascia (indirectly in the investing layer of the cervical fascia), cervical fascia, prevertebral layer, interpterygoid aponeurosis, pharynx, "rideau stylien" (styloid apparatus and associated tissues), and to the tentorium cerebelli (see also this volume, section 2.1.8 and Volume 2, Chapter 4).

Neural connections exist with functions of the temporal lobe, the cerebellum, almost all the cranial nerves (except CN I, CN II, and CN XII), and the internal carotid plexus. Many venous channels run in the temporal bone. The courses of the internal carotid artery, middle meningeal artery, occipital artery, tympanic arteries, and labyrinthine artery are also important.

9.1 The morphology of the temporal bone according to Rohen[9]

There are striking similarities in shape between the embryonic hip bone and the temporal bone: the ilium can be compared with the temporal squama, the ischium and pubis to the mastoid zygomatic processes, and the acetabulum resembles the temporomandibular joint and the external acoustic meatus. For a real understanding of the structures, we need more than just a simple description of similarities between individual elements or homologous features. We need to understand the functional dynamics, including the motions and attitudes seen in the development and growth of the tissue. It is in motion that we gain a deeper understanding, because in motion we find the origin of form.

The temporal bone displays a remarkably similar dynamic to the pelvis, a similar "gesture" or attitude in terms of its polarity as its form unfolds. We see this in the way the ilium opens its surface upward, separating itself from the space around it, rising up and expressing a lightness, while the developing character of the ischium is expressed in a downward thickening of the bone, fortifying, static, and incorporated into the space around it.

Just as the pelvis anchors and balances movements from above and below, so the temporal bone serves to unify these two polarities.

The pelvis establishes and maintains balance upward and downward, and is the point from which the dynamic of motion of the lower limbs originates, reaching out into the space around. In a way the hip joint is the gateway to the world outside. In a corresponding way, the process of hearing brings the inner nature of that world outside into the consciousness, so that the external acoustic meatus is the gateway to inside.

The pneumatization of the petrous part begins in the eighth month of intrauterine development. An epithelial anlage into the middle ear quickly grows and displaces the mesenchyme. This process is complete by the time of birth, but then continues into the inner ear region. In the course of development the petrous part dies off, in effect, to the point where it becomes the hardest, most lifeless bone in the body, which (unlike other intercartilaginous bones) is incapable of any further adaptive or transmutational processes.

9.2 Location, causes, and clinical presentation of osteopathic dysfunctions of the temporal bone

Tip for practitioners

Primary dysfunctions

- Intraosseous: the temporal bone forms part of the cranial base (this portion of the bone has a cartilaginous anlage); and also of the calvaria (this portion has a membranous anlage). At birth, the temporal bone consists of the squamous part with the tympanic ring (tympanic part) and the petrous part. Direct force to the temporal bone, especially during birth or infancy, can give rise to dysfunctions between the petromastoid part/tympanic part, petromastoid part/squamous part, and squamous part/tympanic part.
- Primary traumatic: perinatal, or caused by falls, blows, tooth extraction, whiplash injury, or other effects of force on the sutures; all can lead to motion restrictions of the temporal bone. This can cause compression of the occipitomastoid suture or condylo-squamoso-mastoid pivot point (CSMP), which can result in asynchronous motion between the occipital bone and temporal bone. Falls onto the pelvis can also cause dysfunction of the temporal bone.

Secondary dysfunctions

- Dysfunction of the occipital bone, e.g., in SBS dysfunctions, tension transmitted from the tentorium cerebelli, or extracranial muscle or fascial tension (sternocleidomastoid, trapezius, overall tonicity of the nuchal muscles, etc.) and pelvic dysfunctions, can give rise to motion restrictions of the temporal bone.

9.2.1 Osseous dysfunction (including sutures and other joints)

- **Petrojugular suture and petro-occipital fissure (petrobasilar suture, petro-occipital synchondrosis)**
  - Causes: in connection with the occipital bone: primary traumatic, e.g., in tooth extractions with mouth wide open. Leads to impairment of motion of the temporal bone.
  - Clinical presentation: all functions of structures linked with the temporal bone.
- **Occipitomastoid suture and condylo-squamoso-mastoid pivot point (CSMP)**
  - Causes:
    - In the case of bilateral compression: fall or blow to the occipital squama.
    - In the case of unilateral compression: fall or blow to the side of the occipital squama.
    - Whiplash injury, and sometimes as a result of a direct thrust technique at the back of the head.
    - Secondary to compression of the atlanto-occipital joint or dysfunction of the sphenopetrosal synchondrosis.
  - Sequelae:
    - The effect of unilateral compression may be to force the occipital squama in an anterior direction, the basilar part of the occipital bone in an inferior direction, and the temporal bones into internal rotation. The concave mastoid border of the occipital bone is forced anteriorly and superiorly, wedging it into the convex posterior border of the mastoid part of the temporal bone and moving the mastoid part posteriorly and medially.
    - Compression of the sphenopetrosal synchondrosis may cause opposite motion of the temporal bone relative to the occipital bone, i.e., the occipital bone moves into flexion and the temporal bone into internal rotation.

- Clinical presentation/hypothetical pathology:
  * Abnormal tensions of the tentorium cerebelli.
  * Venous congestion of sinuses (sigmoid sinus).
  * Disturbances in the fluctuation of cerebrospinal fluid.
  * Disturbances of the cerebellum, medulla oblongata, or other centers of the brain, and of the vagus nerve (nausea, vomiting, etc.).
- Sequelae: dysfunction of the SBS and change in the frequency and amplitude of the PRM rhythm, affecting homeostasis of the body overall.

- **Parietomastoid suture**
  - Causes: a fall or blow from above onto the ipsilateral parietal bone.
- **Sphenosquamous suture and sphenosquamous pivot point (SSP)**
  - Causes: primary injury from a fall or blow to the cheek or the ipsilateral mastoid process. Secondary: in connection with the sphenoid bone or hypertonicity of the temporalis muscle (in psychological stress or temporomandibular joint syndrome).
  - Clinical presentation/hypothetical pathology:
    * At the vertical course of the suture: middle meningeal artery, migraine.[5:76,176,282]
    * At the horizontal course of the suture: greater and lesser petrosal nerves. Greater petrosal nerve (to the pterygopalatine ganglion): disturbance of the lacrimal gland, dryness or irritation of the mucosa of the nose, nasopharynx, and palate, allergic rhinitis (pterygopalatine fossa, this volume, section 3.1.2). Lesser petrosal nerve: disturbance of the parotid gland.
    * Functional disturbance of adjacent parts of the brain.
  - Sequelae: dysfunction of the SBS and change in the frequency and amplitude of PRM rhythm, affecting homeostasis of the body overall.
- **Sphenopetrosal synchondrosis**
  - Causes: tooth extraction from the upper jaw can cause ipsilateral dysfunction of the petrosphenoidal ligament, and tooth extraction from the lower jaw can cause contralateral dysfunction of the ligament. Cranial nerves CN III, CN IV, and CN VI (which supply the muscles of the eye) run alongside the body of the sphenoid, near this ligament. CN VI in particular is vulnerable to tensions originating in this ligament.
  - Clinical presentation: disturbances of the eye, fatigue strabismus in young children, etc.
- **Temporozygomatic suture**
  - Causes: a fall or blow to the cheek or SBS dysfunctions.
  - Sequelae: impairment of motion of the zygomatic bone and of the integration between sphenoid and occipital bones.

FURTHER INFORMATION A restriction of the temporozygomatic suture can mean that the zygomatic process of the temporal bone cannot glide outward and inferiorly with the temporal process of the zygomatic bone during the inhalation phase. This would fix the temporal bone in internal rotation during the inhalation phase.
Recall that the zygomatic bone is mainly influenced by the sphenoid and the temporal bone by the occipital bone.

- **Temporomandibular joint** (see Chapter 2)
  - Unilateral and bilateral anomalies of dental occlusion, protrusion and retraction, etc.
  - Disturbances to dental growth.
  - Bruxism (grinding of the teeth).
  - Clicking due to dysfunction of the articular disk.

- "Popping."
- Disturbances of hearing (tinnitus, etc.) or of balance.
- Eye disturbances, taste disturbances.

- **Pharyngotympanic (auditory) tube** (see also Volume 2, section 6.1.2): causes and clinical presentation
  - Internal rotation of the temporal bone → narrowing of the cartilaginous auditory tube → hissing, high-pitched sound.
  - External rotation of the temporal bone → widening of the auditory tube → pulsations, low-pitched sound.

Explanation The sounds heard are probably produced by the blood flow in the internal carotid artery where it forms a bend inside the petrous part of the temporal bone. At this point it is separated from the inner ear only by a thin plate of bone, so that structural changes in this region can cause tinnitus.

9.2.2 Intraosseous dysfunctions

Intraosseous dysfunctions between:

- Petromastoid part/tympanic part.
- Petromastoid part/squamous part.
- Squamous part/tympanic plate.

At birth the temporal bone consists of the squamous part and tympanic ring (tympanic part), and the petrous part. The squamous part and the tympanic part are already partially joined at the time of birth. This gives rise to the petrosquamous fissure, which is a potential site for intraosseous dysfunctions.

The squamous part, petrous part, and styloid process fuse during the first year of life. The mastoid process does not develop until after the second year of life, so cannot yet be palpated in the newborn. The styloid process is still cartilaginous in the newborn, and its proximal and distal parts do not unite until puberty. The mandibular fossa is still shallow at birth and deepens only during the development of the articular tubercle.

Causes Primary injury, by direct force to the temporal bone, especially during birth and infancy. Secondary injury, through dysfunctions of other bones (occipital bone, sphenoid).

Sequelae Reduced pliancy of the bone and functional impairment of all involved structures.

9.2.3 Muscular dysfunction

- **At the mastoid process**
  - Sternocleidomastoid (SCM). (Clinical presentation: headache, abnormal head posture.)
  - Splenius capitis.
  - Digastric (posterior belly).
- **At the styloid process**
  - Stylohyoid. (Clinical presentation: grinding of teeth, pain in the floor of the mouth, pharynx, and larynx.)
  - Styloglossus.
  - Stylopharyngeus.
- **Masticatory muscles**
  - Temporalis: at the temporal fossa.
  - Masseter: at the zygomatic process of the temporal bone.
- **Other muscles**
  - Levator veli palatini: at the inferior opening of the carotid canal that passes through the petrous part.
  - Tensor tympani: the tensor muscle of the tympanic membrane, in the canal for the tensor tympani.
  - Stapedius. (Clinical presentation: abnormal hearing sensitivity.)

9.2.4 Ligamentous dysfunction

- **Petrosphenoidal ligament** (Gruber's ligament) at the sphenopetrosal synchondrosis (see this volume, section 5.2.3).
- **Stylomandibular ligament** Causes: tooth extraction.
- **Stylohyoid ligament**
  - Causes: ossification of the ligament.
  - Sequelae: motion restriction of the hyoid bone.
- **Anterior ligament of the malleus:** from the anterior process of the hammer into the

petrotympanic fissure, from where some fibers run to the spine of the sphenoid and on to the ramus of the mandible, together with the sphenomandibular ligament.

- **Pintus ligament:** irregular occurrence; from the hammer through the petrotympanic fissure to the head of the mandible.
  - Causes: dysfunction of the temporomandibular joint.
  - Clinical presentation: hearing disturbances.

9.2.5 Fascial dysfunctions

See this volume, sections 2.6.4 and 3.2.4, and Volume 2, section 4.2.2.

- Temporal fascia.
- Investing layer of cervical fascia.
- Prevertebral layer of cervical fascia.
- Interpterygoid aponeurosis.
- The “rideau stylien” (styloid apparatus and its adjacent tissues).
- Pharynx.

Causes: muscular, organic disturbances, etc.

Sequelae: motion restrictions of the temporal bone, functional disturbances of involved structures.

9.2.6 Dysfunction of the tentorium cerebelli

- Causes: meningitis, cranial injury, motion restriction, etc.
- Clinical presentation/hypothetical pathology
  - Superior aspect: pain in the eye and the external frontal region.
  - Inferior aspect: pain behind the ear, in the front of the head, and the eye. Obstruction to venous flow in the transverse sinus, sigmoid sinus, inferior and superior petrosal sinuses, headache, and motion restriction of the temporal bone.

9.2.7 Disturbances affecting nerves and parts of the brain

- **Temporal lobe** Causes: dysfunctions in the middle cranial fossa and motion restrictions of the temporal bone, especially internal rotation (IR) of the temporal bone.
- **Cerebellum**
  - Causes: IR of the temporal bone, torsion of the tentorium cerebelli.
  - Clinical presentation: disturbances of balance, of muscle tonus, and of coordination of voluntary muscle activity.
- **Oculomotor (CN III) and trochlear (CN IV) nerves**
  - Causes: dural tensions at the attachment of the tentorium cerebelli to the posterior clinoid process, tensions and stasis at the walls of the cavernous sinus, and dysfunctions at the superior border of the petrous part of the temporal bone.
  - Clinical presentation:
    - CN III, motor: lateral deviation of the eye, horizontal double vision, divergent strabismus, restriction of the line of vision upward, downward, and medially.
    - CN III, autonomic: mydriasis, ptosis, and impairment of the photomotor reflex.
    - CN IV: upward and medial deviation of the eye, vertical or oblique double vision, convergent strabismus.
- **Trigeminal nerve (CN V)** The trigeminal ganglion lies in a dural sac in the trigeminal impression on the anterior surface of the petrous part.
  - Causes: dural tensions affecting the tentorium cerebelli, the meningeal dura of the trigeminal ganglion; change in the position of the temporal bone, tensions and stasis in the wall of the cavernous sinus (CN V_1, V_2).
  - A dysfunction of the temporomandibular joint with tensions at the medial and lateral pterygoid muscles leads to disturbances of the articulation of the sphenoid and palatine bones, which may sometimes affect the pterygopalatine ganglion (CN V_2) in the pterygopalatine foramen.

- Clinical presentation:
  - Trigeminal cave: pain in the facial region.
  - Trigeminal neuralgia, disturbances of sensation affecting the face, functional disturbances of the masticatory muscles, inhibition of the sneezing reflex (CN V_2) or corneal reflex (CN V_1), pain and watering of the eye (CN V_1, some parasympathetic fibers in trigeminal nerve).
- **Abducent nerve (CN VI):** at the apex of the petrous part of the temporal bone, between the petrous part and the petrosphenoidal ligament
  - Causes: cranial nerve VI is particularly vulnerable to tensions arising from the tentorium and petrosphenoidal ligament because of the fibrous link between the nerve and this ligament and the fact that it runs in an osteofibrous canal formed by this ligament and the petrous part of the temporal bone. Stasis and tensions in the wall of the cavernous sinus can also cause disturbances of the abducent nerve.
  - Clinical presentation: fatigue strabismus in young children, horizontal double vision, convergent strabismus, lateral restriction of the line of vision, tendency to hold the head turned to one side to compensate for the functional deficiency.
- **Facial nerve (CN VII) and intermediate nerve (CN VII):** pass through the internal acoustic meatus in the facial canal; unite at the geniculate ganglion; branch at the chorda tympani of sensory fibers and those supplying special sense (taste); main portion passes through the stylomastoid foramen
  - Causes: dural tensions at the internal acoustic meatus and stylomastoid foramen.
  - Clinical presentation:
    - Facial nerve (CN VII): disturbance of facial expression.
    - Intermediate nerve (CN VII): disturbance of saliva secretion, taste disturbances relating to the anterior two-thirds of the tongue, functional disturbance of the lacrimal, nasal, and palatine glands (via the greater petrosal nerve).
- **Vestibulocochlear nerve (CN VIII):** through the internal acoustic meatus to the organs of hearing and balance
  - Causes: dural tensions at the temporal bone and internal acoustic meatus, dysfunction of the petrojugular suture.
  - Clinical presentation: disturbances of hearing, disturbances of balance.
- **Glossopharyngeal nerve (CN IX), vagus nerve (CN X), accessory nerve (CN XI):** at the jugular notch with the intrajugular process
  - Causes: dural tensions at the jugular foramen, dysfunction of the occipital and temporal bones, the occipitomastoid suture, petrojugular suture, and petro-occipital fissure (petrobasilar suture, petro-occipital synchondrosis).
  - Clinical presentation:
    - CN IX: disturbances of taste, dry mouth (parasympathetic fibers supplying the parotid gland), disturbances of swallowing (fibers supplying sensation to the pharynx).
    - CN X: disturbances of cardiac, digestive, and respiratory function, disturbances of speaking and swallowing.
    - CN XI: torticollis.
- **Greater and lesser petrosal nerves:** in the groove of the same name
  - Causes: dural tensions in the groove.
  - Clinical presentation:
    - Greater petrosal nerve: functional disturbance of the lacrimal, nasal, and palatine glands.
    - Lesser petrosal nerve: functional disturbance of the parotid gland.
- **Parasympathetic fibers**
  - Course:
    - Some parasympathetic fibers run together with the facial nerve (CN VII) and innervate part of the internal tympanic membrane.

    * Some parasympathetic fibers run together with the chorda tympani (CN VII) and then on with CN V_3.
    * Some fibers run together with the glossopharyngeal nerve (CN IX) and on to the otic ganglion via the lesser petrosal nerve and then onward with CN V_3.
    * Most together with the vagus nerve (CN X).
  - Interactions can occur between the tympanic membrane and parasympathetic system, e.g., sounds affect the vagus nerve and may produce reactions within the autonomic system.[7:22]
- **Internal carotid plexus**
  - Causes: dural tensions at the carotid canal and foramen lacerum, and changes in position of the apex of the petrous part of the temporal bone, and abnormal tensions of the dura mater at the cavernous sinus.
  - Clinical presentation/hypothetical pathology: disturbances of the sympathetic system.

9.2.8 Vascular disturbances

- **Internal carotid artery**
  - Causes: dural tensions at the carotid canal and at the foramen lacerum, and changes in position of the apex of the petrous part of the temporal bone, and abnormal tensions of the dura mater at the cavernous sinus.
  - The anterior and posterior margins of the foramen lacerum are formed by the posterior border of the greater wing of the sphenoid and the anterior portion of the petrous part of the temporal bone. The foramen lacerum is divided into two by the sphenoidal lingula. It is open on the outside, and closed with fibrocartilage inside. The internal carotid artery lies on this.
  - Clinical presentation/hypothetical pathology: disturbances of the sympathetic system via effect on the internal carotid plexus.
- **Middle meningeal artery**
  - Causes: compression of the sphenosquamous suture and sphenosquamous pivot (SSP), abnormal tensions of the dura mater in the middle cranial fossa.
  - Clinical presentation: migraine and raised intracranial pressure.
- **Occipital artery**
  - Causes: dural tensions in the occipital groove, medial to the mastoid notch.
- **Jugular vein**
  - Causes: dural tensions at the jugular foramen, dysfunction of the occipital and temporal bones, the occipitomastoid suture, petrojugular suture, and petro-occipital fissure (petrobasilar suture; petro-occipital synchondrosis). The jugular foramen resembles a widened suture between the occipital and temporal bones and so can easily be affected by dysfunctions of these bones.
  - Clinical presentation/hypothetical pathology: venous congestion in the cranium, headache, memory disturbances, impairment of brain function.
- **Venous sinuses**
  - **Sigmoid sinus:** in the groove of the same name at the posterior, inferior corner of the petrous part.
  - **Superior petrosal sinus:** in the groove of the same name, on the crest of the posterior border of the petrous part.
  - **Inferior petrosal sinus:** in the groove of the same name, below the opening of the internal acoustic meatus.
  - Causes: change in position of the apex of the petrous part of the temporal bone and abnormal tensions of the tentorium cerebelli.
  - Clinical presentation/hypothetical pathology:
    * Region of the sigmoid sinus → pain behind the ear.
    * Region of the superior petrosal sinus → pain in the temporal region of the head.
    * Venous congestion of regions of the brain → headache, impairment of the relevant function of the brain.

* Venous congestion affecting the eyes → visual disturbances, sensation of pressure.
- Sequelae:
  * Sigmoid sinus: congestion in the confluence of sinuses and superior petrosal sinus.
  * Superior and inferior petrosal sinuses: congestion affecting the cavernous sinus and basilar venous plexus, ophthalmic veins and veins of the medulla, pons, and inferior surface of the cerebellum as well as other regions of the brain.

9.2.9 Disturbances of the endolymphatic ducts

- Causes: tensions at the endolymphatic sac hinder the drainage of endolymph into the dura.
- Clinical presentation: dizziness.

9.3 Diagnosis of the temporal bone

9.3.1 History-taking

The most common symptoms are deafness, tinnitus, dizziness, earache, otitis media, neuralgia (trigeminal neuralgia), migraine, headache, tic douloureux, problems of the temporomandibular joint ("clicking" of the joint, dental malocclusion, pain), and facial nerve paralysis. The temporal bone can also be involved in disturbances of the eye muscles, the nose, the oral cavity, in autism, and in shoulder-hand syndrome (reflex sympathetic dystrophy).

CAUTION Previous injury should always be considered.

9.3.2 Inspection

- Ear: protruding (ER) or close-lying (IR).
- Unilaterally protruding or close-lying ear: torsion or lateroflexion-rotation of the SBS.

9.3.3 Palpation of position

- Mastoid process: posteromedial (ER) or anterolateral (IR).
- Mastoid part of temporal bone: anterolateral (ER) or posteromedial (IR).
- Squamoparietal suture: separated and displaced anterolaterally (ER) or approximated and displaced posteromedially (IR).

9.3.4 Palpation of PRM rhythm

Tip for practitioners

Biomechanical, inhalation phase

Several axes of motion have been described for the temporal bone.[3] One axis runs through the SSP and CSMP.

- There is external rotation of the temporal bone.
- The petrobasilar part moves in a superior and anterior direction.
- The temporal squama moves in a lateral, anterior, and slightly inferior direction.
- The mastoid process moves in a medial, posterior (and superior) direction.
- The mandibular fossa moves in a posteromedial direction.
- The zygomatic process moves in a lateral direction, and inferiorly it also moves in an anterior and inferior direction.

Developmental dynamic, inhalation phase

- The temporal squamae move centrifugally (outward motion).
- The convexity of the temporal squamae becomes less. They become shallower.

If palpation reveals a motion restriction, an impulse in the restricted direction will emphasize the restriction and enable you to sense which structure is the origin of the restriction.

Practitioner: Take up a position at the head of the patient.

Hand position:

- Place your thenar eminences on the mastoid part of the temporal bone on each side.
- Position your thumbs on the anterior tip of the mastoid process on each side.
- Place the palms of your hands on the occiput.
- Clasp your fingers together.
- Rest your elbows on the treatment table (Figure 9.1).

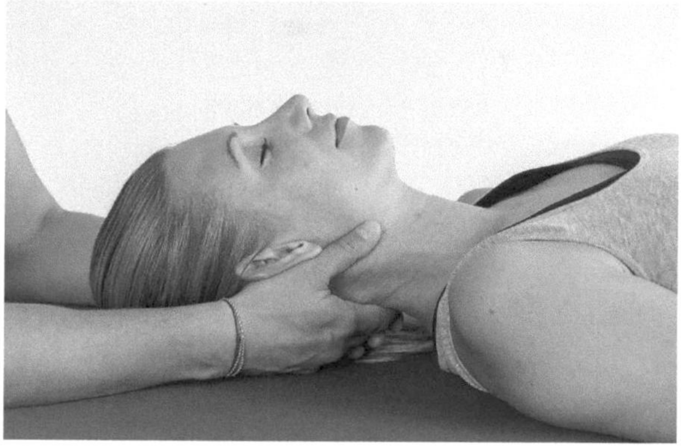

Figure 9.1 Palpation of PRM rhythm of the temporal bone

Biomechanical:

Inhalation phase of PRM rhythm, normal finding (Figure 9.2)

- Your thumbs, resting on the tips of the mastoid processes, will sense a posteromedial motion.
- With the thenar eminences resting on the mastoid part of each temporal bone, you will sense an anterolateral motion.
- The palms of your hands will sense the flexion motion of the occipital bone. (The zygomatic processes move laterally, with an additional anterior and inferior motion of the anterior portion.)

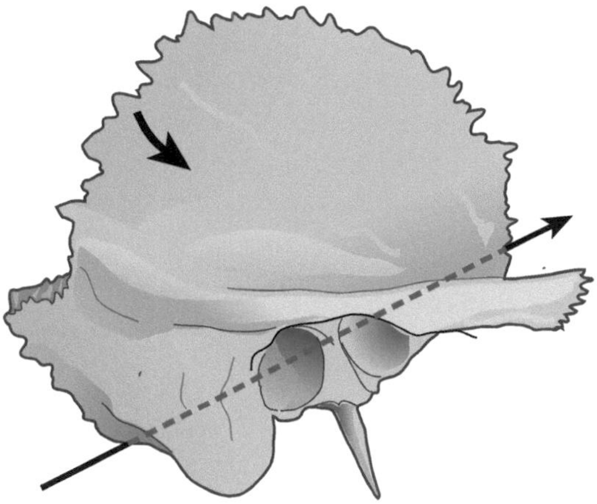

Figure 9.2 Inhalation phase of PRM/biomechanical

Exhalation phase of PRM, normal finding

- Your thumbs, resting on the tips of the mastoid processes, will sense an anterolateral motion.
- With the thenar eminences resting on the mastoid parts of the temporal bones, you will sense a posteromedial motion.
- The palms of your hands will sense the extension motion of the occipital bone. (The zygomatic processes move medially, with an additional posterior and superior motion of the anterior portion.)

Biodynamic, embryological approach: Inhalation phase of PRM, normal finding (Figure 9.3)

- The squamae of the temporal bones move centrifugally (outward motion).

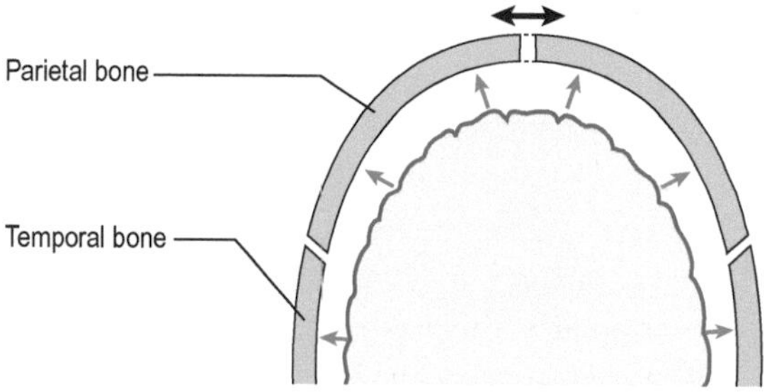

Figure 9.3 Inhalation phase of PRM/developmental dynamic

- The convexity of the squamae becomes less, i.e., they become flatter.

Exhalation phase of PR, normal finding

- The squamae of the temporal bones move in a centripetal direction.
- The convexity of the squamae becomes greater.

Compare the amplitude, strength, ease, and symmetry of the motions of the temporal bones.

Other types of motion of the temporal bone may sometimes occur during external and internal rotation. These provide an indication of any further dysfunctions of the particular temporal bone.

9.3.5 Motion testing

This resembles the palpation of primary respiration except that in motion testing the external and internal rotation motion of the temporal bones is actively induced by the practitioner.

Testing of external and internal rotation

Hand position:

As for palpation of the PRM rhythm (this chapter, section 9.3.4).

Method:

- During the inhalation phase: at the beginning of the inhalation phase, administer an impulse in a posteromedial direction with your thumbs positioned on the tips of the mastoid processes.
- During the exhalation phase: at the beginning of the exhalation phase, administer an impulse in a posteromedial direction with the thenar eminences of your thumbs, positioned on the mastoid parts of the temporal bones.
- Compare the amplitude and ease of motion or the amount of force needed to elicit movement.

Testing external and internal rotation, alternative hand position

Hand position:

- Grasp the zygomatic process of each side between your thumb and index finger.
- Place your middle fingers in the external acoustic meatus of each side.
- Place your ring fingers on the tip of the mastoid process each side.
- Position the little finger of each hand on the mastoid part of the temporal bone.
- Rest both elbows on the treatment table (Figure 9.4).

Method:

During the inhalation phase

- At the beginning of the inhalation phase, administer an impulse in an inferior and lateral direction with your thumbs on the zygomatic processes.
- With your middle fingers in the external acoustic meatus, administer an impulse to ease the temporal bones into anterior rotation and external rotation.
- At the same time, administer a posteromedial impulse with your ring fingers, on the mastoid processes.

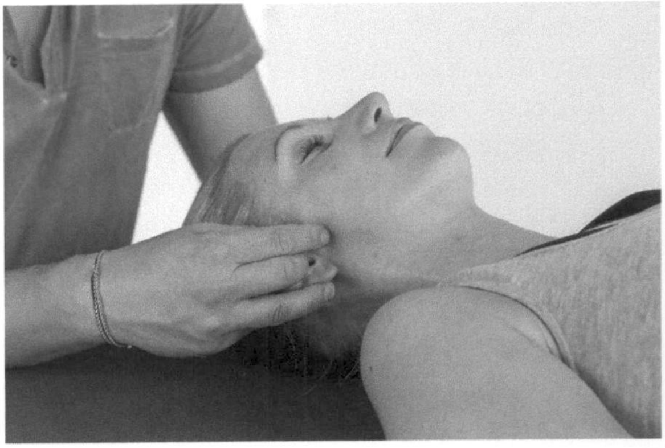

Figure 9.4 Testing external and internal rotation, alternative hand position

During the exhalation phase

- At the beginning of the exhalation phase, administer an impulse in a superior and medial direction with your index fingers on the zygomatic processes.
- With your middle fingers in the external acoustic meatus, administer an impulse to ease the temporal bones into posterior rotation and internal rotation.
- At the same time, administer a posteromedial impulse with your little fingers on the mastoid parts of the temporal bone.

Unilateral testing of external and internal rotation

Hand position:

- Hold the occipital bone in the palm of one hand.
- Position the fingers of the other hand on the temporal bone as described above.
- Rest both elbows on the treatment table (Figure 9.5).

Method:

During the inhalation phase

- At the beginning of the inhalation phase, administer an impulse into flexion with the palm of your hand on the occipital bone.

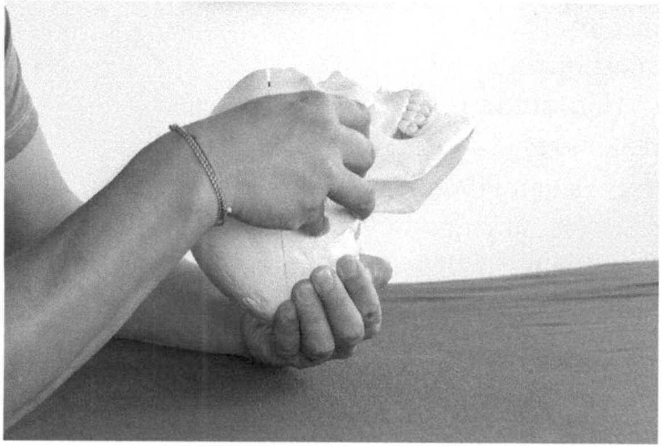

Figure 9.5 Unilateral testing of external and internal rotation (shown on model)

- With your other hand, note the reaction of the temporal bone. Normal finding:
  - External rotation of the temporal bone.
  - Zygomatic process in an inferior, lateral, and anterior direction (thumb and index finger).
  - External acoustic meatus into anterior rotation and external rotation (middle finger).
  - Mastoid process in a posteromedial direction (ring finger).
  - Mastoid part of temporal bone in an anterolateral direction (little finger).

During the exhalation phase

- At the beginning of the exhalation phase, administer an impulse to ease motion into extension with the hand on the occiput.
- With your other hand, sense the reaction of the temporal bone. Normal finding:
  - Internal rotation of the temporal bone.
  - Zygomatic process in a superior, medial, and posterior direction (thumb and index finger).
  - External acoustic meatus into posterior rotation and internal rotation (middle finger).
  - Mastoid process in an anterolateral direction (ring finger).
  - Mastoid part of the temporal bone in a posteromedial direction (little finger).

Compare the amplitude and ease of motion and the amount of force needed to elicit movement.

Test of anterior and posterior rotation

Hand position:

- Grasp the zygomatic process of each side between your thumb and index finger.
- Place your middle finger in the external acoustic meatus on each side.
- Position the ring finger each side anterior to the mastoid process.

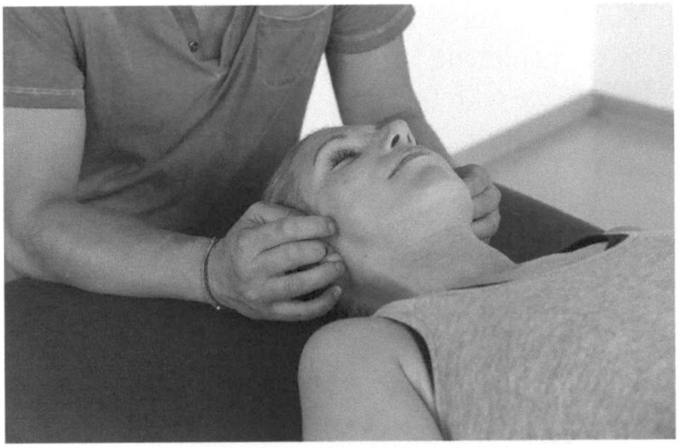

Figure 9.6 Test of anterior and posterior rotation

- Position the little finger each side posterior to the mastoid process.
- Rest both elbows on the treatment table (Figure 9.6).

Method:

During the inhalation phase

- At the beginning of the inhalation phase, administer an impulse in an inferior direction with your thumbs on the zygomatic processes.
- With your middle fingers in the external acoustic meatus, administer an impulse to ease the temporal bones into anterior rotation.
- At the same time, with the ring fingers and little fingers on the mastoid processes, administer an impulse in a superior direction.

During the exhalation phase

- At the beginning of the exhalation phase, administer an impulse in a superior direction with the index fingers on the zygomatic processes.
- With the middle fingers in the external acoustic meatus, administer an impulse to ease the temporal bones into posterior rotation.
- At the same time, with the ring fingers and little fingers on the mastoid processes, administer an impulse in an inferior direction.

Compare the amplitude and ease of motion and the strength needed to elicit movement.

9.4 Treatment of the temporal bone

9.4.1 Intraosseous dysfunctions

Indication: Primary intraosseous dysfunctions, especially those due to direct force to the temporal bone during birth and in infancy, or secondary intraosseous dysfunctions.

Petromastoid part/tympanic part (right), according to Frymann

Hand position:

- Hold the occipital bone in your left hand, with your fingertips resting on the mastoid part and mastoid process.
- Place the little finger of your right hand in the external acoustic meatus (Figure 9.7).[1]

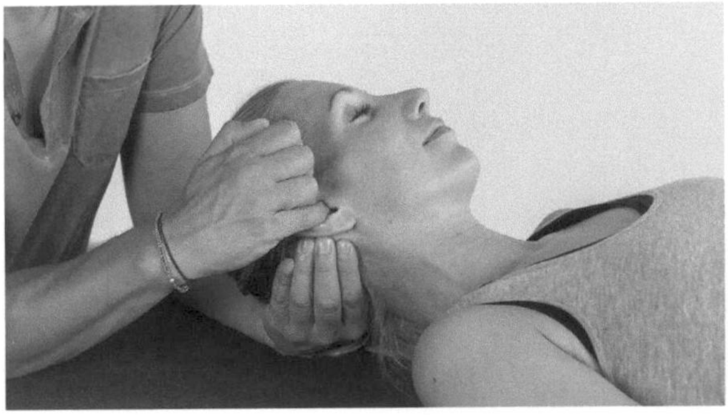

Figure 9.7 Petromastoid part/tympanic part (right)

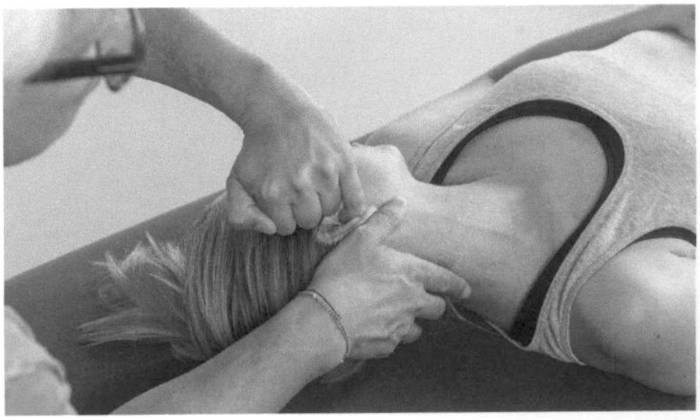

Figure 9.8 Petromastoid part/tympanic part. Alternative hand position

Alternative hand position:

- The patient's head is turned to the left.
- Right hand
  - ▸ Place your thumb on the mastoid process.
  - ▸ Place the thenar eminence on the mastoid part of the temporal bone.
  - ▸ Hold the occipital bone in the remaining fingers of that hand.
- Left hand: place the little finger of your left hand in the external acoustic meatus (Figure 9.8).

Petromastoid part/squamous part (right)

Hand position:

- Hold the occipital bone in your left hand, with your fingertips resting on the mastoid part and mastoid process.
- Rest the index and middle fingers of your right hand, and also your ring finger if necessary, on the squamous part (Figure 9.9).

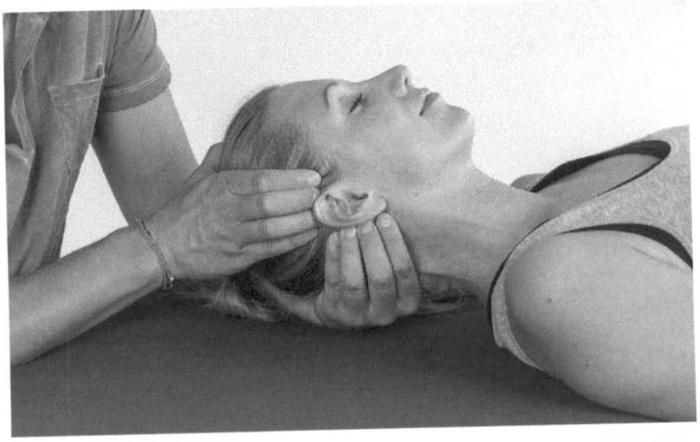

Figure 9.9 Petromastoid part/squamous part (right)

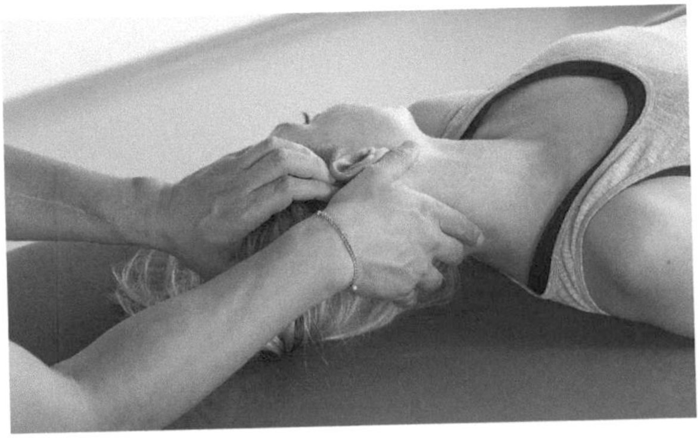

Figure 9.10 Petromastoid part/squamous part. Alternative hand position

Alternative hand position:

- The patient's head is turned to the left.
- Right hand
  - ▸ Place your thumb on the mastoid process.
  - ▸ Place the thenar eminence on the mastoid part of the temporal bone.
  - ▸ Hold the occipital bone in the remaining fingers of that hand.
- Left hand: rest the index and middle fingers of your left hand, and also your ring finger if necessary, on the squamous part (Figure 9.10).

Squamous part/tympanic part (right)

Hand position:

- The patient's head is turned to the left.
- Rest the index and middle fingers of your left hand, and also your ring finger if necessary, on the squamous part.
- Place the little finger of your right hand in the external acoustic meatus (Figure 9.11).

Method:

Direct technique

- Guide both portions of the bone in the direction of restricted motion until you reach the motion barrier.

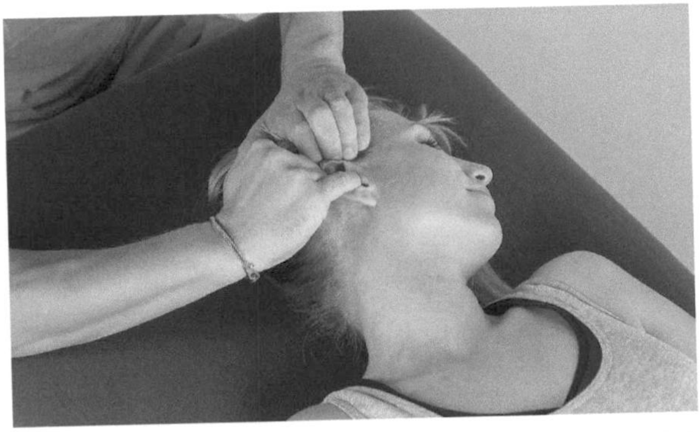

Figure 9.11 Squamous part/tympanic part (right)

- Hold this position until tissue release or a still point occurs.

Indirect technique

- Move both portions of the bone in the direction of the dysfunction, i.e., the direction of greater motion (direction of ease).
- Establish the PBMT and PBFT (the position that achieves the best possible balance between these two portions of the bone).
- Maintain this position until the tissues relax and mobility improves.

9.4.2 Molding

Indication: Asymmetrical convexity or flattening at the ossification centers.

Hand position: With the fingertips of one hand close beside each other, place them on the squama (Figure 9.12).

NOTE—IMPORTANT Gently release the adjacent bones from the temporal bone before beginning to apply this technique.

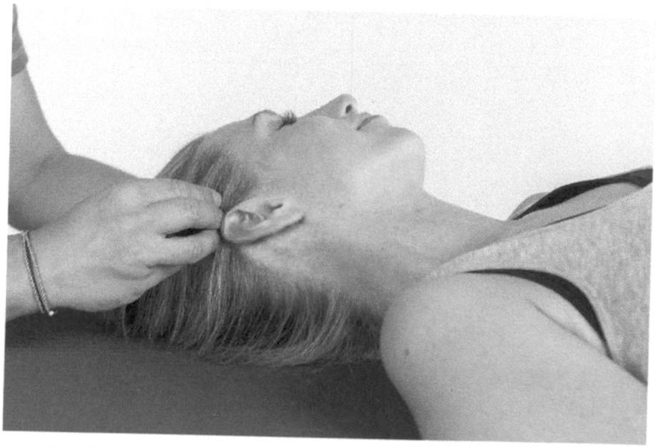

Figure 9.12 Molding

Method:

To treat convexity

- Administer centrifugal impulses with your fingers, to flatten the site of the convexity.
- You may supplement this with a fluid impulse to direct energy toward the borders of the temporal bone.
- Establish PBMT, PBFT.

To treat a flattening of the bone

- Administer centripetal impulses aimed at raising the profile at the flattened site.
- You may supplement this with a fluid impulse to direct energy toward the ossification center from the occipitomastoid suture of the opposite side.
- Establish PBMT, PBFT.

To treat torsion tensions

- Administer an impulse with your fingers, in the direction of the restricted motion.
- Establish PBMT, PBFT.

9.4.3 Dysfunction in external and internal rotation, unilateral

Practitioner: Take up a position at the head of the patient.

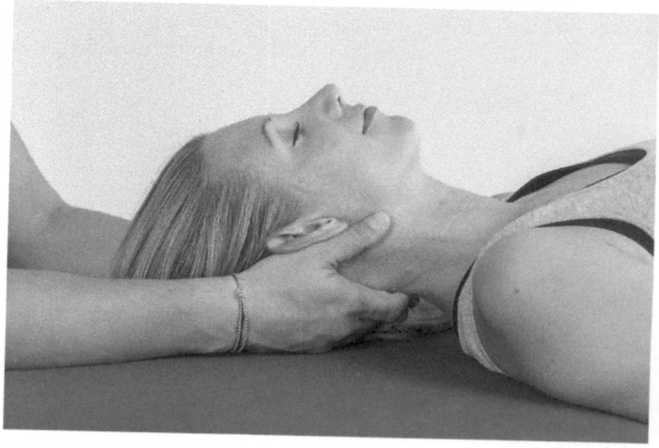

Figure 9.13 Dysfunction in external and internal rotation, unilateral

Dysfunction in external and internal rotation, unilateral

Hand position:

- Place the thenar eminences of your thumbs bilaterally on the mastoid parts of the temporal bone.
- Place your thumbs on the anterior tips of the mastoid processes each side.
- Place the palms of your hands on the occipital bone, with your fingers interclasped posteriorly at the upper cervical vertebrae (this also applies to Figures 9.15–9.18).
- Rest both elbows on the treatment table.

Dysfunction in external and internal rotation, unilateral, alternative hand position

Hand position:

- Hand on the same side as the affected temporal bone.
  - Grasp the zygomatic process between your thumb and index finger.
  - Place your middle finger in the external acoustic meatus.
  - Place your ring finger on the mastoid process.
  - Your little finger should rest on the mastoid part of the temporal bone.
- Hold the occiput in your other hand (Figure 9.14).

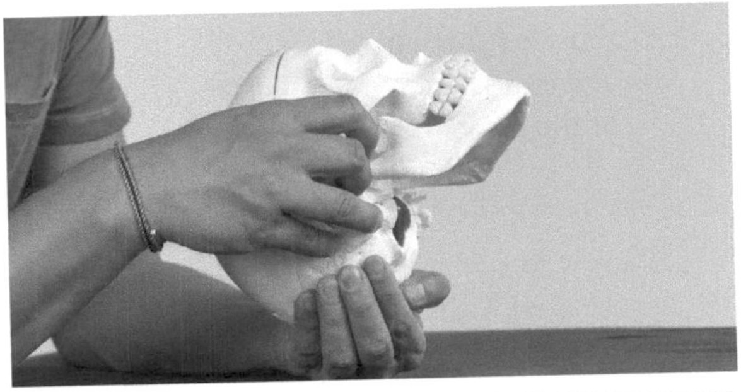

Figure 9.14 Dysfunction in external and internal rotation, unilateral. Alternative hand position

Dysfunction in external rotation, unilateral (right)
Motion restriction in direction of internal rotation

Method:
Indirect technique

- In the inhalation phase, follow the occipital bone into flexion with your left hand.
- At the same time, follow with your right thumb the tip of the mastoid process as it moves posteromedially (external rotation; Figure 9.15).
- Establish the PBMT and PBFT between the temporal bone and the occipital bone.
- Maintain the PBT until a correction of the abnormal tension has been achieved and stabilized by the inherent homeostatic forces (PRM rhythm, etc.).
- Breathing assistance: ask the patient to hold an inhalation for as long as possible at the end of an in-breath. They may also perform plantar flexion of the opposite (left) foot at the same time. Repeat for several breathing cycles.
- You may supplement this with a fluid impulse to direct energy toward the affected temporal bone with your opposite (left) hand.

This technique can also be carried out in harmony with PRM rhythm. During the inhalation phase, administer an impulse to ease the occipital bone into flexion and right temporal bone into external rotation. During the exhalation phase, passively

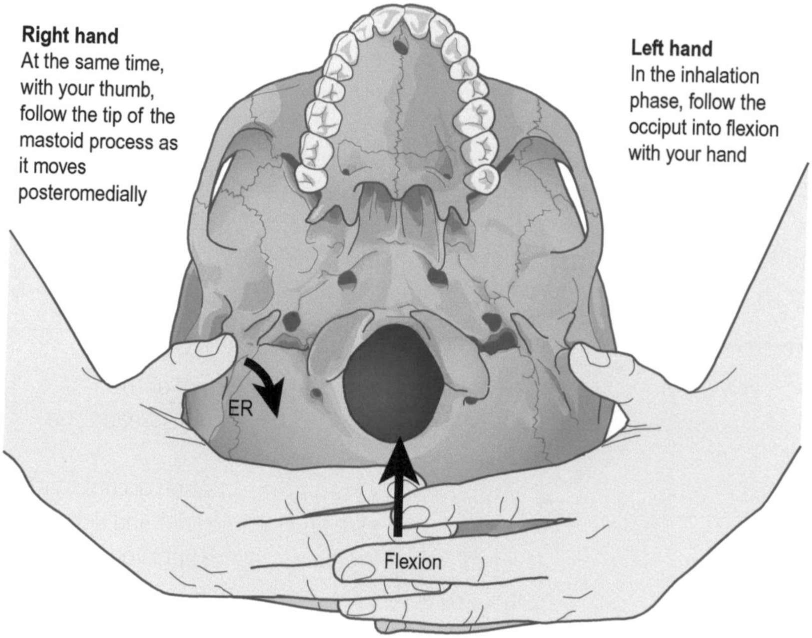

Right hand
At the same time, with your thumb, follow the tip of the mastoid process as it moves posteromedially
Left hand
In the inhalation phase, follow the occiput into flexion with your hand
ER
Flexion

Figure 9.15 Dysfunction in external rotation (right). Indirect technique

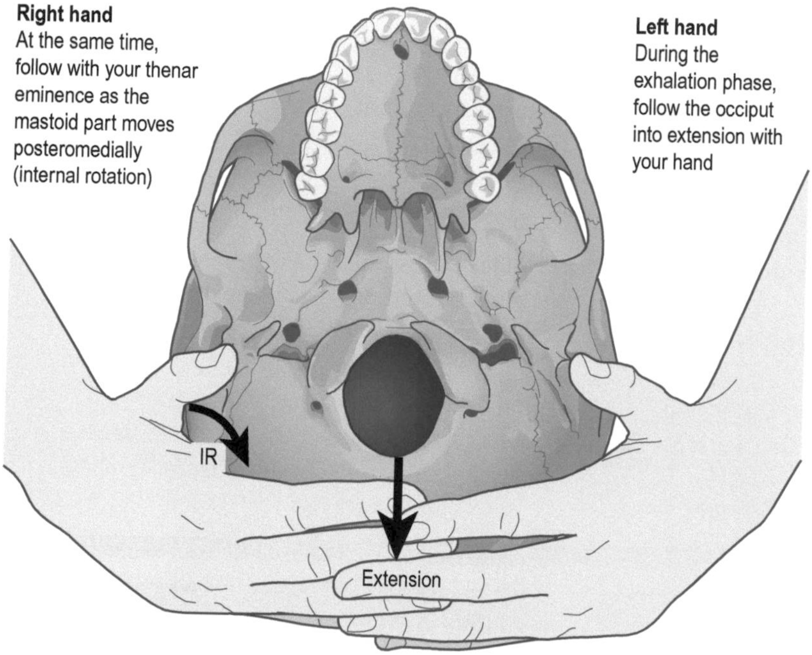

Right hand
At the same time, follow with your thenar eminence as the mastoid part moves posteromedially (internal rotation)
Left hand
During the exhalation phase, follow the occiput into extension with your hand
IR
Extension

Figure 9.16 Dysfunction in internal rotation (right). Indirect technique

follow the motion of these two bones. Continue until the mobility of the temporal bone in the direction of internal rotation improves.

Direct technique

- See dysfunction in internal rotation (right), indirect technique (below, and see Figure 9.16).

Dysfunction in internal rotation, unilateral (right)
Motion restriction in the direction of external rotation

Method:

Indirect technique

- In the exhalation phase follow the occipital bone into extension with the palms of both hands, or with your left hand.
- At the same time, with the thenar eminence of your right thumb, follow the mastoid part of the temporal bone in a posteromedial direction (internal rotation) (Figure 9.16).
- Establish the PBMT and PBFT.
- Breathing assistance: ask the patient to hold an exhalation for as long as possible at the end of an out-breath. They may also perform dorsal flexion of the opposite (left) foot at the same time. Repeat for several breathing cycles.
- You may supplement this with a fluid impulse to direct energy toward the affected temporal bone with your opposite (left) hand.

This technique can also be carried out in harmony with PRM rhythm. During the inhalation phase, passively follow the motion of these two bones. During the exhalation phase, administer an impulse to ease the occipital bone into extension and the right temporal bone into internal rotation. Continue until the mobility of the temporal bone in the direction of external rotation improves.

Direct technique

- See dysfunction in external rotation (right), indirect technique (and see Figure 9.15).

9.4.4 Dysfunction in external and internal rotation, bilateral

The technique described here is an indirect one. However, a direct technique can be used instead if necessary (e.g., when treating newborns and young children).

Practitioner: Take up a position at the head of the patient.

Hand position:

- Place the thenar eminences of each hand bilaterally on the mastoid parts of the temporal bones.
- Place your thumbs on the anterior tips of the mastoid process of each side.
- Place the palms of your hands on the occiput.
- Interclasp your fingers.
- Rest both elbows on the treatment table.

Dysfunction in external rotation, bilateral
Motion restriction in the direction of internal rotation

Method:

- Indirect technique: during the inhalation phase, follow with your thumbs the tips of the mastoid processes as they move in a posteromedial direction (external rotation). Follow the occipital bone into flexion with the palm of your hand (Figure 9.17).
- Establish the PBMT and PBFT.
- Breathing assistance: ask the patient to hold an inhalation for as long as possible at the end of an in-breath. They may also perform plantar flexion of both feet at the same time. Repeat for several breathing cycles.

This technique can also be carried out in harmony with PRM rhythm. During the inhalation phase, administer an impulse to ease the temporal bones into external rotation. During the exhalation phase,

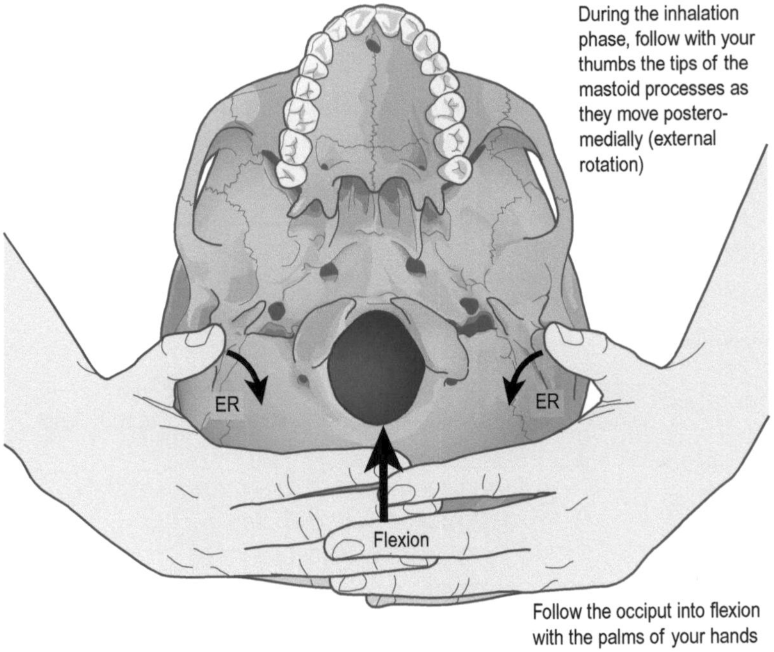

During the inhalation phase, follow with your thumbs the tips of the mastoid processes as they move postero-medially (external rotation)
ER
ER
Flexion
Follow the occiput into flexion with the palms of your hands

Figure 9.17 Dysfunction in external rotation, bilateral. Indirect technique

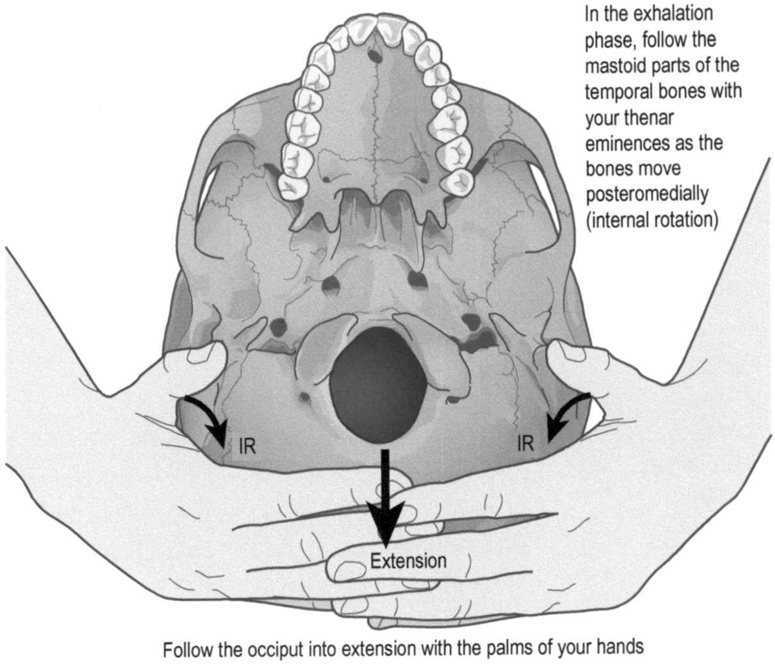

In the exhalation phase, follow the mastoid parts of the temporal bones with your thenar eminences as the bones move posteromedially (internal rotation)
IR
IR
Extension
Follow the occiput into extension with the palms of your hands

Figure 9.18 Dysfunction in internal rotation, bilateral. Indirect technique

passively follow the motion of the two bones. Continue until the mobility of the temporal bones in the direction of internal rotation improves.

Dysfunction in internal rotation, bilateral
Motion restriction in the direction of external rotation

Method:

- Indirect technique: during the exhalation phase, follow the posteromedial motion of the mastoid parts of the temporal bones (internal rotation) with your thenar eminences. Follow the occipital bone into extension with the palms of your hands (Figure 9.18).
- Establish the PBMT and PBFT.
- Breathing assistance: ask the patient to hold an exhalation for as long as possible at the end of an out-breath. They may also perform dorsal extension of both feet at the same time. Repeat for several breathing cycles.

This technique can also be carried out in harmony with PRM rhythm. During the inhalation phase, passively follow the motion of the two bones. During the exhalation phase, administer an impulse to ease the temporal bones into internal rotation. Continue until the mobility of the temporal bones in the direction of external rotation improves.

Vitalist approach: See EV-4 technique (this volume, section 4.4.3).

9.4.5 Dysfunction in anterior and posterior rotation, unilateral

The technique described here is an indirect one. However, a direct technique can be used as necessary.

Hand position:

- Right hand
  - ▸ Grasp the zygomatic process between your thumb and index finger.
  - ▸ Place your middle finger in the external acoustic meatus.
  - ▸ Position your ring finger anterior to the mastoid process.
  - ▸ Position your little finger posterior to the mastoid process.
- Hold the occiput in your left hand.

Dysfunction in anterior rotation, unilateral (right)
Motion restriction in the direction of posterior rotation

Method:

- Indirect technique
  - ▸ Right hand:
    - ◉ During the inhalation phase, induce anterior rotation of the temporal bone (Figure 9.19).
    - ◉ Administer an impulse in an inferior direction with the thumb on the zygomatic process.
    - ◉ With the middle finger in the external acoustic meatus, administer an impulse to anterior rotation.
    - ◉ With the ring finger on the mastoid process, administer an impulse in a superior direction.
  - ▸ Monitor with your left hand.
- Establish the PBMT and PBFT between the temporal bone and the occiput.
- Breathing assistance: ask the patient to hold an inhalation for as long as possible at the end of an in-breath. They may also perform plantar flexion of both feet at the same time. Repeat for several breathing cycles.

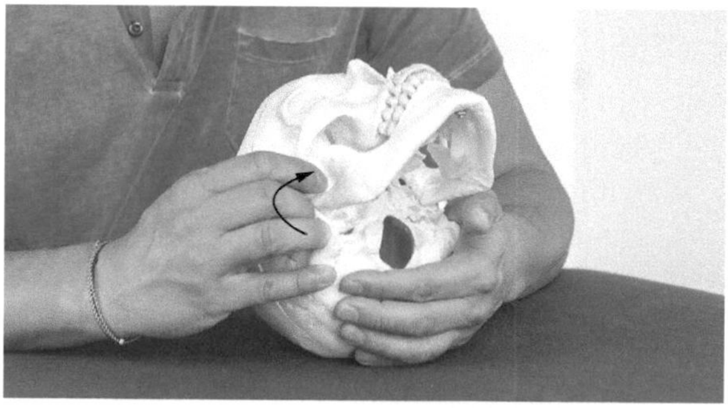

Figure 9.19 Dysfunction in anterior rotation, unilateral (right). Indirect technique

Dysfunction in posterior rotation, unilateral (right)
Motion restriction in the direction of anterior rotation

Method:

- Indirect technique
  - Right hand:
    - During the exhalation phase, induce posterior rotation of the temporal bone (Figure 9.20).
    - With the thumb on the zygomatic process, administer an impulse to ease it in a superior direction.
    - With the middle finger in the external acoustic meatus, administer an impulse into posterior rotation.
    - With the ring finger on the mastoid process, administer an impulse to ease it in an inferior direction.
  - Monitor with your left hand.
- Establish the PBMT and PBFT between the temporal bone and occipital bone.
- Breathing assistance: ask the patient to hold an exhalation for as long as possible at the end of an out-breath. They may also perform dorsal flexion of both feet at the same time. Repeat for several breathing cycles.

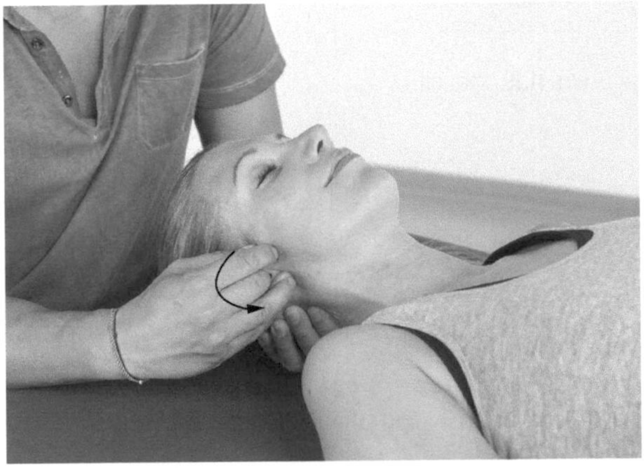

Figure 9.20 Dysfunction in posterior rotation, unilateral (right). Indirect technique

9.4.6 Dysfunction in anterior and posterior rotation, bilateral

The technique described here is an indirect one. However, a direct technique can be used if necessary.

Hand position:

- Grasp the zygomatic processes between thumb and index finger.
- Place your middle fingers in the external acoustic meatus each side.
- Position your ring fingers anterior to the mastoid processes.
- Position your little fingers posterior to the mastoid processes (Figure 9.21).

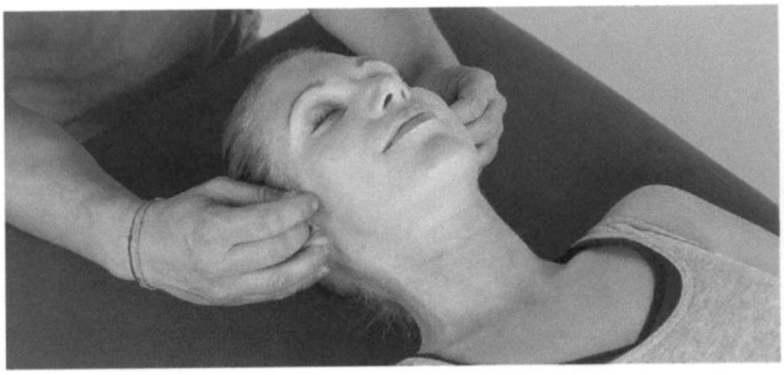

Figure 9.21 Dysfunction in anterior and posterior rotation, bilateral

Dysfunction in anterior rotation, bilateral
Motion restriction in the direction of posterior rotation

Method:

- Indirect technique
  - At the beginning of the inhalation phase, induce rotation of both temporal bones in an anterior direction.
  - With your thumbs on the zygomatic processes, administer an impulse in an inferior direction.
  - With your middle fingers in the external acoustic meatus, administer an impulse into anterior rotation.
  - At the same time administer a superiorly directed impulse with your ring fingers on the mastoid processes.

- Establish the PBMT and PBFT.
- Breathing assistance: ask the patient to hold an inhalation for as long as possible at the end of an in-breath. They may also perform plantar flexion of both feet at the same time. Repeat for several breathing cycles.

> **Tip for practitioners**
>
> This technique can also be used to treat superior vertical strain of the SBS.

Dysfunction in posterior rotation, bilateral
Motion restriction in the direction of anterior rotation

Method:

- Indirect technique
  - At the beginning of the exhalation phase, induce rotation of both temporal bones in a posterior direction.
  - With the thumbs on the zygomatic processes, administer an impulse in a superior direction.
  - With your middle fingers in the external acoustic meatus, administer an impulse into posterior rotation.
  - At the same time, administer an impulse in an inferior direction with the ring finger on the mastoid processes.
- Establish the PBMT and PBFT.
- Breathing assistance: ask the patient to hold an exhalation for as long as possible at the end of an out-breath. They may also perform dorsal extension of both feet at the same time. Repeat for several breathing cycles.

> **Tip for practitioners**
>
> This technique can also be used to treat inferior vertical strain of the SBS.

9.4.7 Temporal bone lift technique

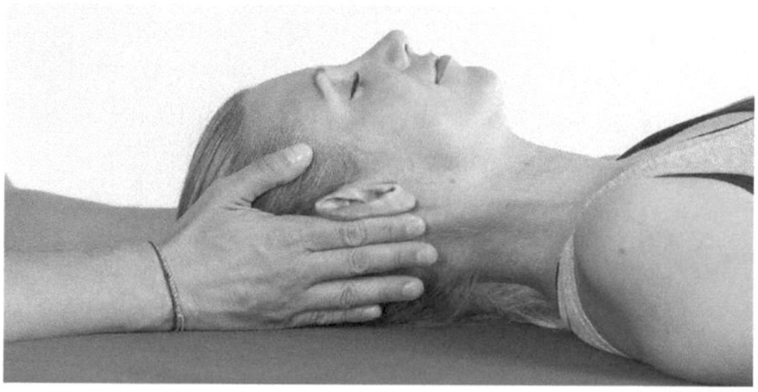

Figure 9.22 Temporal bone lift technique

Indication: Tensions of the tentorium cerebelli, disturbances of the drainage of the inferior and superior petrosal sinuses, restrictions of the sutures of the temporal bone, etc.

Hand position: Place your index fingers on the mastoid processes. Rest your other fingers on the patient's head in a relaxed way (Figure 9.22).

Method:

- Administer gentle cephalad traction with your index fingers on the mastoid processes.
- Permit all motions/tissue unwinding of the temporal bones, without reducing the gentle traction.
- You can sense the various stages of tissue release: first the sutural tensions, then the elastic and collagenous tensions of the tentorium cerebelli (a sensation like cement, or like a rubber band or chewing gum).
- Once release of the tension patterns in the tentorium occurs (floating sensation), you can slowly reduce the cephalad traction, and your hands can be released.

> **CAUTION** Never remove your hands suddenly when performing the release technique, as this could cause dysfunctions.

9.4.8 Sutural dysfunctions

Indication: These occur as a result of compression, often traumatic, which may be primary or secondary. Sequelae: dysfunctions of the other bones, intracranial membranes, nerves, and parts of the brain, or vascular disturbances.

Petro-occipital fissure (petrobasilar suture; petro-occipital synchondrosis)

Suture margin: The lateral borders of the base of the occipital bone form a ridge that articulates with a groove on the posterior, inferior portion of the petrous part of the temporal bone (turning and sliding motion).

Suture type: Synchondrosis.

Indication: Restricted mobility of the temporal bones and resulting functional disturbances.

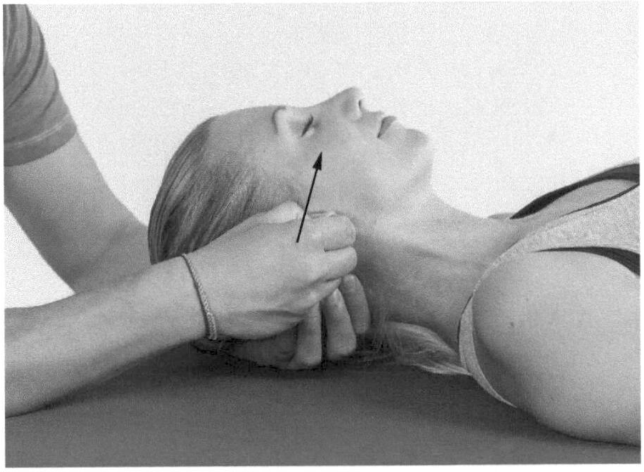

Figure 9.23 Petro-occipital fissure (petrobasilar suture; petro-occipital synchondrosis) and petrojugular suture. General technique

Petrojugular suture

Suture margin: The jugular process articulates with the jugular articular surface of the petrous part of the temporal bone. This is a pivot point for the transmission of motion from the occipital bone to the temporal bone.

Suture type: Synchondrosis.

Indication: Restricted mobility of the temporal bones and resulting functional disturbances.

General technique, e.g., right

Hand position:

- Right hand on the temporal bone on the affected side
  - ▸ Place the thumb in the external acoustic meatus.
  - ▸ Position your index and middle fingers behind the ear lobe, as close as possible to the temporal bone.
  - ▸ Grasp the antitragus and ear lobe with your thumb and fingers.
- Place your left hand across the occiput with your fingers pointing to the right.

Method: (in the sense of disengagement)[3]

- Administer traction to the temporal bone in an anterior direction (Figure 9.23).
- Hold the occiput in position.
- Without reducing the traction, permit all motions/tissue unwinding of the bones that arise.

Specific technique, e.g., right

Hand position:

- Right hand on the temporal bone on the affected side
  - ▸ Grasp the zygomatic process with your thumb and index finger.

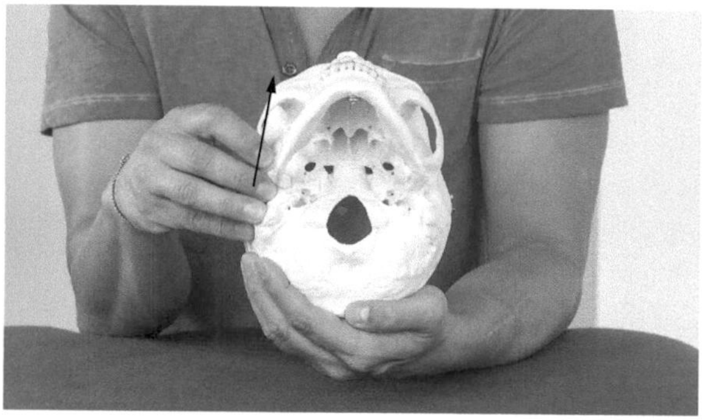

Figure 9.24 Petro-occipital fissure (petrobasilar suture; petro-occipital synchondrosis) and petrojugular suture. Disengagement

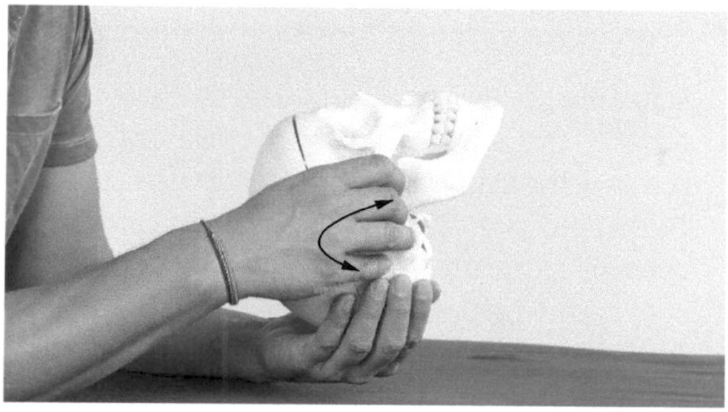

Figure 9.25 Petro-occipital fissure (petrobasilar suture; petro-occipital synchondrosis). Specific technique

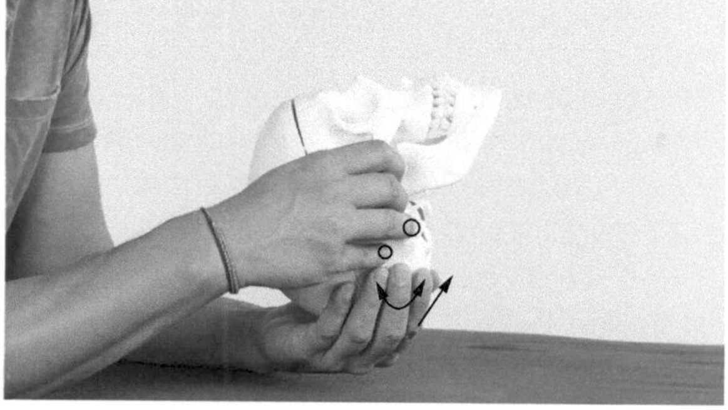

Figure 9.26 Petrojugular suture. Specific technique

- ▸ Place your middle finger in the external acoustic meatus.
- ▸ Place your ring finger on the mastoid process.
- ▸ Place your little finger on the mastoid part of the temporal bone.
- Place your left hand across the occiput with your fingers pointing to the right (Figures 9.24, 9.25, and 9.26).

Disengagement

Method:

- Begin by releasing the temporal bone from the occiput by means of disengagement, by administering gentle, anterior traction on the temporal bone while holding the occipital bone in position (Figure 9.24).
- Maintain the disengagement while seeking the PBMT and PBFT at the suture between the occiput and temporal bone.

To treat the petro-occipital fissure (petrobasilar suture; petro-occipital synchondrosis)

Method:

- Move the occiput in a lateral direction, to the opposite side (to the left), and hold it there (Figure 9.25).
- Then, with the fingers of your right hand, seek the PBMT and PBFT somewhere between the anterior and posterior rotation of the temporal bone.
- Also follow the occipital bone into flexion or extension depending on the tensions present, in order to establish the PBMT.

To treat the petrojugular suture

Method:

- Move the occipital bone laterally, to the opposite side (to the left), and hold it there (Figure 9.26).

- Then seek the PBMT and PBFT somewhere between the external and internal rotation of the temporal bone.
- For external rotation, administer pressure in a medial and posterior direction with your ring finger on the mastoid process.
- For internal rotation, administer pressure in a medial and posterior direction with the little finger on the mastoid part of the temporal bone.
- Also follow the occiput into flexion or extension, according to the tensions present, in order to establish the PBMT.

NOTE PBMT and PBFT for both sutures is normally sought simultaneously. The procedure has been subdivided here for the purpose of instruction only.

Alternative technique, opposite physiological motion according to Magoun (right)

Hand position: As for previous technique.

Method: Opposite physiological motion:

- Move the occiput laterally, to the opposite side (to the left), and hold it there (Figure 9.27).
- During the exhalation phase, go with the occiput into extension and hold it there.

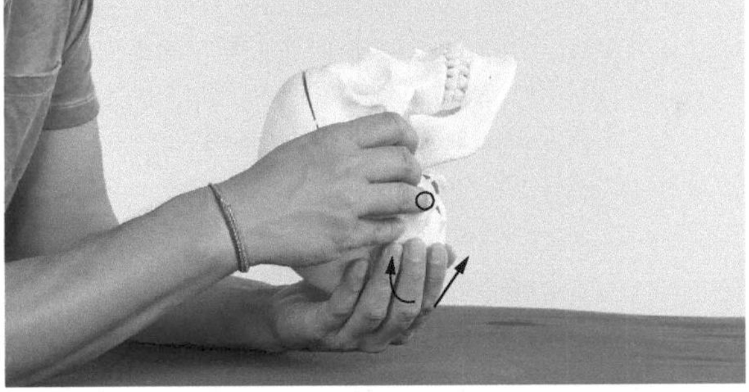

Figure 9.27 Alternative technique for the petro-occipital fissure (petrobasilar suture; petro-occipital synchondrosis) (right): opposite physiological motion according to Magoun

- During the inhalation phase, go with the right temporal bone into external rotation and hold it there: with your ring finger, administer pressure in a medial and posterior direction to the mastoid process. With your thumb and index finger, administer pressure in a lateral and inferior direction on the zygomatic process.
- Hold this position until release of the petro-occipital fissure (petrobasilar suture; petro-occipital synchondrosis) occurs.
- Conclude by resynchronizing the motion of the temporal bone and occiput with the PRM rhythm.

Occipitomastoid suture

Suture margin: The concave mastoid border of the occipital bone articulates with the convex posterior border of the mastoid part of the temporal bone. The suture margin of the occipital bone is normally oriented outward in the superior portion and internally oriented in the inferior portion. The changeover point is called the condylo-squamoso-mastoid pivot point (CSMP).

Suture type: Irregular suture.

The occipital bone and mastoid part of the temporal bone normally move in opposing directions to each other: in the inhalation phase the border of the occiput moves in an anterior direction, while the border of the mastoid part slides posterior.

Compression of this suture can prevent the suture margins from moving in opposite directions in this way. If that happens the temporal bone is carried along with the border of the occiput in the inhalation phase, moving it into internal rotation. In the exhalation phase the temporal bone is then moved into external rotation.

Indication: Disturbances at the tentorium cerebelli, sinus congestion (sigmoid sinus), disturbances of fluctuation of CSF, disturbances of the cerebellum, medulla oblongata, and vagus nerve.

NOTE A dysfunction of the occipitomastoid suture is often the result of compression of the atlanto-occipital joint. The atlanto-occipital joint should therefore be freed first (this volume, section 4.4.1). This often has the effect of releasing the dysfunction of the occipitomastoid suture as well.
A dysfunction of the petrosphenoidal (sphenopetrosal) fissure (suture) can be involved in a restriction affecting the occipitomastoid suture.

Hand position:

- Place the thumbs anterior to the mastoid processes.
- Place the thenar eminences on the mastoid parts of the temporal bones.
- Rest the other fingers on the occipital bone (Figure 9.28).

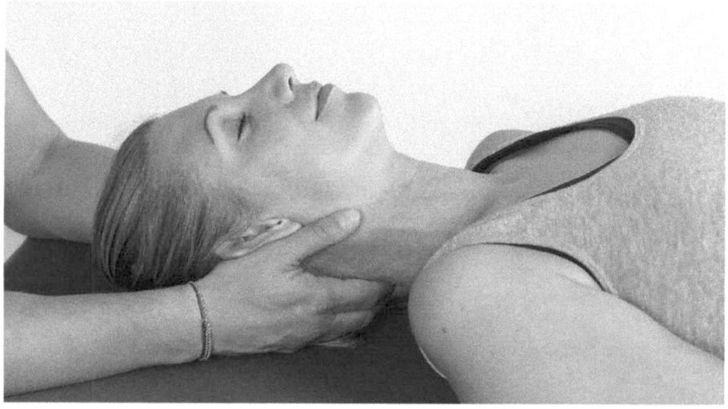

Figure 9.28 Occipitomastoid suture

Temporal bone in internal rotation (right), indirect technique

Method:

Indirect technique

- With the thenar eminence on the dysfunctional side, administer pressure in a medial and posterior direction to the mastoid part of the temporal bone (IR).
- With the other fingers, guide the occipital bone laterally, away from the suture, and posteriorly, into extension (Figure 9.29).
- Breathing assistance: ask the patient to hold an exhalation for as long as possible at the end of an out-breath.
- Establish the PBMT and PBFT.
- Maintain the PBT until a correction of the abnormal tension has been achieved and stabilized by the inherent homeostatic forces (PRM rhythm, etc.).
- A fluid impulse may be used to direct energy from the opposite frontal tuber.

Direct technique

- During the inhalation phase, administer pressure in a medial and posterior direction

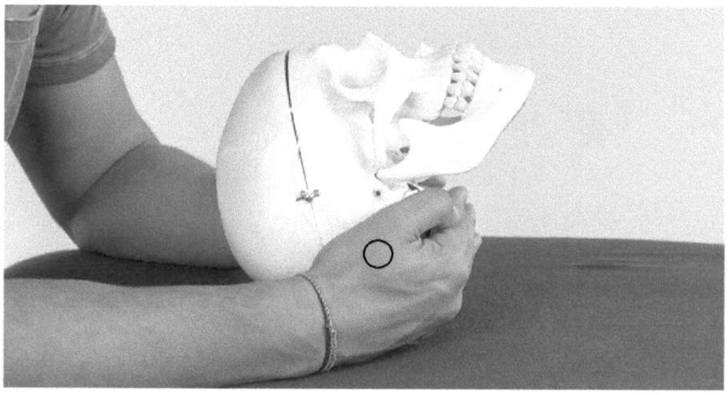

Figure 9.29 Occipitomastoid suture. Indirect technique, right temporal bone in internal rotation

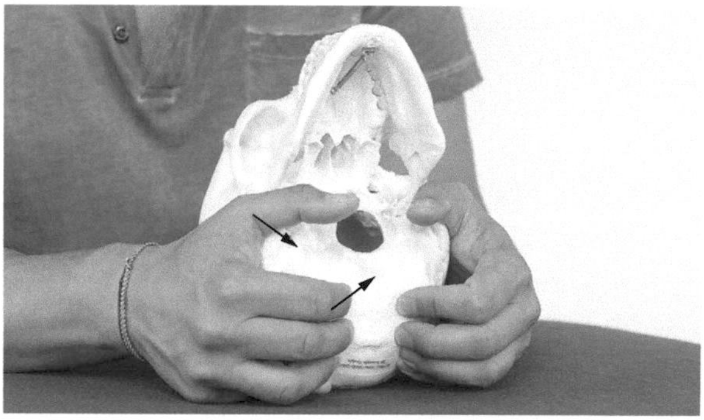

Figure 9.30 Occipitomastoid suture. Direct technique, right temporal bone in internal rotation

to the mastoid process with the thumb on the dysfunctional side (ER).

- With the other fingers, guide the occipital bone laterally, away from the suture, and anteriorly, into flexion (Figure 9.30).
- This draws the suture margins away from each other, which has the effect of opening the suture, especially the posterior portion.
- Breathing assistance: ask the patient to hold an inhalation for as long as possible at the end of an in-breath.
- Establish the PBMT and PBFT.
- A fluid impulse may be performed to direct energy from the opposite frontal tuber.

Tip for practitioners

The indirect technique is usually applied first, followed by the direct technique.

Temporal bone in external rotation, right

For a temporal bone in external rotation, the details are the exact opposite of the above.

Method:

Indirect technique

- The thumb on the dysfunctional side applies pressure in a medial and posterior direction to the mastoid process (ER).
- The other fingers guide the occipital bone posteriorly into extension.

Direct technique

- With the thenar eminence on the dysfunctional side, exert pressure in a medial and posterior direction to the mastoid part of the temporal bone (IR).
- With the other fingers, move the occipital bone anteriorly, into flexion.

Alternative technique, opposite physiological motion according to Magoun

Indirect technique

Method: Indirect technique, temporal bone in internal rotation

- With the thenar eminence on the dysfunctional side, administer pressure in a medial and posterior direction to the mastoid part of the temporal bone (IR).
- With the other fingers, move the occipital bone anteriorly, into flexion (Figure 9.31).
- Breathing assistance: ask the patient to hold an exhalation for as long as possible at the end of an out-breath.
- Establish the PBMT and PBFT.
- A fluid impulse may be used to direct energy from the opposite frontal tuber.

Method: Indirect technique, temporal bone in external rotation

- With the thumb on the dysfunctional side, administer pressure in a medial and posterior direction (ER).
- With the other fingers, guide the occipital bone posteriorly into extension.
- Breathing assistance: ask the patient to hold an inhalation for as long as possible at the end of an in-breath.
- A fluid impulse may be used to direct energy from the opposite frontal tuber.

The direct technique then follows.

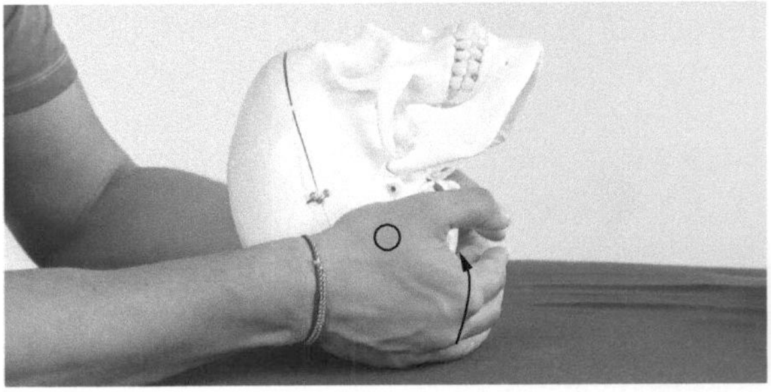

Figure 9.31 Occipitomastoid suture. Alternative technique, opposite physiological motion. Indirect technique, right temporal bone in internal rotation

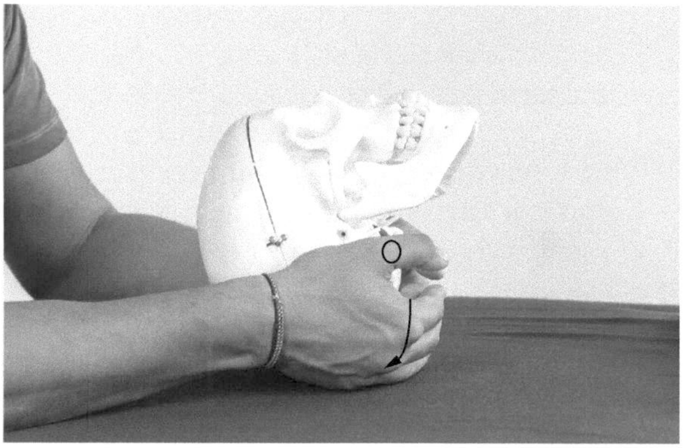

Figure 9.32 Occipitomastoid suture. Alternative technique, opposite physiological motion. Direct technique, right temporal bone in internal rotation

Method:

Direct technique, temporal bone in internal rotation

- With the thumb on the dysfunctional side, administer pressure in a medial and posterior direction (ER) (Figure 9.32).
- With the other fingers, guide the occipital bone posteriorly into extension.
- Breathing assistance: ask the patient to hold an inhalation for as long as possible at the end of an in-breath.
- Establish the PBMT and PBFT.
- A fluid impulse may be used to direct energy from the opposite frontal tuber.

Direct technique, temporal bone in external rotation

- With the thenar eminence on the dysfunctional side, administer pressure in a medial and posterior direction to the mastoid part of the temporal bone (IR).
- With the other fingers, move the occipital bone anteriorly, into flexion.
- Breathing assistance: ask the patient to hold an exhalation for as long as possible at the end of an out-breath.
- Establish the PBMT and PBFT.
- A fluid impulse may be performed to direct energy from the opposite frontal tuber.

Parietomastoid suture

Suture margin: In the anterior quarter of the parietal bone, the mastoid process of the temporal bone is wedged into the parietal. In the second quarter of the parietal, the mastoid part has a more outward-facing border, which lies on the parietal bone. The posterior half of the mastoid part often has an inward-facing border. Overall, this is very irregular.

Suture type: Irregular, more squamous than serrate.

Patient: The patient's head should be turned to the side opposite the dysfunction.

Hand position:

- Place the hand on the side of the dysfunction on the temporal bone. Your thumb should lie on the mastoid process, near the parietomastoid suture.
- Place the other hand on the parietal bone as follows: place the thumb on the parietal bone near the suture.

Method:

- With the thumb on the parietal bone, administer pressure to the bone combined with cephalad traction.
- With the thumb on the mastoid process, administer caudad traction (Figure 9.33).

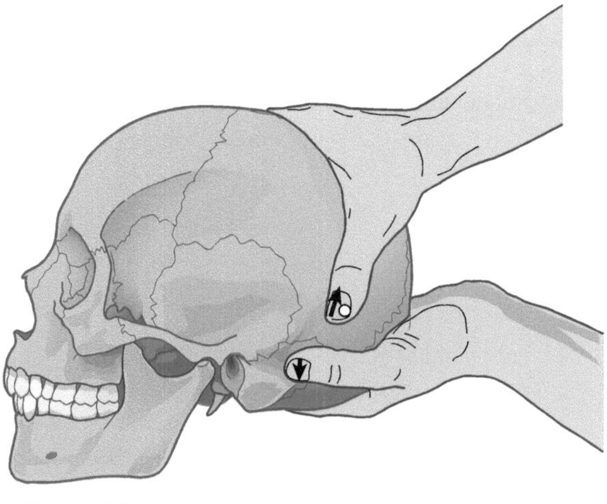

Figure 9.33 Parietomastoid suture

- Permit all motions/tissue unwinding that arise.
- Establish the PBMT and PBFT.
- A fluid impulse may be performed to direct energy from the opposite frontal tuber.

Alternative technique for a temporal bone in internal rotation, right

Patient: Supine, with head slightly turned to the opposite side.

Hand position:

- Place the hand on the side of the dysfunction on the temporal bone as follows: position your thumb anterior to the mastoid process. Position the thenar eminence on the mastoid part of the temporal bone, immediately beside the parieto-mastoid suture.
- Place your other hand on the parietal bone as follows: position your thumb on the parietal bone near the parietomastoid suture. Hold the roof of the skull with the fingers (Figure 9.34).

Method:

Indirect technique

- Hand on the parietal bone. During the exhalation phase, use the thumb next to the parietomastoid suture to begin to move that part of the parietal bone in an inferior, medial, and posterior direction (IR).
- Hand on the temporal bone. At the same time, with the thenar eminence, follow the mastoid part of the temporal bone in a posteromedial direction (IR).
- Establish the PBMT and PBFT.

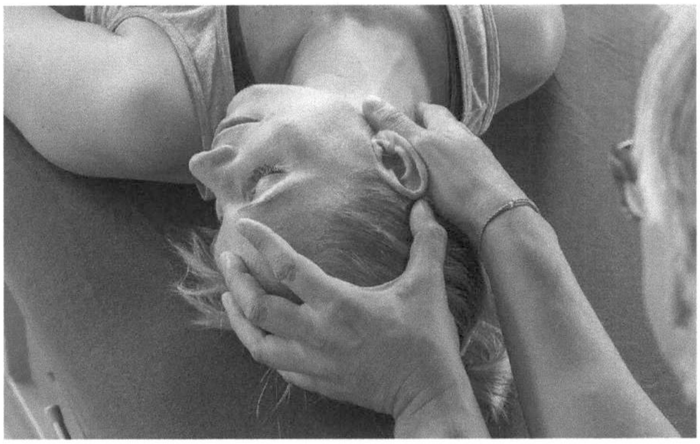

Figure 9.34 Parietomastoid suture. Alternative technique for a temporal bone in internal rotation

Direct technique

- Hand on the parietal bone. During the inhalation phase, begin to administer anterior and cephalad traction (disengagement) with your thumb.
- Hand on the temporal bone. At the same time, gently move the temporal bone downward to release it from the parietal bone (disengagement). Also follow the tip of the mastoid process in a posteromedial direction, using your thumb (ER).
- Permit all motions/tissue unwinding that arise.
- Establish the PBMT and PBFT.

Squamoparietal suture

Suture margin: Parietal border of the squamous part of the temporal bone: internally facing margin; squamous border of the parietal bone: externally facing margin.

Suture type: Squamous suture.

Patient: The patient's head should be turned toward the opposite side.

Hand position:

- Place the hand on the same side as the dysfunction on the temporal bone as follows
  - Position your thumb on the squama, beside and parallel to the squamoparietal suture.
  - Position your other fingers on the patient's neck, pointing caudad.
  - Arrange your thumb and fingers at right angles to each other.
- Place your other hand on the parietal bone as follows
  - Place your thumb on the parietal bone, beside and parallel to the squamoparietal suture.

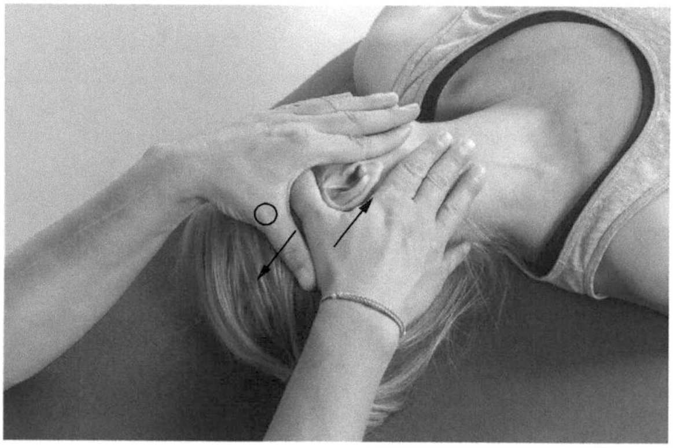

Figure 9.35 Squamoparietal suture

- ▸ Point the other fingers caudad.
- ▸ Arrange your thumb and fingers at right angles to each other.

Method:

- Disengagement (Figure 9.35)
  - ▸ Administer medial pressure with the thumb on the parietal bone, together with cephalad traction.
  - ▸ With the thumb on the temporal bone, administer caudad traction.
  - ▸ Permit all motions/tissue unwinding that arise.
- Establish the PBMT and PBFT.
- A fluid impulse may be used to direct energy from pterion on the opposite side.

Alternative technique for a temporal bone in internal rotation, right

Patient: The patient's head should be turned toward the opposite side to the dysfunction.

Hand position:

- Place the hand on the side of the dysfunction on the temporal bone as follows
  - ▸ Position your thumb on the squama, beside and parallel to the squamoparietal suture.

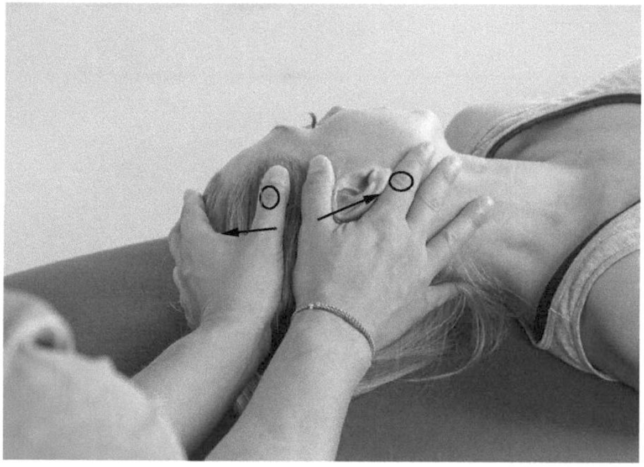

Figure 9.36 Squamoparietal suture. Alternative technique for a temporal bone in internal rotation

  - ▸ Position your index finger on the mastoid process.
- Place your other hand on the parietal bone as follows
  - ▸ Place your thumb on the parietal bone, beside and parallel to the squamoparietal suture.
  - ▸ Hold the roof of the skull with your fingers.

Method: Direct technique, during the exhalation phase (Figure 9.36)

- With the thumb on the parietal bone, by the squamoparietal suture, administer pressure in a medial direction (IR).

Direct technique, during the inhalation phase (Figure 9.36)

- With the thumb on the parietal bone, by the suture, perform a cephalad movement, without reducing the medial pressure.
- At the same time, with the index finger on the mastoid process, administer pressure in a posterior and medial direction. With the thumb on the squama of the temporal bone, perform a lateral, anterior, and inferiorly directed movement (ER).
- Permit all motions/tissue unwinding that arise.
- Establish the PBMT and PBFT.

Sphenosquamous suture: sphenosquamous pivot (Cant hook) technique

Suture margin

- The anterior and inferior border of the squamous part of the temporal bone articulates with the posterior border of the greater wing.
- The suture margin belonging to the temporal bone faces inward along its superior and anterior half. The inferior half faces outward. The suture margins of the sphenoid correspond. The point where the bevel changes is called the sphenosquamous pivot point (SSP).

Suture type: Squamoserrate.

Indication: Migraine, disturbances of the lacrimal gland, parotid gland, nasal mucosa, pharynx, and palate.

Patient: The patient's head should be turned to the opposite side to the dysfunction.

Practitioner: Take up a position beside the patient's head, on the opposite side to the dysfunction.

Hand position:

- Place the hand on the side of the dysfunction on the temporal bone as follows
  - ► Grasp the zygomatic process with your thumb and index finger.
  - ► Place your middle finger in the external acoustic meatus.
  - ► Position your ring finger on the mastoid process.
  - ► Position your little finger on the mastoid part of the temporal bone.
- Place the other hand on the sphenoid as follows
  - ► Position your little finger intraorally on the outside of the lateral pterygoid plate.
  - ► Position your middle and ring fingers on the greater wing (Figure 9.37).

Method:

During the inhalation phase

- Disengagement (Figure 9.38)
  - ► With your thumb and index finger, follow the zygomatic process as it moves in a lateral, anterior, and inferior direction. With your ring finger, follow the mastoid process in a posterior and medial direction (ER).
  - ► Hold the temporal bone in external rotation.
  - ► Also administer gentle posterior traction to the temporal bone.
  - ► At the same time, with your middle and ring fingers, administer medial pressure and anteriorly directed traction to the greater wing.
  - ► Permit all motions/tissue unwinding that arise.
  - ► Continue to perform the disengagement until you sense a release at the suture.
- Without reducing the disengagement, establish the PBMT and PBFT.
- A fluid impulse may be performed to direct energy from the opposite parietal tuber.

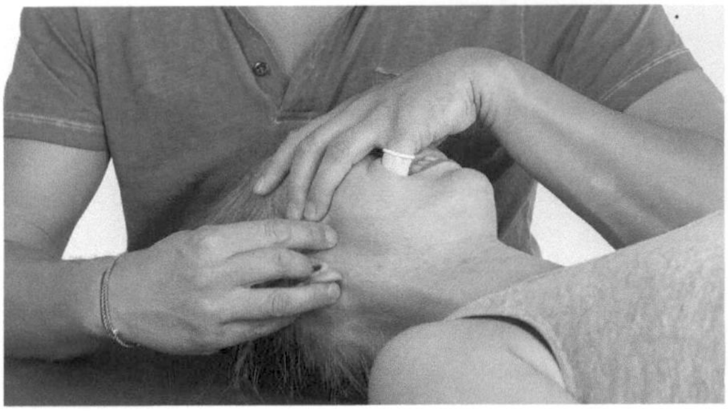

Figure 9.37 Sphenosquamous pivot technique

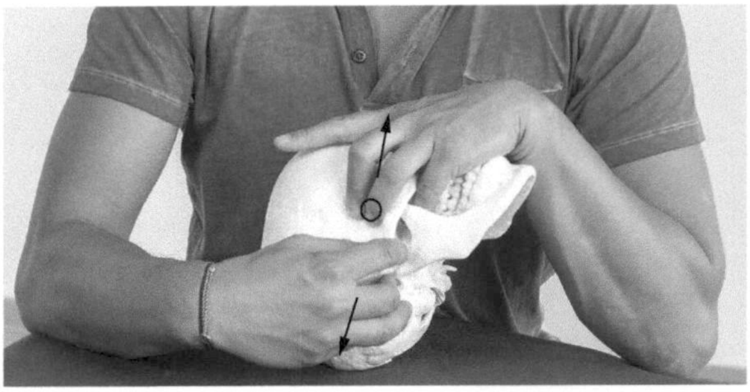

Figure 9.38 Sphenosquamous pivot technique (shown on model)

Sphenopetrosal synchondrosis (petrosphenoidal fissure)

Suture margin: The lateral part of the posterior wall of the hypophysial fossa articulates with the apex of the petrous part of the temporal bone by way of the petrosphenoidal ligament (Gruber's ligament) of the tentorium cerebelli. Also, the horizontal posterior, inferior border of the greater wing articulates with the anterior portion of the petrous part, although these do not actually join: between them lies the foramen lacerum, and they form the anterior and posterior border of the foramen opening.

Indication: Disturbances of the nerves supplying the muscles of the eye.

Hand position: The initial position is as for the technique for the sphenosquamous suture (see above).

Method:

- Disengagement (Figure 9.39)
  - ▸ With the middle and ring fingers on the greater wing, administer pressure in a medial direction and anteriorly directed traction.
  - ▸ Also administer traction in an inferior direction to release the sphenopetrosal synchondrosis (below the SSP).
  - ▸ With your thumb and index finger, follow the zygomatic process in a lateral, anterior, and inferior direction. With your ring finger, follow the mastoid process in a posterior and medial direction (ER).
  - ▸ Hold the temporal bone in external rotation.
- Without reducing the disengagement, establish the PBMT and PBFT between the sphenoid and the temporal bone.
- Maintain the PBT until a correction of the abnormal tension has been achieved and stabilized by the inherent homeostatic forces (PRM rhythm, etc.), and the motion of the sphenoid and the temporal bone has stopped.

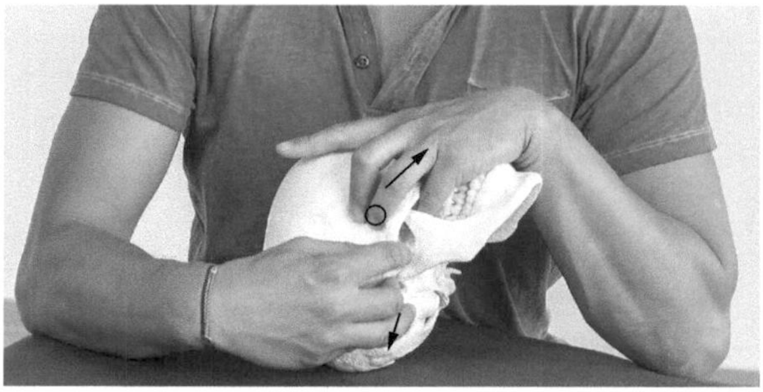

Figure 9.39 Sphenopetrosal synchondrosis (petrosphenoidal fissure)

Alternative technique according to E. Lay

Patient: The patient's head should be turned to the opposite side to the dysfunction.

Practitioner: Take up a position beside the patient's head, on the opposite side to the dysfunction.

Hand position:

- Place the hand on the side of the dysfunction on the temporal bone as follows
  - ▸ Grasp the zygomatic process with your thumb and index finger.
  - ▸ Place your middle finger in the external acoustic meatus.

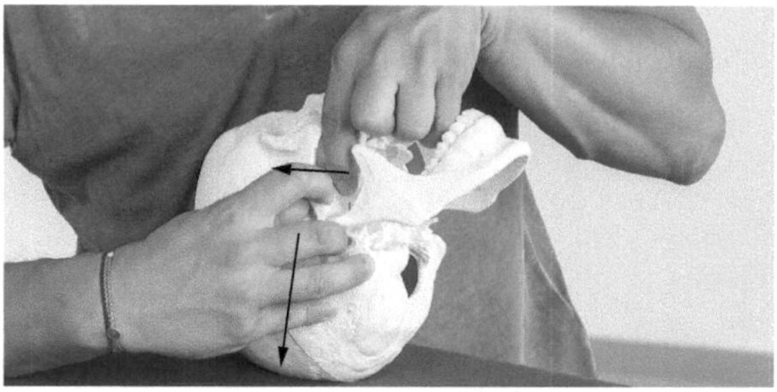

Figure 9.40 Sphenopetrosal synchondrosis. Alternative technique according to E. Lay (shown on model)

- ▸ Position your ring finger on the mastoid process.
- ▸ Position your little finger on the mastoid part of the temporal bone.
- Place your other hand on the sphenoid as follows: place your index finger intraorally, with the phalanx of the finger against the upper molars. The tip of the finger should be bent and placed on the outside of the lateral pterygoid plate (Figure 9.40).

Method:

- Disengagement
  - ▸ Ask the patient to bite together.
  - ▸ At the same time, move the pterygoid process in a superior direction with your index finger; the temporal bone is moved gently posterior (Figure 9.41).
- Without lessening the posterior traction, establish the PBMT (probably moving into IR) and PBFT at the temporal bone.
- Maintain the PBT until a correction of the abnormal tension has been achieved and stabilized by the inherent homeostatic forces (PRM rhythm, etc.), and the motion of the sphenoid and the temporal bone has stopped.
- At this point the patient's teeth can be unclenched.
- The temporal bone will probably now move into ER. Follow this motion.

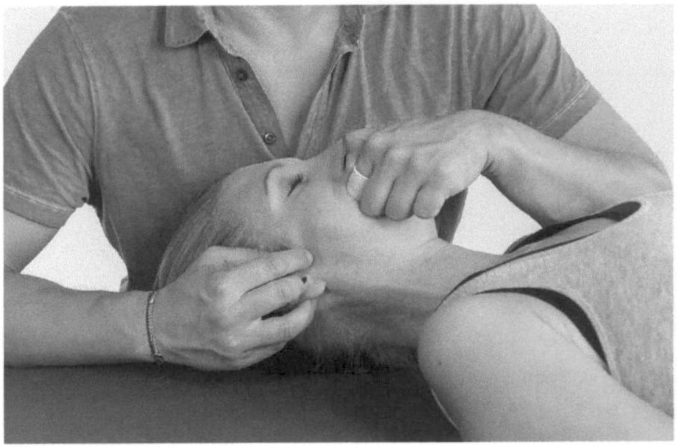

Figure 9.41 Sphenopetrosal synchondrosis. Alternative technique according to E. Lay

Temporozygomatic suture

Suture margin: The process of the temporal bone articulates with the process of the zygomatic bone. In the superior two-thirds of the suture, the temporal bone has an outward-facing border, overlain by the zygomatic bone; in the inferior third of the suture the bevel is the reverse.

Suture type: Serrate suture.

Patient: The patient's head should be turned to the side opposite to the dysfunction.

Practitioner: Take up a position beside the patient's head, on the opposite side to the dysfunction.

Hand position:

- Place the cranial hand on the temporal bone as follows
  - ▸ Grasp the zygomatic process with your thumb and index finger.
  - ▸ Place your middle finger in the external acoustic meatus.
  - ▸ Position your ring finger on the mastoid process.
  - ▸ Position your little finger on the mastoid part of the temporal bone.
- Hand on the zygomatic bone: grasp the temporal process of the zygomatic bone with the thumb and index finger of your caudal hand (Figure 9.42).

Method:

- Disengagement (Figure 9.43)
  - ▸ With the index finger and thumb on the temporal bone, administer traction in a posterior direction.
  - ▸ With the index finger and thumb on the zygomatic bone, administer traction in an anterior direction.

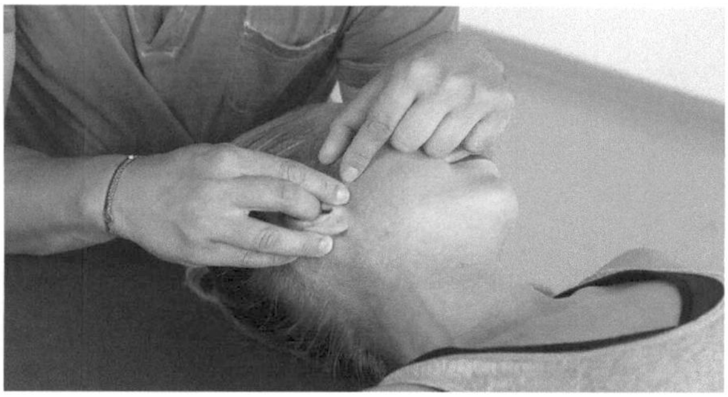

Figure 9.42 Temporozygomatic suture

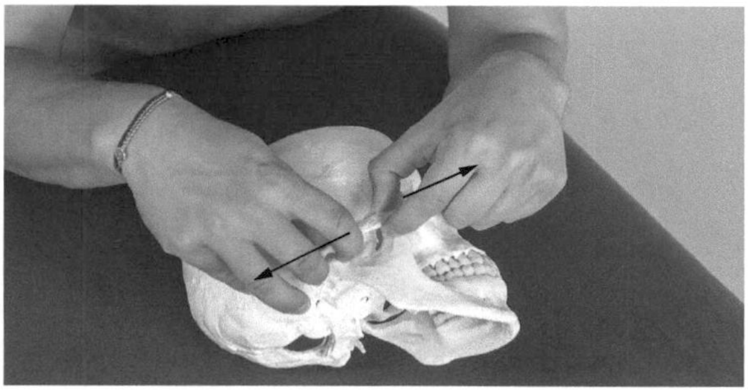

Figure 9.43 Temporozygomatic suture (shown on model)

  - Permit all motions/tissue unwinding that arise.
- Direct technique
  - Without reducing the disengagement, move the temporal bone into ER.
  - Move the zygomatic process of the temporal bone in a lateral, anterior, and inferior direction.
  - Move the little finger on the mastoid part of the temporal bone in a posterior, medial direction.
- Establish the PBMT and PBFT at the zygomatic bone.
- As you conclude the technique, you should bring the motion of the zygomatic bone back into synchrony with that of the temporal bone, in harmony with the PRM rhythm.
- During the inhalation phase, go with the temporal bone and the zygomatic bone into ER, and during the exhalation phase, go with the temporal bone and zygomatic bone into IR.
- A fluid impulse may be used to direct energy from asterion on the opposite side.

Gehin's pivot technique for the temporal bone

Indication: Disturbance between the anterior and posterior parts of the neurocranium, disturbance between the roof and base of the skull, all disturbances of the ears and TMJ, disturbances of the trigeminal and glossopharyngeal nerves.

Hand position: Sutherland's cranial vault hold (this volume, section 5.3.3).

Method:

For all the following regions, first separate your ring finger and little finger (Figure 9.44):

1. Petrobasilar suture (petro-occipital fissure). In addition, administer pressure in a **medial** (slightly oblique) direction with your ring fingers.

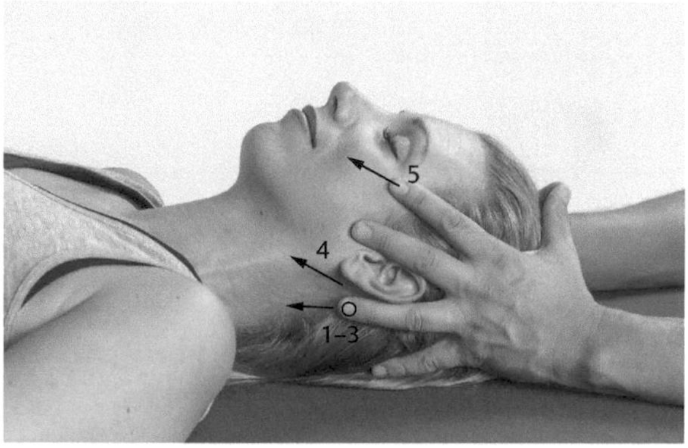

Figure 9.44 Gehin's pivot technique for the temporal bone

2. Petrojugular suture. Administer pressure with your ring fingers in a **medial** and then caudad direction.
3. Occipitomastoid suture. Administer pressure with your ring fingers in a **caudad** and then medial direction.
4. Transition zone between the parietomastoid suture and the squamoparietal suture. Administer traction with your ring fingers in the direction of the sternum.
5. Sphenosquamous suture. Administer traction in a caudad and anterior direction with your index fingers.
6. Petrosphenoidal fissure (suture). Perform a circumduction movement with your middle fingers.

9.4.9 Technique for the auditory ossicles

Indication: Tinnitus, deafness, syringitis.

Patient: Jaw relaxed; masticatory surfaces of the teeth not in contact.

Practitioner: Take up a position at the head of the patient.

Hand position: Place the tip of the index finger on the tragus.

Method:

- Indirect technique With the index finger, administer pressure on the tragus in the direction of the external acoustic meatus (Figure 9.45).
- Without reducing the gentle pressure, rotate the index finger in an anterior or posterior direction and establish the PBMT.
- As you do so, direct your attention to the tympanic membrane, the tissue tension of the tympanic cavity in the middle ear, and to the auditory ossicles.

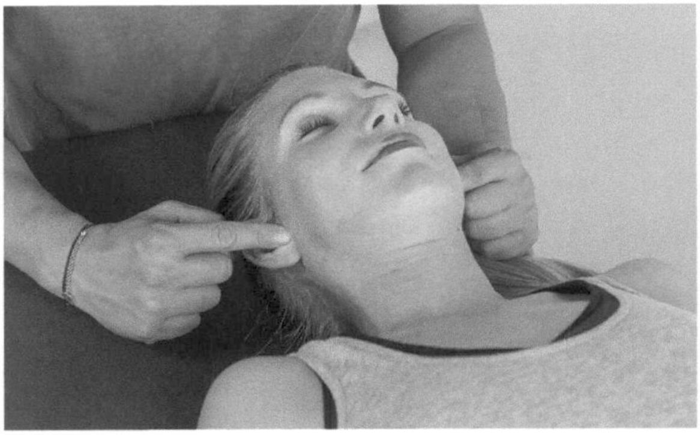

Figure 9.45 Technique for the auditory ossicles

- You may also follow the rotating motions/tissue unwinding that arise.
- A fluid impulse may be directed from pterion on the opposite side.

9.4.10 Dural techniques

J. E. Upledger's "ear pull" technique

Indication: Tensions and fibrosis of the tentorium cerebelli, restrictions of the sutures of the temporal bone, disturbances of the ear or of balance, hindrances to the drainage of the superior and inferior petrosal sinuses, dysfunction at the foramen lacerum.

Hand position:

- Place your thumbs in the external acoustic meatus of each ear.
- Place your index and middle fingers behind the ear lobes, as close as possible to the temporal bones.
- Grasp the antitragus and lobe of each ear with your thumb and fingers.

Method:

- Apply traction in an oblique, lateral, and posterior direction, roughly in a continuous line with the petrous parts (Figure 9.46).

- Gently, very slowly, increase the amount of force. A slightly greater application of force can sometimes be needed to release restrictions of the temporal bone, but this must always be kept below the point where the tissue reacts to the force of the traction and contracts against it.
- While administering the traction you can make constant slight adjustments to the angle of pull to correspond to the tension pattern of the tentorium and the sutures.
- Permit all motions/tissue unwinding of the tentorium by following the motions passively with your hands, without reducing the gentle traction.
- This traction first releases the sutural joint surfaces between the petrous part and the corresponding joint surfaces of the sphenoid and occipital bone, followed by the various membranous tensions of the tentorium (osseous release, elastic/collagen membrane and fluid release).

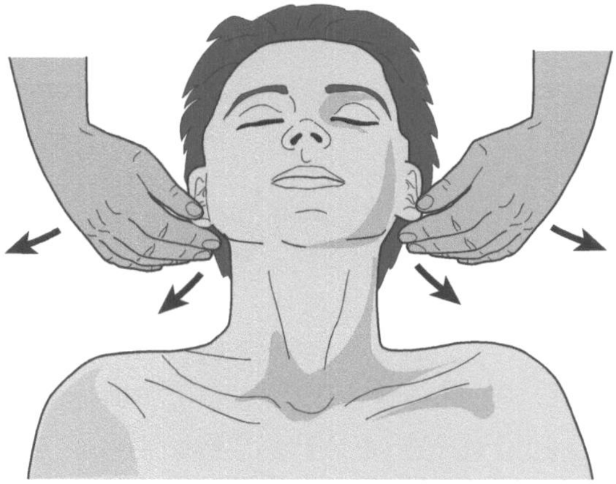

Figure 9.46 J. E. Upledger's "ear pull" technique

- When the tentorium has been released from its tension patterns, you can gradually relax the lateroposterior traction and then remove your hands.

CAUTION When performing the release technique, never remove your hands suddenly from the bone. Doing so can cause dysfunctions.

9.4.11 Specific testing and technique for the falx cerebri and falx cerebelli

Practitioner: Take up a position at the head of the patient, at an angle of 45° to the head.

Patient: Head slightly turned.

Hand position:

- Place the index finger of one hand on the occiput, as close as possible to the foramen magnum and lying along the midline. Place your thumb on the parietal bone, along the midline, in an extended line with your index finger. Your middle finger and thumb are placed on the patient's head on the course of the falx cerebelli and falx cerebri.
- Position the middle finger and thumb of the other hand along the midline in an extended line with the middle fingers and thumb of the other hand.
- Your thumbs meet on the roof of the skull. Your middle fingers and thumb follow the course of the falx cerebri (Figure 9.47).
- In the region of the anterior attachment of the falx, project your attention via your index fingers to the inferior attachment of the falx by the crista galli.

Method:

- **Testing** First, passively sense the tension patterns. Then, using both hands, carry out mobilization in the caudad and cephalad, anterior and posterior directions, and between your two hands positioned posterior and anterior, working in the same and in the opposing direction (rotation, torsion, lateral shifting, etc.). Evaluate the adaptation in the region of the falx cerebri and falx cerebelli.

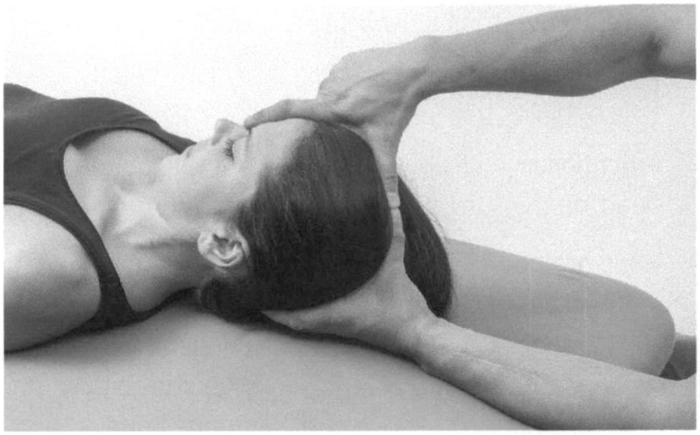

Figure 9.47 Specific testing and technique for the falx cerebri and falx cerebelli. (Liem, T. [2018] *Kraniosakrale Osteopathie. Ein praktisches Lehrbuch,* 7th ed. Stuttgart: Thieme. Photographer: Thomas Möller, Ludwigsburg)

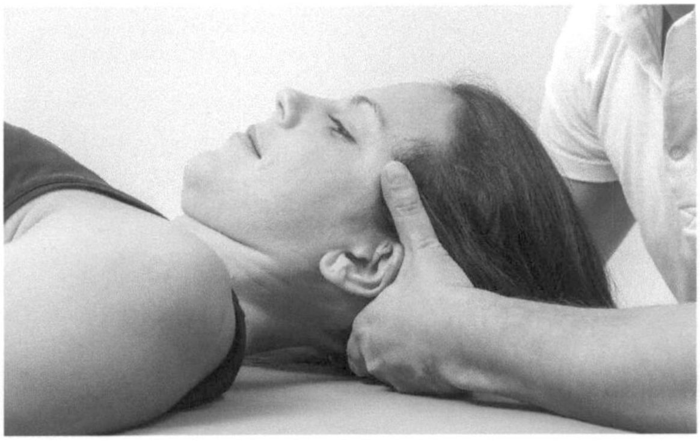

Figure 9.48 Treatment of the tentorium cerebelli. (Liem, T. [2018] *Kraniosakrale Osteopathie. Ein praktisches Lehrbuch,* 7th ed. Stuttgart: Thieme. Photographer: Thomas Möller, Ludwigsburg)

- If you detect a restriction, carry out mobilization, recoil, or low thrust in the direction of the restriction (direct technique), or indirect technique.
- If by your palpation you sense any local points of tension at the attachments of the falx cerebri or falx cerebelli, or if the patient has indicated them by pointing a finger at the spot, release these. To do so, carry out a local fascial release with both thumbs at the point concerned.
- Use anteroposterior and craniocaudal rhythmic compression and decompression to energize sinus lymph flow.

9.4.12 Treatment of the tentorium cerebelli

Practitioner: At the head of the patient.

Hand position:

- Place the index fingers of your two hands on each side of the patient's head, with your fingertips touching in the region of the inion.
- Align your index fingers each side along the course of the groove for the transverse sinus.
- Place your thumbs in an extended line with your index fingers.
- Position them bilaterally on the parietomastoid suture, the region along the superior border of the petrous part of the temporal bone and the greater wing of the sphenoid (Figure 9.48).

Method:

- **Testing** First, passively sense the tension patterns. Then, using both hands, carry out mobilization in the anterior and posterior, medial and lateral directions, and that of your two hands, working in the same and in the opposing direction (flexion, extension, rotation, torsion, lateral shifting, right anterior/left posterior and the reverse, etc.). Evaluate the adaptation in the region of the falx cerebri and falx cerebelli.
- If you detect a restriction, carry out mobilization, recoil, or low thrust in the direction of the restriction (direct technique), or indirect technique.
- If by your palpation you sense any local points of tension at the attachments of the tentorium cerebelli, or if the patient has indicated them by pointing a finger at the spot, release these. To do so, carry out a local fascial release with both thumbs at the point concerned.
- Use anteroposterior and mediolateral rhythmic compression and decompression to energize sinus lymph flow.

9.4.13 Fluid/electrodynamic techniques

H. I. Magoun's "Pussy-foot" technique

Effect and indication:

- Induction of transverse fluctuation through movement of the tentorium; this is brought about by induction of motion at the temporal bones.
- Energizing technique: stimulation of PRM rhythm and enhancement of its amplitude.
- Calming technique: sedation of PRM rhythm and reduction in the amplitude, e.g., to calm excited, nervous, anxious patients.
- In severe dysfunctions of the body.
- In restrictions of the temporal bone sutures.
- In chronic sidebending-rotation dysfunctions of the spheno-occipital (sphenobasilar) synchondrosis (SBS).
- According to Lippincott, lateral motion of the cerebrospinal fluid can restore a harmonious rhythm to the fluctuation.[4:22]
- According to Magoun,[6] this technique is also indicated for insomnia, over-excitement, hypertension, spasms of cerebral vessels, headache, epilepsy, hypertonicity, shock (of the CNS) following injury, excessive fluctuations from iatrogenic causes as a result of overstimulation of the centers in the medulla oblongata and the cranial nerve nuclei on the floor of the fourth ventricle.[5:87]

Practitioner: Take up a position at the head of the patient.

Hand position:

- Position the thenar eminences bilaterally on the mastoid parts of the temporal bones.
- Place your thumbs bilaterally on the anterior tips of the mastoid processes.
- Position your other fingers under the upper cervical vertebrae and interclasp your fingers.
- Rest both elbows on the treatment table.

Method:

- Externally rotate the temporal bone of one side, by transferring your weight onto the elbow of that same side. This has the effect of moving the thumb on the mastoid process in a medial and posterior direction.
- As you transfer your weight from your other elbow, you move the other temporal bone into internal rotation (Figure 9.49). Your hand automatically moves in such a way that you exert medial and posterior pressure with the thenar eminence on the mastoid part of the temporal bone.
- Internal rotation of the right temporal bone/external rotation of the left temporal bone and external rotation of the right temporal bone/internal rotation of the left temporal bone.
- Change direction in step with PRM rhythm, so that you alternate the movement of the temporal bones, moving them in opposite directions to each other. If you are unable to sense the PRM rhythm, you can alternate the movement in time with pulmonary breathing instead.
- Once the motion restriction has been released and the PRM rhythm has taken over the induction of opposite motion, just follow passively and wait for the opposite motion to come to rest.
- After a short pause, a natural symmetrical motion will re-establish itself, of its own accord.

Tip for practitioners

Lippincott instructs the practitioner to roll the middle fingers back and forth to create the movement of the thumbs that induces the external and internal rotation of the temporal bones.[4]

- Energizing technique: the method is the same as for the "pussy-foot" technique described above, except that the rhythm of the opposite (external and internal rotation) motion in the rhythm of pulmonary breathing is accelerated and the amplitude of the motion performed is increased.

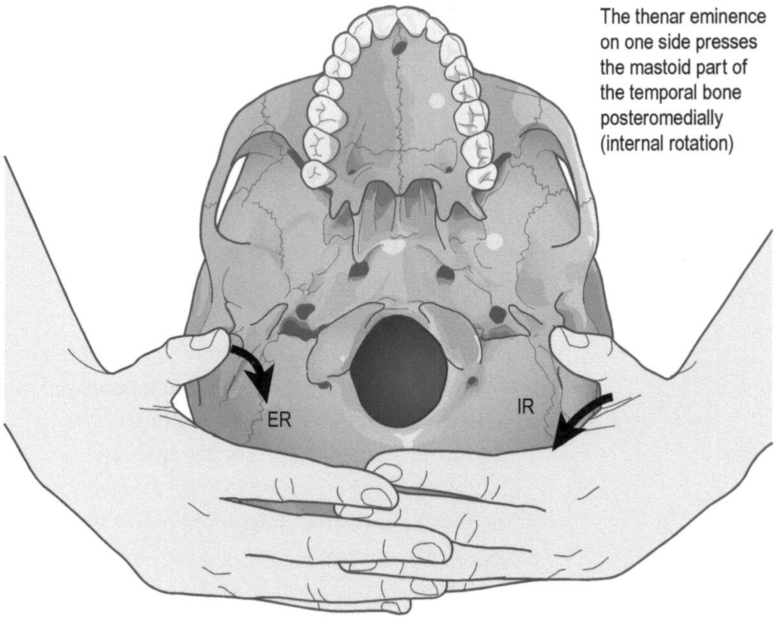
The thenar eminence on one side presses the mastoid part of the temporal bone posteromedially (internal rotation)
ER
IR
...while the thumb on the other side presses the mastoid process posteromedially (external rotation)

Figure 9.49 H. I. Magoun's "pussy-foot" technique

- Calming technique: the method is the same as for the "pussy-foot" technique described above, except that the rhythm of the opposite (external and internal rotation) motion and the amplitude with which it is performed are reduced.

Alternative method:
Perform the procedure at the sacrum or another cranial bone.

Vitalist approach: See EV-4 technique (this volume, section 4.4.3).

Tip for practitioners

This technique stimulates the sympathetic nervous system. When performed more gently, this technique can bring about deeper breathing on the part of the patient and release restrictions at the occipitomastoid suture. It can also be used at the end of a treatment session to neutralize undesired effects of therapy.

W. G. Sutherland's "Father Tom" reanimation technique

Effect: Forces the entire craniosacral system and the body as a whole into flexion/external rotation/inhalation phase.[7]

Indication: Shock; life-threatening situations, when the PRM rhythm has become almost undetectable. In anesthetic-induced breathing disturbances in newborns.

Practitioner: Take up a position at the head of the patient.

Hand position:

- Place the thenar eminences bilaterally on the mastoid parts of the temporal bones.
- Rest the thumbs on the anterior tips of the mastoid processes.
- Interclasp your other fingers under the upper cervical vertebrae (i.e., position of fingers not as appears in Figure 9.49; see also Figure 9.13).

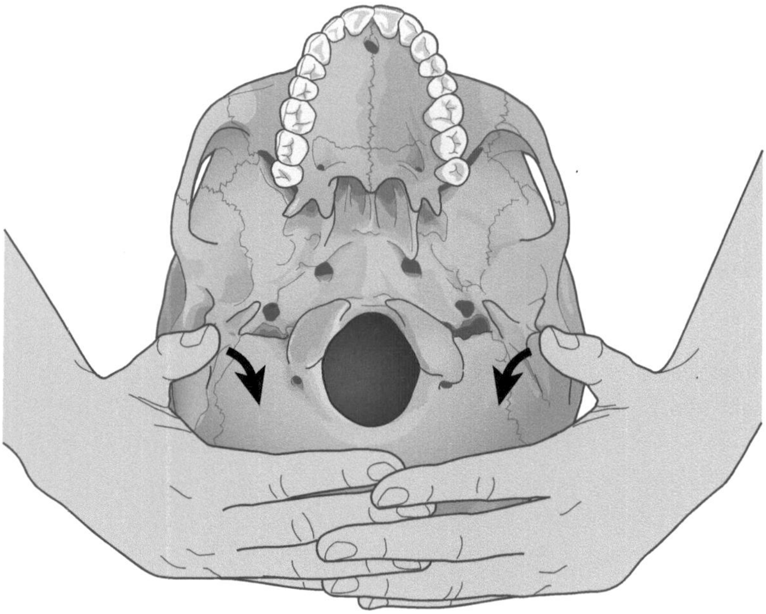

Figure 9.50 W. G. Sutherland's "Father Tom" reanimation technique

Method:

- Bring both temporal bones into external rotation by pressure of your thumbs in a medial and posterior direction on the tips of the mastoid processes (Figure 9.50).
- Maintain this pressure for a few seconds and then release it. Repeat several times until the rhythm can once more be sensed and pulmonary breathing resumes.

NOTE This is the only craniosacral technique for which very strong force is applied! If necessary this technique can be combined with other reanimation techniques. When doing this, bring the temporal bones into external rotation during the inhalation phase. The gentler version differs from the reanimation technique in that less force is used.

9.4.14 Auditory tube technique

See Volume 2, section 6.4.2.

9.5 References

1 Frymann, V. M. and Nordell, B. E. (1981) 'Effects of temporal manipulation of respiration.' *J. Am. Osteopath. Assoc. 80*, 751.

2 Kravchenko, T. I. (1996) 'The principles of osteopathic techniques efficacy monitoring.' In: *The First Russian-French Symposium: Fundamental Aspects of Osteopathy*. 1.–2.7.96, St. Petersburg.

3 Liem, T. (2018) *Kraniosakrale Osteopathie. Ein praktisches Lehrbuch*, 7th Ed. Stuttgart: Thieme.

4 Lippincott, R. C. and Lippincott, H. A. (1995) *A Manual of Cranial Technique*, 2nd Ed. Indianapolis, IN: Cranial Academy.

5 Magoun, H. I. (1951) *Osteopathy in the Cranial Field*. Kirksville: Journal Printing Company.

6 Magoun, H. I. (1976) *Osteopathy in the Cranial Field*, 3rd Ed. Kirksville: Journal Printing Company.

7 Ohanian, M. (1994) *Father Tom et asthme*. Paris: Mémoire.

8 Tomatis, A. A. (1987) *Der Klang des Lebens*. Reinbek: Rowohlt.

9 Rohen, J. W. (2002) *Morphologie des menschlichen Organismus*, 2nd Ed. Stuttgart: Verlag Freies Geistesleben, p. 370.

10.1 The morphology of the frontal bone 372

10.2 Location, causes, and clinical presentation of dysfunctions of the frontal bone 372
10.2.1 Osseous dysfunction 372
10.2.2 Intraosseous dysfunction 373
10.2.3 Muscular dysfunction 373
10.2.4 Fascial dysfunction 373
10.2.5 Dysfunction at the falx cerebri 373
10.2.6 Disturbances of nerves and parts of the brain 373
10.2.7 Vascular disturbances 374

10.3 Diagnosis of the frontal bone 374
10.3.1 History-taking 374
10.3.2 Inspection 374
10.3.3 Palpation of the position 374
10.3.4 Palpation of PRM rhythm 374
10.3.5 Motion testing 376

10.4 Treatment of the frontal bone 376
10.4.1 Intraosseous dysfunction 376
10.4.2 Dysfunction in external rotation 377
10.4.3 Dysfunction in internal rotation 378
10.4.4 Dural techniques 379
10.4.5 Sutural dysfunctions 381

10.5 References 388

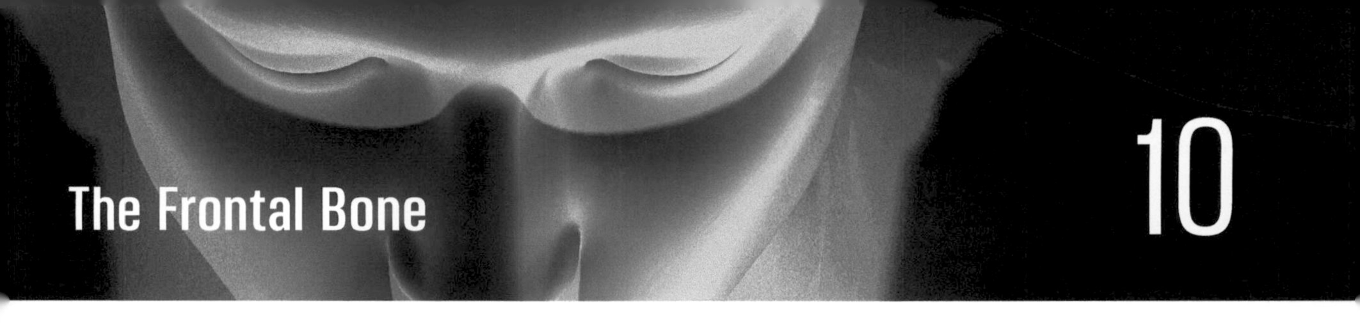

The Frontal Bone

10

The frontal bone is unpaired. The metopic suture is not always ossified in adults. Even when it is closed, there is assumed to be a degree of intraosseous elasticity in the sense of internal and external rotation in the two parts of the frontal squama. The bone helps form the anterior cranial fossa, orbits, and upper airways. There are neural relations with the frontal lobe, the sensory innervation of upper third of the face (cranial nerve V1), the nose, the sphenoidal sinus, and the posterior ethmoidal cells (anterior and posterior ethmoidal nerve); there are muscle connections to the eyes and the masticatory system. The falx cerebri has an anterior attachment to the frontal bone.

10.1 The morphology of the frontal bone

The motion dynamics of the frontal bone with its plate-like structure correspond to those of the shoulder blade, which is also plate-like. Just as the shoulder blade enables the arm to be raised above the space that lies horizontally about it, so the frontal bone reflects the human self in the concept developed by Rohen, and expresses in spatial terms the connection with the world of the mind and spirit.

10.2 Location, causes, and clinical presentation of dysfunctions of the frontal bone

Tip for practitioners

Primary dysfunctions

- Intraosseous: direct effect of force to the frontal bone, especially during birth and in infancy.
- Primary traumatic injury: during early childhood and beyond, falls or blows or other force to the sutures can lead to motion restrictions of the frontal bone and surrounding bones.

Secondary dysfunctions

- Secondary motion restriction of the frontal bone can be caused by dysfunction of the sphenoid, e.g., SBS dysfunctions or transmission of tension via the falx cerebri.

10.2.1 Osseous dysfunction

- **Coronal suture**
  - Sequelae: restriction of mobility of the SBS, frontal bone, and parietal bone.
  - Clinical presentation: functional impairment of the corresponding parts of the brain, e.g., precentral gyrus and postcentral gyrus.
- **Sphenofrontal suture**
  - Sequelae: a fall or blow to the suture can restrict the mobility of the SBS.
- **Frontoethmoidal suture**
  - Sequelae: restriction of mobility of the ethmoid bone; especially, restriction of the falx cerebri; also dysfunction of the anterior and posterior ethmoidal nerves.
- **Frontomaxillary suture**
  - Sequelae: restriction of mobility of the maxilla, especially dysfunction of the frontal process.
  - Clinical presentation: according to Sutherland, this leads to narrowness in the nasal conchae.[2]
- **Frontozygomatic suture**
  - Clinical presentation: disturbance of the orbits, resulting in visual disturbances.
- **Frontonasal suture**
  - Causes: falls or blows to the suture can restrict the mobility of the nasal bone.

- **Frontolacrimal suture**
  - Sequelae: restriction of mobility of the lacrimal bone.

10.2.2 Intraosseous dysfunction

Clinical presentation: impairment of function of the related parts of the brain and the frontal sinus.

10.2.3 Muscular dysfunction

- Traumatic injury in infancy can lead to disturbances of the muscles of the eye by affecting cranial nerves III, IV, and VI. Contact between the superior oblique muscle of the eye and the frontal bone is created by a connective tissue loop at the trochlear fovea.
- Unilateral spasm of the anterior part of the temporalis muscle can move or restrict the frontal bone to one side.

10.2.4 Fascial dysfunction

Temporal fascia: e.g., in dysfunction of the jaw or via fascial continuities with other body tissues.

10.2.5 Dysfunction at the falx cerebri

- Causes: in dysfunctions of the frontal bone, especially involving the ethmoid bone (frontoethmoidal suture).
- Clinical presentation: congestion in the anterior portion of the superior sagittal sinus with functional disturbances in the corresponding parts of the brain; pain in the ipsilateral eye.[1]

10.2.6 Disturbances of nerves and parts of the brain

- **Frontal lobe**
  - Causes: dysfunctions of the frontal bone and dysfunctions in the anterior cranial fossa.
  - Clinical presentation: personality changes; irresponsible and inappropriate behavior; functional disturbances of the intellect, voluntary motor function, expression, and olfactory center.
- **Olfactory nerve** (CN I)
  - Causes: dysfunctions of the frontal bone, especially the frontoethmoidal suture and the cribriform plate of the ethmoid bone.
  - Clinical presentation: disturbances of the sense of smell.

Symptoms affecting the following nerves as a result of dysfunctions of the frontal bone occur rarely:

- **Frontal nerve** (CN V_1), **supraorbital nerve, lateral and medial branches**
  - Causes: dysfunction of the frontal bone, especially disturbances located at the roof of the orbit, the supraorbital foramen, and the frontal notch (foramen).
  - Clinical presentation: disturbances of sensation and pain affecting the skin of the forehead, the upper eyelid, the mucosa of the frontal sinus, and connective tissue membrane.
- **Lacrimal nerve** (CN V_1)
  - Causes: dysfunction of the frontal bone, especially disturbances affecting the lateral wall of the orbit.
  - Clinical presentation: disturbances of sensation and pain affecting the skin of the lateral corner of the eye; disturbance of the lacrimal gland (parasympathetic fibers from the pterygopalatine ganglion and sympathetic fibers from the internal carotid plexus supplying the lacrimal gland run via the lacrimal nerve).
- **Nasociliary nerve** (CN V_1)
  - Causes: dysfunction of the frontal bone, especially disturbances at the medial wall of the orbit and tensions of the common tendinous ring (anulus of Zinn) (origin of recti muscles of the eye).
  - Clinical presentation: disturbances of sensation and pain affecting the mucosa of the frontal sinus, and in the region of the ethmoidal cells and anterior part of the nasal cavity, disturbance of pupil dilation (sympathetic fibers supplying the dilator pupillae muscle).

10.2.7 Vascular disturbances

- **Superior sagittal sinus**
  - Causes: dysfunction of the frontal bone, especially along the sinus, at the foramen cecum and frontal crest.
  - Clinical presentation: superior sagittal sinus and the veins draining into this: pain in the frontoparietal region and region of the eye.

Symptoms affecting the following blood vessels, caused by dysfunctions of the frontal bone, occur rarely.

- **Ophthalmic artery**
  - Clinical presentation: disturbances at the wall of the orbit, the lacrimal gland, the external muscles of the eye, and sometimes the eyeball.
- **Supraorbital and supratrochlear arteries**
  - Clinical presentation: disturbances of the skin and the muscles of the frontal region.

10.3 Diagnosis of the frontal bone

10.3.1 History-taking

- Headache affecting the frontal region.
- Inflammation of the paranasal sinuses.
- Disturbances of the eye.
- Abnormalities of social behavior.
- Previous traumatic injury.

10.3.2 Inspection

- Metopic suture: indented (ER) or convex (IR).
- Forehead: sloping (ER) or prominent (IR).
- More pronounced vertical supranasal furrow (IR of the affected side).
- Lateral corner: displaced anteriorly (ER) or posteriorly (IR).
- Bregma: indented, e.g., in the case of primary traumatic injury through force to bregma, or prominent.
- Frontal tuber: convex or flat (intraosseous dysfunction).

10.3.3 Palpation of the position

See under Inspection, section 10.3.2 above.

10.3.4 Palpation of PRM rhythm

Tip for practitioners

Biomechanical approach, inhalation phase

Flexion and external rotation of the frontal bone occur. The rotation is organized around two vertical axes running through the frontal tubers.

- The metopic suture flattens.
- The glabella moves in a posterior and superior direction.
- The zygomatic process of the frontal bone moves in an anterior, inferior, and lateral direction.
- Bregma sinks downward.
- The ethmoidal notch widens in its posterior portion, and descends.

Developmental dynamic, inhalation phase

- Expansive force is anteriorly directed.
- The motion is centrifugal (outward).
- Convexity lessens.

If a motion restriction is discovered on palpation, an impulse in the restricted direction can be induced. This will emphasize the restriction and enable you to sense more easily which structure is the origin of the motion restriction.

Practitioner: Take up a position at the head of the patient.

Hand position:

- Place your ring fingers on the outside of the zygomatic processes of the frontal bone.
- Position your little fingers alongside the ring fingers.
- Place your middle and index fingers to the side, by the midline of the frontal bone.
- Your thumbs should be either crossed or touching, posteriorly (Figure 10.1).

Biomechanical:

Inhalation phase of PRM, normal finding (Figure 10.2)

- With your ring fingers of the zygomatic processes of the frontal bone, you will sense motion in an anterior, lateral, and inferior direction.
- Your index fingers on the metopic suture sense a flattening.
- Overall, the frontal bone flattens and becomes more sloping.

Exhalation phase of PRM, normal finding

- The ring fingers on the zygomatic processes of the frontal bone sense motion in a posterior, medial, and superior direction.
- Your index fingers on the metopic suture sense increasing convexity.
- Overall, the frontal bone becomes steeper and more vertical.

Developmental dynamic:

Inhalation phase of PRM, normal finding (Figure 10.3)

- Your hands on the frontal bone sense an expansive, anteriorly directed force.
- The motion is centrifugal (outward). Convexity decreases.

Exhalation phase of PRM, normal finding

- Your hands on the frontal bone sense a retractive, posteriorly directed force. The motion is centripetal. Convexity increases.

Compare the amplitude, strength, ease, and symmetry of the motions of the frontal bone.

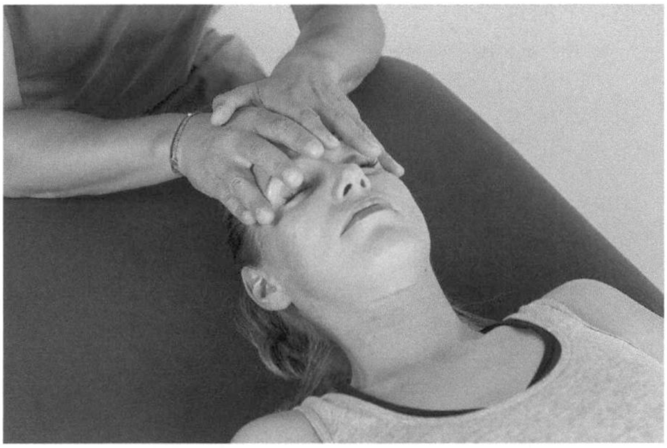

Figure 10.1 Palpation of PRM rhythm of the frontal bone

Other types of motion of the frontal bone may sometimes occur during external and internal rotation. These provide an indication of further dysfunctions of the frontal bone.

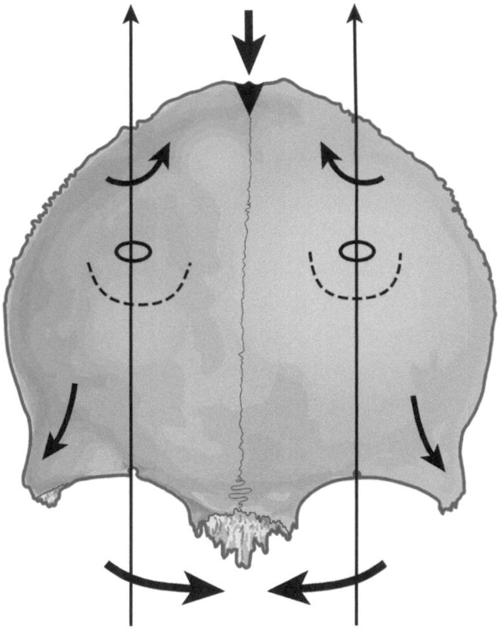

Figure 10.2 Inhalation phase of PRM/biomechanical

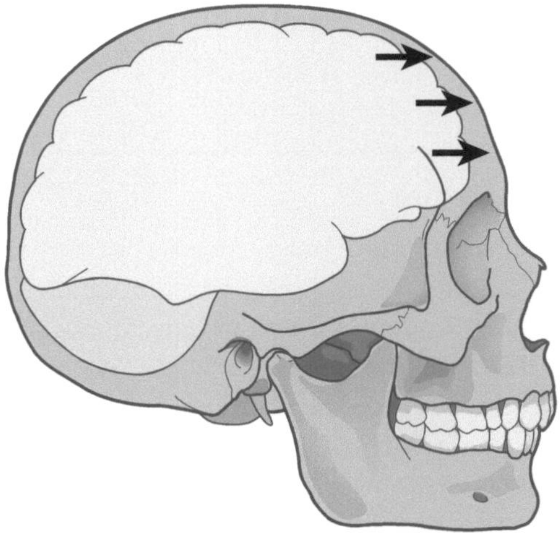

Figure 10.3 Inhalation phase of PRM/developmental dynamic

10.3.5 Motion testing

Hand position: See palpation of PRM rhythm (section 10.3.4).

Testing of external and internal rotation

Method:

During the inhalation phase

- At the beginning of the inhalation phase, administer a posteriorly directed impulse with your index fingers on the metopic suture.
- With your ring fingers on the zygomatic processes of the frontal bone, administer an impulse in an anterior, lateral (and inferior) direction.

During the exhalation phase

- At the beginning of the exhalation phase, administer an impulse in a posterior, medial (and superior) direction with the ring fingers on the zygomatic processes of the frontal bone.

Compare the amplitude and ease of motion and the degree of force needed to elicit motion.

Testing of flexion and extension motion

Method:

During the inhalation phase

- At the beginning of the inhalation phase, administer an impulse with your hands aimed at imparting a more shallow-angled slope to or flattening the frontal bone.

During the exhalation phase

- At the beginning of the exhalation phase, administer an impulse with your hands aimed at making the frontal bone more vertical.

Compare the amplitude and ease of motion or the degree of force needed to elicit motion.

NOTE External rotation and flexion of the frontal bone can be tested at the same time, as can internal rotation and extension.

10.4 Treatment of the frontal bone

10.4.1 Intraosseous dysfunction

Molding

Indication: Asymmetric convexity or flattening, and torsion tensions at the ossification centers, usually as a result of birth trauma or a fall in early childhood.

Hand position: Placing the fingertips of one hand close together, position them on the frontal tuber (Figure 10.4).

NOTE It is important to release the surrounding bones gently from the frontal bone before beginning this technique.

Method:

In the case of a convexity

- Administer centrifugal impulses with your fingers, aimed at flattening the site.
- This treatment may be augmented by using a fluid impulse to direct energy toward the borders of the frontal bone.
- Establish PBMT, PBFT.

In the case of flattening

- Administer centripetal impulses with your fingers, aimed at making the flattened site more prominent.
- This treatment may be augmented by using a fluid impulse to direct energy from the opposite occipito-mastoid suture toward the center of the frontal tuber.
- Establish PBMT and PBFT.

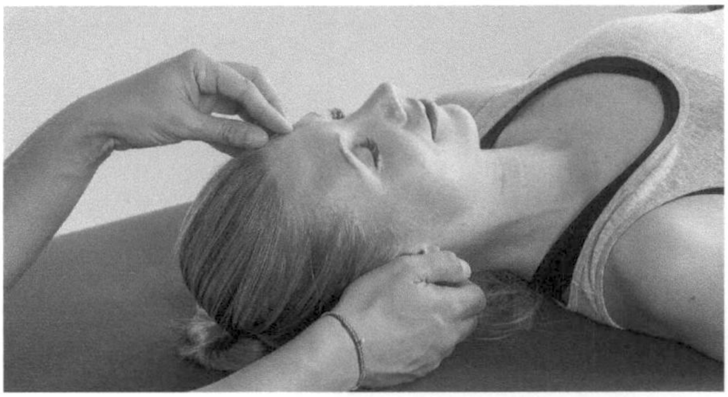

Figure 10.4 Molding of the frontal bone

In the case of torsional tensions

- Administer an impulse with your fingers in the direction of the restriction.
- Establish PBMT and PBFT.

Spreading the metopic suture

Indication: Compression of the suture by transverse forces during the birth process.

Practitioner: Take up a position at the head of the patient.

Hand position: Cross your thumbs over the metopic suture, so that they rest next to the suture on the opposite sides of the frontal bone. Place the palms of your hands laterally on the roof of the skull each side (Figure 10.5).

Alternative hand position: Place the fingers of both hands bilaterally on the metopic suture (Figure 10.6).

Method:

- Disengagement
  - ▸ Administer diverging lateral traction with your fingers, so as to spread the metopic suture.
  - ▸ Permit all motions/tissue unwinding that arise.
- Establish PBMT and PBFT.
- Maintain the PBT until a correction of the abnormal tension has been achieved and stabilized by the inherent homeostatic forces (PRM rhythm, etc.).
- This treatment may be augmented by using a fluid impulse to direct energy from inion.

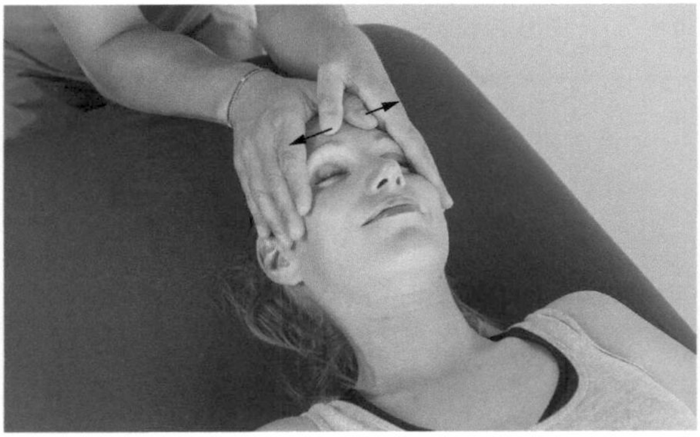

Figure 10.5 Spreading of the metopic suture

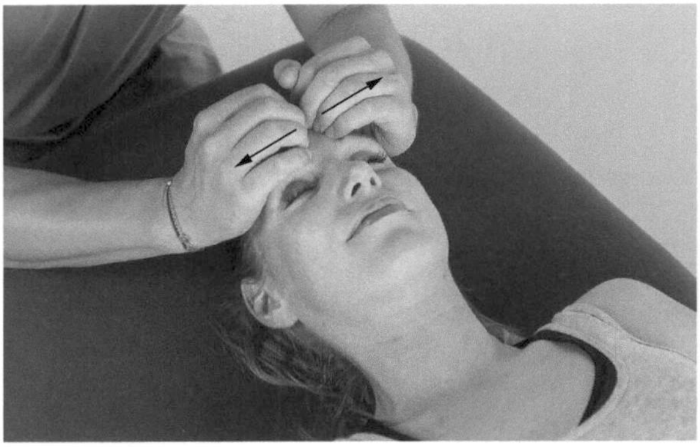

Figure 10.6 Spreading of the metopic suture. Alternative hand position

10.4.2 Dysfunction in external rotation

Restricted internal rotation of the frontal bone.

Hand position:

- Place your ring fingers on the outside of the zygomatic processes of the frontal bone. Grasp these securely from outside with your in-bent fingers, to provide a firm hold.
- Place your little fingers beside your ring fingers.
- Position your middle and index fingers laterally adjacent to the midline of the frontal bone.
- Your thumbs should lie posteriorly, either crossed or touching.

Indirect technique, frontal bone spread technique

Method:

- At the beginning of the inhalation phase, begin to apply gentle posteriorly directed pressure with your index fingers on the midline of the frontal bone (ER).
- With your ring fingers, administer an impulse in an anterior, lateral (and inferior) direction to the zygomatic processes of the frontal bone (ER; Figure 10.7).
- This reduces the anteroposterior diameter of the falx, reducing the membrane tension.
- Try to find the position in which the membrane tension on the frontal bone is most balanced (PBMT).
- Maintain the PBMT until a correction of the abnormal tension has been achieved and stabilized by the inherent homeostatic forces (PRM rhythm, etc.).
- Breathing assistance: ask the patient to hold an inhalation at the end of an in-breath for as long as possible.
- A fluid impulse may be directed from the inion or further caudad in the midline.

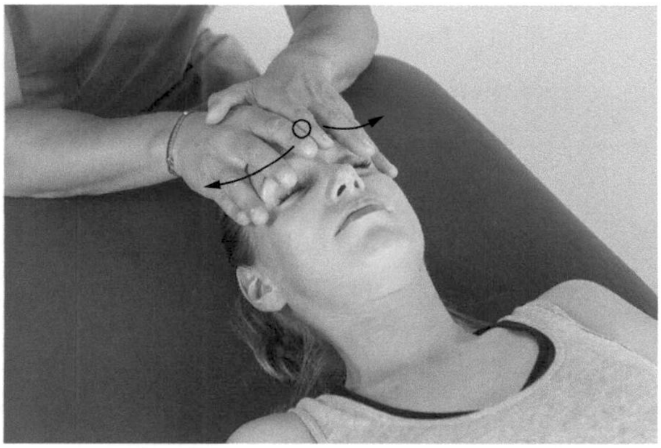

Figure 10.7 Dysfunction in external rotation. Indirect technique. Frontal bone spread technique

Direct technique

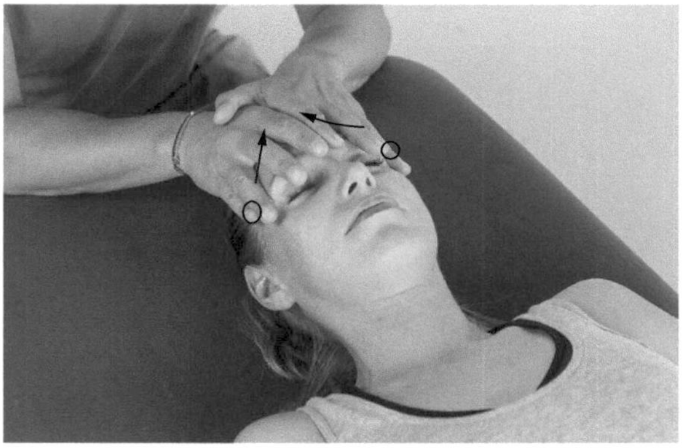

Figure 10.8 Dysfunction in external rotation. Direct technique

Method:

- At the beginning of the exhalation phase, begin to administer an impulse in a posterior, medial (and superior) direction with your ring fingers on the zygomatic processes of the frontal bone (IR; Figure 10.8).
- Maintain the PBMT until no further release can be sensed, or the fluctuation of the cerebro-spinal fluid has stopped and the frontal bone wants to move into external rotation.
- Breathing assistance: ask the patient to hold an exhalation for as long as possible at the end of an out-breath.
- A fluid impulse may be used to direct energy from the inion or further caudad in the midline.

Vitalist approach: See EV-4 technique (section 4.4.3).

10.4.3 Dysfunction in internal rotation

Restricted external rotation of the frontal bone.

Method:

Indirect technique

- At the beginning of the exhalation phase, begin to administer an impulse in a posterior, medial

(and superior) direction with your ring fingers on the zygomatic processes of the frontal bone (IR).
- Maintain the PBMT until no further release can be sensed, or the fluctuation of CSF has stopped and the frontal bone wants to move into external rotation.
- Breathing assistance: ask the patient to hold an exhalation at the end of an out-breath for as long as possible.
- A fluid impulse may be used to direct energy from inion or further caudad in the midline.

Direct technique, frontal bone spread technique
- At the beginning of the inhalation phase, begin to administer a posteriorly directed impulse with your index fingers on the metopic suture (ER).
- With your ring fingers on the zygomatic processes of the frontal bone, administer an impulse in an anterior, lateral (and inferior) direction (ER).
- Maintain the point of balance until no further release can be sensed, or the fluctuation of the CSF has stopped and the frontal bone wants to move into internal rotation.
- Breathing assistance: ask the patient to hold an inhalation for as long as possible at the end of an in-breath.
- A fluid impulse may be directed from inion or further caudad in the midline.

10.4.4 Dural techniques

Frontal bone lift technique

Indication: In combination with the spread technique: tensions and fibrosis of the falx cerebri, disturbances of the drainage of the superior and inferior sagittal sinuses, restrictions of the sutures of the frontal bone, rhinitis, sinusitis, functional disturbances of the sense of smell.

Hand position: Use the same position as for the spread technique.

Method:
- During the exhalation phase, begin to apply gentle pressure in a medial direction (Figure 10.9a) with the ring fingers on the lateral surface of the frontal bone so as to release it from the sphenoid (IR).
- As soon as the frontal bone begins to move anteriorly you can relax the medial pressure of your ring fingers.
- Replace this pressure with an anterior, slightly cephalad traction (Figure 10.9b). This traction is very gentle; it must remain below the threshold where the tissue begins to react by countercontracting. Induce the anterior traction by pressing your elbows slightly down into the table, so that your fingers lift anterior.
- The weight of the skull is enough to hold the occiput, the posterior attachment of the falx, in position on the table.
- At each release of the tissues, seek the new motion barrier of the frontal bone in the anterior direction.
- Permit all motions/tissue unwinding of the frontal bone that arise, without reducing the gentle traction.
- You can sense the various stages of tissue release: first the sutural tensions, then the elastic and collagenous tensions of the falx cerebri (a sensation like cement, or a rubber band, or chewing gum).
- When the falx has been freed from its tension patterns (floating sensation), you can slowly reduce the anterior traction and remove your hands.

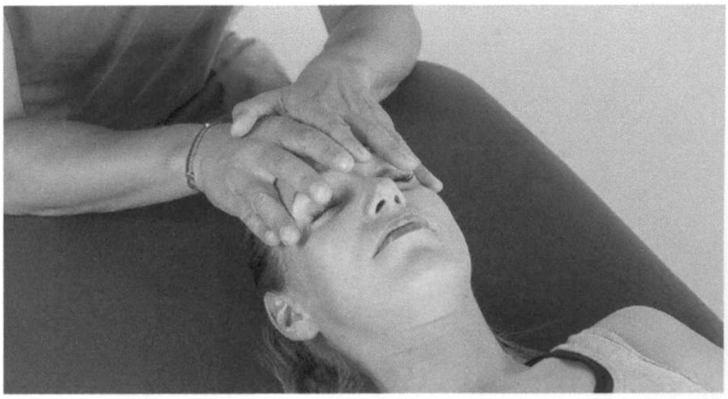

Figure 10.9 Frontal bone lift technique. (a) Medial pressure. (b) Anterior and slightly cephalad traction

NOTE—IMPORTANT In the lift technique, the traction applied imitates the tension that is present, with an additional 5 g beyond the current degree of tension.
Never remove your hands suddenly from the bone during the technique.
Always take care to position your hands accurately. Failure to do so would mean that at best the technique would be ineffective. In the worst case, especially if your fingers are on the sutures, this could worsen or even give rise to symptoms.

Tip for practitioners

As an alternative you may assist the flexion and extension motions of the frontal bone (in harmony with the PRM) during the gentle anterior traction.

Alternative hand position for the frontal bone lift technique I

Hand position: Place the ball of your little fingers bilaterally behind the edges of the temporal lines and behind the zygomatic processes of the frontal bone. Interclasp your fingers and support your elbows on the table slightly caudad and lateral to your hands (Figure 10.10).

Method:

- Apply gentle medial pressure with the ball of your hands on the sides of the frontal bone. V. M. Frymann refined this method by drawing her fingertips apart laterally to produce the gentle medial compression. This internal rotation of the frontal bone causes a disengagement of the sutural articulations with the sphenoid.

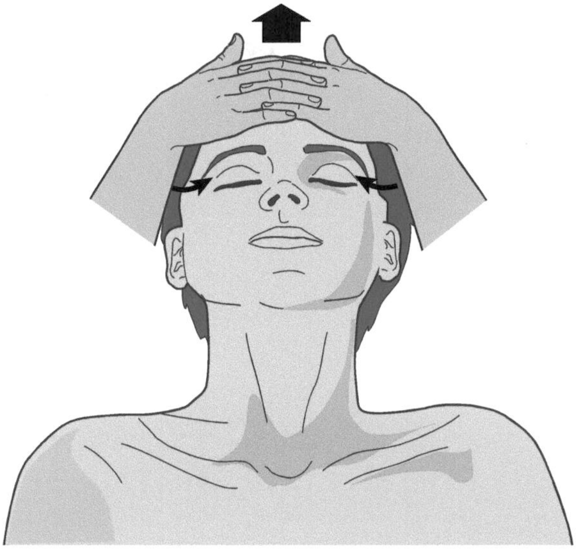

Figure 10.10 Alternative hold for the frontal bone lift technique I

- When the frontal bone begins to move slightly in an anterior direction, the cranial bones have released from each other.
- Then administer anterior traction to the frontal bone and so to the falx cerebri. An alternative way of performing this traction is to stretch your fingers gently in an anterior direction.

Alternative hand position for the frontal bone lift technique II
Fronto-occipital cranial hold

Hand position: Hold the frontal bone with your upper hand, with your fingers pointing caudad. With your lower hand, hold the occipital bone, fingers also pointing caudad (Figure 10.11).
This hold offers the advantage that you can check the nuchal muscles and the whole of the cranium together. The disadvantage, especially if you have small hands, is first that you cannot grasp the frontal bone adequately, and second, that the

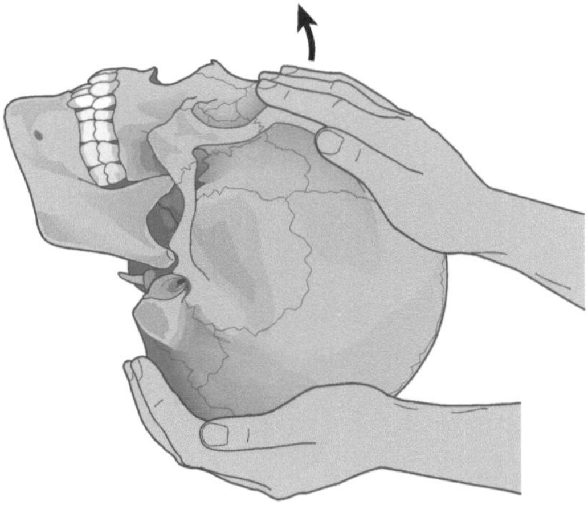

Figure 10.11 Alternative hold for the frontal bone lift technique II

anterior traction force applied to the frontal bone is generally more awkward and involves more tension of the hands and shoulders.

In this method, as previously, the anterior traction is induced by pressing the elbows in the direction of the table.

10.4.5 Sutural dysfunctions

Sphenofrontal suture, Cant hook technique

Suture margin: Greater wing: inward facing margin (L-shaped); frontal bone: outward-facing margin (rocking motion; limits sphenoid motion). Lesser wing: usually outward-facing border; frontal bone: usually lies above (gliding motion).

Suture type: Squamoserrate suture.

Aim: To free the L-shaped joint surface of the greater wing from the frontal bone. This dysfunction is common. Also to release the lesser wing from the frontal bone.

Practitioner: Take up a position beside the head of the patient, on the side opposite to the dysfunction.

Hand position:

- Caudal hand
  - Place your little finger intraorally, laterally on the pterygoid process. It will sometimes be necessary to ask patients to move their jaw to that side to make room for your finger.
  - Position your index and middle finger externally on the greater wing on the side being treated.
  - Place your thumb on the outside of the opposite greater wing if possible.
- Cranial hand
  - Position your middle finger (or index finger) laterally on the frontal bone on the side of the dysfunction (directly above the sphenofrontal suture).
  - Position your thumb laterally on the frontal bone on the opposite side. Do not move it; it provides the fixed point around which the motion is organized. It should be touching the thumb of the other hand.

Suture between the greater wing of the sphenoid and the frontal bone

Method:

- Disengagement (Figure 10.12)
  - With your caudal hand, hold the sphenoid in place.
  - Do not move the thumb on the side opposite the dysfunction. It is the hub around which the motion is organized.
  - During the inhalation phase, begin to apply traction in a superior and very slightly anterior direction (disengagement of the frontal bone from the greater wing) with the middle finger on the frontal bone.
  - Without reducing the gentle disengagement, permit all motions/unwinding of the frontal bone that arise.
- Establish the PBMT and PBFT.
- A fluid impulse may be used to direct energy from the opposite parietal tuber.

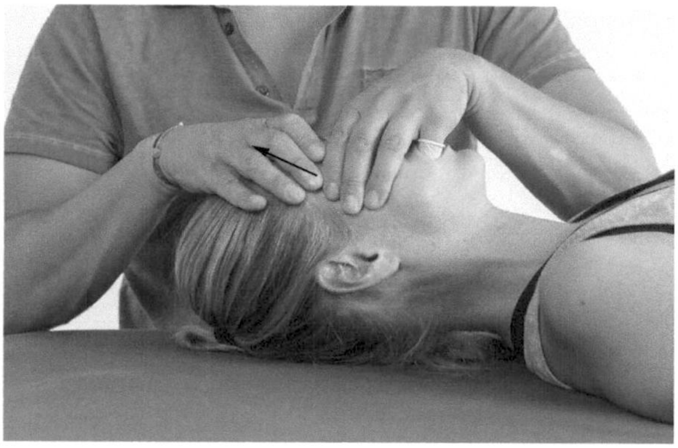

Figure 10.12 Sphenofrontal suture. Cant hook technique. Suture between the greater wing of the sphenoid and the frontal bone

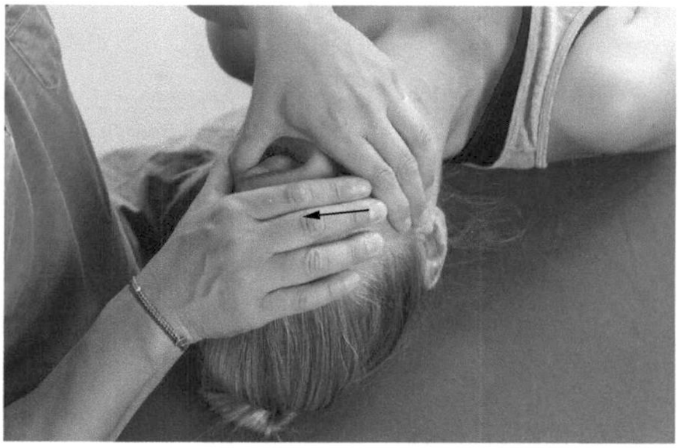

Figure 10.13 Sphenofrontal suture. Cant hook technique. Suture between the lesser wing of the sphenoid and the frontal bone

Alternative option: without reducing the gentle disengagement, assist the flexion and extension motions of the greater wings in harmony with the PRM rhythm, either in synchrony with the flexion and extension motions of the frontal bone or as opposite physiological motion (flexion of the sphenoid with extension of the frontal bone and vice versa).

Suture between the lesser wing of the sphenoid and the frontal bone

Method:

- Disengagement (Figure 10.13)
  - With your caudal hand, hold the sphenoid in place.
  - Do not move the thumb on the opposite side to the dysfunction. It is the hub around which the motion is organized.
  - During the inhalation phase, begin to administer anterior traction (disengagement of the frontal bone from the lesser wing) with the middle finger on the frontal bone.
  - Without reducing the gentle disengagement, permit all motions/tissue unwinding of the frontal bone that arise.
- Establish the PBMT and PBFT.
- A fluid impulse may be used to direct energy from the opposite lambdoid suture.

Alternative option: without reducing the gentle disengagement, assist the flexion and extension motions of the lesser wings of the sphenoid in harmony with the PRM rhythm, either in synchrony with the flexion and extension motions of the frontal bone or as opposite physiological motion (flexion of the sphenoid with extension of the frontal bone and vice versa).

Sphenofrontal suture, alternative technique with cranial vault hold

Hand position:

- Place your index fingers laterally on the frontal bone and on the zygomatic processes of the frontal bone.
- Place your middle fingers laterally on the greater wings of the sphenoid.
- For small children: place your ring fingers and little fingers on the lateral parts of the occiput.
- For adults: place your ring fingers on the mastoid process.

Method:

- Disengagement (Figure 10.14)
    - During the inhalation phase, begin to administer traction in a posterior direction with your ring fingers on the lateral parts of the occiput. This applies posterior traction to the sphenoid (via the anterior attachment of the tentorium to the sphenoid).
    - Additionally, apply posterior traction with your middle fingers on the greater wings.
- Take care: the greater wing has an inward-facing border at the sphenofrontal suture. Medial pressure to the greater wing compresses the suture.
    - Administer anterior traction with your index fingers on the frontal bone.
    - Permit all motions/tissue unwinding that arise.
- Without reducing the disengagement, establish PBMT between the sphenoid, occipital bone, and frontal bone at the position in which the abnormal joint tensions are in the best possible state of balance one to another.
- Maintain the PBMT until a correction of the abnormal tension has been achieved and stabilized by the inherent homeostatic forces (PRM rhythm, etc.), and the motion of the sphenoid and the frontal bone has stopped.

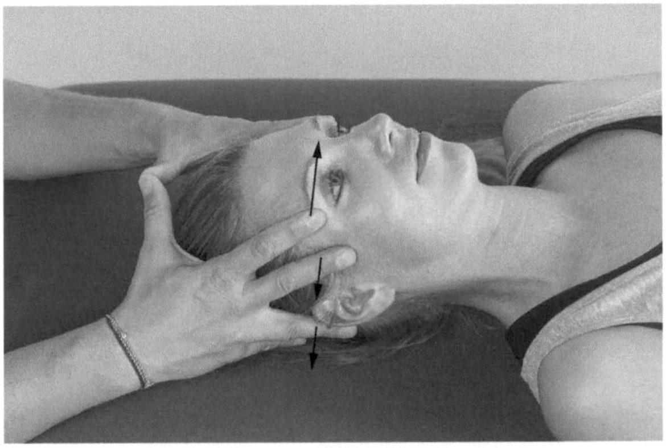

Figure 10.14 Sphenofrontal suture. Alternative technique

Coronal suture (left)

Suture margin:

- Medial: frontal bone: inward-facing margin; parietal bone: outward-facing margin.
- Lateral: frontal bone: outward-facing margin; parietal bone: inward-facing margin.

Suture type: Squamoserrate suture.

Indication: Restricted mobility of the SBS, frontal bone, and parietal bone with functional impairment of the corresponding regions of the brain.

Patient: The patient's head should be turned to the opposite side to the dysfunction.

Practitioner: Take up a position beside the patient's head on the opposite side to the dysfunction.

Hand position:

- Place the index and middle fingers of your left hand on the parietal bone, near the coronal suture. Position your index finger medially to the pivot point and your middle finger laterally to it.
- Place the index and middle fingers of your right hand on the frontal bone, near the coronal suture. Position the index finger medially to the pivot point and your middle finger laterally to it.

Method:

- Disengagement (Figure 10.15)
    - Hand on the frontal bone: administer anteriorly directed traction on the frontal bone with your index and middle fingers. Also apply pressure to the bone with the middle finger positioned below the pivot point.
    - Hand on the parietal bone: administer posterior traction on the frontal border of the parietal bone with your index and middle fingers. Also apply pressure on the bone with the index finger positioned above the pivot point.

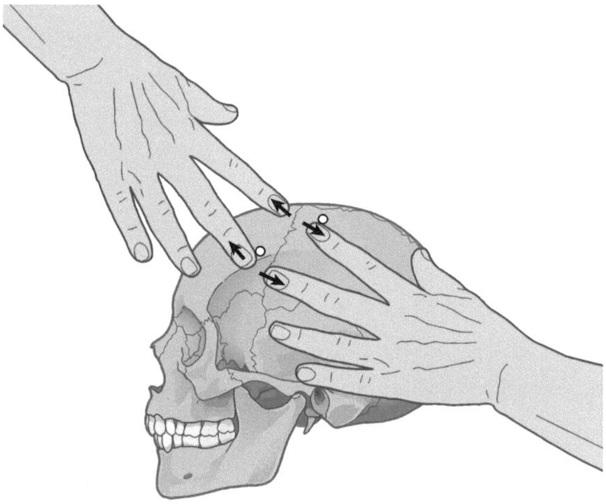

Figure 10.15 Coronal suture (left)

- Without reducing the gentle disengagement, permit all motions/unwinding of the frontal bone that arise.
- Establish PBMT and PBFT between the frontal bone and parietal bone at the position in which the abnormal tensions in the joint are in the best possible state of balance with each other.
- A fluid impulse may be used to direct energy from the opposite asterion.

Coronal suture (left), alternative technique

Patient: Supine.

Practitioner: Take up a position beside the patient's head, on the opposite side to the dysfunction.

Hand position:

- Hold the parietal bone in your cranial hand
  - Your index finger should point toward pterion.
  - Your middle finger should point toward the zygomatic process of the temporal bone.
  - Your ring finger should point toward asterion.
  - Place the basal joints of your fingers on the axis of motion of the parietal bone, so that the basal joint of your index finger lies on the pivot point of the coronal suture.
- Place your caudal hand on the frontal bone
  - Position your index, middle, and ring fingers directly anterior to the coronal suture and pointing toward it.
  - Your middle finger should be on the pivot point of the coronal suture.

Method:

- Disengagement (Figure 10.16)
  - Administer posterior traction on the frontal border of the parietal bone. At the same time apply pressure to the medial part of the frontal border.
  - Administer anterior traction to the parietal margin of the frontal bone. At the same time apply pressure to the lateral part of the parietal margin of the frontal bone with your ring finger.
  - Without reducing the gentle disengagement, permit all motions/unwinding of the frontal bone that arise.
- Establish the PBMT and PBFT.
- A fluid impulse may be used to direct energy from the opposite asterion.

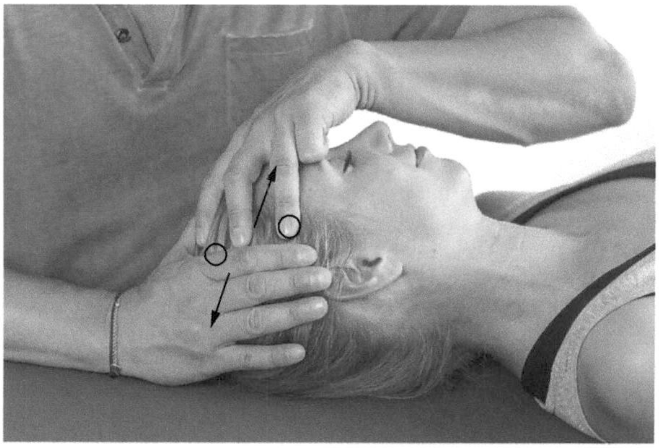

Figure 10.16 Coronal suture. Alternative technique

Frontomaxillary suture, Cant hook technique

Suture margin: The lateral portion of the nasal part articulates with the frontal process of the maxilla.

Suture type: Serrate suture.

Practitioner: Take up a position beside the patient's head, on the opposite side to the dysfunction.

Hand position:

- Cranial hand
  - Span the frontal bone with your cranial hand.
  - Place your middle finger laterally on the frontal bone on the side of the dysfunction (directly above the frontozygomatic suture).
  - Position your thumb laterally on the frontal bone on the opposite side.
- Caudal hand
  - Place your index finger on the frontal process of the maxilla.
  - Place your middle finger externally (Figure 10.17) or intraorally (Figure 10.18) on the lateral surface of the alveolar part of the maxilla.

Method:

- Disengagement
  - Caudal hand: hold the maxillary bone in position with your index and middle fingers.
  - Cranial hand: do not move the thumb on the opposite side to the dysfunction. It is the fixed point around which the motion is organized. With your index finger, administer traction in a superior direction to the lateral part of the frontal bone (disengagement of the frontal bone from the maxilla).
  - Without reducing the gentle disengagement, permit all motions/unwinding of the frontal bone that arise.
- Establish PBMT and PBFT.
- A fluid impulse may be used to direct energy from the opposite parietal bone.

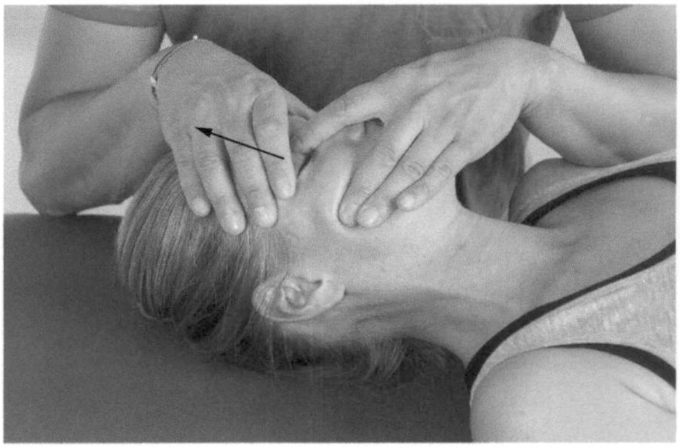

Figure 10.17 Frontomaxillary suture: Cant hook technique

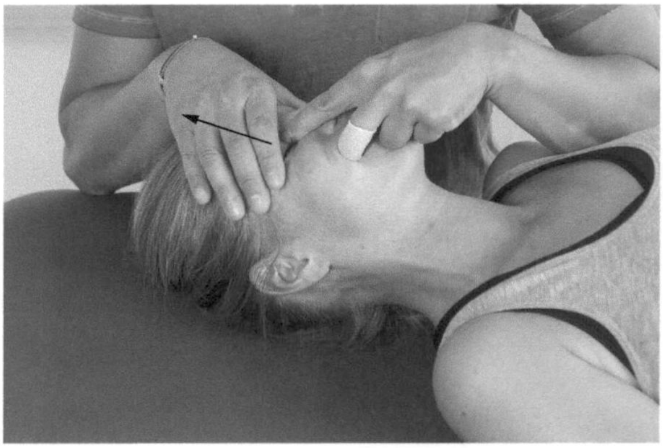

Figure 10.18 Frontomaxillary suture: Cant hook technique. Middle finger on the alveolar part of the maxilla, intraorally

Frontozygomatic suture, Cant hook technique

Suture margin: The zygomatic process articulates with the frontal process of the zygomatic bone.

Suture type: Serrate suture.

Indication: Disturbances of the orbits leading to visual disturbances.

Practitioner: Take up a position beside the patient's head, on the opposite side to the dysfunction.

Hand position:

- Cranial hand
  - Span the frontal bone between thumb and index finger.
  - Place your index or middle finger laterally on the frontal bone on the side of the dysfunction (directly above the frontozygomatic suture).
  - Place your thumb laterally on the frontal bone on the opposite side.
- Caudal hand
  - Grasp the frontal process of the zygomatic bone with your thumb and index finger (Figure 10.19). (Alternatively you may hold the zygomatic bone with your thumb from inside [intraorally] and your index finger from outside [Figure 10.20].)

Method:

- Cranial hand: do not move the thumb on the opposite side to the dysfunction. It is the fixed point around which the motion is organized.
  - With the index finger or middle finger of your cranial hand, administer traction in a superior direction on the zygomatic process of the frontal bone.
  - Without reducing the gentle disengagement, permit all motions/unwinding of the frontal bone that arise.
  - At each release of the tissue, seek the new limit to motion of the frontal bone in the superior direction on the side of the dysfunction.
- Direct technique: in the case of a restriction of the frontozygomatic suture with a dysfunction of the frontal bone in internal rotation.
  - Guide the frontal bone into flexion and external rotation.
  - During the inhalation phase, gently move the frontal process of the zygomatic bone laterally with your thumb and index finger.
  - Breathing assistance: ask the patient to hold an inhalation for as long as possible at the end of an in-breath. Repeat for several breathing cycles.
- Establish PBMT: maintain the gentle disengagement. At the same time follow the zygomatic bone into the position in which the tension between IR and ER is in the best possible state of balance.
- At the end of the technique, the motion of the zygomatic bone should be resynchronized with the motion of the frontal bone, in harmony with the PRM rhythm.
- A fluid impulse may be used to direct energy from the opposite parietal tuber.

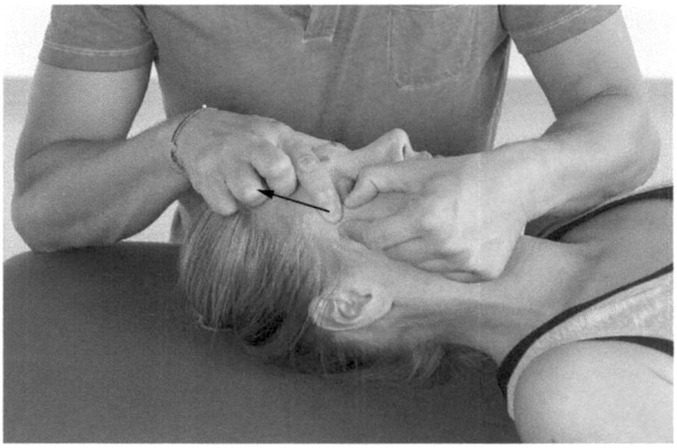

Figure 10.19 Frontozygomatic suture: Cant hook technique

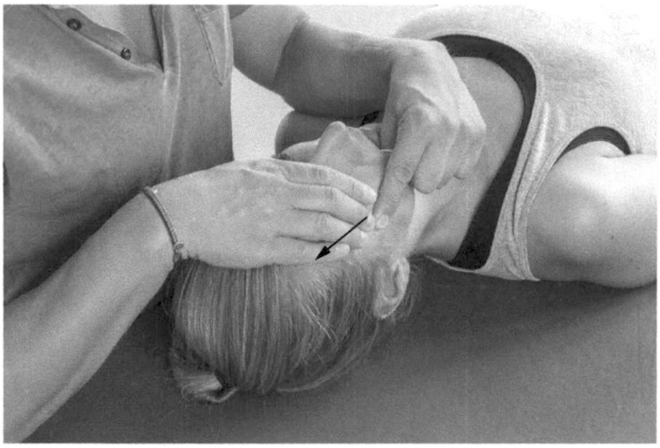

Figure 10.20 Frontozygomatic suture: Cant hook technique, intraoral hold

Frontoethmoidal suture

- See technique to treat the cribriform plate (section 7.4.6).
- See frontal bone spread and frontal bone lift techniques (above).

Indication: Motion restriction of the ethmoid bone, and especially of the falx cerebri, and dysfunction of the anterior and posterior ethmoidal nerves.

Frontonasal suture

Indication: Restricted mobility of the nasal bone due to falls or blows to the suture.

Practitioner: Take up a position at the head of the patient.

Hand position:

- Cranial hand
  - Place your thumb and index finger on the superciliary arch of the frontal bone.
  - Place the basal joint of the index finger on the glabella (the area between the superciliary arches).
- Caudal hand: grasp the two nasal bones with your thumb and index finger.

Method:

- Disengagement
  - During the inhalation phase, begin to apply a more angled tilt to the frontal bone (flexion) with your index and middle finger, while applying posterior and superior pressure to glabella with the basal joint of your index finger (ER).
  - Hold the frontal bone in flexion and ER.
  - At the same time, move the nasal bones caudad (Figure 10.21).
  - Without reducing the gentle traction, permit all motions/unwinding of the frontal and nasal bones that arise.
- Establish the PBMT and PBFT.

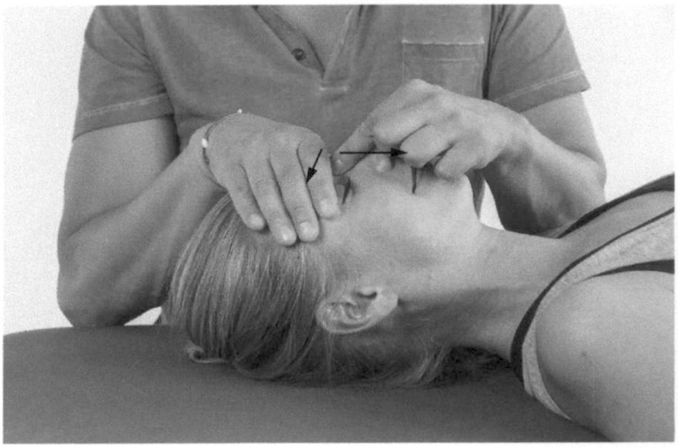

Figure 10.21 Frontonasal suture

- Breathing assistance: ask the patient to hold an inhalation for as long as possible at the end of an in-breath. Repeat for several breathing cycles.

NOTE Alternatively you may administer impulses easing the nasal bone into ER and IR in harmony with PRM rhythm, without reducing the disengagement.

Frontolacrimal suture

Practitioner: Take up a position beside the head of the patient.

Hand position:

- Place the index and middle fingers of your cranial hand on the superior orbital margin, as close as possible to the frontolacrimal suture.
- Place the index finger of your caudal hand on the lacrimal bone.

Method:

- Disengagement
  - During the inhalation phase, begin to apply a more angled tilt to the frontal bone (flexion) with your index and middle finger, and to apply posterior and superior pressure to the glabella (ER).

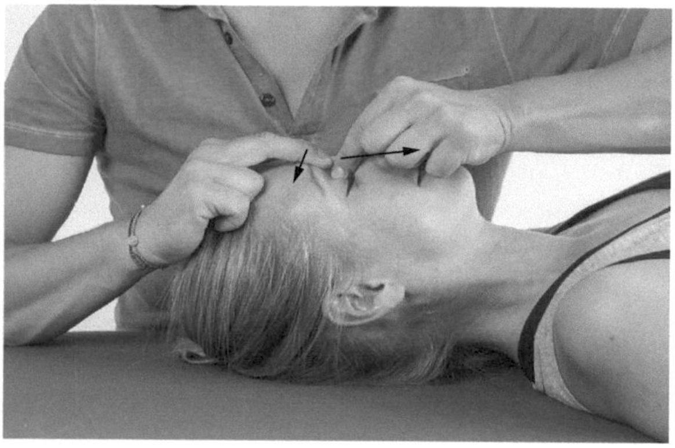

Figure 10.22 Frontolacrimal suture

- ► Hold the frontal bone in flexion and ER.
- ► At the same time, move the lacrimal bone caudad (Figure 10.22).
- ► Without reducing the gentle traction, permit all motions/unwinding of the lacrimal bone that arise.
- Establish the PBMT and PBFT.

NOTE Alternatively you may administer impulses easing the lacrimal bone into ER and IR in harmony with the PRM rhythm, without reducing the disengagement.

Bregma

See section 11.4.6.

10.5 References

1 Liem, T. (2018) *Kraniosakrale Osteopathie. Ein praktisches Lehrbuch*, 7th Ed. Stuttgart: Thieme.

2 Sutherland, W. G. (1944) 'The cranial bowl.' *J. Am. Osteopath. Assoc. 1944*, 348–353.

11.1 The morphology of the parietal bones and cranial vault according to Rohen 390

11.2 Location, causes, and clinical presentation of dysfunctions of the parietal bones 390
11.2.1 Osseous dysfunctions 390
11.2.2 Intraosseous dysfunction 391
11.2.3 Muscular dysfunction 391
11.2.4 Fascial dysfunctions 391
11.2.5 Dysfunctions of the falx cerebri and the tentorium cerebelli 391
11.2.6 Disturbances of nerves and parts of the brain 391
11.2.7 Vascular disturbances 391

11.3 Diagnosis of the parietal bone 392
11.3.1 History-taking 392
11.3.2 Inspection 392
11.3.3 Palpation of position 392
11.3.4 Palpation of PRM rhythm 392
11.3.5 Motion testing 394

11.4 Treatment of the parietal bones 394
11.4.1 Intraosseous dysfunctions 394
11.4.2 Dysfunction in external rotation 394
11.4.3 Dysfunction in internal rotation 396
11.4.4 Dural techniques 396
11.4.5 Sinus techniques 398
11.4.6 Sutural dysfunctions 398

11.5 References 403

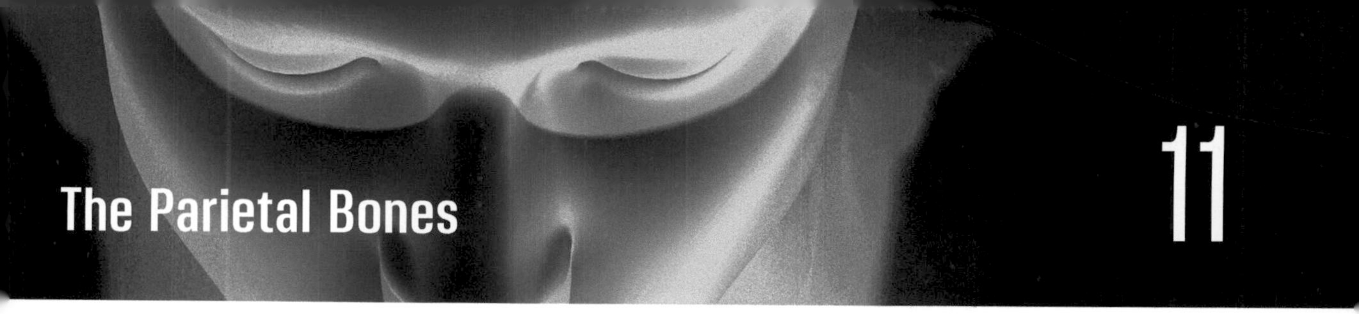

11 The Parietal Bones

The paired parietal bones belong to the roof of the skull, and undergo membranous ossification. There are fascial relations with the temporalis muscle and the falx cerebri. Another significant feature relates to the mastoid angle of the parietal bone; the course of the sigmoid sinus runs alongside it, and the tentorium cerebelli has an attachment there. Other important relations are to the parietal lobe, meningeal artery, and superior sagittal sinus.

11.1 The morphology of the parietal bones and cranial vault according to Rohen[4]

The parietals, like the rest of the roof of the skull, undergo membranous ossification from outside in a similar way to the compact substance of the long bones. The difference is that the process begins from an ossification center in the bones of the calvaria, rather than as a surrounding "sleeve" of bone. Rays of bone spread outward, linking the ossification centers in the shape of a pentagon, which Rohen sees as expressing dominating strength of form.

Whereas the powers of the will in the case of the limbs find their outworking in movement, in the case of the head this outworking is in the powers of thought. These powers of the will can be found on the skull's exterior and reflected in the brain within, which Rohen sees as a complete reversal from the limbs to the head region.

Stone[5] sees the parietal bone as exhibiting the energetic polar reflexes of the sides of the body.

11.2 Location, causes, and clinical presentation of dysfunctions of the parietal bones

Tip for practitioners

Primary dysfunctions

- Intraosseous: direct force to the parietal bone, especially pre- or perinatally or in infancy.
- Primary traumatic injury: during early childhood and beyond, falls, blows, or other effects of force to the sutures can lead to motion restrictions of the parietal bone and its surrounding bones. Falls onto the feet or pelvis can also affect the parietal bone.

Secondary dysfunction

- Secondary motion restriction of the parietal bones can arise due to dysfunctions of the occipital bone, temporal bone, temporomandibular joint (via the temporalis muscle), or SBS dysfunctions of transmission of tension via the falx cerebri. The most common secondary dysfunction is internal rotation of the parietal bone.

11.2.1 Osseous dysfunctions

Simultaneously occurring motion restrictions of the parietal bones and the thoracic cage are quite frequently found.

- **Coronal suture**
    - Sequelae: restriction of mobility of the SBS, frontal bone, and parietal bone.
    - Clinical presentation: functional impairment of the corresponding parts of the brain, e.g., precentral and postcentral gyrus.

- **Sagittal suture, bregma, and lambda**
  - Causes: a fall, blow, or other force to the suture:
    - Force to bregma → compression in the anterior region of the sagittal suture.
    - Force to vertex → compression in the central region of the sagittal suture.
    - Force to lambda → compression in the posterior region of the sagittal suture.
  - Occurrence: frequently in asthmatic, hyperactive children or children with sleep disturbances.
  - Clinical presentation/hypothetical pathology: disturbances of drainage in the superior sagittal sinus with functional disturbances in the corresponding parts of the brain, e.g., precentral and postcentral gyrus; pain in the frontoparietal and eye regions; sometimes spasticity in the case of severe compression.
  - Sequelae:
    - Force to bregma: posterior displacement of the occipital condyles and lateral movement of the posterior inferior angles of the parietal bones.
    - Force to vertex: ER of the temporal bones and flexion dysfunction of the SBS.
    - Force to lambda: impaction of the occipital condyles into the atlas and flexion dysfunction of the occipital bone and SBS, and ER of the temporal bones.
  - **Lambdoid suture** The squamoserrate suture type prevents the bones from overlapping but can be compressed by a fall or blow.
  - **Squamoparietal suture** Causes: a blow or fall from above onto the ipsilateral parietal bone; severe hypertonicity of the temporalis muscle.
  - **Parietomastoid suture/sphenoparietal suture** Causes: a blow or fall from above onto the ipsilateral parietal bone.

11.2.2 Intraosseous dysfunction

Clinical presentation/hypothetical pathology: functional impairment of the parietal lobe.

11.2.3 Muscular dysfunction

Temporalis muscle

- Causes: include dysfunction of the temporomandibular artery.
- Sequelae: restriction of mobility of the parietal bone and squamoparietal suture.

11.2.4 Fascial dysfunctions

The **temporal fascia** and **superficial layer** are affected.

11.2.5 Dysfunctions of the falx cerebri and the tentorium cerebelli

- Causes: motion restriction, sutural compression, and change in position of the parietal bone, especially in conjunction with the occipital bone, temporal bone, and dysfunctions of the SBS.
- Clinical presentation/hypothetical pathology
  - **Falx cerebri:** disturbances of drainage in the superior sagittal sinus with functional disturbances in the corresponding parts of the brain; pain along the falx cerebri.[1]
  - **Tentorium cerebelli:** congestion in the transition from the transverse sinus/sigmoid sinus at the parietomastoid suture.

11.2.6 Disturbances of nerves and parts of the brain

Parietal lobe

- Causes: motion restriction, sutural compression, and change in position of the parietal bone, especially in conjunction with the occipital bone, temporal bone, and dysfunctions of the SBS.
- Clinical presentation/hypothetical pathology: functional impairment of the motor and sensory centers, disturbances of attention in the field of visual and tactile perception,[3] aggressive behavior.

11.2.7 Vascular disturbances

- **Middle meningeal artery**
  - Causes: dysfunction of the parietal bone and sphenoparietal suture (especially

in the case of compression of the sphenosquamous suture between the temporal bone and sphenoid).
    - Clinical presentation/hypothetical pathology: migraine and raised intracranial pressure.
- **Superior sagittal sinus**
    - Causes: compression of the sagittal suture, dysfunction of the parietal bones.
    - Sequelae: the greatest number of arachnoid villi is to be found in the superior sagittal sinus. Disturbances can affect the fluctuation of cerebrospinal fluid.
    - Clinical presentation/hypothetical pathology: pain in the frontoparietal and eye regions.
- **Sigmoid sinus**
    - Causes: compression of the parietomastoid suture.
    - Clinical presentation/hypothetical pathology: signs and symptoms of congestion; pain in the temporal region.
- **Middle meningeal veins:** at the internal surface of the bone.

11.3 Diagnosis of the parietal bone

11.3.1 History-taking

- Headache, especially in the parietal region.
- Idiopathic epilepsy.
- Previous traumatic injury.

11.3.2 Inspection

- Mastoid angle: anterolateral (ER) or posteromedial (IR).
- Squamosal border: anterolateral (ER).
- Sagittal suture: flattened (ER), e.g., as a result of traumatic force, or convex (IR).
- Lambdoid suture: indented (ER), e.g., as a result of primary traumatic force, or convex (IR).
- Coronal suture: depressed at bregma and displaced laterally in an anterior and outward direction (ER) or elevated at bregma and displaced laterally in a posterior and inward direction (IR).
- Parietal tuber: convex or flat (intraosseous dysfunction).

11.3.3 Palpation of position

See under Inspection, section 11.3.2.

11.3.4 Palpation of PRM rhythm

Tip for practitioners

Biomechanical, inhalation phase

There is external rotation of the parietal bone around an axis running from posterior/external/inferior to anterior/internal/superior.

- Bregma and lambda descend.
- The sagittal suture descends, its two margins shift away from each other, more markedly posterior than anterior.
- The sphenoidal angle moves in an outward and anterior direction.
- The squamosal border moves in an outward and anterior direction.
- The mastoid angle moves in an outward and anterior direction.

Developmental dynamic, inhalation phase

- The expansive force is in a cephalad, lateral direction.
- The motion is centrifugal (outward).
- The convexity decreases.

Tip for practitioners

If palpation reveals a motion restriction, an impulse can be administered in the direction of restricted motion. This will emphasize the restriction and enable you to sense more easily which structure accounts for the origin of the motion restriction.

Indication: Tensions and fibrosis of the falx, disturbances of drainage of the superior and inferior sagittal sinuses and of the lateral ventricles, restrictions of the sutures of the parietal bone; according to Magoun, in the case of idiopathic epilepsy, where the suture is frequently fixed in the extension position.[2]

Hand position:

- Place the palms of both hands on the parietal tubers.
- Cross your thumbs to lie on the parietal bone on the opposite side.
- Place your index fingers on the sphenoidal angles (anterior inferior angles of the parietal bones).
- Position your middle fingers above the roots of the zygomatic processes of the temporal bones.
- Position your ring fingers on the mastoid angles (posterior inferior angles of the parietal bones).
- Place the basal or proximal joints of your index, middle, and ring fingers on the parietal bones. Position them on the lateral borders of the parietal bones (Figure 11.5).

Method:

- **Indirect technique** (Figure 11.6)
  - At the beginning of the inhalation phase, begin to administer gentle caudad and lateral pressure with the pads of your thumbs so that the sagittal suture spreads and descends. This reduces the membrane tension in the craniocaudal course of the falx.
  - At the same time, with the basal or proximal joints of your fingers, administer an anterior and lateral impulse to the inferior and lateral borders of the parietal bones.
  - Establish the PBMT of the parietal bones—the position in which the tension of the dural membrane is in the best possible state of balance—and the PBFT.
  - Maintain the PBT until a correction of the abnormal tension has been achieved and stabilized by the inherent homeostatic forces (PRM rhythm, etc.), and the motion of the parietal bone has stopped.
- Breathing assistance: ask the patient to hold an inhalation for as long as possible at the end of an in-breath.
- A fluid impulse may be used to direct energy from inion or further caudad in the midline.

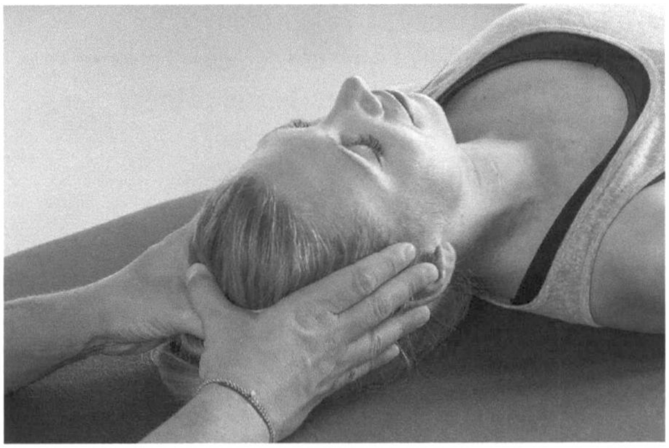

Figure 11.5 Dysfunction in external rotation, parietal spread technique

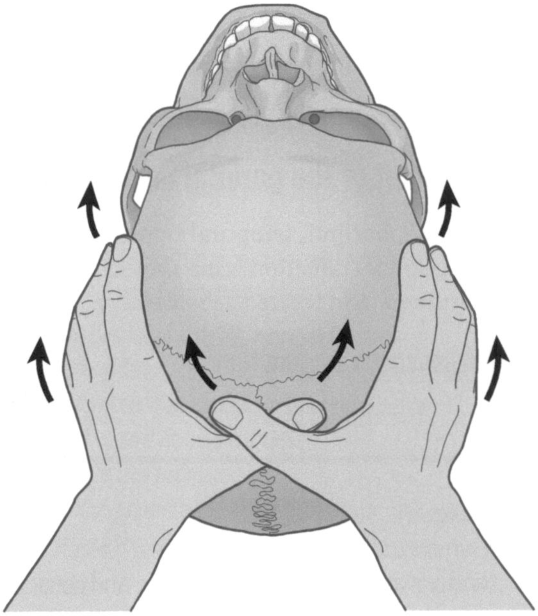

Figure 11.6 Dysfunction in external rotation, parietal spread technique (diagram)

NOTE If this technique is used for the release of the sagittal suture, it is considered to be a direct technique, as the impulse is designed to produce motion in the direction of the restriction.

Vitalist approach: See EV-4 technique (this volume, section 4.4.3).

11.4.3 Dysfunction in internal rotation

Motion restriction in the direction of external rotation.

Hand position: See dysfunction in external rotation above (section 11.4.2), except that, now, the tips of your thumbs should touch each other at the sagittal suture, but without resting on the suture.

Method:

Indirect technique: at the beginning of the exhalation phase, begin to administer a posteromedial impulse with the palms of your hands at the inferior and lateral borders of the parietal bones (Figure 11.7).

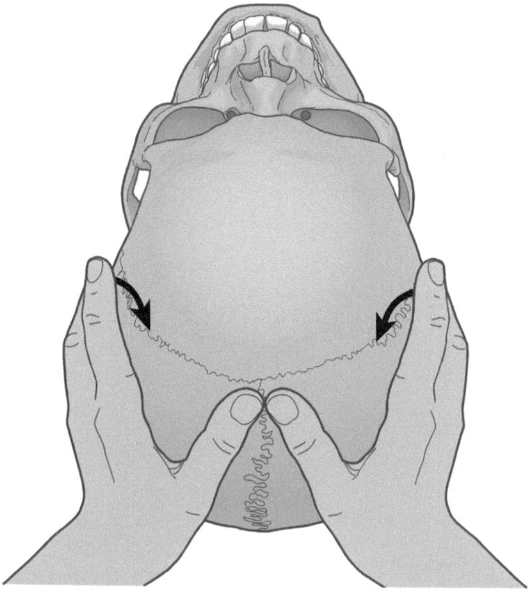

Figure 11.7 Dysfunction in internal rotation

- Establish PBMT and PBFT.
- Breathing assistance: ask the patient to hold an exhalation for as long as possible at the end of an out-breath.
- A fluid impulse may be used to direct energy from the inion or further caudad in the midline.

NOTE Internal rotation dysfunctions of the parietal bones are frequently caused by a dysfunction of the sagittal suture, so this treatment should be followed by a direct technique.

Vitalist approach: See EV-4 technique (this volume, section 4.4.3).

11.4.4 Dural techniques

Parietal lift technique

Indication: In combination with the spread technique: tensions and fibrosis of the falx cerebri, disturbances of drainage of the superior and inferior sagittal sinuses, restrictions of the sutures of the parietal bone; according to Magoun also insomnia and hypertonus.[3]

Hand position: The hand position is the same as for the spread technique (section 11.4.2) except that the tips of your thumbs should touch each other at the sagittal suture, but without resting on the suture.

Method:

- During the exhalation phase, begin to administer gentle medial pressure with your index, middle, and ring fingers on the inferior lateral borders of the parietal bones, to release them from the temporal bones (IR; Figure 11.8).
- As soon as the parietal bones begin to move cephalad (release of the parietal bones from

the temporal bones), you can relax the medial pressure of your fingers. Replace this with cephalad traction with your fingers. This traction is very gentle. It always remains below the threshold at which the tissue reacts by countercontracting.

- At the same time, without reducing the cephalad traction, you can administer slight posterior traction to release the parietal bones from the frontal bone, and then slight anterior traction to release the parietal bones from the occipital bone (Figure 11.9).

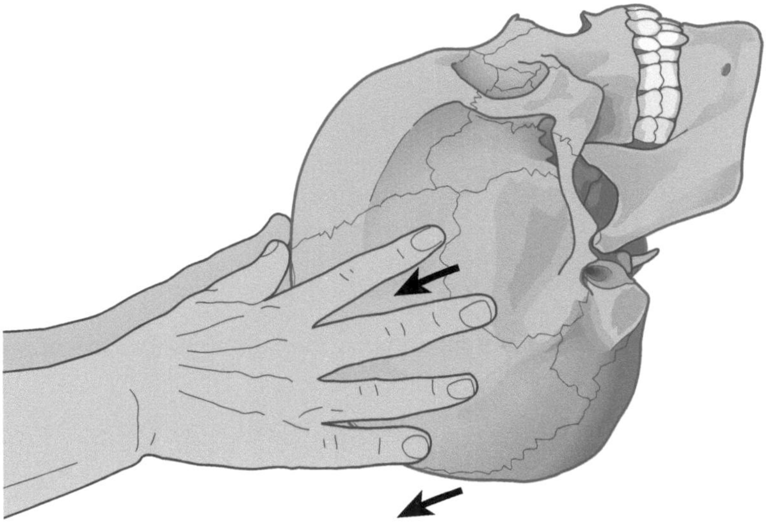

Figure 11.8 Parietal lift technique

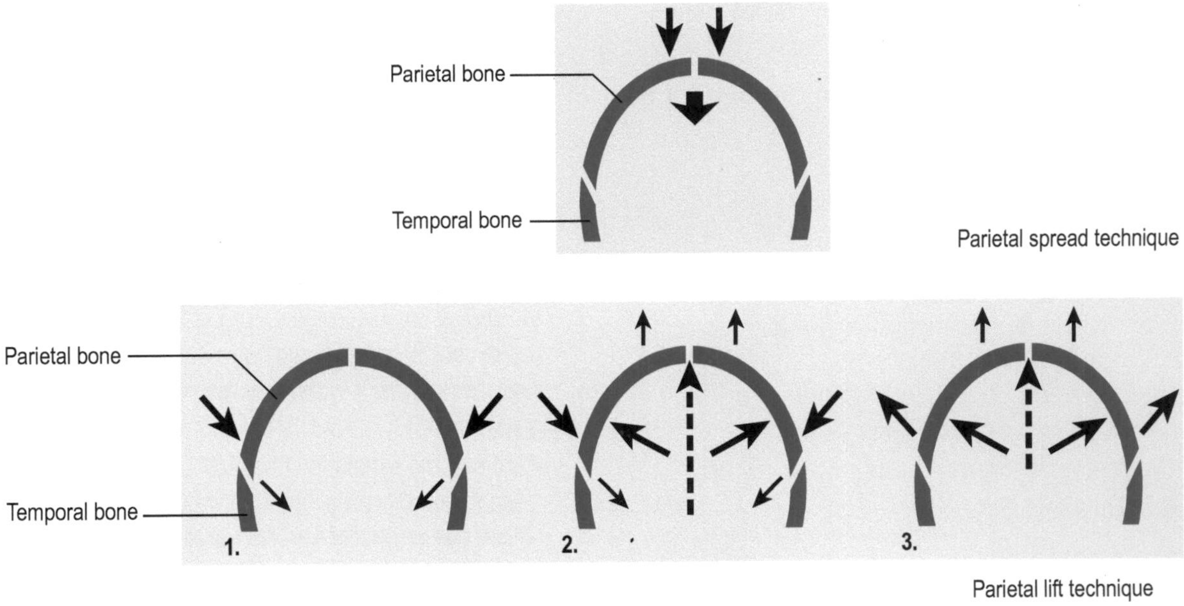

Figure 11.9 Diagrammatic representation of the parietal spread and lift technique

- At each release of the tissue, seek the new limit to motion of the parietal bones in the cephalad direction.
- Permit all motions/tissue unwinding of the frontal bone, without reducing the gentle traction.
- You will be able to sense the various stages of tissue release: first the sutural tensions, then the elastic and collagenous tensions of the falx cerebri (a sensation like cement, or a rubber band, or chewing gum). When the falx has been released from its tension patterns (floating sensation), the hands can be removed.

NOTE The traction applied in the lift technique should imitate the tension that is present, plus about 5 g.
Never remove your hands suddenly from the bone during the technique.
Always take care to position your hands accurately. Failure to do so would mean that, at best, the technique would be ineffective. In the worst case, especially if your fingers are on the sutures, this could worsen or even give rise to symptoms.

Tip for practitioners

Another option is to assist the flexion and extension motions of the parietal bones (in harmony with the PRM rhythm) during the gentle cephalad and slightly posterior traction.

11.4.5 Sinus techniques

Technique for the superior sagittal sinus

Special technique for the superior sagittal sinus and alternative technique for a dysfunction in internal rotation.

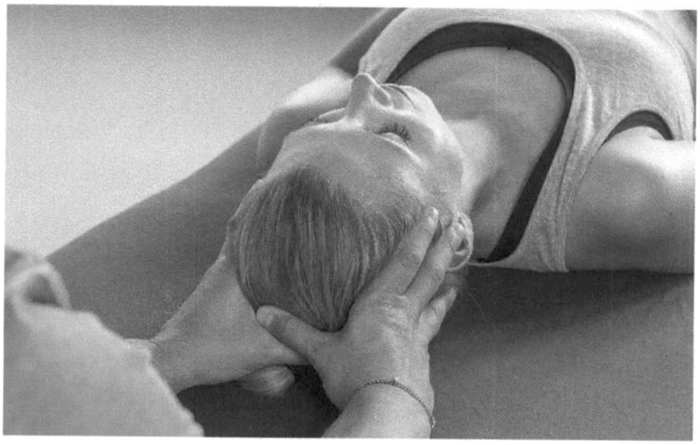

Figure 11.10 Technique for the superior sagittal sinus (and sagittal suture)

Hand position: As for the parietal spread technique (section 11.4.2), except that the thumbs are placed at the posterior end of the sagittal suture at the level of lambda (Figure 11.10).

Method:

- During the inhalation phase, administer gentle caudad, lateral pressure with your thenar eminences to the sagittal borders of the parietal bones, so that the suture spreads and descends.
- When release of the suture location occurs, shift your thumbs a little further anterior and begin again with the same procedure until you reach the end of the suture at bregma.

11.4.6 Sutural dysfunctions

Sphenoparietal suture, Cant hook technique

Suture margin: Sphenoidal angle of the parietal bone: outward-facing margin. Greater wing of the sphenoid: inward-facing margin.

Suture type: Squamous suture.

Practitioner: Take up a position beside the patient's head, on the opposite side to the dysfunction.

Hand position:

- Caudal hand
  - Place your little finger intraorally, laterally positioned on the pterygoid process.
  - Position your middle finger externally on the greater wing on the side of the dysfunction.
  - If possible place your thumb externally on the greater wing on the opposite side to the dysfunction.
- Cranial hand
  - Span the parietal bones with your thumb and your index and/or middle finger.
  - Position your middle finger on the sphenoidal angle of the parietal bone on the side of the dysfunction (Figure 11.11).

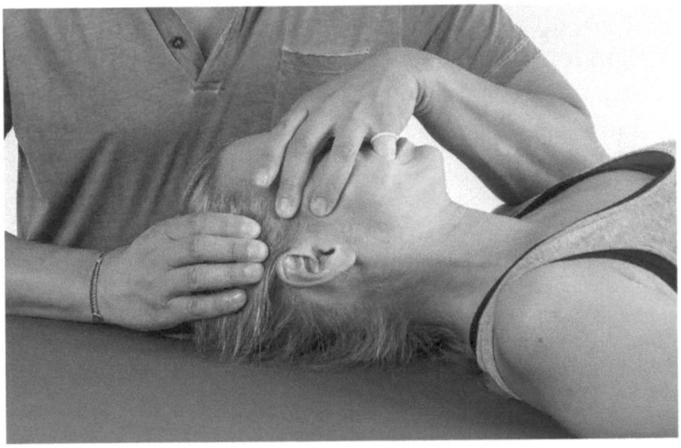

Figure 11.11 Sphenoparietal suture. Cant hook technique

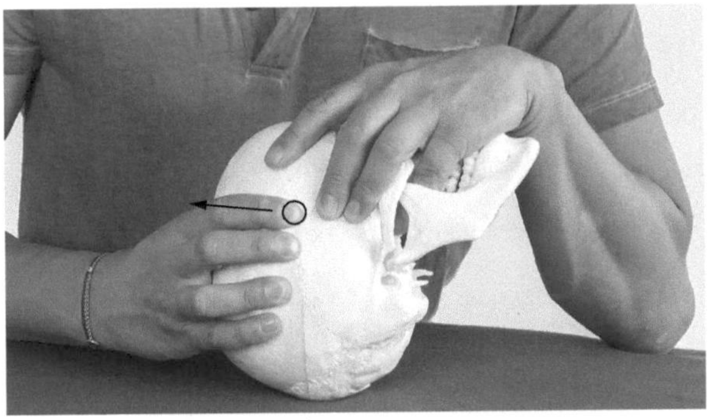

Figure 11.12 Sphenoparietal suture. Cant hook technique (shown on model)

Method:

- Disengagement
  - Hold the sphenoid in position with your caudal hand.
  - Apply medial pressure and superiorly directed traction on the sphenoidal angle of the parietal bone with the index finger of your cranial hand (Figure 11.12).
  - Without reducing the disengagement, permit all motions/unwinding of the parietal bone that arise.
- Establish PBMT and PBFT between the sphenoid and the parietal bone.
- A fluid impulse may be used to direct energy from the opposite lambdoid suture or caudal to it.

Alternative technique

Practitioner: Take up a position at the head of the patient.

Hand position: Place the ball of your two little fingers on the sphenoidal angles of the parietal bones. Interclasp your fingers and support your elbows on the table slightly caudad and lateral to your hands.

Method:

- Disengagement
  - During the exhalation phase, apply medial pressure with the ball of your little fingers on the sphenoidal angles of the parietal bones (Figure 11.13). Induce this pressure by drawing your fingertips apart laterally. The internal rotation of the parietal bones causes the disengagement of the sutural articulations with the sphenoid.
  - During the next inhalation phase, move the sphenoidal angles cephalad, without reducing the medial pressure.
  - Without reducing the disengagement, permit all motions/unwinding of the parietal bones that arise.
  - At each release of the tissues, seek the new limit to motion of the parietal bones in the superior direction.

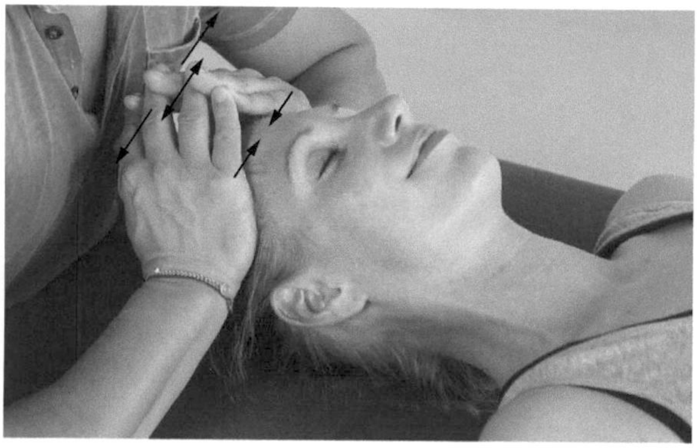

Figure 11.13 Sphenoparietal suture. Alternative technique

- Establish PBMT and PBFT.
- A fluid impulse may be used to direct energy from the opposite lambdoid suture or caudad to it.

Technique for the lambdoid suture (e.g., right)

Suture margin: The suture margin of the occipital bone is inward-facing in its upper medial half, while the lower lateral half is outward-facing.
Suture type: Squamoserrate suture.
Practitioner: Take up a position on the opposite side to the suture that is to be treated.
Hand position:

- Place your hands on the right-hand side of the cranium, on top of each other and with your fingers pointing posterior/caudad.
- Position the index and middle fingers of your left hand on the parietal bone anterior to the suture.
- Position the index and middle fingers of your upper hand posterior to the suture, on the occipital bone.

Method:

- With the fingers on the parietal bone, administer traction in an anterior direction. Also apply pressure to the bone (occipital border of the parietal bone) with the index finger above the pivot point.
- With the fingers on the occipital bone, administer posterior traction. Also apply pressure to the bone (parietal border of the occipital bone) with the index finger below the pivot point (Figure 11.14).

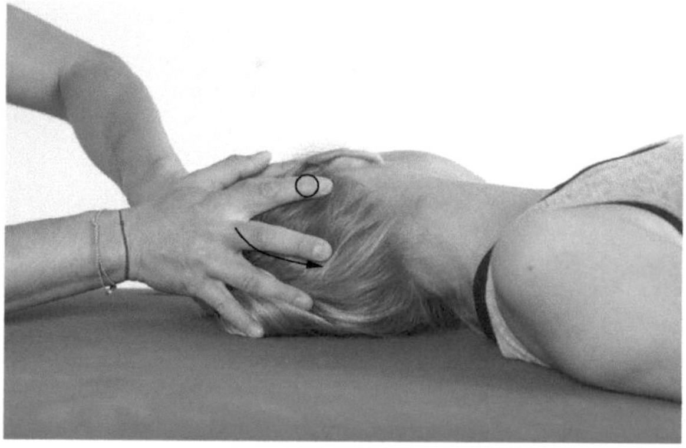

Figure 11.14 Technique for the lambdoid suture (right)

- Then establish PBMT and PBFT and maintain this until release of the suture occurs and mobility improves.
- A fluid impulse may be used to direct energy from the opposite frontal tuber or from pterion.

Technique for the sagittal suture

This technique corresponds to the parietal spread technique (see section 11.4.2).

Suture margin: The digits become longer toward the rear of the suture. This means that spreading of the suture can be wider here than at the front.
Suture type: Denticulate suture.
Indication: Compression resulting from a fall, blow, or other effect of force causes disturbances of drainage in the superior sagittal sinus, with functional disturbances in the corresponding regions of the brain, pain in the frontoparietal region and eye region, and asthma, hyperactivity, and sleep disturbances in childhood.
Hand position: Place your thumbs, crossing, on the parietal bones. Place your fingers on the sides of the parietal bones.

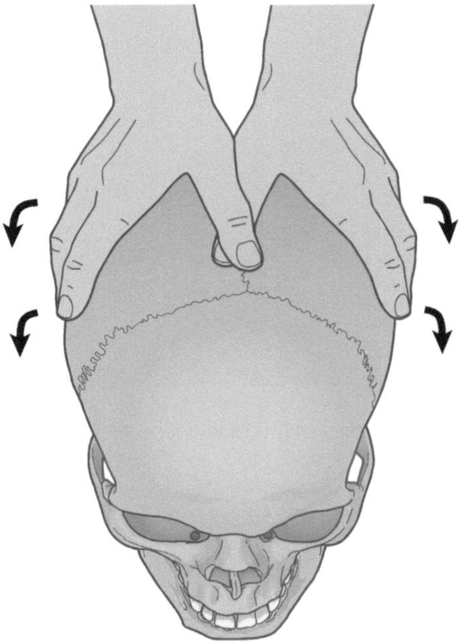

Figure 11.15 Technique for the sagittal suture

Method:

- During the inhalation phase, begin to administer caudad and lateral traction with your thumbs on the sagittal borders of the parietal bones (Figure 11.15).
- Establish PBMT and PBFT.
- A fluid impulse may be used to direct energy from the inion or further caudad in the midline.

Bregma

Suture margin: At bregma: frontal bone: inward-facing margin; parietal bone: outward-facing margin.
Practitioner: Take up a position at the head of the patient.
Hand position:

- Place your index finger on the frontal bone.
- Place your thumbs next to the sagittal suture, crossing, and each resting on the opposite parietal bone.
- Place your other fingers on the side of the cranium.

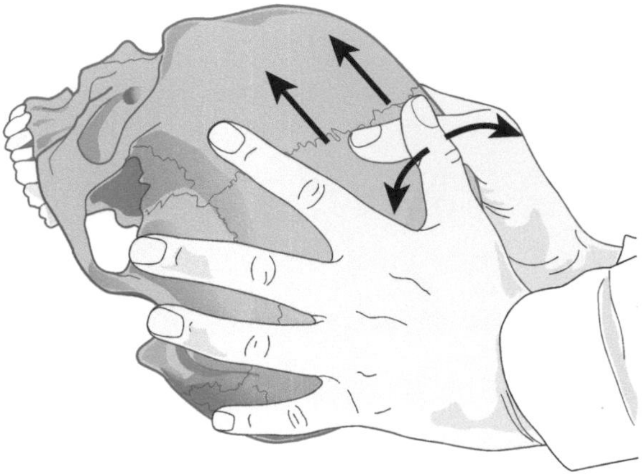

Figure 11.16 Bregma

Method:

- Disengagement
  - With your index fingers, move the frontal bone in an anterior direction.
  - At the same time, move the parietal bones posterolaterally with your thumbs (Figure 11.16).
  - Without reducing the gentle disengagement, permit all motions/unwinding of the frontal bone that arise.
  - With each release of the tissues, seek the new limit to motion of the frontal bone in the anterior direction and of the parietal bones in the posterior and lateral direction.
- Establish PBMT and PBFT.
- A fluid impulse may be used to direct energy from inion or further caudad in the midline.

Lambda

Suture margin: At lambda: occipital bone: inward-facing margin; parietal bone: outward-facing margin.
Hand position: Place your thumbs next to the sagittal suture, crossing, so that each rests on the opposite parietal bone.

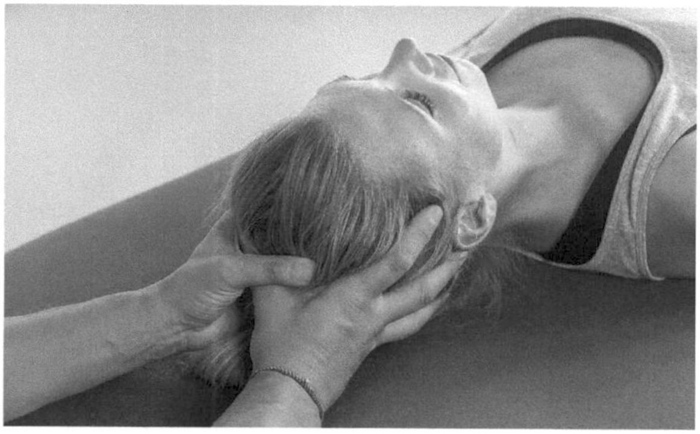

Figure 11.17 Lambda

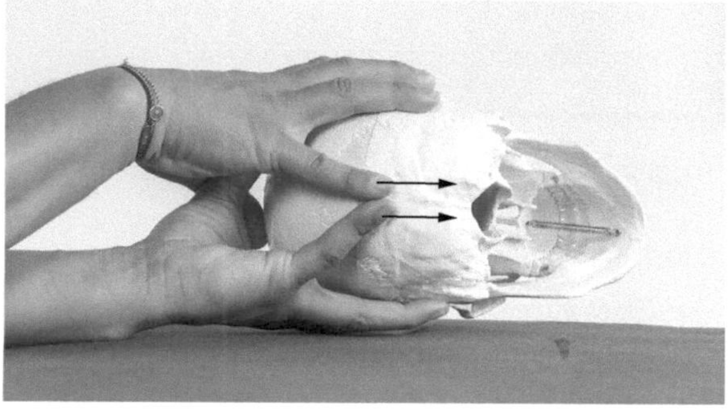

Figure 11.18 Lambda (shown on model)

- Position your little fingers on the occipital squama, fingertips touching.
- Place your other fingers on each side of the cranium, on the parietal bones (Figure 11.17).

Method:

- With your little fingers, move the occipital bone caudad (Figure 11.18).
- At the same time, guide the parietal bones in an anterior and lateral direction with your thumbs.
- Your other fingers should remain passive.
- Without reducing the gentle disengagement, permit all motions/unwinding of the parietal bones that arise.
- At each release of the tissues, seek the next limit to anterolateral motion of the parietal bones and to caudad motion of the occipital bone.
- Establish PBMT and PBFT.

Alternative hand position (the three-finger technique)
Place the index and middle fingers of one hand on the two parietal bones, and the thumb of the same hand on the occipital bone. Simultaneously move the thumb caudad and the middle and index fingers in an anterior and lateral direction.

Pterion

Sutures: Four bones overlie each other at this point. Working outward, these are: the frontal bone, parietal bone, sphenoid, and temporal bone.

Hand position:

- Place all your fingers close to the pterion.
- Place your index finger on the frontal bone.
- Place your thumb on the parietal bone.
- Place your middle finger on the sphenoid.
- Place your ring finger on the temporal bone.

Method:

- With your index finger, apply gentle pressure to the frontal bone together with anterior and superior traction (Figure 11.19).
- When the frontal bone begins to disengage from the other bones, apply gentle pressure with your thumb on the parietal bone, together with traction in a superior and slightly posterior direction.

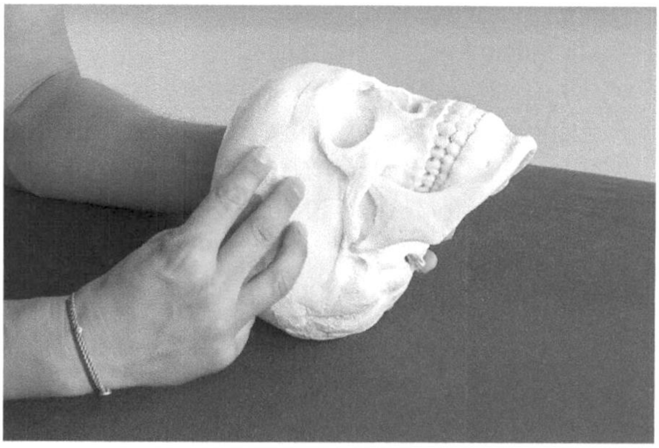

Figure 11.19 Pterion

- When the parietal bone begins to disengage from the other bones, apply gentle pressure with your middle finger on the sphenoid, together with anterior and slightly caudad traction.
- When the sphenoid begins to disengage from the other bones, apply caudad and posterior traction with your ring finger on the temporal bone.
- End by administering centrifugal traction with all your fingers to the bones.
- Establish PBMT and PBFT.

Asterion

Sutures: Three bones overlap at this point; working outward, these are: the occipital bone, temporal bone, and parietal bone.
Patient: The patient's head should be turned to the opposite side.
Hand position:

- Place all your fingers close to the asterion.
- Place your thumb on the parietal bone.
- Place your index finger on the temporal bone.
- Place your middle finger on the occipital bone (Figure 11.20).

Method:

- Apply gentle pressure to the occipital bone with your middle finger, together with posterior traction.
- Then apply pressure to the parietal bone with the thumb positioned there, together with cephalad traction.
- Then with your index finger on the temporal bone, together with your middle finger and thumb, administer centrifugal traction to the bones.
- Establish PBMT and PBFT.

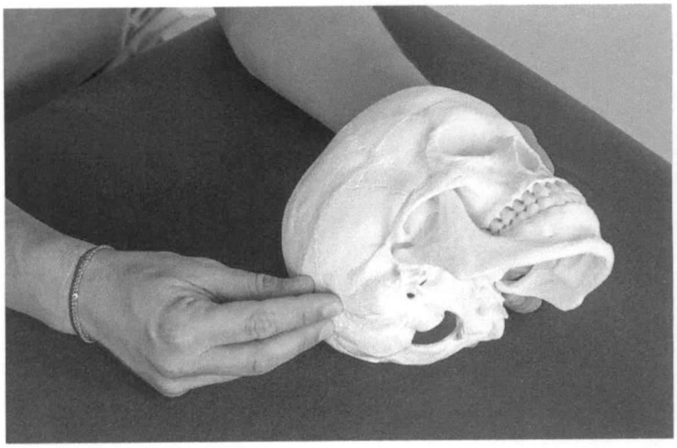

Figure 11.20 Asterion

Coronal suture

See this volume, section 10.4.5.

Squamoparietal suture and parietomastoid suture

See this volume, section 9.4.8.

11.5 References

1 Liem, T. (2018) *Kraniosakrale Osteopathie. Ein praktisches Lehrbuch*, 7th Ed. Stuttgart: Thieme.
2 Magoun, H. I. (1951) *Osteopathy in the Cranial Field*, 1st Ed. Kirksville: Journal Printing Company, p. 147.
3 Magoun, H. I. (1976) *Osteopathy in the Cranial Field*, 3rd Ed. Kirksville: Journal Printing Company, p. 176.
4 Rohen, J. W. (2002) *Morphologie des menschlichen Organismus*, 2nd Ed. Stuttgart: Verlag Freies Geistesleben, p. 387.
5 Stone, R. (1994) *Polaritätstherapie*, 2nd Ed. Hugendubel, p. 207.

12.1 The morphology of the maxillae according to Rohen 406

12.2 Location, causes, and clinical presentation of maxillary dysfunctions 406
12.2.1 Osseous dysfunctions 407
12.2.2 Muscular dysfunction 407
12.2.3 Disturbances of the nerves 407
12.2.4 Vascular disturbances 408
12.2.5 Ocular disturbances 408

12.3 Diagnosis of the maxilla 408
12.3.1 History-taking 408
12.3.2 Inspection 408
12.3.3 Palpation of position 408
12.3.4 Palpation of PRM rhythm 409
12.3.5 Motion testing 411

12.4 Treatment of the maxillae 411
12.4.1 Rotation dysfunction of the maxillae 411
12.4.2 Dysfunction in external and internal rotation 412
12.4.3 Global rotation dysfunction about a vertical axis 415
12.4.4 Global lateral strain 415
12.4.5 Decompression of the maxillary complex 416
12.4.6 Sutural dysfunctions 417

12.5 References 422

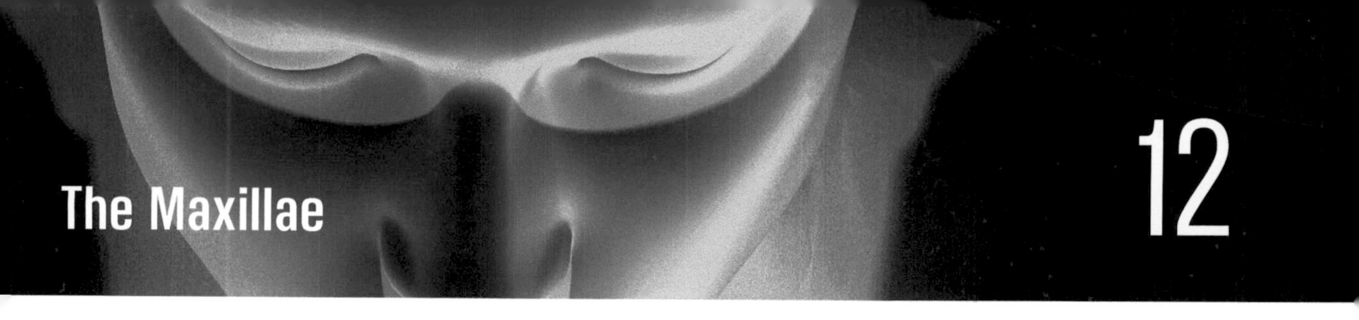

12 The Maxillae

The maxilla is a paired bone and, in shape, a very irregular bone. It is the central bone of the viscerocranium. It contributes to the lateral wall of the nasal cavity, and most of the floor of the nasal cavity and the hard palate. It also forms most of the inferior wall (floor) of the orbit.

The alveolar process is important to the act of chewing. Masticatory forces are transmitted from the sockets of the canines into the medial superior rim of the orbit via the frontal process.

The maxilla has a necessary role, together with the tongue, in speaking. It also contributes to the nasal cavities, oral cavity, and orbit, and their functions.

A number of facial muscles attach at the maxilla, and branches of the maxillary nerve (CN V_2) run through and alongside the bone.

According to Sutherland, local injury and dental procedures often cause dysfunctions of the maxilla, leading to disturbances in nasal, postnasal, and pharyngeal regions.[3]

12.1 The morphology of the maxillae according to Rohen[1]

The dynamics of motion of the upper limbs is reflected in the global organization of the maxilla.

Upright posture endows the upper limbs with the full range of movement between above and below. For Rohen, two primal gestures are manifested in the hand: the grasp of the fist, taking action in the world, in the earthly sphere, and the open hand, expressing a gesture of opening up and of receiving.

This paradoxical motion dynamic is also apparent in the design of the maxilla, with its four processes.

The narrow, upwardly sweeping frontal process corresponds to the open hand and has a role in forming the nasal root, which is located in the region of greatest concentration of ego consciousness. In enclosing the nasal cavity, it also plays a role in the rhythmic system.

At the base, the maxilla develops into the alveolar process. This structure accommodates the teeth and is thus involved in chewing, that is, in the processing of material aspects. The gesture of the fist is discernible in the alveolar process.

Midway between these two polarities we find the medially oriented palatine process and the laterally oriented zygomatic process. For Rohen, the palatine process is the diaphragm of the head in that it separates the oral cavity from the nasal cavity, while the zygomatic process links the viscerocranium with the neurocranium.

However, the integrative expressivity of the maxilla is achieved only through its being supported, rearward, vis-à-vis the cranial base via the zygomatic bone, and upward, vis-à-vis the roof of the skull via the frontal bone.

For Stone,[2] the maxilla reflects polarity reflexes of the anterior pelvis and of the hips laterally.

12.2 Location, causes, and clinical presentation of maxillary dysfunctions

> **Tip for practitioners**
>
> **Primary dysfunctions**
> - Intraosseous.
> - Traumatic injury: falls, blows, tooth extraction, poor chewing habits, or other effects of force to the maxilla can cause restrictions of the upper jaw and surrounding bones, especially the palatine bone and also the pterygopalatine ganglion.

> **Secondary dysfunctions**
> - Due to dysfunction of the sphenoid, e.g., SBS dysfunctions (torsion of the SBS leads to relative restriction of the maxilla in internal and external rotation), dental braces, myofascial tension.
> - Developmental disturbances of the cranial base at the embryonic stage lead to disturbances of development of the maxilla.

12.2.1 Osseous dysfunctions

A high palatine arch (IR of maxilla) with vertical alignment of the frontal process is usually combined with narrow nasal cavities and disturbances of the nasal septum. This can lead to functional impairment of the vascular, neural, and lymphatic structures, as well as to mouth breathing, nasal problems, etc.

- **Frontomaxillary suture.**
- **Ethmoidomaxillary suture** Sequelae: dysfunctions of the maxilla have a usually direct influence on the mobility of the ethmoid bone, and may even lead to motion restriction of the SBS.
- **Zygomaticomaxillary suture**
    - Causes: falling, or blows to the face.
    - Clinical presentation/hypothetical pathology: orbital disturbance, disturbance of the maxillary sinus resulting in sinusitis.
- **Lacrimomaxillary suture.**
- **Transverse palatine suture.**
- **Palatomaxillary suture** Causes: a fall or blow to the face often causes compression of the suture.
- **Nasomaxillary suture.**
- **Vomeromaxillary suture.**
- **Conchomaxillary suture.**
- **Median palatine suture**
    - The mobility of the median palatine suture is often restricted by the use of dental braces.
    - Sequelae: reduced capacity to absorb masticatory forces, especially in the case of bruxism.
- **Incisive suture** This suture, between the incisive bone (premaxilla) and the maxilla, ossifies between the 12th and the 18th month of life. It is often motion-restricted, due either to early traumatic influences or to the use of dental braces.
- **Inferior orbital fissure** The infraorbital nerve and the inferior ophthalmic vein, which runs into the pterygoid venous plexus, are among the structures that pass through the fissure. Narrowness of the fissure can impair venous drainage.
- **Disturbances of bite.**
- **Dental malocclusions** Causes: SBS dysfunction, dysfunction of the incisive suture, faulty nutrition, poor corrective dentistry, and dental surgery.

12.2.2 Muscular dysfunction

Although the maxilla is the site of attachment of many minor muscles, dysfunctions of these muscles affecting the upper jaw are not often encountered. To give one example, spasm of the **masseter** could be capable of moving the upper jaw in a posterior direction. Other masticatory muscles may affect the maxilla in connection with a dysfunction of the temporomandibular joint.

12.2.3 Disturbances of the nerves

- **Maxillary nerve (V_2)** The maxillary nerve emerges through the foramen rotundum into the pterygopalatine fossa, where it subdivides further.
- **Infraorbital nerve (V_2)**
    - Runs through the inferior orbital fissure into the infraorbital canal, and on through the infraorbital foramen.
    - Clinical presentation: e.g., following injury to the orbital floor: disturbances of sensitivity, or pain in the skin of the midfacial region, and in the mucosa and teeth of the upper jaw.

- **Superior alveolar nerves (V_2)**
  - The branches supplying the teeth and gingivae of the upper jaw lead off from the infraorbital nerve in the pterygopalatine fossa, and then run in the alveolar canals on the back of the infratemporal surface.
  - Clinical presentation: toothache and painful gums.
- **Greater palatine nerves** Clinical presentation: disturbances of sensitivity and pain in the mucosa of the hard palate.
- **Sympathetic fibers**
  - From the deep petrosal nerve, via the pterygopalatine ganglion, the sensory root of the pterygopalatine ganglion, the maxillary nerve, the zygomatic nerve to the lacrimal nerve (lacrimal gland).
  - Clinical presentation: disturbance of the lacrimal gland.
- **Zygomatic nerve** Clinical presentation: disturbances of sensitivity and pain in the skin around the temporal and zygomatic bones.
- **Pterygopalatine ganglion**
  See this volume, sections 3.1.3 and 3.2.3.
- Clinical presentation: secretory disturbances of the lacrimal gland and of the nasal and palatine mucosa, with reduced resistance to infection of mucosa of the nose, oral cavity, and pharynx, possibly ocular disturbances and olfactory impairment (due to dryness of the nasal mucosa).

12.2.4 Vascular disturbances

- **Infraorbital artery and vein** Metabolic disturbance of the front teeth, the bones, and the gingivae of the upper jaw.
- **Anterior superior alveolar arteries** Metabolic disturbance of the front teeth.
- **Posterior superior alveolar artery** Functional disturbance of the maxillary sinus and upper molars, and of the bones and gingivae of the upper jaw.
- **Descending palatine artery** In the greater palatine canal; functional disturbance of the pharyngeal mucosa, gingivae of the anterior teeth, and soft palate. Effects may be seen in the retromandibular and facial veins.

12.2.5 Ocular disturbances

Displacement of the eye, e.g., following traumatic injury to the orbital floor.

12.3 Diagnosis of the maxilla

12.3.1 History-taking

- Nasal, oral, or pharyngeal symptoms.
- Ocular symptoms.
- Dental malocclusions, disturbances of bite.
- Sometimes, allergic rhinitis and asthma via the pterygopalatine ganglion.
- Dental braces.

12.3.2 Inspection

- Nasolabial fold: deep (ER) or shallow (IR).
- Incisors: posteriorly positioned and widely spaced, while the remaining upper teeth appear inclined to the side (ER).
- Incisors: anteriorly positioned and close together, while the remaining teeth appear inclined inward (IR).
- Anterior teeth: protruding (possibly intraosseous dysfunction, IR of the premaxilla).
- Canine: prominent, if the incisive bone is in ER and the maxilla in IR.
- Canine: posteriorly shifted, if the incisive bone is in IR and the maxilla in ER.

12.3.3 Palpation of position

- Orbital process: tilted (ER) or straight (IR).
- Palatine process: lowered (ER) or elevated (IR).
- Alveolar process: externally rotated (ER) or vertically aligned (IR).

12.3.4 Palpation of PRM rhythm

Tip for practitioners

Biomechanical approach, inhalation phase

- External rotation of the maxilla occurs around two vertical axes running through the frontal processes of the maxilla.
- The maxilla moves in synchrony with the frontal bone.
- The zygomatic process of the maxilla moves in a superior, anterior direction.
- The median palatine suture and arch of the palate descend.
- The alveolar process widens on the lateral side.
- The intermaxillary suture moves posterior.

Developmental dynamic, inhalation phase

- The expansive force is in an anterior and inferior direction.

If palpation reveals a restriction, the practitioner may induce an impulse in the direction of the restriction. This will emphasize it, making it easier to sense from which structure it originates.

Hand positions:

- **Palpation of the PRM rhythm of the maxilla** Take up a position at the head of the patient. Position your index fingers on both sides of the nose, on the alveolar arches of the two maxillae. Place the other fingers beside the index fingers, on the alveolar arches of the two maxillae (Figure 12.1).
- **Alternative hand position I** Take up a position at the head of the patient. Place your index fingers intraorally, and your thumbs externally on the alveolar arches of the two maxillae. Grasp the alveolar arches with your thumbs and index fingers (Figure 12.2).

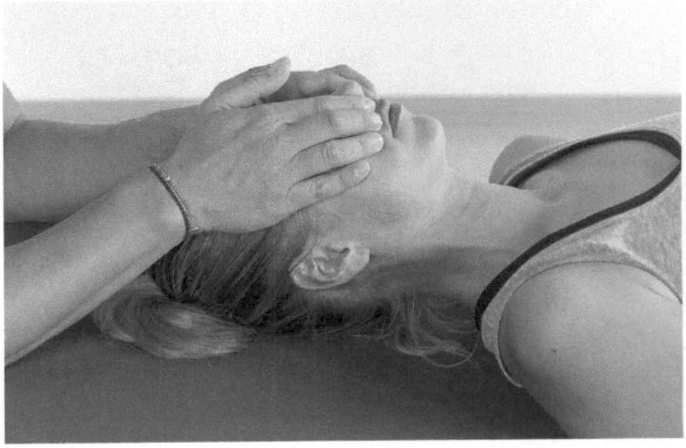

Figure 12.1 Palpation of PRM rhythm of the maxillae

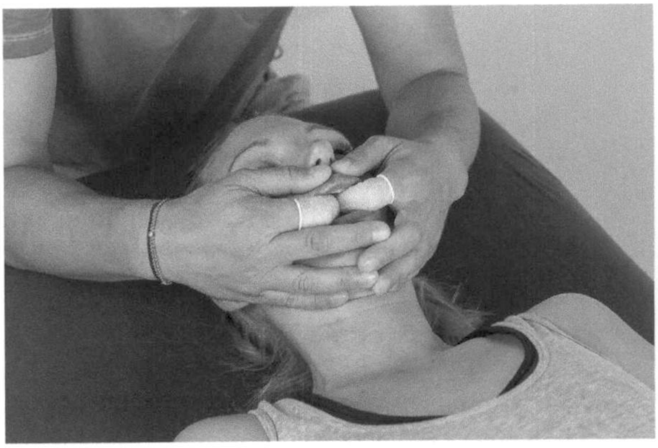

Figure 12.2 Alternative hand position I

- **Alternative hand position II** Take up a position beside the patient's head. Grasp the greater wings with the middle finger and thumb of your cranial hand. Place the index finger and middle finger of the other hand on the upper teeth on each side (Figure 12.3).
- **Alternative hand position III, unilateral** Take up a position beside the patient's head, on the opposite side to the one being tested. Place the index finger of your caudal hand intraorally on the alveolar part. Place the index finger of your cranial hand on the frontal process of the maxilla (Figure 12.4).

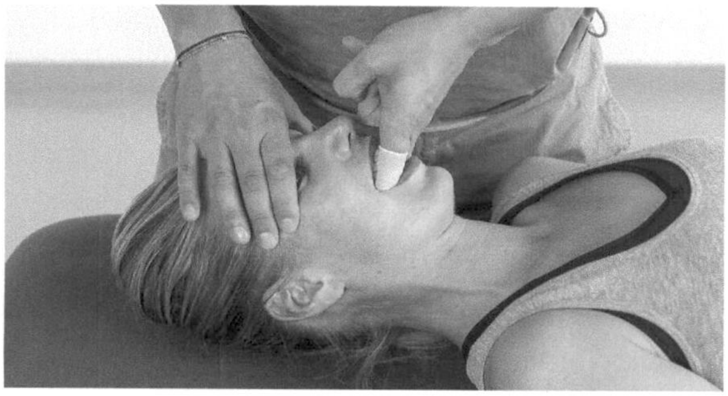

Figure 12.3 Alternative hand position II

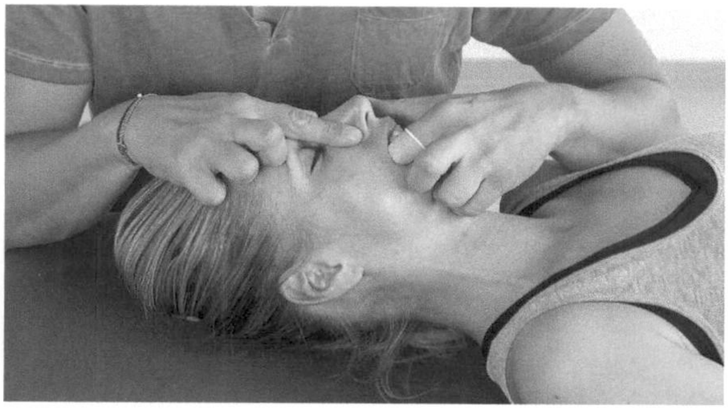

Figure 12.4 Alternative hand position III, unilateral

Biomechanical:

Inhalation phase of PRM, normal finding (Figure 12.5)

- The alveolar arch widens on the lateral side.
- The intermaxillary suture moves posterior.
- The arch of the palate moves down.

Exhalation phase of PRM, normal finding

- The alveolar arch narrows on the lateral side.
- The intermaxillary suture moves anterior.
- The arch of the palate moves cephalad.

Biodynamic/embryological approach:

Inhalation phase of PR, normal finding (Figures 12.6, 12.7)

- The hands may perceive a force in an anterior, inferior direction on the maxillae.

Exhalation phase of PRM, normal finding

- The hands may perceive a force in a posterior, superior direction on the maxillae.

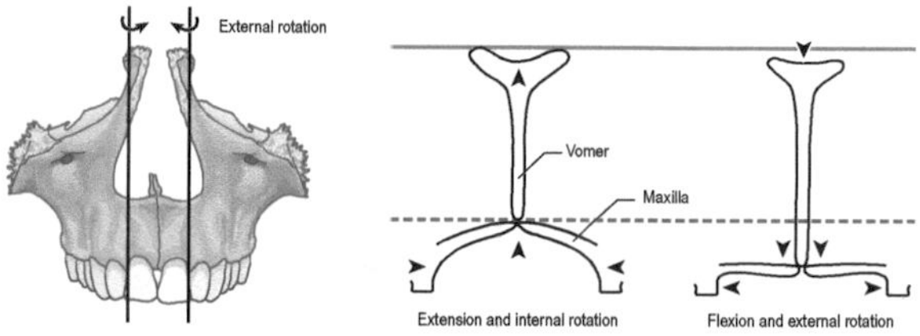

Figure 12.5 PRM inhalation phase/biomechanical approach

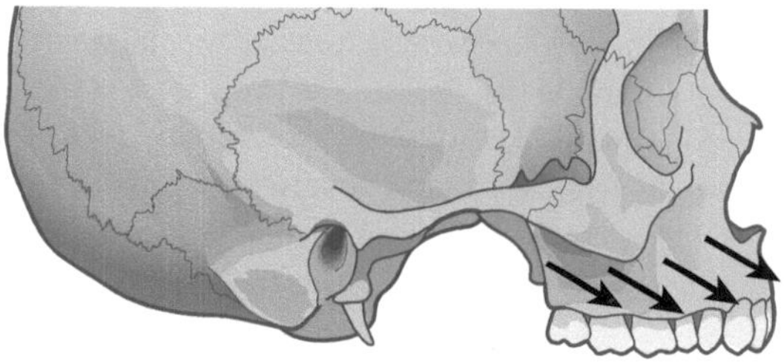

Figure 12.6 PRM inhalation phase/developmental dynamic

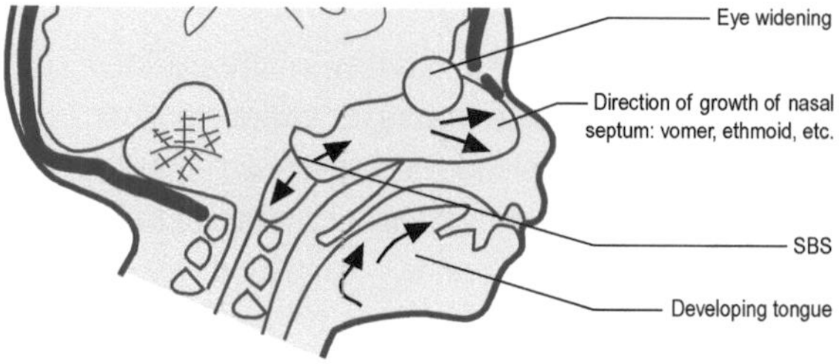

Figure 12.7 PRM inhalation phase/developmental dynamic. Effects on the maxillary complex

Compare the amplitude, strength, ease, and symmetry of the motion of the maxillae.
Other types of motion of the maxillae may sometimes occur during external and internal rotation. These provide an indication as to further dysfunctions of the particular maxilla involved.
Maxillary dysfunctions may be unilateral or bilateral, symmetrical or asymmetrical.

12.3.5 Motion testing

This differs from palpation of the PRM rhythm only in one respect: the external and internal rotation of the frontal bone and maxilla are now actively induced by the practitioner.

Hand position:
See palpation of PRM rhythm (section 12.3.4).

Method: Testing of external and internal rotation:

During the inhalation phase

- At the beginning of the inhalation phase, with your index fingers, direct an impulse in a posterior direction on the intermaxillary suture.
- At the same time, deliver a laterally directed impulse on the posterior region of the alveolar arches with your other fingers.

During the exhalation phase

- At the beginning of the exhalation phase, with your ring fingers and little fingers, deliver a medially directed impulse on the posterior region of the alveolar arches.
- At the same time, follow the intermaxillary suture anterior with your index fingers.

Compare the amplitude and the ease of the respective maxillary motion, or the force needed to induce motion.

12.4 Treatment of the maxillae

12.4.1 Rotation dysfunction of the maxillae

Maxilla lift and spread technique

Aim: Freedom of motion of the maxilla, release of the ethmoidomaxillary, lacrimomaxillary, and ethmoidolacrimal sutures, and freedom of motion of the perpendicular plate.

Practitioner: Take up a position at the head of the patient.

Hand position:

- Place your hands either side of the patient's head.
- Place your thumbs on the outside, on or slightly above the alveolar arches of the maxillae. Your thumbs should be medially oriented.
- Place your index fingers intraorally on the alveolar arches of the maxillae.
- This means that you are in effect grasping the maxilla between your index finger and thumb, from inside and outside (Figure 12.8).

Method:

- With your thumb and index finger, administer traction to the two maxillary bones in the anterior and caudad direction (Figure 12.9). This frees the maxillae from the ethmoid bone. (The medial border of the orbital surface of the maxilla is released from the bottom of the ethmoidal cells, the posterior border of the maxillary frontal process is freed from the anterior of the ethmoidal labyrinth, and the ethmoidal crest on the medial side of the maxilla is released from the middle nasal concha of the ethmoid.)
- When you perceive a release at the ethmoidomaxillary suture, you can go on to spread the maxillae away from one another.
- Without reducing the anterior and caudad traction, instead induce external rotation of the maxillae.
- Administer posterior pressure on the intermaxillary suture with your thumbs.

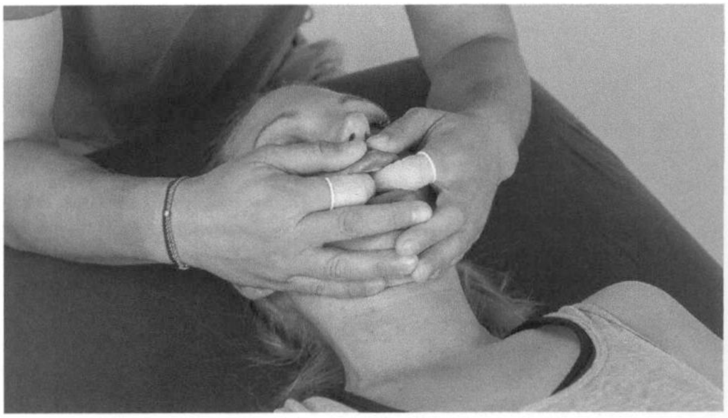

Figure 12.8 Maxilla lift and spread technique

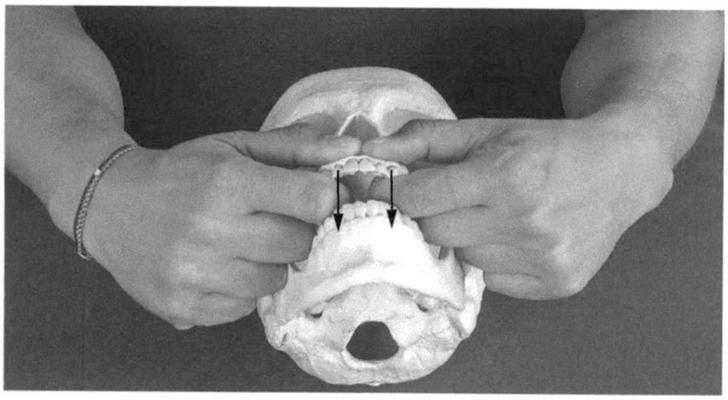

Figure 12.9 Maxilla lift and spread technique (shown on model)

- With your index fingers, guide the alveolar arches in a lateral and anterior direction.
- Establish PBMT and PBFT.

Alternative technique to treat an internal rotation dysfunction of the maxillae

Aim: Freedom of motion of the maxilla, release of the ethmoidomaxillary suture, and freedom of motion of the perpendicular plate.

Practitioner: Take up a position beside the patient's head.

Hand position:

- Cranial hand: span the greater wings with your thumb and middle or index finger.
- Caudal hand: place your middle and index fingers against the upper teeth, one on each side.

Method:

- During the inhalation phase, give an impulse via the greater wings to induce flexion (caudad impulse).
- At the same time, spread apart the fingers resting on the upper teeth (external rotation of the maxillae; Figure 12.10; see also Figure 12.3).
- During the exhalation phase, passively follow the motion of the cranial bones.
- Repeat this procedure for a few cycles, until the mobility of the maxillae increases.

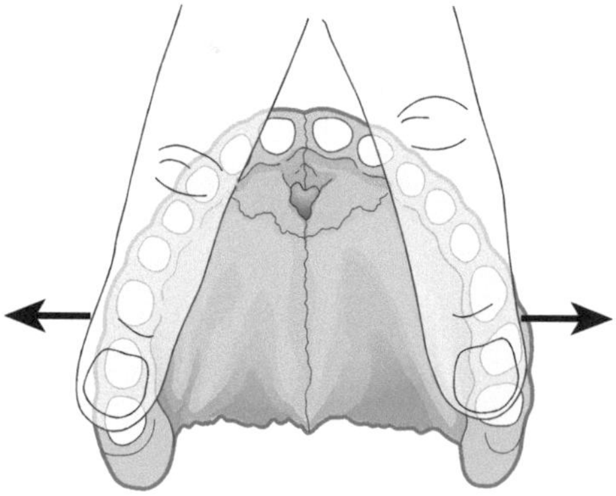

Figure 12.10 Alternative technique to treat an internal rotation dysfunction of the maxillae

12.4.2 Dysfunction in external and internal rotation

Dysfunction in external rotation, bilateral

Practitioner: Take up a position at the head of the patient.

Hand position:

- Position your index fingers each side of the nose, on the alveolar arches of the two maxillae.
- Place the other fingers beside the index fingers on the alveolar arches of the two maxillae.

Method:

Direct technique

- Administer slight, laterally directed traction on the maxillae with your fingers (disengagement).
- At the beginning of the exhalation phase, with your ring fingers and little fingers, deliver a medially directed impulse on the posterior region of the alveolar arches (IR).
- At the same time, follow the intermaxillary suture anterior with your index fingers (Figure 12.11).
- Establish PBMT and PBFT.
- Maintain the PBT until a correction of the abnormal tension has been achieved and the inherent homeostatic forces (PRM rhythm, etc.) have established the correction.

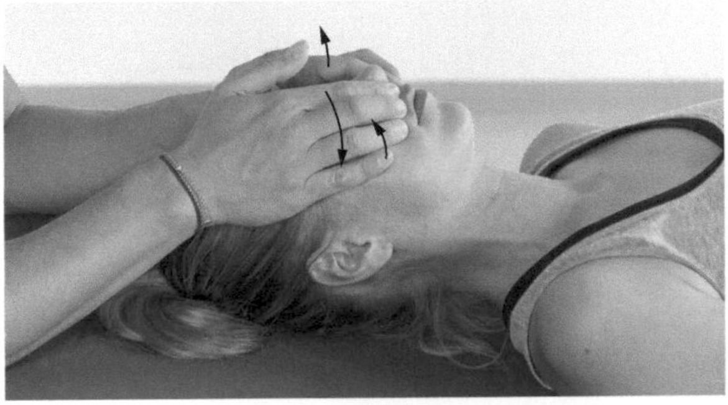

Figure 12.11 External rotation dysfunction, bilateral: direct technique

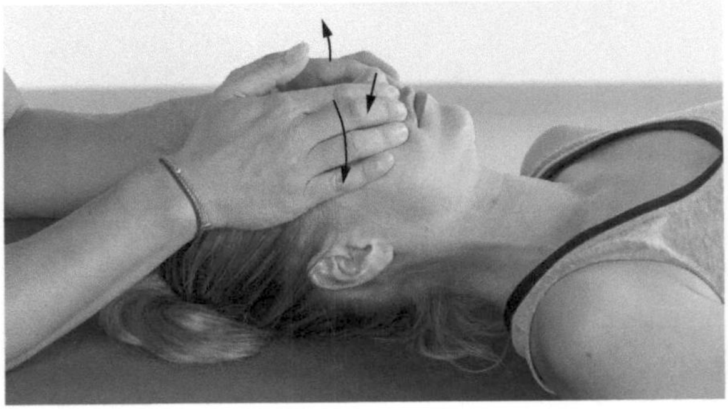

Figure 12.12 Internal rotation dysfunction, bilateral: direct technique

Indirect technique

- Administer slight, laterally directed traction on the maxillae with your fingers (disengagement).
- At the beginning of the inhalation phase, deliver an impulse in the posterior direction with your index fingers on the intermaxillary suture (ER).
- At the same time, deliver a laterally directed impulse with your ring fingers and little fingers to the posterior region of the alveolar arches (ER).
- Establish PBMT and PBFT.

Vitalist approach: See EV-4 technique (this volume, section 4.4.3).

Dysfunction in internal rotation, bilateral

Hand position:
As for dysfunction in external rotation, bilateral (see above).

Method:

Direct technique

- Administer slight, laterally directed traction on the maxillae with your fingers (disengagement).
- At the beginning of the inhalation phase, with your index fingers on the intermaxillary suture, deliver an impulse posterior (ER).
- At the same time, deliver a laterally directed impulse on the posterior region of the alveolar arches with your ring fingers and little fingers (ER; Figure 12.12).
- Establish PBMT and PBFT.

Indirect technique

- Administer slight, laterally directed traction on the maxillae with your fingers (disengagement).
- At the beginning of the exhalation phase, with your ring fingers and little fingers, deliver a medially directed impulse on the posterior region of the alveolar arches (IR).
- At the same time, your index fingers follow the intermaxillary suture in the anterior direction (IR).
- Establish PBMT and PBFT.

Alternative hand position I for dysfunction in external and internal rotation

Practitioner: Take up a position at the head of the patient.

Hand position: Place your index fingers intraorally and your thumbs externally on the alveolar arches of the two maxillae. Grasp the alveolar arches with your thumbs and index fingers.

Method: For dysfunction in **external rotation**.

Direct technique:

- The method already described (dysfunction in external rotation, bilateral, direct) may be supplemented by applying cephalad pressure to the palatine processes of the maxillae using the index fingers (IR; Figure 12.2).

Indirect technique:

- The method already described (dysfunction in external rotation, bilateral, indirect) may be supplemented by encouraging the lowering of the palatine processes of the maxillae using the index fingers (ER).

Method: For dysfunction in **internal rotation**.
Direct technique:

- The method already described (dysfunction in internal rotation, bilateral, direct) may be supplemented by encouraging the lowering of the palatine processes of the maxillae using the index fingers (ER).

Indirect technique:

- The method already described (dysfunction in internal rotation, bilateral, indirect) may be supplemented by applying cephalad pressure to the palatine processes of the maxillae using the index fingers (IR).

Alternative hand position II for dysfunction in external and internal rotation

Practitioner: Take up a position beside the patient's head.

Hand position:

- Cranial hand: span the greater wings with your middle or index finger and your thumb.
- Caudal hand: place the index finger and middle finger of this hand against the upper teeth, one on each side (Figure 12.3).

Method: For dysfunction in **external rotation**.
Direct technique:

- The greater wings are moved into extension.
- Move the index finger and middle finger resting on the teeth closer together (IR).

Indirect technique:

- Go with the greater wings into flexion.
- Spread apart the index finger and middle finger resting on the teeth (ER).

Method: For dysfunction in **internal rotation**.
Direct technique:

- The greater wings are moved into flexion.
- Spread apart your index finger and middle finger on the teeth (ER).

Indirect technique:

- Follow the greater wings into extension.
- Move the index finger and middle finger resting on the teeth closer together (IR).

Dysfunction in external rotation, unilateral: direct technique

Practitioner: Take up a position beside the patient's head, on the opposite side to the dysfunction.

Hand position:

- Cranial hand: span the greater wings with your thumb and your middle or index finger.
- Caudal hand: place your ring finger or middle finger on the alveolar arches. Place your index finger on the frontal process of the maxilla.

Method:

- Direct technique
  - ▸ Using your ring or middle finger, deliver an impulse in the medial direction on the posterior region of the alveolar arches (IR).
  - ▸ At the same time, using your index finger on the frontal process, deliver an impulse in the vertical alignment direction (IR; Figure 12.13).
- Establish PBMT and PBFT.
- A fluid impulse may be used to direct energy from the opposite lambdoid suture.

Vitalist approach: See EV-4 technique (this volume, section 4.4.3).

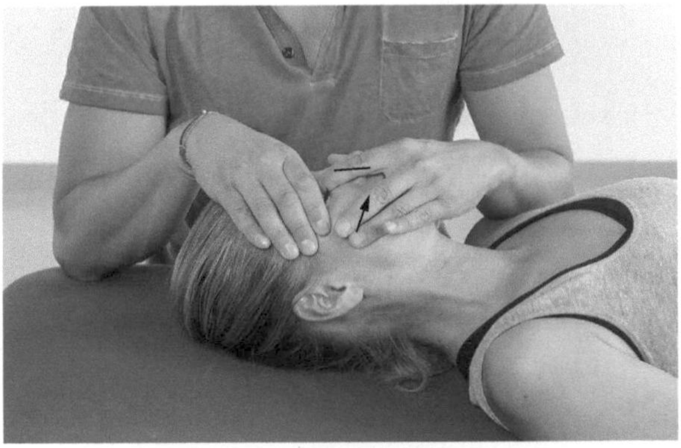

Figure 12.13 External rotation dysfunction, unilateral: direct technique

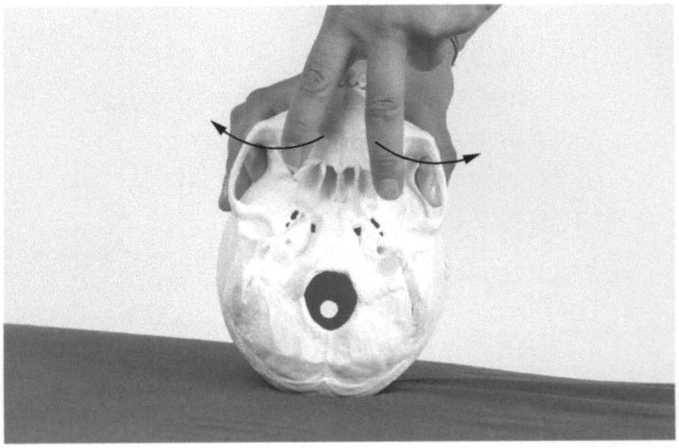

Figure 12.14 Global rotation dysfunction about a vertical axis

12.4.3 Global rotation dysfunction about a vertical axis

Possible cause: Effect of a force from the side on the maxilla. The maxillae move in conjunction with the palatine bones and the sphenoid.

Possible sequelae: Lateral strain of the SBS.

Practitioner: Take up a position beside the patient's head.

Hand position:

- Cranial hand: span the greater wings with your thumb and middle or index finger.
- Caudal hand: place the middle finger and index finger of one hand against the upper teeth, each side.

Motion test: With your index and middle fingers, induce a global rotation of the two maxillae while holding the sphenoid firmly in the neutral position. Compare the amplitude and ease of the maxillary global rotation.

Method: The sphenoid is held firmly in the neutral position.

Exaggeration:

- With your index and middle fingers, induce global rotation of the two maxillae in the direction of greater motion (of ease) (Figure 12.14).

Direct technique:

- With your index and middle fingers, induce global rotation of the two maxillae in the direction of the restriction.
- Establish the PBMT and PBFT.

12.4.4 Global lateral strain

Possible cause: Effect of a force from the side on the maxilla. The maxillae move relative to the palatines and sphenoid.

Sequelae: Curvature of the nasal septum, including the vomer.

Practitioner: Take up a position beside the patient's head.

Hand position:

- Cranial hand: span the greater wings with your thumb and middle or index finger.
- Caudal hand: place the index and middle finger of one hand against the upper teeth on each side.

Motion test: Using your index finger and middle finger, carry out global lateral strain of the two

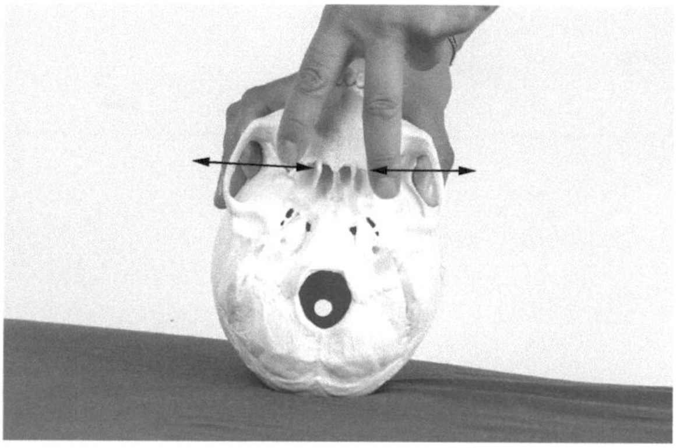

Figure 12.15 Global lateral strain. Exaggeration: encourage motion of the maxilla in the direction of greater motion (of ease). Direct technique: encourage motion of the maxilla in the direction of the restriction

maxillae, while holding the sphenoid firmly in the neutral position. Compare the amplitude and ease of the maxillary global lateral strain.

Method: The sphenoid is held firmly in the neutral position.

Exaggeration:

- Using your index and middle fingers, induce a lateral shifting of the two maxillae in the direction of greater motion (of ease) (Figure 12.15).

Direct technique:

- With your index and middle fingers, induce a lateral shifting of the two maxillae in the direction of the restriction (Figure 12.15).
- Establish PBMT and PBFT.

12.4.5 Decompression of the maxillary complex

Decompression of the maxillary complex I

Indication: Dysfunction of the pterygopalatine ganglion following a fall or a blow to the face, compression of the sphenopalatine and palatomaxillary sutures.

Practitioner: Take up a position beside the patient's head.

Hand position:

- Cranial hand: span the greater wings with your thumb and middle or index finger.
- Caudal hand: place the index and middle finger of this hand on the upper teeth on each side and hook them firmly on the posterior surface of the maxillary alveolar arches. Place your thumb externally, beneath the nose, on the intermaxillary suture.

Method:

- During the inhalation phase, go with the greater wings into flexion and hold them in the flexion position.
- At the same time, administer traction on the maxilla in an anterior direction with your thumb, index finger, and middle finger (Figure 12.16).
- Decompression occurs first of all at the palatomaxillary suture, and then at the pterygopalatine suture.
- Without reducing the decompression movement, permit all motions and unwinding of the maxillary complex.
- With each release of the tissues, seek the new limit of motion of the maxillary complex in the anterior direction.
- Establish PBMT and PBFT.
- A fluid impulse may be used to direct energy from the opposite parietal tuber.

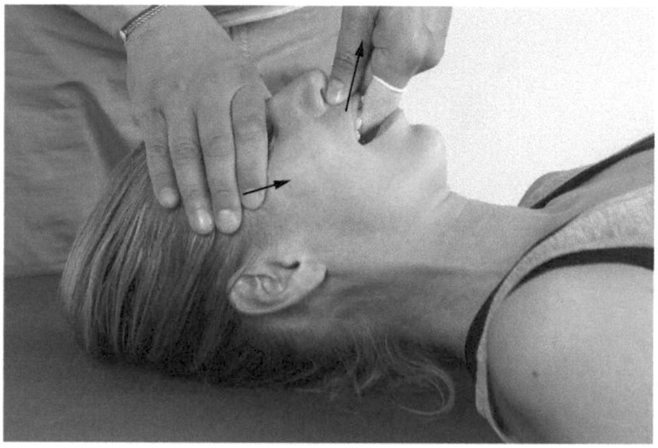

Figure 12.16 Decompression of the maxillary complex I

Decompression of the maxillary complex II

Aim: To release the frontomaxillary, palatomaxillary, pterygopalatine, and incisive sutures.

Hand position:

- Cranial hand: span the greater wings with your thumb and middle or index finger. Place the basal joint of your index finger on the frontal bone glabella.
- Caudal hand: position your index finger intraorally, immediately behind the incisors. Place your thumb externally, beneath the nose, on the intermaxillary suture. Grasp the incisive bone with these two fingers.

Method:

- Cranial hand: hold the greater wings and the frontal bone firmly in the neutral position.
- At the same time, with the index finger and thumb of your caudal hand, administer traction in an anterior, inferior direction at an angle of about 45° (Figure 12.17).
- This frees the frontomaxillary, palatomaxillary, and pterygopalatine sutures. Decompression of the incisive suture also occurs (section 12.4.6).
- Establish PBMT and PBFT.

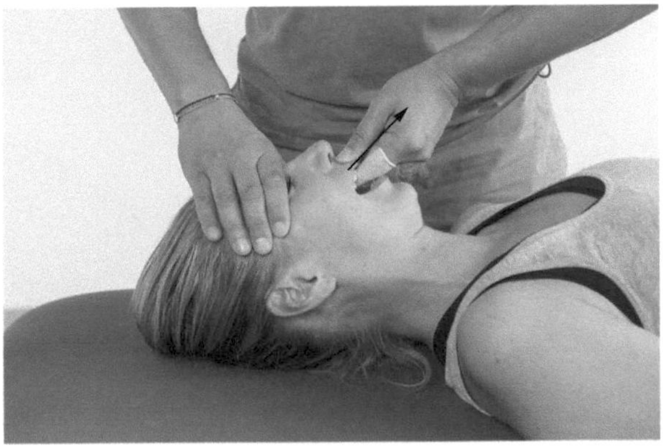

Figure 12.17 Decompression of the maxillary complex II

12.4.6 Sutural dysfunctions

Transverse palatine suture

Suture margin: Posterior margin of the palatine process of the maxilla: superior-facing margin; anterior margin of the horizontal plate of the palatine bone: inferior-facing margin (Figure 12.20).

Suture type: Serrate suture.

Indication: Disturbances of sensitivity and pain in the mucosae of the hard and soft palate resulting from falls or blows to the upper jaw, impairment of the greater and lesser palatine nerves.

Practitioner: Take up a position beside the patient's head.

Hand position:

- Cranial hand: span the greater wings with your thumb and middle or index finger.
- Caudal hand: place your index finger intraorally, unilaterally on the palatine process of the maxilla, immediately behind the anterior incisors. Position your middle finger intraorally, unilaterally on the horizontal plate of the palatine bone, immediately behind the transverse palatine suture.

Method:

- Direct technique (Figures 12.18 and 12.19)
  - ▸ During the exhalation phase, go with the greater wings into extension and hold them there.

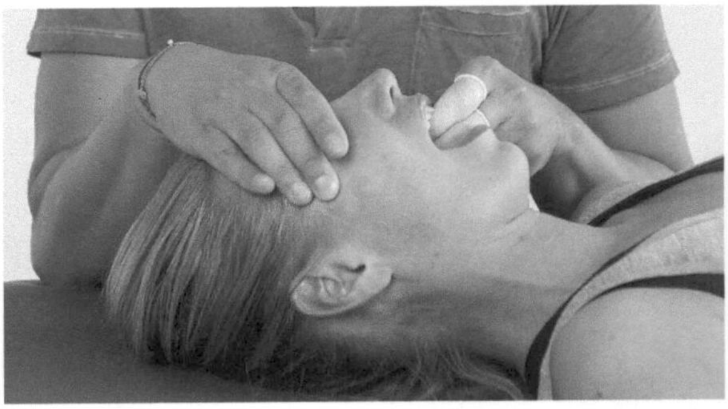

Figure 12.18 Transverse palatine suture

- ▸ Caudal hand: apply pressure in the superior direction with your two fingers. This moves the horizontal plate of palatine bone in a superior direction and the posterior margin of the horizontal plate of the maxilla inferior.
- Establish PBMT and PBFT.
- A fluid impulse may be used to direct energy from the opposite lambdoid suture.

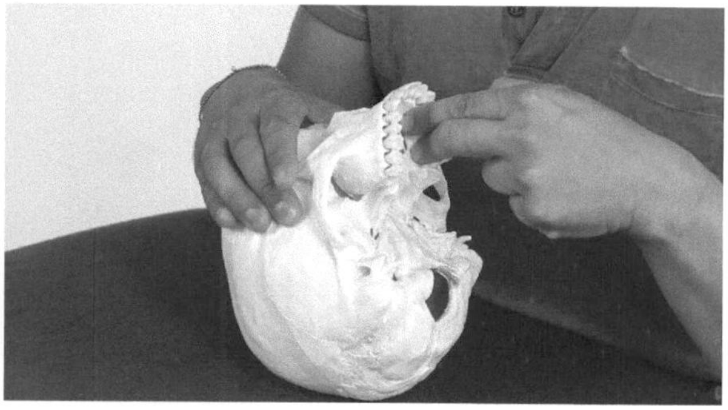

Figure 12.19 Transverse palatine suture (shown on model)

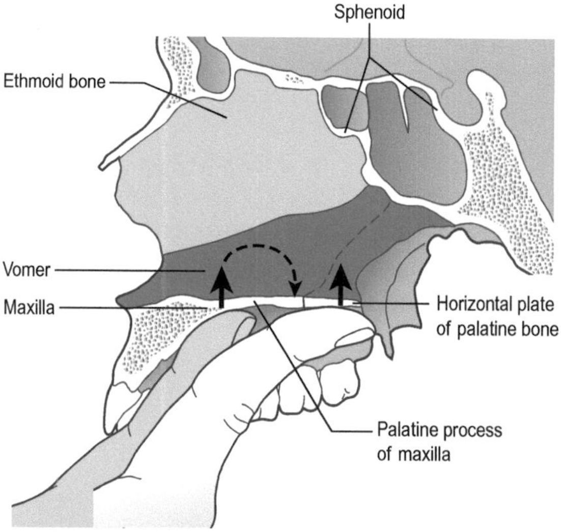

Figure 12.20 Transverse palatine suture. Solid arrows: impulse from the fingers on to the maxilla and palatine bone. Dotted arrow: cranially directed pressure from the index finger on the anterior region of the maxillary palatine process causes the posterior region to move caudad

Palatomaxillary suture

Suture margin: The posterior medial aspect of the orbital surface of the maxilla articulates with the anterior part of the orbital process of the palatine bone. The posterior margin of the maxillary sinus articulates with the lateral edge of the perpendicular plate of the palatine bone. The lower, rough surface of the posterior border of the maxilla articulates with the pyramidal process of the palatine bone.

Suture type: Plane suture, irregular.

Indication: This suture is frequently disturbed by falls or blows to the face.

Practitioner: Take up a position beside the patient's head, on the same side as the dysfunction.

Hand position:

- Cranial hand: span the greater wings with your thumb and your middle or index finger.
- Caudal hand: place your index finger intraorally, on the horizontal plate of the palatine bone, immediately behind the transverse palatine suture. Place the distal phalanx of your middle finger intraorally, on the posterior surface of the maxillary alveolar arch. The middle phalanx of the middle finger lies on the first molar.

Method:

- Direct technique (Figures 12.21 and 12.22)

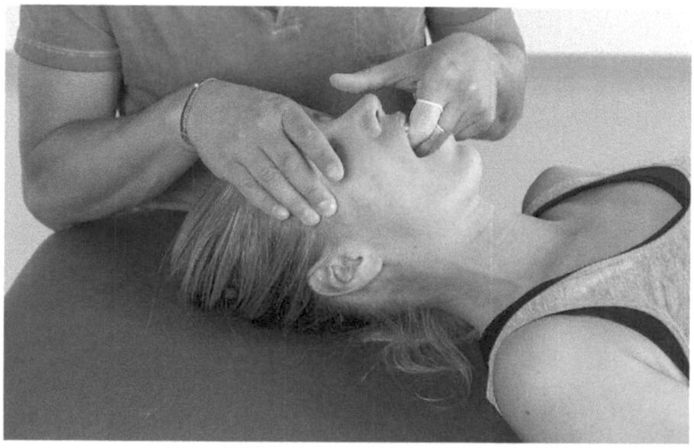

Figure 12.21 Palatomaxillary suture

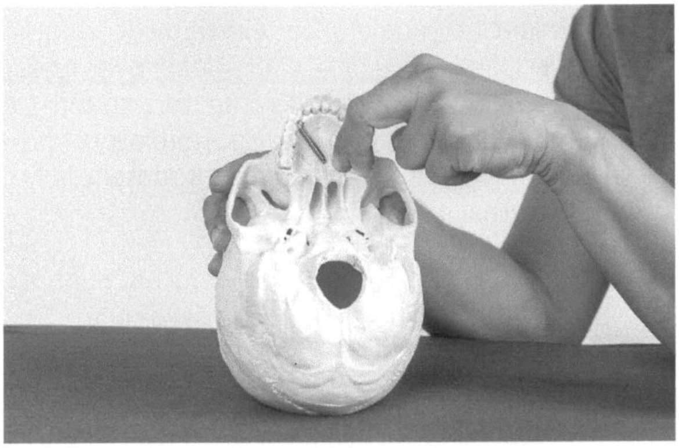

Figure 12.22 Palatomaxillary suture (shown on model)

- ▸ During the exhalation phase, go with the greater wings into extension in the cranial direction and hold them there.
- ▸ At the same time, with the index finger of your caudal hand, apply pressure in a superior direction and traction medially on the horizontal plate (IR).
- ▸ During the subsequent inhalation phase, hold the position of the sphenoid and palatine bone.
- ▸ At the same time, move the alveolar arch of the maxilla laterally and slightly anteriorly with your middle finger (ER).
- ▸ Without reducing the gentle traction, permit all motions/unwinding of the maxilla.
- ▸ With each release of the tissues, seek the new limit of motion of the alveolar arch on the side of the dysfunction in the lateral direction (ER).

- Establish PBMT and PBFT.
- A fluid impulse may be used to direct energy from the opposite lambdoid suture.

Frontomaxillary suture

Suture margin: The frontal process of the maxilla articulates with the outer lateral portion of the nasal part of the frontal bone (see also this volume, section 10.4.5).

Suture type: Serrate suture.

Practitioner: Take up a position beside the patient's head.

Hand position:

- Cranial hand: span the frontal bone with your thumb and middle finger or index finger, and hook them firmly laterally on the frontal bone. Place the basal joint of your index finger on glabella, above the frontomaxillary suture.
- Caudal hand: grasp the frontal processes of the maxillae with your thumb and index finger, beneath the frontomaxillary sutures (Figure 12.23).

Alternative hand position:

- Cranial hand: span the frontal bone with your thumb and middle finger or ring finger, and hook them firmly laterally on the frontal bone.
- Caudal hand: place your thumb intraorally, behind the anterior incisors. Position your index and middle finger either side of the frontal processes of the maxillae (Figure 12.24).

Method:

- Disengagement
  - ▸ During the inhalation phase, go with the frontal bone into external rotation and hold it there.
  - ▸ At the beginning of the inhalation phase, using the basal joint of your index finger, begin to apply slight pressure in a posterior direction on the midline of the frontal bone and traction in a superior direction (ER).

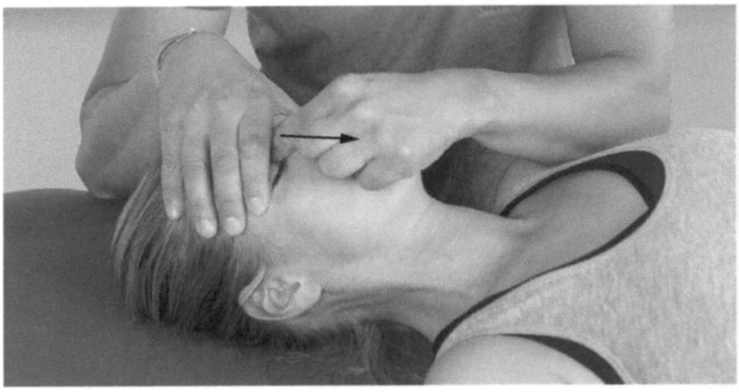

Figure 12.23 Frontomaxillary suture

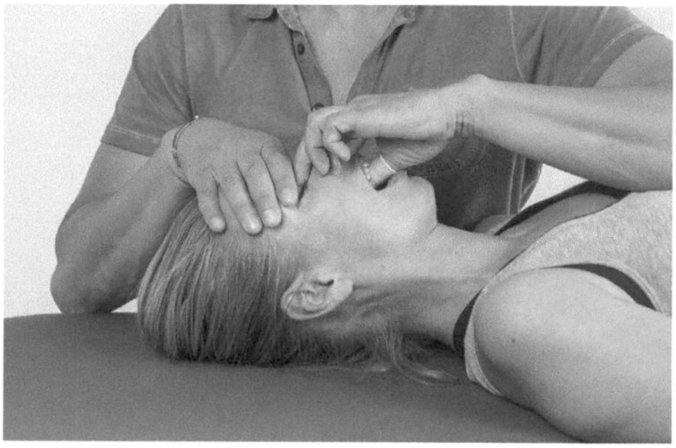

Figure 12.24 Frontomaxillary suture. Alternative hand position

- ▸ Using your thumb and middle finger or index finger, deliver an impulse on the zygomatic processes of the frontal bone in an anterolateral direction (ER).
- ▸ The overall effect is to move the frontal bone into a flattened position (flexion).
- ▸ Hold the frontal bone firmly in place in flexion and ER.
- ▸ At the same time, with the index finger and thumb, administer traction caudad on the frontal processes of the maxillae.
- ▸ Without reducing the gentle disengagement, permit all motions/unwinding of the maxillae.
- ▸ With each release of the tissues, seek the new limit of motion of the frontal processes in an inferior direction.

- Establish PBMT and PBFT.
- A fluid impulse may be used to direct energy from the opposite occipital squama.

Incisive suture

Aim: To release the incisive bone (premaxilla) from the maxilla.

Diagnosis: When an incisive bone is in ER and the maxilla in IR, the canine tooth is usually prominent. When the incisive bone is in IR and the maxilla in ER, the canine tooth is usually posteriorly shifted.

Indication: Restricted mobility following the effects of early traumatic injury, or use of dental braces.

Practitioner: Take up a position beside the patient's head.

Hand position:

- Cranial hand: span the greater wings with your thumb and middle finger or index finger.
- Caudal hand: position your index finger intraorally on the incisive bone, immediately behind the anterior incisors. Place your thumb externally, beneath the nose, on the intermaxillary suture.

Method:

- Disengagement
    - ▸ Hold the greater wings firmly in the neutral position.
    - ▸ At the same time, administer traction in an anterior direction with the index finger and thumb of your caudal hand (Figure 12.25).
    - ▸ Without reducing the gentle disengagement, permit all motions/unwinding of the incisive bone that arise.
    - ▸ With each release of the tissues, seek the new limit of motion of the incisive bone in an anterior direction.
- A fluid impulse may be used to direct energy from the lambda.

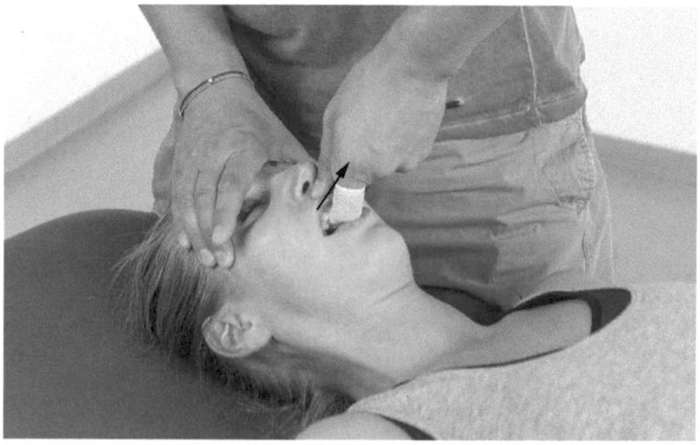

Figure 12.25 Incisive suture

Zygomaticomaxillary suture

Suture margin: The zygomatic process of the maxilla articulates with the anterior and inferior border of the zygomatic bone.

Suture type: Irregularly formed suture.

Indication: Disturbance to the orbits due to a fall or a blow to the face; also disturbance of the maxillary sinus with sinusitis.

Practitioner: Take up a position beside the patient's head, on the opposite side to the dysfunction.

Hand position:

- Caudal hand: place the index finger intraorally on the inner surface of the zygomatic bone. Your thumb is placed externally, against the zygomatic bone, so that you grasp the zygomatic bone between thumb and index finger.
- Cranial hand: place the palm of your hand passively on the frontal bone. Position your index finger along the course of the frontal process of the affected maxilla (Figure 12.26).

Alternative hand position:

- Cranial hand: grasp the zygomatic bone with your thumb and index finger. Position your thumb on the orbital border of the zygomatic bone. Position your index finger on the inferior border of the zygomatic bone.
- Caudal hand: your index finger is placed intraorally beneath the zygomatic process of the maxilla (Figure 12.27).

Method:

- Disengagement: with your caudal hand, administer traction in the lateral direction on the zygomatic bone. As you do this, hold the maxilla firmly in position with the index finger of the cranial hand.
- Establish PBMT: maintain the gentle disengagement. At the same time, follow the zygomatic bone into the position that creates the best possible balance of the tension between the zygomatic bone and maxilla.
- A fluid impulse may be used to direct energy from the opposite lambdoid suture.

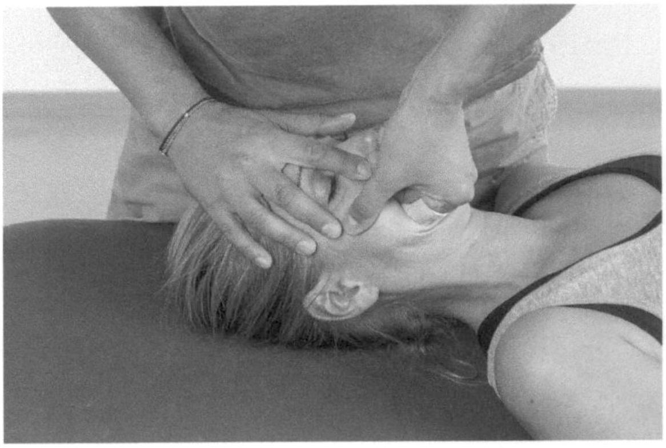

Figure 12.26 Zygomaticomaxillary suture

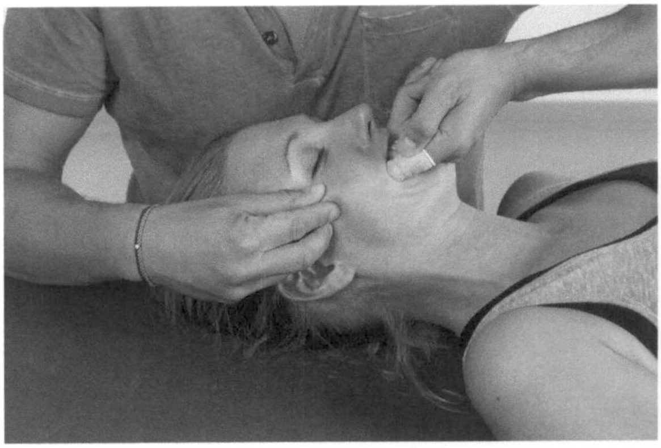

Figure 12.27 Zygomaticomaxillary suture. Alternative hand position

Median palatine suture

Indication: Restricted mobility due to the use of dental braces.

Practitioner: Take up a position beside the patient's head.

Hand position:

- Cranial hand: span the greater wings with your thumb and middle finger or index finger.
- Caudal hand: position your index finger and middle finger intraorally either side, on the two palatine processes of the maxillae anterior to the transverse palatine suture.

Method:

- Disengagement
  - ▶ Hold the greater wings firmly in the neutral position.
  - ▶ At the same time, spread the index finger and middle finger of your caudal hand (Figures 12.28 and 12.29).
  - ▶ Without reducing the gentle disengagement, permit all motions/unwinding of the maxillae.

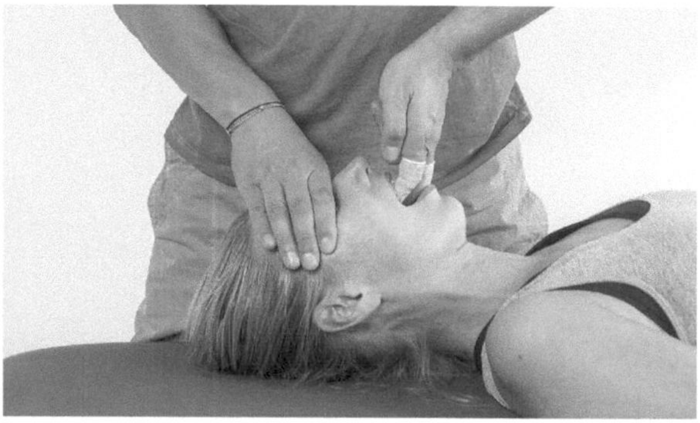

Figure 12.28 Median palatine suture

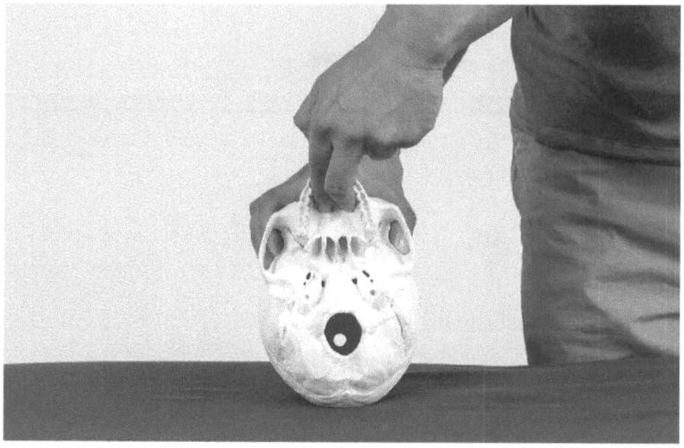

Figure 12.29 Median palatine suture (shown on model)

  - ▶ With each release of the tissues, seek the new limit of motion of the maxillae laterally.
- Establish PBMT and PBFT.
- A fluid impulse may be used to direct energy from inion.
- At the end of the technique, the motion of the maxilla should be re-synchronized with that of the sphenoid in harmony with the PRM rhythm.
- During the inhalation phase, go with the sphenoid and the maxillae into flexion and ER; during the exhalation phase, go with the sphenoid and the maxillae into extension and IR.

Nasomaxillary suture

See this volume, section 15.1.

12.5 References

1 Rohen, J. W. (2002) *Morphologie des menschlichen Organismus*, 2nd Ed. Stuttgart: Verlag Freies Geistesleben, p. 366.

2 Stone, R. (1994) *Polaritätstherapie*, 2nd Ed. Hugendubel, p. 207.

3 Sutherland, W. G. (1944) 'The cranial bowl.' *J. Am. Osteopath. Assoc. 1944*, 348–353.

13.1 Location, causes, and clinical presentation of palatine dysfunctions 424
13.1.1 Osseous dysfunctions 424
13.1.2 Muscular dysfunctions 425
13.1.3 Neural disturbances 425
13.1.4 Vascular disturbances 425

13.2 Diagnosis of the palatine bone 425
13.2.1 History-taking 425
13.2.2 Inspection 425
13.2.3 Palpation of position 426
13.2.4 Palpation of PRM rhythm 426
13.2.5 Motion testing 427

13.3 Treatment of the palatine bones 428
13.3.1 General mobilization of the palatine bones 428
13.3.2 Sutural dysfunctions 429

13.4 Reference 430

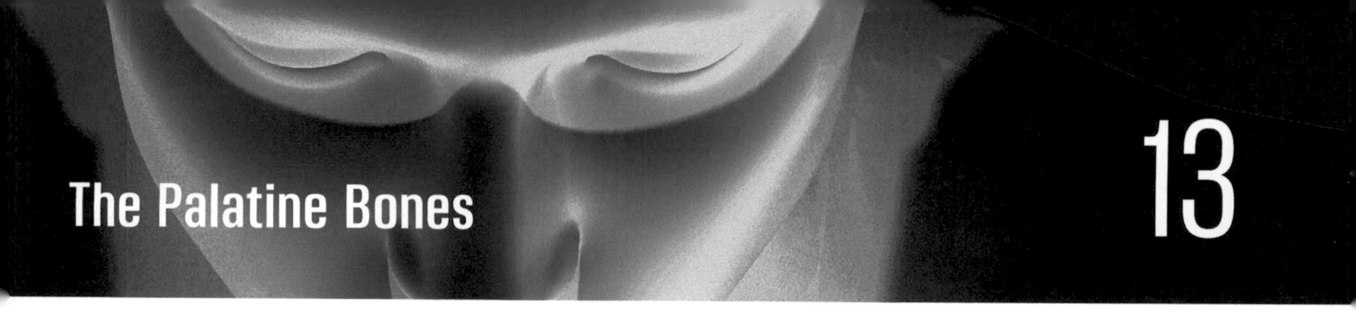

13 The Palatine Bones

The palatine is a paired bone, primarily consisting of a vertical and a horizontal bony plate, which contribute to the nasal septum and floor of the nose. The palatine bone also contributes to the orbit via the small orbital process.

According to Sutherland, the palatine bone mediates between the maxilla and the sphenoid, serving as a "speed reducer." Dysfunctions of this bone are usually secondary to dysfunctions of the maxilla or sphenoid.[1] Muscular connections exist with the masticatory system and palate. Branches of cranial nerve V_2 run along the palatine bone. Another significant feature is that the bone contributes to the pterygopalatine fissure, in which the pterygopalatine ganglion is situated.

13.1 Location, causes, and clinical presentation of palatine dysfunctions

> **Tip for practitioners**
>
> **Primary dysfunctions**
> - Intraosseous.
> - Traumatic injury: due to falls, blows, tooth extraction, poor masticatory habits, or other effects of force on the maxillae. These can lead to motion restrictions of the maxillae and palatine bone, and of the pterygopalatine ganglion.
>
> **Secondary dysfunctions**
> - Due to dysfunction of the sphenoid (e.g., SBS dysfunctions) and of the maxilla.
> - Developmental disturbances of the cranial base during the embryonic stage lead to developmental disturbances of the palatine bone.
> - In the case of TMJ dysfunctions.

13.1.1 Osseous dysfunctions

- **Sphenopalatine suture**
  - The pterygoid notches of the pterygoid processes of the sphenoid articulate with the pyramidal processes of the palatine bones. The pterygoid processes converge anteriorly and separate posteriorly, so that the sphenoid spreads the small palatines in the inhalation phase and moves them into external rotation. According to Sutherland, this slight pendulum motion between the pterygoid processes of the sphenoid and the grooves on the palatines is particularly important for the effective transmission of motion to the palatine and maxillary bones, and also for its function as a "speed reducer." The palatine bone reduces the stronger motion of the sphenoid relative to the maxilla. This mechanism is frequently disturbed, for example in SBS dysfunctions or in traumatic injuries to the face. The consequence is a restriction of the maxillary complex.
  - The inferior lateral surface of the sphenoid articulates with the orbital process.
  - The inferior anterior angle of the body of the sphenoid articulates with the orbital process.
  - The anterior margin of the medial pterygoid plate articulates with the posterior margin of the perpendicular plate of the palatine (the vertical part of the palatine bone).
- **Orbital process** The orbital process enters into the formation of the orbit. Clinical presentation: eye problems (Volume 2, sections 3.1.1 and 3.2).
- **Transverse palatine suture:** see this volume, section 12.4.6.

- **Palatomaxillary suture:** see this volume, section 12.4.6.
- **Vomeropalatine suture:** Sequelae: motion restriction of the vomer and palatine bone.
- **Palatoethmoidal suture:** Sequelae: motion restriction of the ethmoid bone.
- **Median palatine suture:** see this volume, section 12.4.6.

13.1.2 Muscular dysfunctions

Dysfunctions between the pyramidal and pterygoid processes and motion restriction of the palatine bone can arise in cases of severe hypertonicity of the lateral/medial pterygoid muscles.

- **Lateral pterygoid:** on the external surface of the pyramidal process.
- **Medial pterygoid:** on the posterior external margin of the pyramidal process.
- **Tensor veli palatini:** on the lower posterior region of the horizontal plate.

13.1.3 Neural disturbances

- **Pterygopalatine ganglion** (see this volume, sections 3.1.3 and 3.2.3).
  - Causes: blows, falling onto the frontal bone or a zygomatic bone, or onto the upper jaw, may push the small palatine bone into the ganglion, leaving less space for the ganglion and impairing its function.
  - Clinical presentation: functional disturbances of the lacrimal gland, and of the small glands of the nasopharyngeal space and palate, olfactory disturbance due to dryness of the nasal mucosae.
- **Maxillary nerve**
  - The maxillary nerve extends into the orbit from the foramen rotundum via the pterygopalatine fossa and inferior orbital fissure. There it detours the small orbital process of the palatine bone, and then first passes into the maxillary canal before arriving at the surface. This small process of the palatine bone acts like a tension regulator for this nerve, so that it is not subjected to excessive tensile forces during the slight movements of PRM rhythm.
  - Clinical presentation: paresthesia of the mid-facial region, etc.
- **Greater and lesser palatine nerves**
  - Causes: blows or falling onto the upper jaw, resulting in a dysfunction of the transverse palatine suture and palatomaxillary suture.
  - Clinical presentation: disturbances of sensitivity and pain in the mucosa of the hard and soft palate.
- **Pharyngeal branch of the maxillary nerve**
  - Dysfunction in the sphenopalatine suture, particularly in the palatovaginal canal.
  - Clinical presentation: disturbances of sensitivity of the pharyngeal mucosa.

13.1.4 Vascular disturbances

Symptoms in the vessels listed below are only rarely induced solely by palatine dysfunction.

- **Descending palatine artery** (branch of the middle meningeal artery): in the greater palatine canal.
- **Sphenopalatine artery** (branch of maxillary artery): in the sphenopalatine foramen.
- **Ascending pharyngeal artery** (branch of maxillary artery): in the palatovaginal canal.

13.2 Diagnosis of the palatine bone

13.2.1 History-taking

- Nasal symptoms (rhinitis, sinusitis, hay fever).
- Oral or pharyngeal symptoms.
- Ocular symptoms.
- Asthma.

13.2.2 Inspection

- Palate: lowered/flat (ER of maxilla and palatine).
- Palate: elevated (IR of maxilla and palatine).
- Unilaterally lowered or elevated palate: torsion or lateroflexion-rotation of SBS.

13.2.3 Palpation of position

Horizontal plate: lowered (ER) or elevated (IR).

13.2.4 Palpation of PRM rhythm

Tip for practitioners

Biomechanical, inhalation phase

An external rotation of the palatine bone occurs.

- The horizontal plate moves downward.
- The median palatine suture moves downward and posterior.
- The transverse diameter increases.
- The orbital process and sphenoid process move inferior, following the body of the sphenoid.
- The pyramidal process moves outward and in a downward and posterior direction, following the pterygoid process of the sphenoid.
- The sphenoid lowers the palatine bone via the pterygoid process and the vomer.

Developmental dynamic, inhalation phase

- The expansive force is in the anterior and inferior direction.

If palpation reveals a motion restriction, the practitioner may induce an impulse in the direction of the restriction. This will emphasize it, making it easier to sense from which structure it originates.

Practitioner: Take up a position beside the patient's head.

Hand position:

- Cranial hand: span the greater wings with your thumb and your middle or index finger.
- Caudal hand: place your index and middle fingers intraorally, one on either side on the horizontal plates of the palatine bone laterally to the median palatine suture. To position them exactly, slide the fingers along the medial side of the upper molars. Just behind the last molars, position them slightly medially on the hard palate (Figures 13.1 and 13.2).
- For the unilateral test, only the index finger of the caudal hand is positioned intraorally on the horizontal plate of one palatine bone (Figure 13.5).

Biomechanical approach: With your cranial hand, passively follow the motion of the SBS into extension and flexion. With your caudal hand, sense whether the palatine bone moves in harmony with the motion of the SBS.

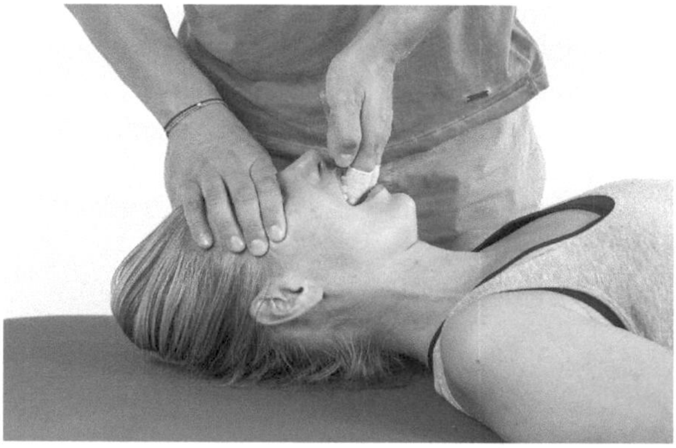

Figure 13.1 Palpation of PRM rhythm of the palatine bones

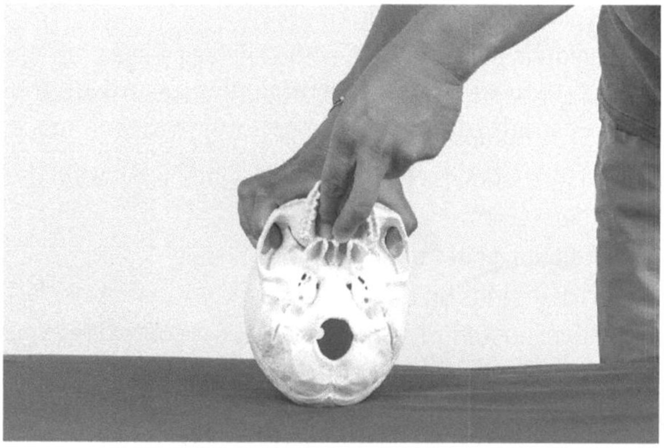

Figure 13.2 Palpation of PRM rhythm of the palatine bones (shown on model)

Inhalation phase, normal finding:

- The horizontal plate moves inferior (and somewhat laterally; Figure 13.3).

Exhalation phase, normal finding:

- The horizontal plate moves superior (and somewhat medially).

Developmental dynamic approach

Inhalation phase, normal finding:

- The hands may perceive a force on the palatines in an anterior, inferior direction (Figure 13.4).

Exhalation phase, normal finding:

- The hands may perceive a force on the palatines in a posterior, superior direction.

Compare the amplitude, strength, ease, and symmetry of the motion of the palatines.

Other types of motion of the palatine bones may sometimes occur during external and internal rotation. These provide an indication as to further dysfunctions of the particular palatine involved.

Palatine dysfunctions may be unilateral or bilateral, symmetrical or asymmetrical.

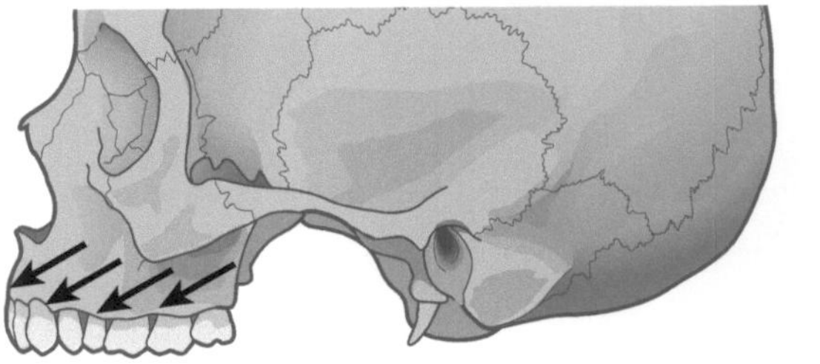

Figure 13.4 PRM inhalation phase/developmental dynamic approach

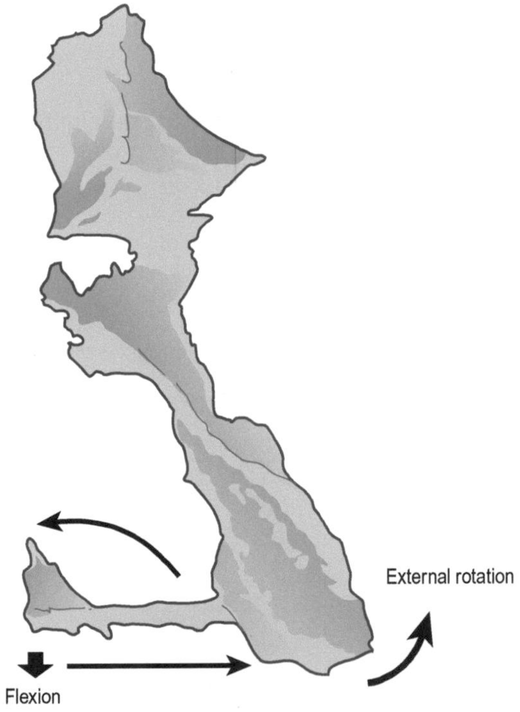

Figure 13.3 PRM inhalation phase/biomechanical approach

13.2.5 Motion testing

Hand position: See palpation of PRM rhythm (section 13.2.4).

Method: Testing of ER and IR.

During the inhalation phase:

- With your middle finger and thumb, deliver an impulse caudad to the greater wings (motion into flexion).
- With the index and middle fingers that are on the horizontal plates, you will perceive a minute inferior motion in response to this pressure.

During the exhalation phase:

- With your middle finger and thumb, deliver an impulse cephalad (motion into extension).
- With the index and middle fingers that are on the horizontal plates, you will perceive a minute superior motion in response to this pressure.

Compare the amplitude and the ease of motion of the palatine under consideration, or the force needed to bring about motion.

13.3 Treatment of the palatine bones

The sphenoid and the maxilla not infrequently need to be corrected before treating the palatine.

13.3.1 General mobilization of the palatine bones

Practitioner: Beside the patient's head.

Hand position:

- Cranial hand: span the greater wings with your thumb and your middle or index finger.
- Caudal hand: place your index finger intraorally on the horizontal plate of the palatine, laterally to the median palatine suture. To position it exactly, slide the index finger along the medial side of the upper molars. Just behind the last molar, position the finger slightly medially on the hard palate (Figure 13.5).

Method:

- Cranial hand: establish the PBMT of the sphenoid. Hold the sphenoid in PBMT.
- Caudal hand
  - With your index finger, apply pressure in a superior direction (release from the maxilla).
  - Then, using your index finger, administer traction in a lateral direction (release from the opposite palatine).
  - Now administer gentle traction medially using your index finger.
- Finally, lower your index finger and administer a degree of traction in an inferior direction.
- At the end of the technique, the motion of the palatine bone should be re-synchronized with the motion of the sphenoid in harmony with the PRM rhythm.
- During the inhalation phase, go with the sphenoid and palatine into flexion and ER (greater wing of the sphenoid inferior, horizontal plate inferior).
- During the exhalation phase, go with the sphenoid and the palatine into extension and IR (greater wing of the sphenoid superior, horizontal plate superior).

CAUTION Proceed only very gently, especially in the case of a cranially directed impulse, as there is otherwise a risk of causing a restriction of the palatine bone.

Alternative hand position

Practitioner: At the head of the patient.

Hand position: Bilateral: position the index fingers of both hands intraorally one on either side, on the horizontal plates of the palatines laterally to the median palatine suture (Figure 13.6).

Method: As for the normal hand position, except that the sphenoid is not involved and the two palatines are mobilized simultaneously.

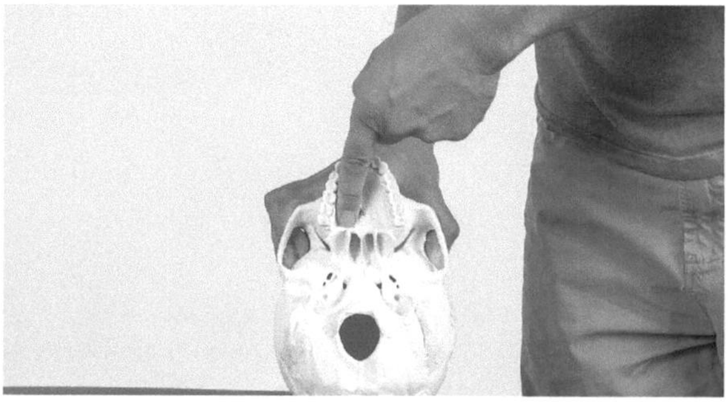

Figure 13.5 General mobilization of the palatine bone

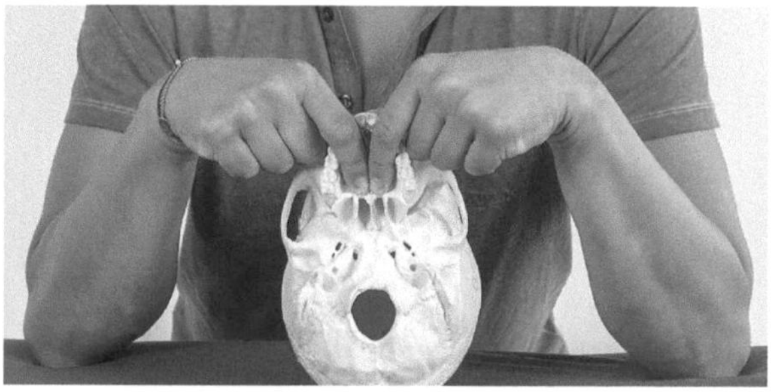

Figure 13.6 General mobilization of the palatine bone. Alternative hand position

13.3.2 Sutural dysfunctions

Sphenopalatine suture

Suture margin:

- The inferior lateral surface of the body of the sphenoid articulates with the sphenoid process of the palatine bone.
- The anterior inferior angle of the body of the sphenoid articulates with the orbital process of the palatine.
- The anterior margin of the medial plate of the pterygoid processes of the sphenoid articulates with the posterior margin of the palatine perpendicular plate.
- The pterygoid notch articulates with the pyramidal process of the palatine.

Suture type (all four joints)**:** Plane suture.

Indication: The technique releases in particular the pterygoid notch of the sphenoid from the pyramidal process of the palatine.

Patient: Supine.

Practitioner: Beside the patient's head, on the opposite side to the dysfunction.

Hand position:

- Cranial hand: span the greater wings with your thumb and your middle or index finger.
- Caudal hand: position the index finger intraorally on the horizontal plate of the palatine (at the height of the last molar) on the dysfunctional side.

Method:

- Disengagement (Figure 13.7)
  - ▸ Move the palatine anterolaterally, to release the pyramidal process from the pterygoid notch.
  - ▸ At the same time, guide the greater wings caudad (flexion).
- Establishing the PBMT
  - ▸ Maintain the disengagement, while at the same time establishing PBMT between the sphenoid and the palatine.
  - ▸ Follow the sphenoid in the direction of greater motion (in the motion axes of flexion/extension, torsion and sidebending-rotation, etc.).
  - ▸ Move it just far enough in these directions for the membrane tensions (between flexion and extension, torsion right and left, etc.) to be in the best possible balance.
  - ▸ Follow the palatine in the direction of greater motion (of ease).
  - ▸ Follow it just far enough in these directions for the tensions on the sphenopalatine suture to be in the best possible balance. This makes it possible for a new tension equilibrium to be established between palatine and sphenoid.
- Establish the PBFT.
- Maintain PBT until the abnormal tension has corrected itself and the inherent homeostatic forces (PRM rhythm, etc.) have established the correction.
- Breathing assistance: the patient can assist as follows: at the end of an in-breath, hold the inhalation for as long as possible, while performing a plantar flexing of both feet. Repeat for several breathing cycles.
- A fluid impulse may be used to direct energy from the opposite parietal tuber.

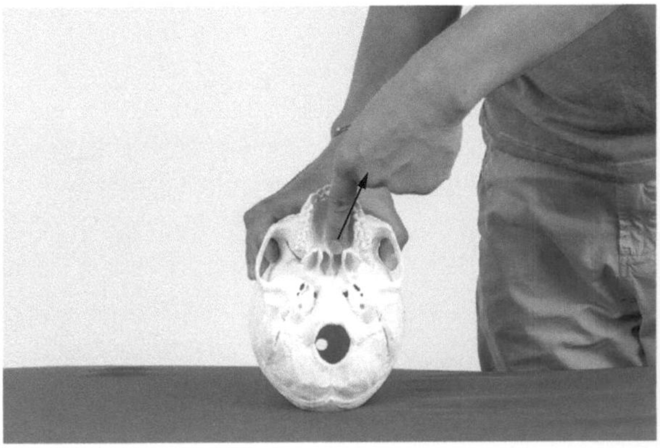

Figure 13.7 Sphenopalatine suture

Median palatine suture

Practitioner: Beside the patient's head.

Hand position:

- Cranial hand: span the greater wings with your thumb and your middle or index finger.
- Caudal hand: position your index and middle fingers intraorally one on either side, on the horizontal plates of the palatines.

Method:

- Disengagement
  - Hold the greater wings firmly in place in the neutral position.
  - Spread the index and middle fingers of your caudal hand to gently disengage the suture (Figure 13.8).
  - Without reducing the gentle disengagement, permit all motions/tissue unwinding of the palatine bones.
  - With each release of the tissues, seek the new limit of motion of the palatines laterally.
- Establishing the PBT
  - Maintain the disengagement while establishing PBMT between the sphenoid and the palatine—the position in which the abnormal tensions in the joints are in the best possible reciprocal balance—and PBFT. Maintain the PBT until the abnormal tension has corrected itself and the inherent homeostatic forces (PRM rhythm, etc.) have established the correction.
  - Breathing assistance: the patient can assist as follows: at the end of an in-breath, hold the inhalation for as long as possible, while performing a plantar flexing of both feet. Repeat for several breathing cycles.

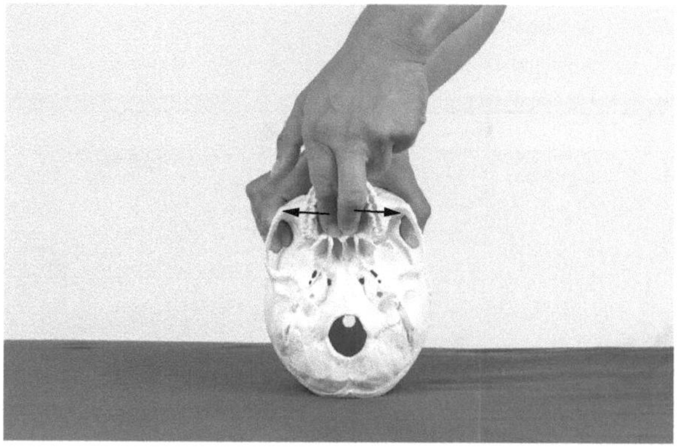

Figure 13.8 Median palatine suture

- A fluid impulse may be used to direct energy from the mid-line.
- At the end of the technique, the motion of the palatine should be re-synchronized with the motion of the sphenoid in harmony with the PRM rhythm.
- During the inhalation phase, go with the sphenoid and the palatines into flexion and ER; during the exhalation phase, go with the sphenoid and the palatines into extension and IR.

Transverse palatine suture and palatomaxillary suture

See this volume, section 12.4.6.

Technique for the cranial nerves

See technique for the pterygopalatine ganglion (Volume 2, section 7.6.2).

13.4 Reference

1 Sutherland, W. G. (1944) 'The cranial bowl.' *J. Am. Osteopath. Assoc. 1944*, 348–353.

14.1 The morphology of the zygomatic bone according to Rohen 432

14.2 Location, causes, and clinical presentation of dysfunctions of the zygomatic bone 432
14.2.1 Osseous dysfunctions 432
14.2.2 Muscular dysfunctions 433
14.2.3 Fascial dysfunctions 433

14.3 Diagnosis of the zygomatic bone 433
14.3.1 History-taking 433
14.3.2 Inspection 433
14.3.3 Palpation of position 433
14.3.4 Palpation of PRM rhythm 433
14.3.5 Motion testing 436

14.4 Treatment of the zygomatic bones 436
14.4.1 Rotation dysfunction 436
14.4.2 Decompression of the zygomatic bone 437
14.4.3 Sutural dysfunctions 437

14.5 References 439

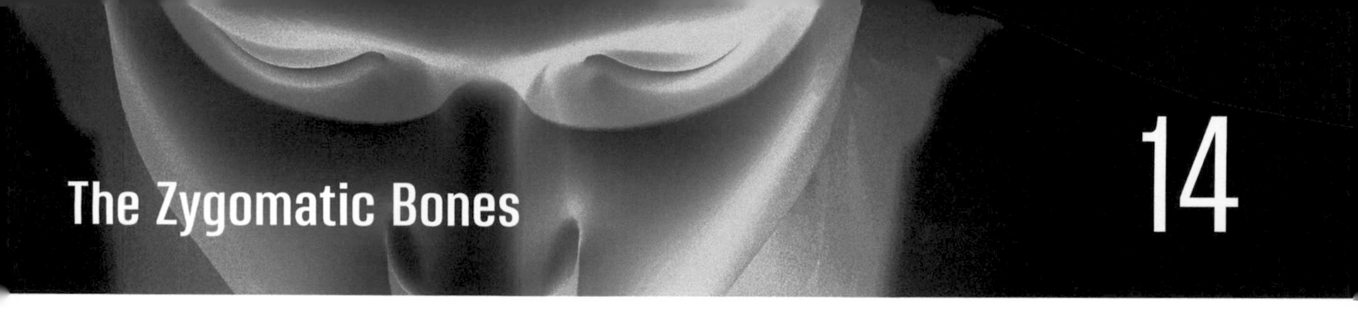

14 The Zygomatic Bones

This is a paired bone, four-cornered in shape. It contributes to the lateral wall of the orbit, and provides an important connection between the viscerocranium and neurocranium. According to Sutherland, like the palatine bone, it mediates between the sphenoid and maxilla and has the effect of a "speed reducer." Influences from the temporal bone are also received here. Frequently, the zygomatic bone is a place where abnormal tensions can be palpated.[2] The bone contributes importantly to the physiognomy of the face.

The zygomatic buttress runs from the molar sockets to the zygomatic bone, and masticatory forces are transmitted from the molar sockets through this, posteriorly to the inferior temporal lines of the frontal bone, anteriorly to the lateral part of the upper wall of the orbit, and along the zygomatic arch.

There are connections to the masticatory muscles and facial muscles. Branches of cranial nerve V_2 course through the region of the zygomatic bone.

14.1 The morphology of the zygomatic bone according to Rohen[1]

In its motion dynamics, the zygomatic bone corresponds to the clavicle. The relationship between the maxilla and the neurocranium, with interposition of the zygomatic bone, is analogous to the separation of the upper limb and thorax by the clavicle. By connecting the maxilla to the frontal and temporal bones, the zygoma links the expressivity of the three bones and thus plays a crucial role in physiognomic expression. It serves to integrate the viscerocranium and neurocranium or, to be more precise, the viscerocranium, roof of the skull, and cranial base. Binocular vision, the means by which we receive an accurate image of our environment, is possible only as a result of the evolutionary forward migration of the eyes; laterally, the zygomatic bone forms a border between the orbit and the temporal sinus.

14.2 Location, causes, and clinical presentation of dysfunctions of the zygomatic bone

> **Tip for practitioners**
>
> **Primary dysfunctions**
> - Intraosseous.
> - Traumatic injury: falls and blows to the zygomatic bone.
>
> **Secondary dysfunctions**
> - As a result of dysfunction of the frontal bone, temporal bone, and maxilla; less frequently due to dysfunction of the sphenoid, and the occipital bone.

14.2.1 Osseous dysfunctions

The zygomatic bone links the bones of the face to the temporal bone via the intermediary of the sphenoid and under the influence of the occipital bone. Its relationship with the four bones which surround it is thus one of integration and balance.

- **Sphenozygomatic suture** Causes: falling onto or a blow to the cheek, and SBS dysfunctions.
- **Temporozygomatic suture**
  - Causes: falling onto or a blow to the cheek, and SBS dysfunctions.
  - The sliding motion of the zygomatic and temporal processes at the temporozygomatic suture integrates the influences of the sphenoid and occipital bone. If the suture

is compressed, the mobility relative to the temporal bone is restricted.
    - Sequelae: impaired mobility of the temporal and zygomatic bones.
    - Restriction of the temporozygomatic suture could result in the zygomatic process of the temporal bone being unable to slide downward and outward with the temporal process of the zygomatic bone during the inhalation phase. This would restrict the temporal bone in internal rotation during the inhalation phase. Recall that the zygomatic bone is largely influenced by the sphenoid; the temporal bone is influenced by the occipital bone.
- **Frontozygomatic suture** Clinical presentation/hypothetical pathology: disturbance to the orbit, resulting in visual disturbances.
- **Zygomaticomaxillary suture**
    - Causes: fall or blow to the face.
    - Clinical presentation/hypothetical pathology: disturbance to the orbit, disturbance of the maxillary sinus, resulting in sinusitis.

14.2.2 Muscular dysfunctions

Masseter Sequelae: restriction of the mobility of the zygomatic bone.

14.2.3 Fascial dysfunctions

Masseteric fascia, temporal fascia

- Causes: tension in the anterior cervicocranial fasciae and dysfunction of visceral structures.
- Sequelae: restriction of the mobility of the zygomatic bone.

14.3 Diagnosis of the zygomatic bone

14.3.1 History-taking

- Fall onto or blow to the zygomatic bone.
- In rare cases, very frequent supporting of the head on the hand at the zygomatic bone can lead to a dysfunction.

14.3.2 Inspection

- Zygomatic bone: prominent (ER) or receding (IR).
- Orbital diameter: enlarged (ER) or reduced (IR).

14.3.3 Palpation of position

- Zygomatic bone: prominent (ER) or receding (IR).
- Eye margin: everted (ER) or inverted (IR).
- Temporozygomatic suture: downward, outward, and slightly anterior (ER), or upward, inward, and slightly posterior (IR).

14.3.4 Palpation of PRM rhythm

Tip for practitioners

Biomechanical, inhalation phase

An external rotation of the zygomatic bone occurs, around two axes: an oblique axis from posterior/outward to anterior/inward, and a vertical axis through the frontal process in a slightly oblique direction, running anterior, downward, and inward.

- The motion of the zygomatic bone is induced by the sphenoid via the greater wings. It is also dependent upon the movement of the frontal bone, maxilla, and temporal bone.
- The orbital surface moves anterior, outward, and slightly downward (influenced by the sphenoid).
- This results in enlargement of the orbit at the diameter running from an inner, upper position to an outer, lower position. The angle between zygomatic bone and frontal bone is also increased.
- The temporal process moves in an outward, downward, and slightly anterior direction, while the zygomatic process of the temporal bone moves outward, downward, and slightly posterior. The sliding motion of the two processes at the temporozygomatic suture integrates the influences of sphenoid and occipital bone.

Developmental dynamic, inhalation phase

- The expansive force is in an anterior, inferior direction.

If palpation reveals a restriction, the practitioner may induce an impulse in the direction of the restriction. This will emphasize the restriction, making it easier to sense from which structure it originates.

Practitioner: Take up a position at the head of the patient.

Hand position:

- Your two thumbs should touch one another and create a fulcrum.
- Position the index fingers, middle fingers, and ring fingers of your two hands each side, on the zygomatic bones. Place your index fingers on the maxillary processes, your middle fingers on the lower margins, and your ring fingers on the posterior margins of the zygomatic bones (Figure 14.1).

Alternative hand position:

- Place your thumbs anterior on the two frontal processes of the zygomatic bones (on the orbital margins).
- Place your index fingers on the posteroinferior margins of the two zygomatic bones.
- Position your middle fingers posterior on the frontal processes of the two zygomatic bones (on the posterosuperior margins; Figures 14.2 and 14.3).

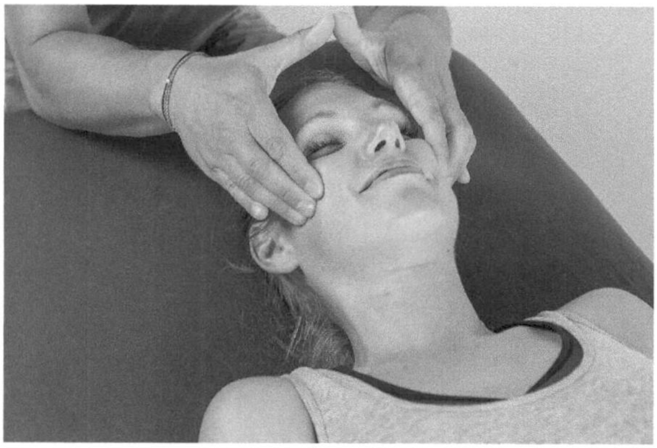

Figure 14.1 Palpation of PRM rhythm of the zygomatic bones

Biomechanical approach:
Inhalation phase of PRM, normal finding: external rotation (Figure 14.4)

- The maxillary process moves in a lateral, anterior, and slightly superior direction.
- The frontal process moves anterolaterally.
- The posteroinferior margin moves inferiorly and medially.

Exhalation phase of PRM, normal finding: internal rotation

- The maxillary process moves in a medial, posterior, and slightly inferior direction.
- The frontal process moves posteriorly and medially.
- The posteroinferior margin moves superiorly and laterally.

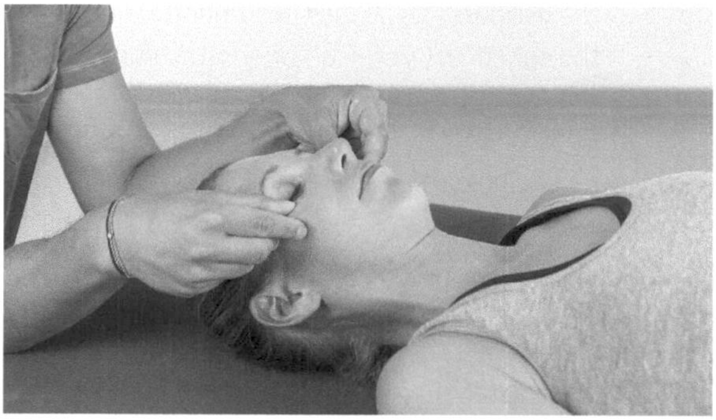

Figure 14.2 Palpation of PRM rhythm of the zygomatic bones. Alternative hand position

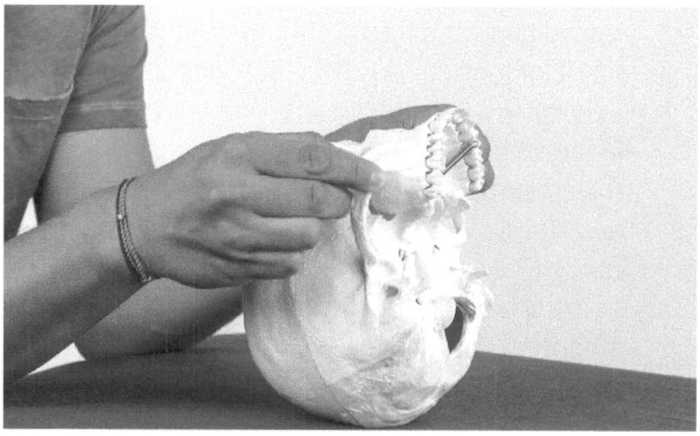

Figure 14.3 Palpation of PRM rhythm of the zygomatic bones. Alternative hand position (shown on model)

Developmental dynamic approach:
Inhalation phase of PRM, normal finding (Figure 14.5):

- The zygomatic bone and maxilla move in an anterior, inferior direction.

Exhalation phase of PRM, normal finding:

- The zygomatic bone and the maxilla move in a posterior, superior direction.

Compare the amplitude, strength, ease, and symmetry of the motion of the zygomatic bone. Other types of zygomatic bone motion may sometimes occur during external and internal rotation. These provide an indication as to further dysfunctions of the particular zygomatic bone involved. Zygomatic bone dysfunctions may be unilateral or bilateral, symmetrical or asymmetrical.

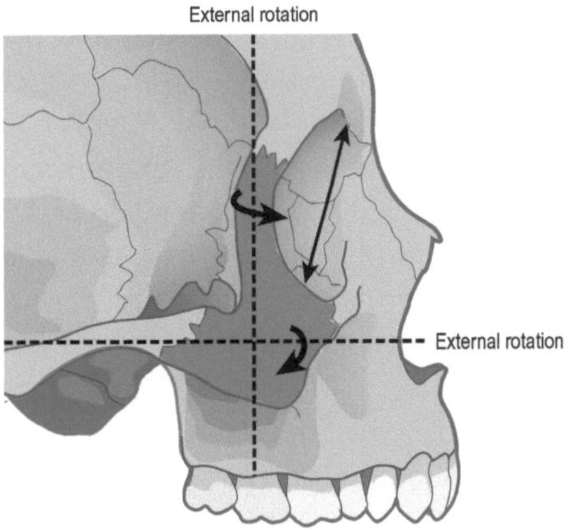

Figure 14.4 PRM inhalation phase/biomechanical approach

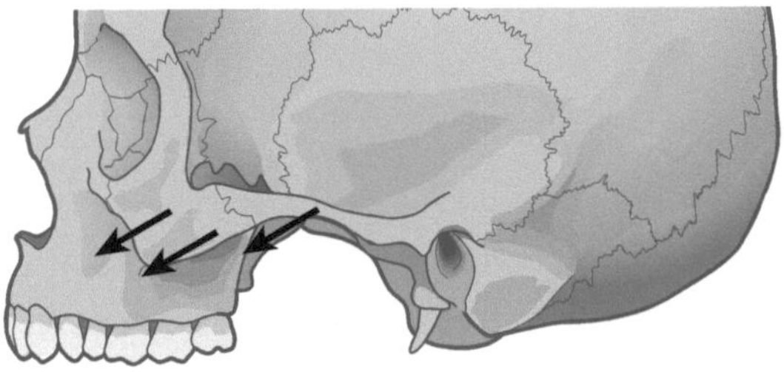

Figure 14.5 PRM inhalation phase/developmental dynamic approach

Alternative hand position, unilateral

Practitioner: Take up a position at the head of the patient on the side to be tested.

Hand position:

- Cranial hand: span the greater wings with your thumb and your middle or index finger.
- Caudal hand: position your index finger intraorally on the inner surface of the zygomatic bone. Place your thumb on the outer surface of the zygomatic bone (Figure 14.6).

Method: With your cranial hand, passively follow the motion of the SBS into extension and flexion. With your caudal hand, sense whether the zygomatic bone moves in harmony with the motion of the SBS.

Inhalation phase, normal finding: external rotation

- The maxillary process moves in an anterolateral and slightly superior direction.
- The frontal process moves anterolaterally.

Exhalation phase, normal finding: internal rotation

- The maxillary process moves in a medial, posterior, and slightly inferior direction.
- The frontal process moves in a posterior and medial direction.

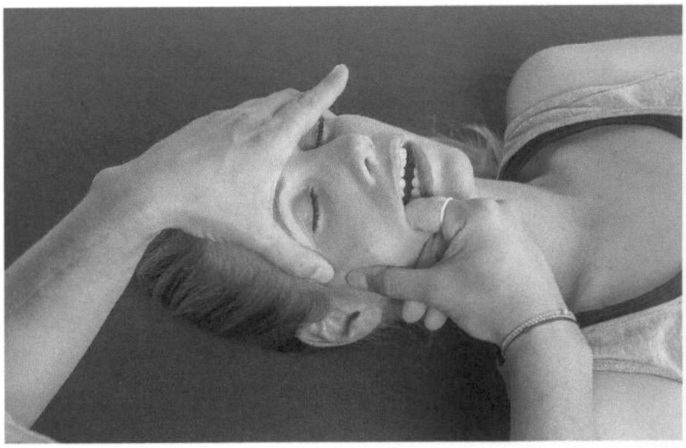

Figure 14.6 Palpation of PRM rhythm of the zygomatic bones. Alternative hand position, unilateral

14.3.5 Motion testing

Hand position:
See palpation of PRM rhythm above (section 14.3.4).

Method: Testing of external rotation and internal rotation.

During the inhalation phase:
- On the frontal processes and maxillary processes, direct an impulse in an anterolateral direction.
- On the inferior margin of the zygomatic bone, direct an impulse medially and superior.

During the exhalation phase:
- On the frontal processes and maxillary processes, direct an impulse medially and posterior.
- On the inferior margin of the zygomatic bone, direct an impulse laterally and inferior.

Compare the amplitude and the ease of motion, or the force needed to bring about motion at the zygomatic bones.

14.4 Treatment of the zygomatic bones

14.4.1 Rotation dysfunction

Practitioner: Take up a position at the head of the patient, somewhat over to the side of the dysfunction.

Hand position:
- Hand on the frontal bone: span the frontal bone with your thumb and middle finger (and/or index finger), by hooking them firmly around the outside of the zygomatic processes of the frontal bone.
- Hand on the zygomatic bone on the dysfunctional side: position your index finger on the orbital margin. Place your middle finger on the posteroinferior margin of the zygomatic bone (Figure 14.7).

Alternative hand position:
- Hand on the frontal bone: span the frontal bone with your thumb and middle finger (and/or index finger), by hooking them firmly around the outside of the zygomatic processes of the frontal bone.
- Hand on the zygomatic bone on the dysfunctional side: position your index finger intraorally on the inferior margin of the zygomatic bone. Place your thumb externally, on the zygomatic bone. Grasp the zygomatic bone with your two fingers (Figure 14.8).

Method:
- Establishing the PBMT
  - ▸ With the hand that is on the frontal bone, passively follow the motion of the frontal bone into extension and flexion.

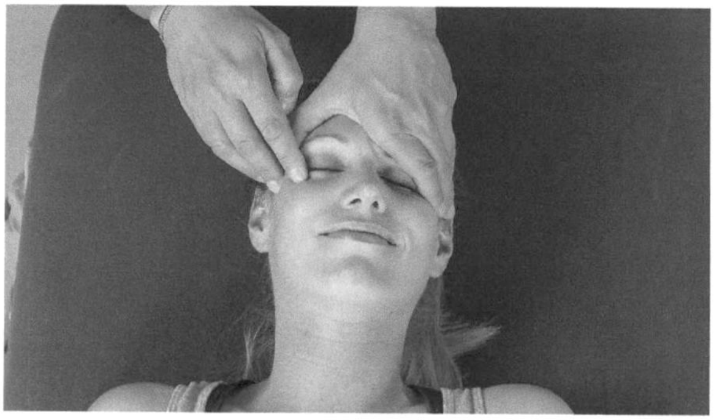

Figure 14.7 Rotation dysfunction

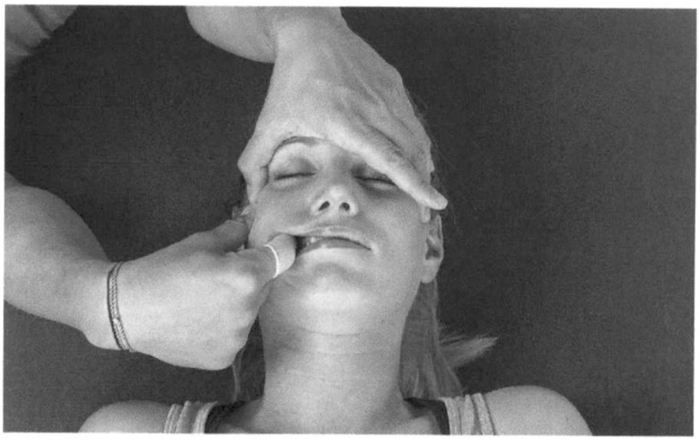

Figure 14.8 Rotation dysfunction. Alternative hand position

- ▸ During the inhalation phase, follow the ER of the zygomatic bone. The index finger on the frontal process and maxillary process follows laterally and anteriorly. The middle finger on the lower margin follows inferiorly and medially.
- ▸ During the exhalation phase, follow the IR of the zygomatic bone. The index finger on the maxillary process follows in a medial, posterior, and slightly inferior direction. The middle finger on the frontal process follows posteriorly and medially.
- ▸ The PBMT is the position between ER and IR in which the abnormal tensions on the joints are in the best possible reciprocal balance.

- Establish PBFT.
- Maintain the PBT until a correction of the abnormal tension has been achieved and the inherent homeostatic forces (PRM rhythm, etc.) have established the correction.
- At the end of the technique, the motion of the zygomatic bone should be re-synchronized with the sphenoid motion in harmony with the PRM rhythm.
- During the inhalation phase, go with the sphenoid and the palatine bones into flexion and ER; during the exhalation phase, go with the sphenoid and the palatine bones into extension and IR.

Vitalist approach: See EV-4 technique (this volume, section 4.4.3).

14.4.2 Decompression of the zygomatic bone

Practitioner: Take up a position beside the patient's head, on the same side as the dysfunction.

Hand position:

- Cranial hand: span the frontal bone with your thumb and ring finger. Also position your thumb on the greater wing on the affected side, and your index finger on the frontal process of the maxilla on the affected side.

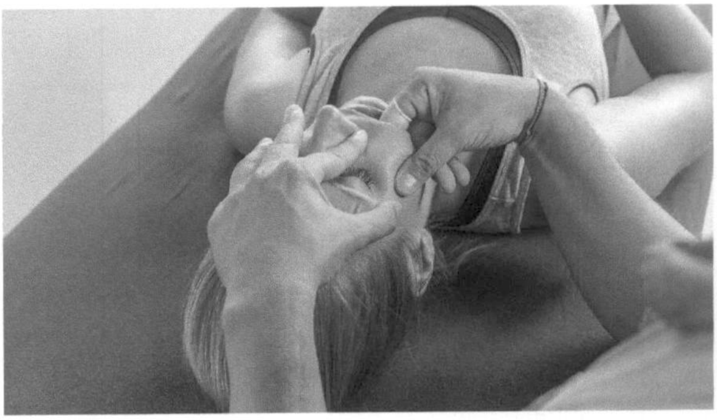

Figure 14.9 Decompression of the zygomatic bone

- Caudal hand: place your index finger intraorally, on the lower margin of the zygomatic bone. Place your thumb externally, on the zygomatic bone. Grasp the zygomatic bone with your two fingers.

Method:

- Hold the frontal bone and sphenoid and the maxilla firmly in the neutral position. While doing this, administer laterally directed traction on the zygomatic bone (Figure 14.9).
- Without reducing the traction, permit all motions/tissue unwinding.
- Establish PBMT, PBFT.

14.4.3 Sutural dysfunctions

Sphenozygomatic suture

Suture margin: The anterior-directed process of the zygomatic bone articulates with the anterior border of the greater wing.

Suture type: Serrate suture.

Practitioner: Take up a position beside the patient's head, on the opposite side to the dysfunction.

Hand position:

- Cranial hand: span the greater wings with your thumb and middle finger. Place your index finger on the zygomatic process of the frontal bone.

- Caudal hand: grasp the frontal process of the zygomatic bone with your thumb and index finger.

Method:
- Disengagement
  - ▸ Cranial hand: hold the sphenoid firmly in the neutral position. Similarly, hold the affected side of the zygomatic process of the frontal bone in position with your index fingers.
  - ▸ Caudal hand: at the same time, administer traction on the zygomatic bone caudad with your thumb and index finger (Figure 14.10).
  - ▸ Without reducing the traction, permit all motions/tissue unwinding.
- Direct technique
  - ▸ A dysfunction in ER is treated by going with the sphenoid into the extension position during the exhalation phase and holding it there.
  - ▸ A dysfunction in IR is treated by going with the sphenoid into flexion during the inhalation phase and holding it there.
- Establishing the PBT
  - ▸ Maintain the gentle disengagement while you establish PBMT of the zygomatic bone—the position between ER and IR in which the abnormal tensions on the joints are in the best possible reciprocal balance—and PBFT.
  - ▸ Maintain the PBT until a correction of the abnormal tension has been achieved and the inherent homeostatic forces (PRM rhythm, etc.) have established the correction.
- At the end of the technique, the motion of the zygomatic bone and of the sphenoid and frontal bones should be synchronized, in harmony with the PRM rhythm.
- During the inhalation phase, go with the zygomatic bones, sphenoid, and frontal bone into flexion and external rotation; in the exhalation phase, go with the bones into extension and internal rotation.
- A fluid impulse may be used to direct energy from the opposite lambdoid suture or caudad of it.

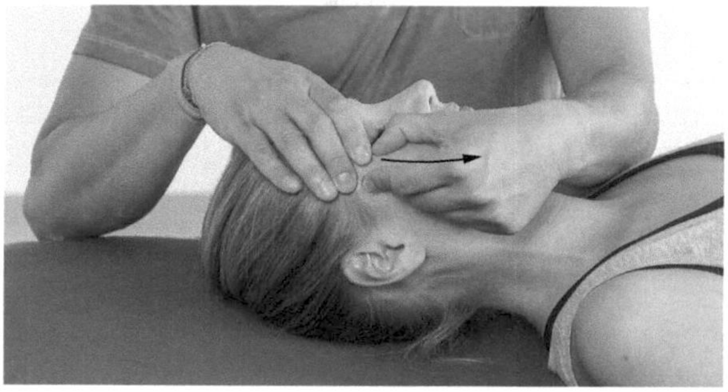

Figure 14.10 Sphenozygomatic suture

Tip for practitioners

An exaggeration technique may be indicated, rather than a direct technique. For a dysfunction in external rotation, go with the sphenoid into flexion during the inhalation phase and hold it there. In the case of a dysfunction in internal rotation, go with the sphenoid into extension during the exhalation phase and hold it there.

Alternative hand position

Patient: The patient's head is turned toward the opposite side from the dysfunction.

Practitioner: Take up a position beside the patient's head, on the same side as the dysfunction.

Alternative hand position:
- Cranial hand: span the greater wings with your thumb and middle finger.
- Caudal hand: grasp the zygomatic bone, by placing your thumb externally on the zygomatic bone, and your index finger on the zygomatic bone from inside (intraorally) (Figure 14.6).

Temporozygomatic suture

Suture margin: The posterior-directed temporal process of the zygomatic bone articulates with the zygomatic process of the temporal bone.

Suture type: Serrate suture.

Patient: The patient's head is turned toward the opposite side from the dysfunction.

Practitioner: Take up a position beside the patient's head, on the opposite side from the dysfunction.

Hand position:

- Cranial hand on the temporal bone
  - Grasp the zygomatic process with your thumb and index finger.
  - Position your middle finger in the external acoustic meatus.
  - Place your ring finger on the mastoid process.
  - Place your little finger on the mastoid part.
- Caudal hand on the zygomatic bone: grasp the temporal process of the zygomatic bone with your index finger and thumb.

Method:

- Disengagement
  - Administer traction posterior with the index finger and thumb that are on the temporal bone.
  - Administer traction anterior with the index finger and thumb that are on the zygomatic bone (Figure 14.11).
  - Permit all motions/tissue unwinding that occur.
  - Maintain this position until you sense a release of tension at the suture.
- Direct technique: hold the zygomatic bone gently in position. During the inhalation phase, go with the temporal bone into an external rotation and hold it there.
- Establish the PBMT, PBFT.
- At the end of the technique, the motion of the zygomatic bone should be re-synchronized with that of the temporal bone in harmony with the PRM rhythm.
- During the inhalation phase, go with the temporal bone and zygomatic bone into ER; during the exhalation phase, go with the temporal bone and zygomatic bone into IR.
- A fluid impulse may be used to direct energy from the opposite lambdoid suture or caudad to it.

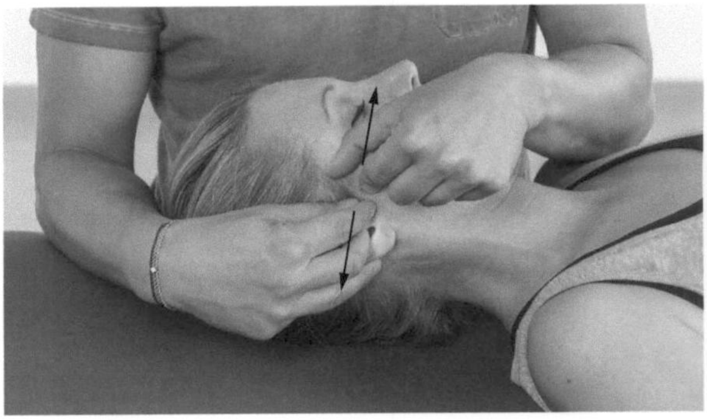

Figure 14.11 Temporozygomatic suture

Frontozygomatic suture

See this volume, section 10.4.5.

Indication: Disturbances of the orbits and visual disturbances.

Zygomaticomaxillary suture

See this volume, section 12.4.6.

Indication: Disturbances of the orbits and disturbances of the maxillary sinus with sinusitis.

14.5 References

1 Rohen, J. W. (2002) *Morphologie des menschlichen Organismus*, 2nd Ed. Stuttgart: Verlag Freies Geistesleben, p. 367.

2 Sutherland, W. G. (1944) 'The cranial bowl.' *J. Am. Osteopath. Assoc. 1944*, 348–353.

15.1 The nasal bones 442
15.1.1 Causes of dysfunctions 442
15.1.2 Diagnosis 442
15.1.3 Treatment of the nasal bones 443

15.2 Lacrimal bones 445
15.2.1 Causes of dysfunctions of the lacrimal bones 445
15.2.2 Diagnosis 445
15.2.3 Treatment of the lacrimal bones 446

15.3 Inferior nasal concha 448

Nasal Bones, Lacrimal Bones, Inferior Nasal Concha

15

The paired nasal bone has contact with the frontal bone, maxilla, and ethmoid bone. The paired lacrimal bone contributes to the medial wall of the orbit and lateral nasal wall. The inferior nasal concha is a plate of bone, concave on the medial side; it provides the inferior continuation of the nasolacrimal canal.

15.1 The nasal bones

15.1.1 Causes of dysfunctions

Tip for practitioners

Primary dysfunctions The primary cause as a rule is traumatic injury due to blows, falls, or a too tightly fitting spectacle frame.

Secondary dysfunction Due to dysfunction of the maxilla and of the frontal bone.

15.1.2 Diagnosis

History-taking

- Disturbance of nasal secretion and nasal breathing.
- Previous traumatic injuries.

Inspection and palpation of position

- Asymmetric nasal bones.
- Nasal bone cranial sutures tender to pressure.

Palpation of PRM rhythm

The nasal bone moves around a vertical axis. It is influenced by the frontal bone and maxilla. In the inhalation phase, it rotates slightly outward relative to the frontal process of the maxilla. The internasal suture moves posteriorly.

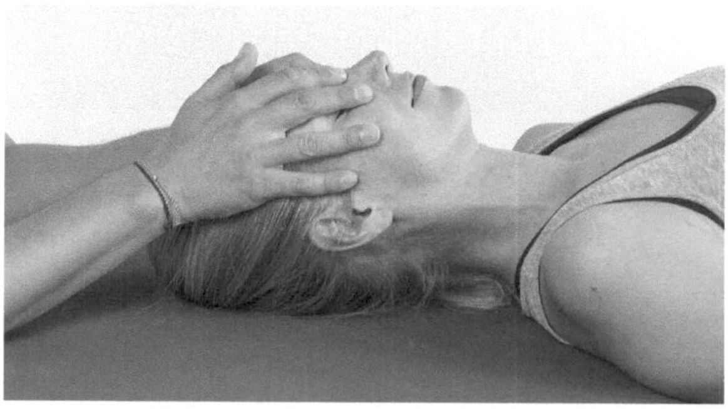

Figure 15.1 Palpation of PRM rhythm of the nasal bones

Practitioner: Take up a position at the head of the patient.

Hand position: Position your index fingers on both sides of the nose, one on each nasal bone. Rest the other fingers passively on the cranium (Figure 15.1).

Alternative hand position: The practitioner should take up a position beside the patient's head:

- Cranial hand: place your cranial hand on the frontal bone with your middle finger on the metopic suture, immediately above the frontonasal suture. Your index and ring fingers lie next to the middle finger.
- Caudal hand: place your thumb and index finger one on either side, on the nasal bones (Figure 15.3).

Biomechanical approach

Inhalation phase, normal finding: external rotation

- The internasal suture moves posterior (Figure 15.2).

Exhalation phase of the PR, normal finding: internal rotation

- The internasal suture moves anterior.

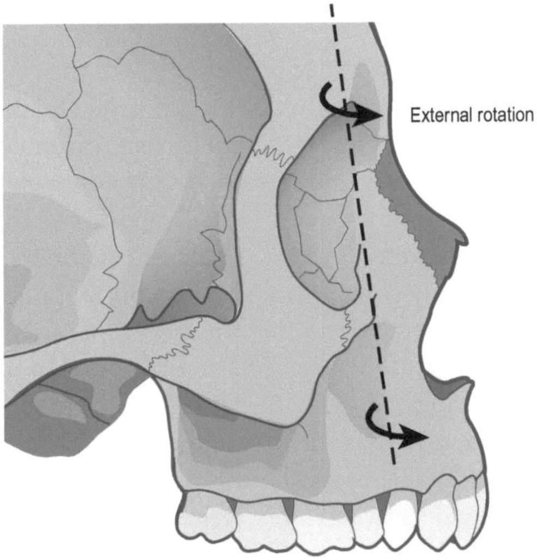

Figure 15.2
Inhalation phase of PRM/biomechanical

Compare the amplitude, strength, ease, and symmetry of the motion of the nasal bones.

Other types of motion of the nasal bones may sometimes occur during external and internal rotation. These provide an indication as to further dysfunctions of the particular nasal bone involved.

Nasal bone dysfunctions may be unilateral or bilateral, symmetrical or asymmetrical.

Motion testing

This differs from palpation of PRM rhythm in one feature only: external and internal rotation of the nasal bone are now actively induced by the practitioner in harmony with the PRM rhythm. Compare the amplitude and the ease of motion of the nasal bone under consideration, or the force needed to bring about motion.

15.1.3 Treatment of the nasal bones

When treating a nasal bone, it is usually necessary to treat the maxilla and frontal bone also.

Global technique to treat the nasal bones

Practitioner: Take up a position beside the patient's head.

Hand position:

- Cranial hand: place your cranial hand on the frontal bone with your middle finger on the metopic suture, immediately above the frontonasal suture. Place your index finger and ring finger next to the middle finger.
- Caudal hand: place your thumb and index finger one on each nasal bone (Figure 15.3).

Method:

- Register the cranial motions of the frontal bone with your hand resting passively on the frontal bone.
- During the inhalation phase, deliver an impulse into ER with the thumb and index finger that are on the nasal bones.
- During the exhalation phase, deliver an impulse into IR with the thumb and index finger that are on the nasal bones.

Vitalist approach: See EV-4 technique (this volume, section 4.4.3).

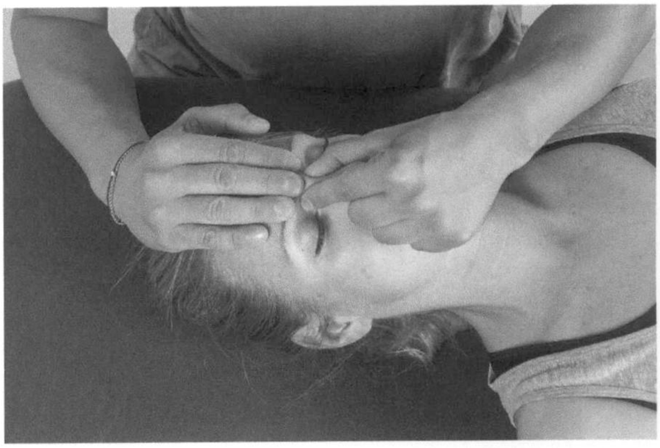

Figure 15.3 Global technique to treat the nasal bones

Technique for the frontonasal suture

Suture margin: The superior border of the nasal bone articulates with the medial portion of the nasal part of the frontal bone (serrate suture). The bony ridge of the nasal bone (nasal crest) articulates with the medial pointed projection (nasal spine) of the frontal bone (plane suture).

Practitioner: Take up a position beside the patient's head.

Hand position:

- Cranial hand: place your cranial hand on the frontal bone. Position your index and middle fingers immediately above the frontonasal suture.
- Caudal hand: place your thumb and index finger, one on each nasal bone (Figure 15.4).

Alternative position of the cranial hand I: Grasp the frontal bone at the zygomatic processes with your thumb and index finger. The basal joint of your index finger rests on glabella (Figure 15.5).

Alternative position of the cranial hand II, according to Magoun: Position your middle finger on the glabella. Place your index and ring fingers alongside the metopic suture (Figure 15.6).

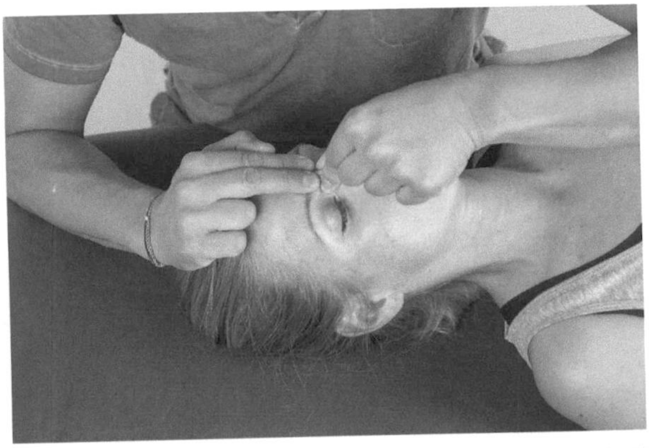

Figure 15.4 Technique for the frontonasal suture

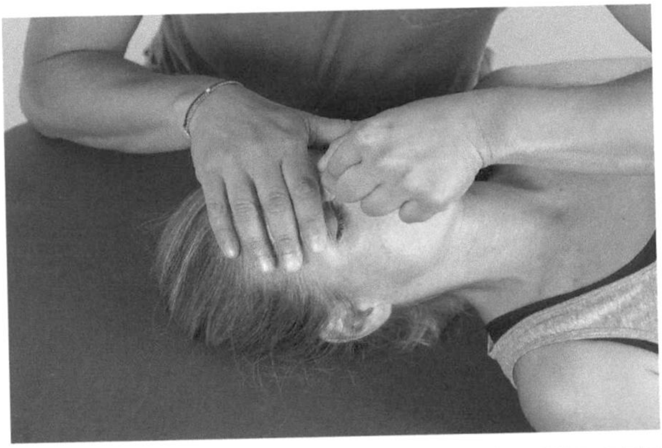

Figure 15.5 Technique for the frontonasal suture. Alternative hand position

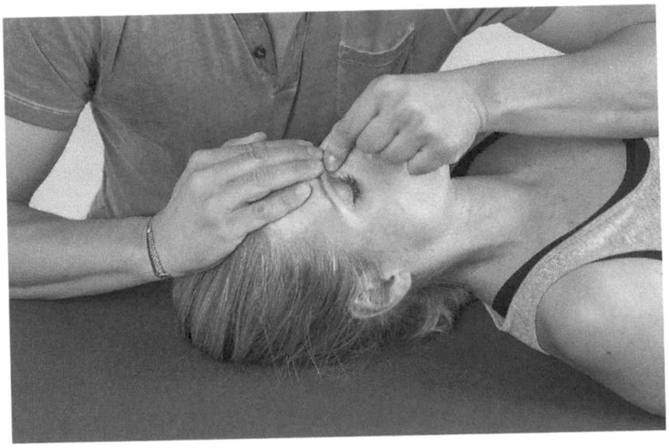

Figure 15.6 Frontonasal suture. Magoun's alternative hand position

Method: Disengagement

- Administer gentle traction cephalad on the frontal bone.
- At the same time administer traction caudad on the nasal bones.
- Permit all motions/tissue unwinding that occur.

Technique for the nasomaxillary suture

See also maxilla lift and spread technique, this volume, section 12.4.1 and section 12.4.6.

Technique for the internasal suture

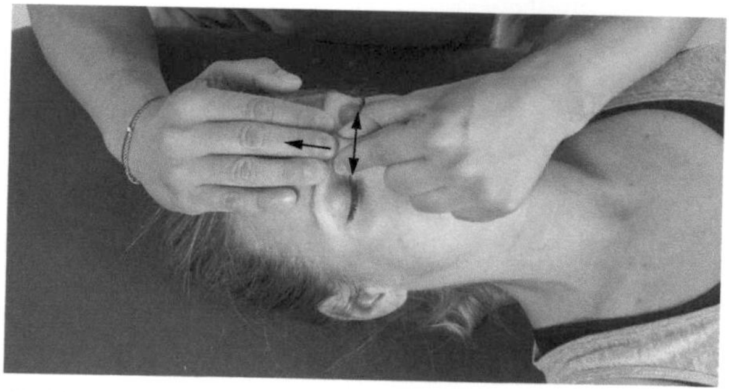

Figure 15.7 Technique for the internasal suture

Practitioner: Take up a position beside the patient's head.

Hand position:

- Cranial hand: place your cranial hand on the frontal bone with your middle finger on the metopic suture, immediately above the frontonasal suture. Your index and ring fingers lie next to the middle finger.
- Caudal hand: place your thumb and index finger one on each nasal bone.

Method: Disengagement

- Administer gentle traction cephalad on the frontal bone (Figure 15.7).
- Maintain this traction while spreading the nasal bones away from one another.
- Permit all motions/tissue unwinding that occur.

15.2 Lacrimal bones

The lacrimal is a paired bone. It forms part of the medial wall of the orbit and lateral nasal wall.

15.2.1 Causes of dysfunctions of the lacrimal bones

Tip for practitioners

Primary dysfunctions: Traumatic injury due to blows or falling.

Secondary dysfunction: Due to dysfunction of the maxilla, frontal bone, or ethmoid.

15.2.2 Diagnosis

History-taking

- Disturbance of lacrimation (nasolacrimal duct).
- Possibly also disturbances of motion at the orbit, or disturbances of the ethmoidal cells.

Palpation of PRM rhythm

Tip for practitioners

Biomechanical approach, inhalation phase:
The lacrimal bone is influenced by the maxilla, frontal bone, and ethmoid and, via these bones, by the sphenoid.

- During the inhalation phase it rotates slightly outward relative to the frontal process of the maxilla.
- The nasolacrimal duct enlarges.

Developmental dynamic, inhalation phase:

- Rotation of the lacrimal bone, during which its inferior portion moves in a lateral direction.

Practitioner: Take up a position beside the patient's head on the side to be tested.

Hand position: Place your cranial hand on the frontal bone. Place the index finger of your caudal hand on the lacrimal bone (Figure 15.8).

Biomechanical:

Inhalation phase, normal finding: external rotation

- The lateral margins move anterolaterally (Figure 15.9).

Exhalation phase, normal finding: internal rotation

- The lateral margins move in a posterior and medial direction.

Developmental dynamic:
Inhalation phase, normal finding:

- Rotation of the lacrimal bone, during which its inferior portion moves in a lateral direction (Figure 15.10).

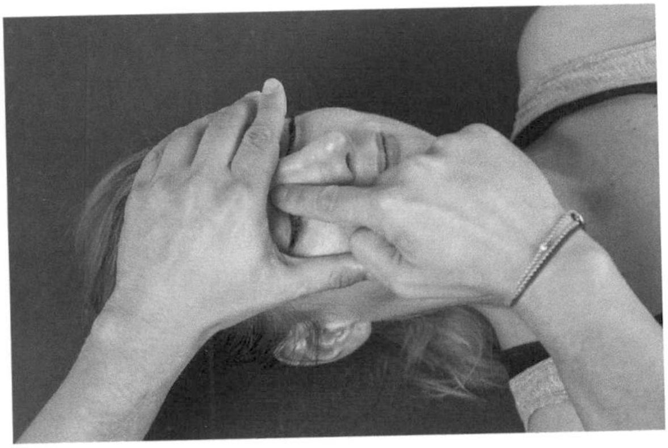

Figure 15.8 Palpation of PRM rhythm of the lacrimal bones

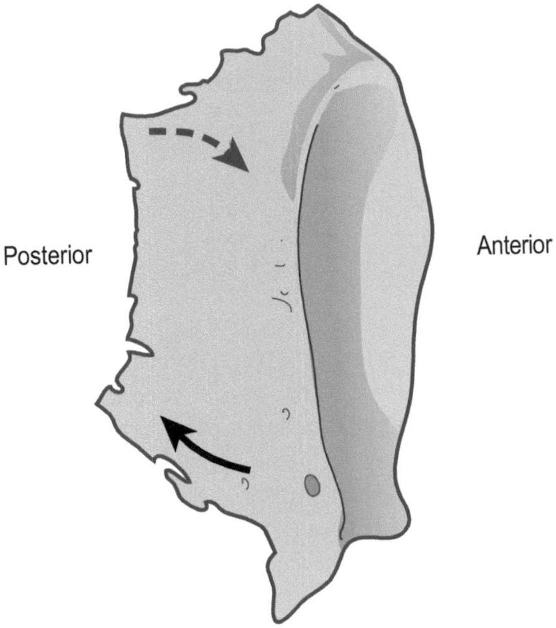

Figure 15.10 Inhalation phase of PRM/developmental dynamic approach

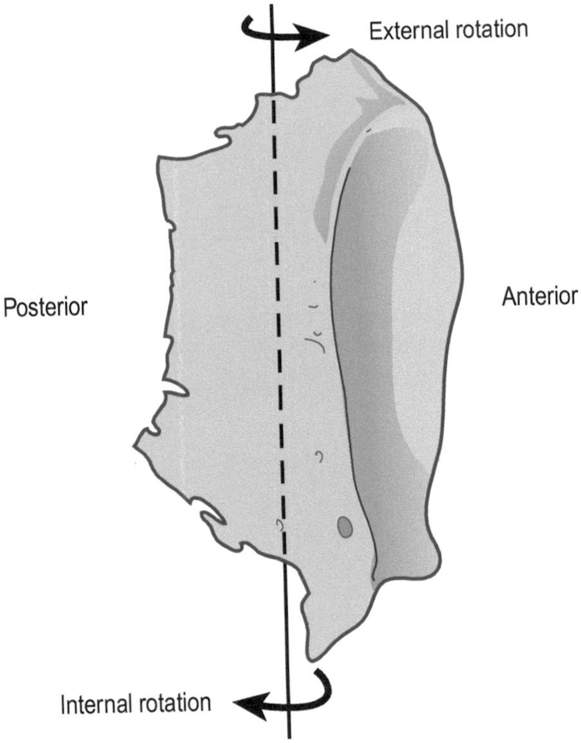

Figure 15.9 Inhalation phase of PRM/biomechanical approach

Exhalation phase, normal finding:

- Rotation of the lacrimal bone, during which its inferior portion moves in a medial direction.

Motion test

This differs from palpation of PRM rhythm only in one feature: the external and internal rotation of the lacrimal bone are now actively induced by the practitioner in harmony with PRM rhythm.

15.2.3 Treatment of the lacrimal bones

When treating a lacrimal bone it is usually necessary to treat the maxilla and the frontal bone also.

Global technique to treat the lacrimal bones

Practitioner: Take up a position beside the patient's head, on the side of the dysfunction.

Hand position:

- Place your cranial hand across the frontal bone. Position the index and middle fingers of your cranial hand on the upper orbital margins, as close as possible to the frontolacrimal suture.
- Place the index finger of your caudal hand on the lacrimal bone (Figure 15.11).

Method:

- Register the cranial motion of the frontal bone with your hand resting passively on it.
- During the inhalation phase, with your index finger, direct an impulse into ER on the lacrimal bone.
- During the exhalation phase, with your index finger, direct an impulse into IR on the lacrimal bone.

Alternative method: During the inhalation phase, with your index and middle fingers, begin to tilt the frontal bone (flexion), while applying pressure on the glabella in a posterior and superior direction with the basal joint of your index finger (ER). Hold the frontal bone in flexion and ER, while directing impulses into ER and IR of the lacrimal bone in harmony with the PRM rhythm.

Vitalist approach: See EV-4 technique (this volume, section 4.4.3).

Technique for the frontolacrimal suture

Suture margin: The upper part of the lacrimal bone articulates with the anterior quadrant of the ethmoidal notch.

Suture type: Squamous suture.

Hand position: See global technique for the lacrimal bones (above).

Method:

- Disengagement
  - ► During the inhalation phase, with your index and middle fingers, begin to tilt the frontal bone (flexion), while applying pressure on the glabella in a posterior and superior direction with the basal joint of your index finger (ER; Figure 15.12).
  - ► Hold the frontal bone in flexion and ER.
  - ► At the same time move the lacrimal bone caudad.
  - ► Permit all motions/tissue unwinding of the lacrimal bone that occur.
  - ► With each release of the suture, seek the new limit of motion of the frontal bone in the direction of external rotation and flexion.
- Establish PBMT and PBFT.
- A fluid impulse may be used to direct energy from the occipital bone.

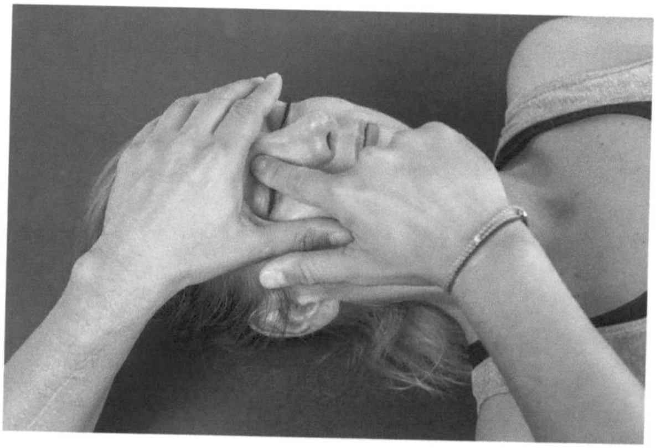

Figure 15.11 Global technique to treat the lacrimal bones

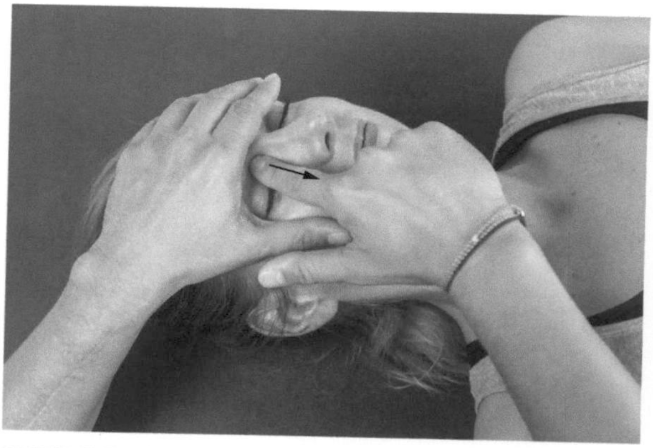

Figure 15.12 Technique for the frontolacrimal suture

Ethmoidolacrimal and lacrimomaxillary sutures

See maxilla lift and spread technique, this volume, sections 7.4.5 and 12.4.1.

15.3 Inferior nasal concha

The inferior nasal concha is a plate of bone, concave on the medial side; it provides the inferior continuation of the nasolacrimal canal.

Tip for practitioners

Primary dysfunctions Traumatic injury due to blows, surgery to the nose.

Secondary dysfunction Due to dysfunction of the maxilla, palatine bone, and ethmoid bone, deviation of the nasal septum.

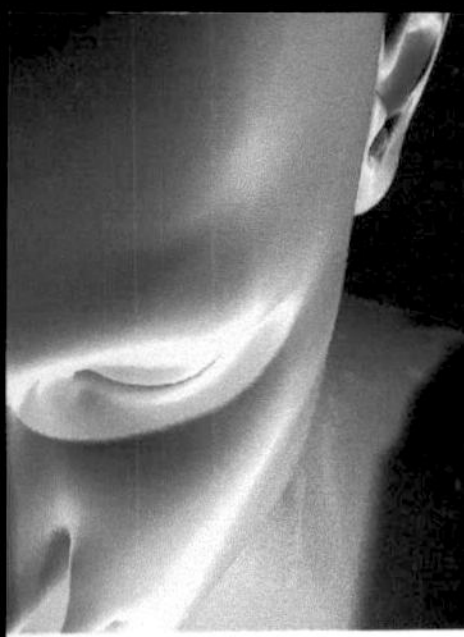

GLOSSARY

A number of important concepts of cranial osteopathy are explained here. These explanations look back in large part to the original writings of W. G. Sutherland and the first edition of Magoun's *Osteopathy in the Cranial Field* (1951), on which Sutherland collaborated and which he approved. seen from the modern perspective, matters have changed, yet it is helpful to present his understanding if we are to comprehend the origins and significance of his approach; indeed, the roots of cranial osteopathy. It may be that some of his chosen terminology is based on palpatory experience and was used to clarify certain palpatory approaches to his students. It is also helpful to know about the original concepts and their importance to create understanding in the cranial field of osteopathy and to understand its ongoing development.

"Automatic shifting suspension fulcrum"

Sutherland chose this term to describe a functional area on the course of the straight sinus, where the falx cerebri, falx cerebelli, and tentorium cerebelli unite. It is also called Sutherland's fulcrum. It is a movable point of rest for the reciprocal tension membrane in the cranium and spinal canal. In order to ensure the balance of membranous motion and tension equally in all directions, the membranes need to operate from a fulcrum, a point of rest. If this fulcrum is to shift automatically, it must be in "suspension" so that any pressure or pull can be evenly distributed in the dural membranes.

Sutherland writes that the changing position of the automatic shifting suspension fulcrum can be palpated at the beginning of respiration, and that a sense of warmth arises from the fluctuation of the CSF.[12:215,15:285]

Balance/Equilibrium

The normal state of acting and reacting between different parts within the body.[14:245]

Sutherland writes that the movements of the tide or fluctuation in their entirety derive from a "balance" between two points on a given scale, a point where the mechanism is motionless, exactly at the "neutral point."[13]

Balance point

See Point of balance.

"Be still and know"

Sutherland often used this biblical quotation (from Psalm 46:10) to make clear the significance of a particular attitude of consciousness during palpation, and also to indicate a particular fulcrum/point of balance between inspiration and expiration (inhalation and exhalation) of the PRM in the fluctuation of the fluids.[14:16,285]

Bent twigs

An expression frequently used by Sutherland, referring to the saying "as the twig is bent, so doth the tree incline." It is intended to show how the slightest tensions in the cranium or spine of a newborn or young child can develop into visible asymmetries as the structures increase in size with the progressive growth of the child.[14:286]

Biodynamics

This concept is particularly used by the osteopath J. Jealous. Inherent self-regulatory and self-correcting forces are employed to achieve correction. These forces possess intelligence, the capacity for decision, and goal-direction. See "Breath of Life" and "potency." Examination: this is mainly carried out by passive sensing. Correction: the "Breath of Life" performs and directs the correction.[4]

Biomechanics

Sutherland's theories 1936–1948. The SBS was seen as the primary location of dysfunctions. Mechanical approach: bones, sutures, membranes, and axes of motion (sutural; membranous). Definition of the five structures of the PRM: motility (inherent motion) of the brain and spinal cord, fluctuation of the cerebrospinal fluid (CSF), mobility of the intracranial and intraspinal membranes, mobility of the cranial bones, and involuntary mobility of the sacrum between the pelvic bones. Examination: mainly by active motion testing, but also by passive sensing. Correction: mechanical; the practitioner performs the correction. Inherent self-regulating forces were hardly mentioned or defined. No use of "potency" or the "Breath of Life."

"Breath of Life"

The Breath of Life is described as the fluid in the cerebrospinal fluid, as "liquid light," "potency," and A. T. Still's "highest known element"; as something that disperses the darkness when it is switched on.[12:347] It is the first spark, the release of the involuntary motion, something that releases the motion,[12:142f.] something invisible in the cerebrospinal fluid,[12:191;14:5] something in the motion of the tides, not the breath of air,[14:5] comparable with the lightning that shines through the cloud without touching it. Sutherland also sees the breath of life as "transmutation" (q.v.).[14:34] Sutherland frequently used a quotation from the Bible to show that the breath of life was not to be confused with the air: "The Lord God...breathed into his nostrils the breath of life, and man became a living being" (*Genesis* 2:7).[14:35]

Cant Hook technique

This is a technique that operates by means of leverage. Here, a hand position to the side enables one part to act as a fulcrum for the movement of another, like the hinge of a door, e.g., release of the frontosphenoidal suture: one hand spans the frontal bone between the thumb and index or middle finger; the thumb on one side acts as the fixed point and the fingers lift the frontal bone on the other.[14:286]

Core link

The structural and functional link of the reciprocal tension membrane (the spinal dura mater as the continuation of the cranial dura mater) that connects the occiput with the sacrum, and thus the cranium with the pelvis. Each pole reciprocally affects the other. According to Sutherland,[12:224–226, 344f., 350] it is via this link that the involuntary, inherent cranial motion is transmitted to the sacrum.[7]

Cranio-rhythmic impulse

This concept was introduced only after Sutherland's death, and was intended to denote simply the physiological involuntary and rhythmic fluctuation of the cerebrospinal fluid, as a palpable motion of expansion and retraction of the cranium, unassociated with the primary respiratory mechanism. The term was coined by the psychiatrists and osteopaths Woods and Woods to enable other physicians to palpate and evaluate this motion without having to confront the notion of the primary respiratory mechanism. According to both Woods and Woods and Magoun, the CRI is shown by palpation and by electronic measurements to have a frequency of 10–14 cycles per min.[19] Sutherland himself never specified a frequency. According to Magoun the CRI can still be palpated even after death (for up to about 15 min).[9] He states that it influences the physiological centers of the body, including pulmonary breathing.

Fluctuation of the cerebrospinal fluid

According to Sutherland and Magoun, the fluctuation of the cerebrospinal fluid, together with the structures that produce and resorb it (choroid plexus; arachnoid granulations), is partly responsible for the fourth rhythm that can be palpated at the cranium, the CRI, or craniosacral rhythm.[10:35] For Sutherland, the motion of the brain causes a rhythmic change in shape of the cerebral ventricles, so causing fluctuation of the CSF.[14] The fluctuation of the CSF consists in rhythmic phases of filling and emptying of the ventricles, and is characterized by specific intra- and extracranial directions of flow. The intracranial and intraspinal membranes continue along the nerve exit points of the cranium and vertebral column, and it is along these nerve sheaths that CSF is able to reach the extracranial system. There are also exchange processes in the lymphatic system. According to Sutherland and Magoun, these exchange processes have great physiological significance,[10:56] and this fluctuation can be palpated[12:215]). The motion of the intracranial dural membranes exerts a pressure on the CSF, causing motion of the fluid.[10:56] The inherent motility of the nervous system moves the CSF. There is a fluctuation in volume caused by the increase in size of the ventricles and subarachnoid space.[10:16f.] This can be influenced by compression of the fourth ventricle.[12:272] Sutherland emphasizes that it is the fluid fluctuation that leads the structures being treated to a membranous point of balance during therapy.[10:73] Some misunderstandings have arisen concerning the concept of the fluids; these appear to stem from the fact that Sutherland initially used the term to describe bioelectric phenomena, whereas other osteopaths used it to refer to the dynamics of fluids. In this book, the term fluids generally refers to the palpatory qualities of fluids in the body; electromagnetic and bioelectric phenomena in the body will generally be referred to by the term "potency" or "electrodynamics" (point of balanced electrodynamic tension, PBET).[7] State of research: pulsations of the CSF of various frequencies have been found. New findings relating to the dynamics of the CSF dating roughly from the decade of 2010 onward place earlier assumptions in a more nuanced light. The connection between this and the hypothesis of primary respiration or the craniosacral rhythm has not been explained.

"Fluid drive"

The PRM has a "fluid drive" brought about by the activity of the cerebrospinal fluid.[12:298] The concept is frequently used in practice to express the hydrodynamic relationship between the CSF, interstitial fluid, and lymph.

Frequency of the PRM rhythm

Sutherland did not specify any particular data regarding this rhythm. Different data exist as to the PRM rhythm or craniosacral rhythm; a selection is given here. The list below gives only a selection of possible rhythms: 10–14 cycles per min, a 4–6 second cycle (Magoun, Traube-Hering oscillation);[20] 6–12 cycles per min: a 5–10 second cycle (Upledger;[16:18] 8–12 cycles per min: a 5–7.5 second cycle (Becker, Upledger;[1:120] 2.5 cycles per min: a 24 second cycle (Jealous[2]); 6–10 cycles per 10 min: a 60–100s cycle (Becker's slow (large) tide, Mayer oscillation;[1:122f.] 1 cycle per 5 min: a 300 second cycle (Liem[5]). A rhythm of 1 cycle in around 33 min (2000s cycle) has also been recorded, by Lewer-Allen, Bunt et al., in the brain. No recorded data based on palpation of this rhythmic pattern presently exist. Personal experience of palpation does also seem to offer some evidence of very slow impulses of expansion and retraction, but these results tend to be inconsistent and irregular, and no continuous rhythmicity could be palpated. Kiviniemi et al. describe three types of pulsation in the CSF:[3] (1) Cardiovascular pulsations: these are the most rapid, at 0.8–1.2 Hz. They bring about a negative change in the MREG signal in peri-arterial regions, which extends centrifugally to cover the entire brain. (2) Respiratory pulsations: these are centripetal pulses of 0.3 Hz which occur periodically, mainly in perivenous regions. (3) Vasomotor waves: these are the slowest type of pulsation, occurring

at very low frequency (VLF0.001–0.023 Hz and LF 0.023–0.73 Hz). They show unique spatiotemporal patterns of parasympathetic and sympathetic origin.

Fulcrum

See also "Automatic shifting suspension fulcrum." A fulcrum is like a point of rest or movable fixed point.[7] Fulcrums do not only exist in the human body; they are also found elsewhere in Nature. There are bony fulcrums (SBS), membranous fulcrums (Sutherland fulcrum), and fluid fulcrums. Sutherland and Becker have also described spiritual fulcrums.[14:14, 46]

Highest known element

See also "Breath of Life." Still states that this "highest known element" is found in the cerebrospinal fluid. Sutherland repeatedly refers to it. For him, on the basis of practical experience, it is the constant seat of an intelligent potency with the ability to transcend everything else in the body. He uses this potency for diagnosis and therapy.[10:15]

Ligamentous articular strain

See "Membranous articular strain."

"Long tide"

Becker used this term (also "slow" or "large" tide) to denote the concept of a very slow rhythm. He states that this rhythm enters the body from outside, originating anywhere and spreading through the body. He palpated a rhythm that took 1.5 min to permeate into the body and the same length of time to ebb away.[16]

Membranous articular strain

Sutherland terms dysfunctions and abnormal tensions affecting the joints of the vertebral column and their associated ligaments as "ligamentous articular strain." Dysfunctions affecting the bones of the craniosacral system and their associated intracranial and intraspinal dural membranes (falx cerebri, tentorium cerebelli, falx cerebelli, spinal dura mater) he called "membranous articular strain." These strains can impinge on cerebrospinal fluctuation, cranial arterial and venous perfusion, and the lymphatic drainage of the head and neck. His treatment is therefore above all aimed at a resolution of these imbalances of tension. The treatment principle for the ligamentous and membranous articular types is the same.[14:119–122]

Midline

According to van den Heede it is possible to differentiate between a dorsal "midline" (neural tube), a middle (the former ventral) "midline" (chorda dorsalis to the sphenoid and the ethmoidal cells), and an anterior "midline." Nasion is a reference point for the development of the middle midline, as is the sacrum. The development of the first two midlines induces the formation of a third (anterior) midline, anterior to the former ventral one. This anterior midline draws a line from the nose via the hyoid to the sternum, the xiphoid, and linea alba to the pubic symphysis. It develops through the meeting points of the outstretching dorsoventral growth movement. The hyoid is the balance point of the anterior midline (to the dorsal midline). The heart is the balance point for the fluid middle (previously ventral) midline. Sutherland's fulcrum is the balance point for the dorsal midline. Exchange and memorization occurs in the dorsal "midline," the middle "midline" acts as a support for the body, and in the anterior "midline" the potential body presents itself. According to van den Heede, expansion occurs through the lateralization of the midline; however, the concentric force of the midline is required to provide the polarity to enable lateralization to develop.[6,8]

Molding

Molding is a direct treatment technique which uses the application of external pressure or pull to change the shape or malleability of bony structures. It is mainly used in childhood.

Morphodynamics

This is a concept in osteopathy formulated by Liem, to discuss and describe the influences, interactions, and governing principles of morphological dynamics—or the dynamics of morphology—and the application of these insights in osteopathic practice. The increasing complexity of material form emerging in the course of evolution goes hand in hand with increasingly intricate refinement of energies and inner consciousness. In this phylogenetic and ontogenetic dynamic, matter—including its associated energy fields—is continuously present, through from the external form to the highest possible consciousness—the external objective through to the highest inner subjective. The subjective reality of inner consciousness stands over against the objective reality of the tissue structures and the energies belonging to them; these are embedded in inter-objective and intersubjective realities. The inter-objective realities we can understand as the sociobiological environment; the intersubjective consist of culture and family. If we are adequately to treat the "wholeness" of the person, it is not enough to treat only the tissue correlation; the ability to discover and take account of components of inner consciousness is equally necessary.[6,8]

Motility of the brain

According to Magoun, there is a slow, rhythmic rolling and unrolling of the cerebral hemispheres, which also leads to a dilation and contraction of the cerebral ventricles.[14:52] The other motion described by Magoun is the CRI, or rhythm of the PRM. In the osteopathy, attention is being directed not only to examining these hypotheses, but above all to considering what factors maintain the health of the neural tube.[17] Current state of research: to date, motions of the brain have been demonstrated; however, these have mainly tended to occur in synchrony with contractions of the heart and blood vessels. Less often, slower motions have been found, mainly in CT scans, and also a small number of contractile elements of the neuroglia. Various rhythmicities have been recorded (e.g., Traube-Hering-Mayer oscillation [THM oscillation]). So far, the connection with the motion referred to as PRM rhythms has not been clarified.

Neutral state ("neutral")

See Chapter 1.

Osteopathic "felt sense"

See Chapter 1.

Osteopathic heart-focused palpation

See Chapter 1.

Pivot

See also "Fulcrum" (above). The pivot points of the cranial sutures (these are the points where the bevel of the cranial sutures changes direction) represent a fulcrum, a point of rest or turning for the motion of the cranial bones. They are the place where the inward-facing border meets the outward-facing border of the articulating bones; where there is a change in the direction of inclination of the suture margins. They serve as fulcrums, points of rest or of turning, and are potential bony axes for the movement of the cranial bones. They are often used in treatment as the place where disengagement techniques can be applied, e.g., sphenosquamous pivot (SSP); condylosquamosomastoid pivot point (CSMP).[10:70,118,123]

Point of balance (PBT) (membranous)

See Chapter 1. Magoun defines this as the point in the range of movement of a joint articulation where the membranes are in a state of balance. This is a

point between normal tension, which can be seen in the free range of movement, and the increased tension that results from strains and restrictions, and appears when the joint is moved beyond its natural physiological range of movement.[10:68] The same principle applies to the ligamentous point of balance, e.g., in the joints of the vertebrae. Sutherland says that the reciprocal membranous tension and the fluctuation of the fluids should be kept at "balance point" during treatment.[12:349] The midpoint between inhaling and exhaling is also referred to as a "balance point."[14:14,16] Electromagnetic fields and their interactions with the anatomical tissues of the body can be sensed. The osteopath may, using the principle of the PBT, induce a point of balanced electrodynamic tension (PBET) in the electrodynamic field.[7]

Potency

The "Breath of Life" has "potency," which operates as "the thing that makes it move" and is called intelligent potency, more intelligent than the human mentality.[14:14] The potency in the CSF is also described as an electrical potential, constantly becoming charged and uncharged.[10:72] It can be seen as a fundamental principle in the functioning of the primary respiratory mechanism (PRM).[12:239] Magoun says that it produces a specific, selective fluctuating motion or transfer of energy in the cranium.[10:59] This potency in the fluctuation of the CSF can be used for diagnosis and treatment.[12:220] The potency in the fluid can be directed (see under "fluid drive").[10:59f.]

Primary respiratory mechanism (PRM)

Sutherland chose this term to refer to his concept of a particular physiological approach.[14:289] This referred in particular to an old anatomy text which located all physiological centers, including respiration, in the floor of the fourth ventricle. Sutherland therefore concluded that "primary respiration" begins in the CNS.[12:298] It was called "primary" in the first instance because it was believed to come into existence first, even before pulmonary respiration, and also, according to Sutherland, because of its great importance to the body as a whole. It was referred to as "respiratory" because the PRM, like pulmonary respiration, represents a rhythmic process that has to do with exchange processes. It was held to be an anabolic and catabolic metabolic process. It was a "mechanism" because it was made up of linked, constituent parts whose interaction produced a specific effect.[7,10:16]

Reciprocal tension membrane

Sutherland chose this term to describe the mechanical function of the inner layer of the dura mater, which is a mechanical functional unity. The reciprocal tension membrane in the cranium is organized around Sutherland's fulcrum and regulates the motion and integrity of the cranial bones. In the spinal canal the tension membrane links and coordinates the motion of the cranium and sacrum.[7,14:289]

Rhythms

See also "Breath of Life" and "Frequency." The PRM rhythm appears to be another physiological rhythm of the body, in addition to the respiratory rhythm and cardiac rhythm. However, the source of this rhythm has not so far been explained. A number of other rhythms are also present in the body, e.g., that of the flow of lymph, rhythms in the secretion of hormones, etc.

Speed reducer

Some bones in the cranium have a motion that is greater than that of the bones with which they articulate, e.g., the palatine and the zygomatic bone.[11:347] Sutherland quotes the sphenoid as an example of this; its motion is greater than that of the palatine bones. These in turn have greater motion than the maxillae. The palatine bones act as mediators. The zygomatic bones are a further

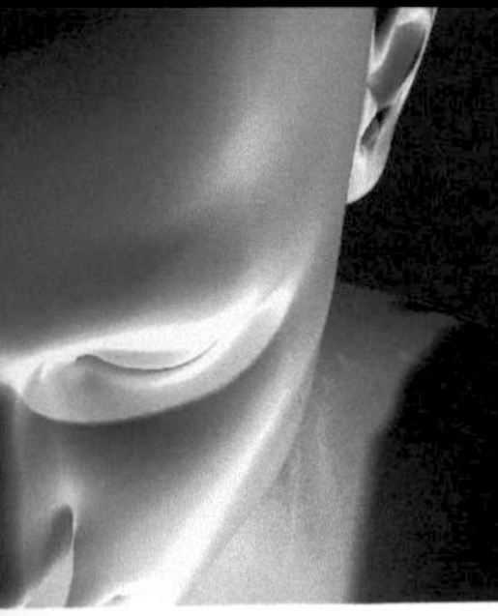

example of speed reducers.[14:78] The importance of the speed reducers appears to be to integrate the motion of various structures with one another.

Spiral motion of the tide

A spiral outward and spiral inward motion of the "tide" has been described.[14:16]

Still point

Sutherland's fulcrum is a still point around which the tension membranes operate.[14:18] A fulcrum is a still point that enables a weight to be lifted.[14:46] The fulcrum of the cerebrospinal fluid or the point when the fluctuation of the CSF stops is called the "still point."[14:135] The craniosacral motion stops.[18:52]

Sutherland fulcrum

See "Fulcrum."

Techniques

Point of balance, exaggeration technique (indirect technique), direct technique, opposite physiological motion, disengagement of joint surfaces, molding, fluctuation, and fluid impulse techniques.[7]

Tide

The "tide" fluctuates like the tides of the sea; not like the motion of the waves but like the ocean. The tide rises during the inhalation phase and ebbs during the exhalation phase. It possesses more "potency" and "intelligence" than any force applied from outside. For the later Sutherland it was essential to perform treatment, not by applying external force, but by allowing the "tide" to work.[14:14f.,166] According to Sutherland, the tide can be directed even from a foot, and even without touching it.[14:168]

Transmutation

The transformation from one form, nature, or substance to another.[14:290]

References

1 Becker, R. E. In: Brooks, R. E. (1997) *Life in Motion: The Osteopathic Vision of Rollin E. Becker.* Portland: Stillness Press.
2 Jealous, J. 'Emergence of originality.' *Kursskript 12*, 35, 36f.
3 Kiviniemi, V., Wang, X., Korhonen, V. et al. (2016) 'Ultra-fast magnetic resonance encephalography of physiological brain activity – glymphatic pulsation mechanisms?' *J. Cereb. Blood Flow Metab. 36*, 6, 1033–1045.
4 Lay, E. M., Cicorda, R. A. and Tettambel, M. (1978) 'Recording of the cranial rhythmic impulse.' *J. Am. Osteopath. Assoc. 78*, 10, 149.
5 Liem, T. (1998) *Vortrag OFM.* München.
6 Liem, T. (2013) *Morphodynamik in der Osteopathi*, 2nd Ed. Stuttgart: Haug.
7 Liem, T. (2018) *Kraniosakrale Osteopathie. Ein praktisches Lehrbuch*, 7th Ed. Stuttgart: Thieme.
8 Liem, T. and van den Heede, P. (2017) *Foundations of Morphodynamics in Osteopathy.* Edinburgh: Handspring.
9 Magoun, H. I. (1951) *Osteopathy in the Cranial Field.* Kirksville: Journal Printing Company.
10 Magoun, H. I. (1976) *Osteopathy in the Cranial Field*, 3rd Ed. Kirksville: Journal Printing Company.
11 Nelson, K. E., Sergueef, N., Lipinski, C. M. et al. (2001) 'Cranial rhythmic impulse related to the Traube-Hering-Mayer oscillation: comparing laser Doppler flowmetry and palpation.' *J. Am. Osteopath. Assoc. 101*, 3, 163–173.
12 Sutherland, W. G. (1998) *Contributions of Thought*, 2nd Ed. Portland: Sutherland Cranial Teaching Foundation.
13 Sutherland, W. G. (1991) Teachings in the *Science of Osteopathy.* Portland: Sutherland Cranial Teaching Foundation.
14 Sutherland, W. G. (1939) *The Cranial Bowl.* Mankato, MN: Free Press Company, p. 56.
15 'The cranial letter.' *Cranial Academy 1994*, 7.
16 Upledger, J. E. and Vredevoogd, J. D. (2016) *Lehrbuch der CranioSacralen- Therapie I*, 7th Ed. Stuttgart: Haug.
17 Wales, L. A. (1987) 'Embryology of the central nervous system.' Lecture III. Attleboro.

18 Wirth-Patullo, V. and Hayes, K. W. (1994) 'Interrater reliability of craniosacral rate measurements and their relationship with subjects and examiners' heart and respiratory rate measurements.' *Phys. Ther. 67*, 10, 1526–1532.

19 Woods, J. M. and Woods, R. H. (1961) 'A physical finding related to psychiatric disorders.' *Journal of the American Osteopathic Association 60*, 988–993.

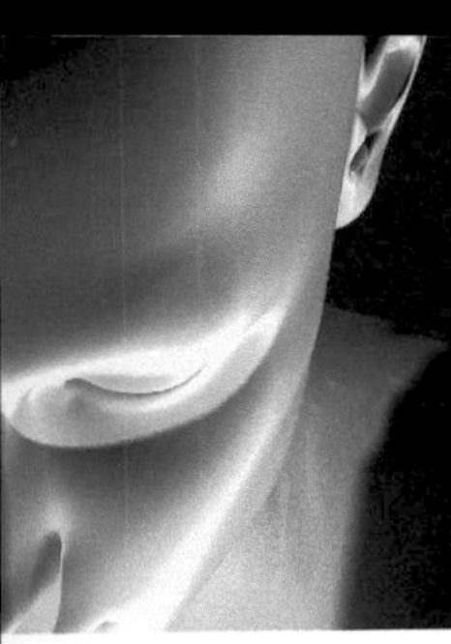

INDEX

A

alveolar bone 203
Angle's classification 72
ankylosis 108
anterior attachment to mandible 33
anterior attachment to temporal bone 33
anterior band 33
anterior girdle and tentorium 287
anterior superior alveolar arteries 29, 95
anteromedial disk displacement 151–3
anxiety 97
arteries
  anterior tympanic 29
  ascending palatine 217
  ascending pharyngeal 217, 425
  auricular 29
  buccal 29
  carotid 19, 90, 158–9, 212, 238, 246, 247, 262, 281, 338
  descending palatine 29, 96, 408, 425
  inferior alveolar 20, 28–9, 96
  inferior thyroid 217, 248
  infraorbital 95
  laryngeal 221
  masseteric 19, 29, 96
  maxillary 19, 28, 29, 246, 247
  meningeal 29, 201, 281, 338–9, 391–2
  mental 96
  mylohyoid branch 96
  occipital 263, 338
  ophthalmic 374
  palatine 29, 96, 217, 246, 408, 425
  posterior superior alveolar 29, 96, 408
  pterygoid canal 29, 211
  sphenopalatine 29, 217, 425
  sublingual 209
  submental 209
  superficial temporal 19, 29, 95
  superior laryngeal artery 217
  superior thyroid 247
  supraorbital 374
  supratrochlear 374
  treatment 246–8
arthrogenous dysfunction 115
articular capsule 17–8, 33
articular disk 16–7, 17
articular tubercle 14, 32
assessment (visual) 101–5
asterion 403
atlanto-occipital joint 262, 264, 266–9
auditory ossicles 365
autonomic nervous system 4–5

B

basal ganglia 36, 95, 295
bilaminar zone 16, 18, 33
body of mandible 20
bottle-fed babies 65
branches
  communicating 201
  dental 29
  ganglionic 212
  glandular 202
  maxillary nerve 245
  meningeal 201
  mylohyoid 29
  nasal 205, 212
  orbital 212
  pharyngeal 212, 425
  pterygoid 29
  sympathetic 202
  tracheal 221
  trigeminal 131
bregma 401
bruxism 43, 64, 170–3
buccal fat pad 20
butterfly hug 5

C

canine guidance 67
cant hook technique 284, 361, 381–2, 385–6, 398–9
capsule, disk, and muscle complex 41–2, 156–7
carotid canal 81
carotid plexus 201
cartilage framework (larynx) 220
cartilaginous growth 41
case report form 102
cementum 203
central nervous system 94–5
central sensitization 92
centric condyle position 67
centric occlusion 67
centric premature contact 67
cerebellum 336
cerebral cortex 36
cerebrospinal fluid 6
cervical plexus 25, 77, 82
cervical spine 82, 241
cervicothoracic transition zone 55
Chapman reflex points 231–2
cheeks 103, 105
chemoreceptors 36
chewing 31, 36, 65
chewing exercises 166–7
childhood (disturbances in early) 222
children
  cranial base-occiput-foramen magnum technique 270
  treating 173–4
chin tip 103–4
chorda tympani 200, 201, 210
chronic stress 97
cingulate gyrus 281
circumlaryngeal technique 244–5
clavicle 88
clicking jaw 78–80
compensatory fascial organization 59
compression
  cranial 117, 118
  fourth ventricle 272–4
  passive compression test 116
  SBS 293, 300
  third ventricle 285–6
  TMJ 145–6, 146
compression release technique 142, 145
condylar process 32, 34, 35, 74–6, 146–54, 153
coordination exercises 164–5
COPA splint 176
cortical regions 296
cover-bite 67
cranial base-occiput-foramen magnum technique 270
cranial vault hold 282, 382–3
craniocervical balance 42
craniomandibular dysfunction (CMD)
  causes 63–4
  clinical features 43–5
  comorbidities 43
  dental occlusion related factors 66–73
  diagnosis 98–134
  differential diagnosis 132–4
  disk-related factors 77–8
  dynamic signs 58–63
  effects on body statics 52–5
  epidemiology 42–3
  exercise programs 161–7
  history-taking 99–101
  locations 64–6
  myogenic 80–1, 82–9
  postural signs 55–8
  primary 65
  secondary 65–6
  self-help for 161–7
  symptoms 99
  symptoms in other regions 100–1
  treatment 134–61
  visual assessment 101–5
cranium development 41
cribriform plate 313–4
cricoarytenoid joint 220
cricoid cartilage 230, 243, 244
cricothyroid joint 220
crossbite 68–9, 168
CSF spaces 296

D

decompensatory fascial organization 59, 60

decompression
- condyles 153, 266–7
- cranial base 307–8
- of maxillary complex 416–7
- SBS 300–1
- TMJ 146–9, 162–3
- vomer 327–8
- zygomatic bones 437

deep bite 67, 170
dental root canal 203
dentin 203
depression 97
depressor labii inferioris 24, 25
deviation of incisor midline 107–8
disk displacement 77–8
disto-occlusion 67
dorsal pattern 52–4
drainage
- deep venolymphatic pharyngeal 248
- ethmoidal cells 317–20
- palatine tonsils 249
- tongue 236

dry lips 170
dura mater 48
dural dysfunctions 91, 293–4
dural techniques 286–7, 365–6, 379–81, 396–8
dynamic balanced tension (DBT) 6–7
dynamic occlusion 66
dysgnathias 169

E

Eagle syndrome 89
ear pull technique 365–6
edge-to-edge bite 68
effleurage of connective tissue/fasciae 142
embryonic development 38
enamel 203
end feel 116
endocrine disturbances 281
endocrine glands 96–7
energy polarity 9
epicranial aponeurosis 91
epiglottis 213
esophageal plexus 223, 227
ethmoid bone 324
- decompression of cranial base 307–8
- diagnosis 305–7
- drainage of ethmoidal cells 317–20
- dysfunction of falx cerebri 304–5
- extension dysfunction 309–10
- flexion dysfunction 309
- intraosseous dysfunctions 307–8
- intraosseous treatment 308
- morphology of 304
- motion testing 307
- nerve disturbances 305
- osseous dysfunction 304–5
- overview 304
- rotation dysfunction of frontal bone 310–1
- rotation dysfunction of maxilla 312–3
- treatment 307–20
- V-spread technique 308

ethmoidal cells 20
ethmoidal labyrinth (lateral masses) 314–7
exercise programs
- craniomandibular dysfunction (CMD) 161–7
- orofacial system 249–56

"exhalation phase" 9
external acoustic meatus 33

F

face (blows to the) 65
falx cerebelli 293, 366–7
falx cerebri 20, 48, 293, 305, 366–7, 373, 391
fascia
- buccopharyngeal 22, 91, 209, 215
- cervical 90, 91, 221, 241, 263, 281
- clavipectoral 91
- deep 22, 26, 91
- dysfunction 90–1
- larynx 221
- masseteric 19, 85, 433
- orbital 280
- parotideomasseteric 91
- pharyngobasilar 213–4, 213–5
- pterygoid 85
- temporal 26, 373, 391, 433

fascial organization 59
fascial testing 62
"Father Tom" reanimation technique 369–70
faucial isthmus 199
"felt sense" 5
flexion test sitting 62
fluid impulse 7
fluid tension 6
fluid/electrodynamic techniques 272–5
foramen ovale 81
foramen rotundum 81, 211
foramen spinosum 81
frenulum 223, 235–6
frontal bone
- clinical presentation presentation of dysfunctions 372–4
- cranial vault hold 382–3
- diagnosis 374–6
- dural techniques 379–81
- dysfunction at the falx cerebri 373
- dysfunction in external rotation 377–8
- dysfunction in internal rotation 378–9
- external and internal rotation 376
- fascial dysfunction 373
- intraosseous dysfunction 373, 376–7
- lift technique 379–81
- molding technique 376–7
- morphology of 372
- motion testing 376
- muscular dysfunction 373
- osseous dysfunction 372–3
- spreading techniques 377, 378
- treatment 376–88
- vascular disturbances 374

frontal bone lift technique 311
frontal bone spread technique 310
frontal gyrus 95
frontal lobe 20, 373
Fukuda test 61
functional triangles 49–51, 61–2

G

Gehin's pivot technique 364–5
genetic factors 98
geniculate ganglion 200, 210
genu vasculosum 16
gingiva 203, 225–6
gliding hinge movement 37
global treatment of TMJ 148–9
glossoptosis 224
glottis 220
gnathology 66
golgi tendon organs 28
gravity lines 45–8, 51–2

H

habitual occlusion 66
"hamster" cheeks 103
hard palate 199
headache 43, 64
heart-focused palpation 4–5
horizontal overbite 67
HPA (hypothalamus–pituitary–adrenal) axis 96
hyoid bone 32, 80, 88, 238–41
hyoid cartilage 230
hypomobility/hypermobility 105
hypothalamus 296

I

immune system 96–7
incisal guidance 67
incisive foramen 81–2
inferior alveolar vein 20
inferior orbital fissure 407
infraocclusion 67
"inhalation phase" 9
intermediate zone 33
internal carotid plexus 212, 262, 281, 338, 338–9

interpterygoid aponeurosis 30, 91, 140, 280
intraosseous dysfunctions 270–2
intraosseous treatment 155
investing layer 281
irritable bowel syndrome 43
isometric contraction 140–1

J

joint sounds 78–80, 131
joints
  atlanto-occipital 262, 264, 266–9
  cricoarytenoid 220
  cricothyroid joint 220
  see also temporomandibular joint (TMJ)
jugular foramen 81, 161, 264

L

lacrimal bones 445–7
lacrimal gland 200
lambda 401–2
lamellated (pacinian) corpuscles 28
laryngeal mobilization 242–5
laryngitis 232
laryngopharynx 214
larynx 220–1, 226–9
larynx questionnaire 228
lateral forced bite 168
lateral pharyngeal bands 220
laterognathia 168
laterotrusion 35–6, 106–7
Laughlin's dysfunction mechanism 69
ligament
  sphenomandibular 19, 34, 36
  stylomandibular 19, 34, 36
ligaments
  and body posture 52–3
  discocondylar 34, 35
  discotemporal 34
  dysfunction 89–90
  larynx 220
  lateral 13, 14, 18–9, 34, 35, 90, 118, 156–7
  lateral collateral 19
  malleus 21, 90, 335
  medial 13, 18, 19
  nuchal 263
  periodontal 203–4, 234–5
  petrosphenoidal 280
  pintus 21, 90, 336
  sphenomandibular 18, 19, 89–90, 119–20, 157, 280
  sphenopetrosal 90, 279
  stylohyoid 18, 211, 335
  stylomandibular 18, 19, 89, 119, 157, 158, 335
  tanaka 21
  temporomandibular joint 18–9
limbic system 95
lingual tonsil 219
lip exercises 254–5
lips function 103
Littlejohn model 45–8
low thrust 7
lower limb (mandible as reflection of) 37
lymphatic drainage 248
lymphatic vessels 29

M

malleus 21
malocclusion 67
mandible 15, 25, 33, 37, 38–41, 73–4, 213
mandibular fossa 14
mandibular head 13–4, 33
manipulation for anteromedial disk displacement 151–3
masticatory force 31
maxilla lift and spread technique 312
maxillae
  clinical presentation of dysfunctions 406–8
  decompression of maxillary complex 416–7
  diagnosis of 408–11
  disturbances of the nerves 407–8
  dysfunction in external and internal rotation 412–5
  global lateral strain 415–6
  global rotation dysfunction 415
  internal rotation dysfunction 412
  lift and spread technique 411–2
  morphology of 406
  motion testing 411
  muscular dysfunction 407
  osseous dysfunctions 407
  overview 15
  PRM rhythm 409–10
  rotation dysfunction 411–2
  sutural dysfunctions 417–22
  treatment 411–22
  vascular disturbances 408
maximum intercuspation 66
mechanoreceptors 28, 36
mediotrusion 35–6
Meersseman test 60–1
mental foramen 82
mesencephalon 295
mesial occlusion 67
methodology (overview) 2–4
Michigan occlusal splint 176–7
microbiome of oral cavity 249
migraine 64
motion barriers 8
mouth breathing 48
mouth closing 34, 105–6
mouth opening 31–4, 65, 105–6, 115, 117–8
multiple hand technique 154
muscle cramp 115, 116
muscle hypertonicity 58, 83–7, 89, 137, 138, 226, 227, 237, 238, 244, 262–3
muscle spasm 86
muscles
  abdominal 52, 54
  adductor 84, 85
  auxiliary 108
  back 57, 64
  buccinator 20, 24, 25, 27, 86, 103, 125, 206, 207, 209
  cervical 57
  chondroglossus 24, 47, 207, 208, 210, 239
  constrictor of pharynx 24, 80, 211, 215, 216, 226, 239, 241, 242, 243, 244, 263
  corrugator supercilii 25
  cricopharyngeus 38
  cricothyroid 38, 220, 227, 233, 242, 243, 245
  depressor anguli oris 24, 25, 123
  digastric 20, 24, 27, 32, 35, 38, 50, 57, 80, 87, 88, 121, 125, 127, 143, 205, 210, 211
  elevator muscles of pharynx 216
  eye 63, 280, 339
  femoris 52, 53
  flexor digitorum profundi 273
  foramen ovale 25, 81, 280
  genioglossus 20, 24, 47
  geniohyoid 20, 24, 47, 80, 88, 206, 210
  hyoglossus 24, 47, 206, 207, 210
  iliopsoas 53
  inferior rectus 20
  infrahyoid 24, 40, 47, 50, 57, 210
  ischiocrural 54
  larynx 25, 220
  lateral pterygoid 13, 15, 22, 23, 27, 32, 33, 35, 36, 40, 47, 75, 83, 84, 85, 93, 108, 120, 121, 124, 126, 129, 138, 139, 144, 145, 163, 164, 425
  lateral rectus 20
  laterotractor 141
  levator labii superioris alaeque nasi 24, 87
  levatores veli palatini 25, 201, 216, 217, 226
  longus capitis 263
  masseter 20, 21, 22, 27, 32, 40, 44, 47, 57, 83, 84, 120, 121, 124, 126, 131, 137–8, 145, 163, 433
  masticatory 15, 27, 41, 44, 54, 65, 69, 73, 74, 82, 83, 120, 121, 136, 163, 171, 280, 335
  medial pterygoid 20, 22–3, 25, 27, 30, 32, 35, 36, 40, 47, 85, 86, 120–1, 125, 127, 139–40, 143, 145, 425
  medial rectus 20
  mentalis 24, 86

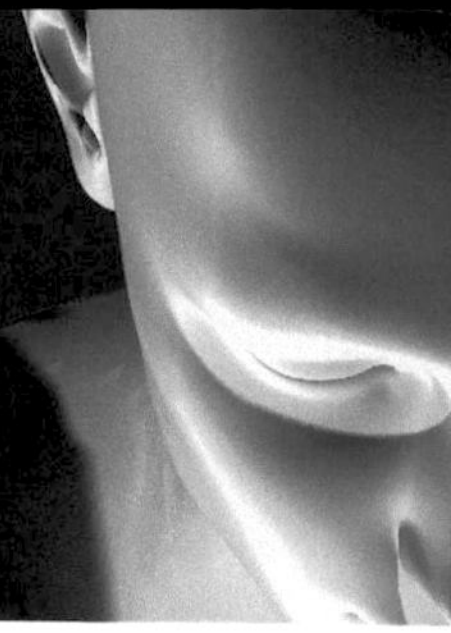

myloglossus 24
mylohyoid 20, 23, 24, 27, 80, 87, 205, 210, 236
nuchal 25, 47, 262, 267
obliquus capitis superior 263
occipitofrontalis 25
omohyoid 24, 88, 210, 236, 238
orbicularis oculi 25
orbicularis oris 25, 86, 254
palatoglossus 24, 206, 207, 208, 209, 217
palatopharyngeus 216, 280
pectoralis major 71
pelvic 53
peribuccal 204
pharyngeal 25
procerus 25
protractor 128, 129, 130, 141
rectus capitis anterior 263
rectus capitis lateralis 263
rectus capitis posterior major and minor 263
semispinalis capitis 262–3
sphenomandibular 23, 86
stapedius 38, 335
sternocleidomastoid 25, 50, 57, 71, 74, 88, 89, 125, 262
sternohyoid 24, 80, 88, 210
sternothyroid 24, 88
styloglossus 24, 47, 206
stylohyoid 24, 50, 57, 80, 87, 125, 210, 211
stylopharyngeus 215, 216
superior oblique 20
superior rectus 20
suprahyoid 23–4, 32, 40, 47, 50, 57, 122, 123, 210, 237, 256
temporalis 20, 21, 21–2, 27, 32, 34, 35, 36, 40, 47, 50, 57, 75, 83, 120, 121, 124, 126, 136, 144, 145, 163, 391
tensor tympani 201, 335
tensores veli palatini 25
thyrohyoid 24, 88, 210
tibialis anterior 53
tongue 24, 206–7, 208–11
trapezius 262
zygomaticus 24, 25, 121, 122, 123, 144, 146
musculus uvulae 217
mylohyoid branch 29
myofascial dysfunction 69

N

nasal bones 442–5
nasal breathing disturbance 65
nasal cavity 20
nasal conchae 219, 448
nasal glands 200
nasal septum 20, 38
nasopharynx 213
nerves
abducent 280, 294, 337
accessory 77, 295, 337
alveolar 20, 27, 28, 93, 94, 95, 201, 204, 205, 408
auricular 160
auriculotemporal 18, 19, 27, 28, 93–4, 201
buccal 27
cervical 36, 223
deep temporal 27, 28, 93
disturbances to 294–6, 305, 336, 373, 391
ethmoidal 205, 305, 372, 387
facial 27, 36, 76, 201, 208, 217, 223, 233, 245, 295, 337, 339
frontal 373
glossopharyngeal 36, 200, 207, 208, 209, 216, 217, 218, 219, 223, 232, 233, 234, 245, 261, 295, 337, 364
hypoglossal 55, 208, 209, 223, 232, 233, 245, 295
infraorbital 20, 27, 94, 245, 407
intermediate 281, 295, 337
intermedius 200, 201, 211
lacrimal 94, 373, 408
laryngeal 221, 227, 245
lateral pterygoid 93
lingual 27, 85, 93, 200, 201, 202, 205, 208, 209, 210
mandibular 21, 22, 23, 27, 28, 30, 39, 93, 217, 233
masseteric 19, 27, 28, 93
maxillary 27, 84, 86, 94, 200, 204, 211, 212, 217, 233, 245, 406, 407, 425
mental 27, 28, 82
mylohyoid 27, 28, 205
nasociliary 305, 373
oculomotor 294, 336
olfactory 20, 294, 305, 373
ophthalmic 100, 305
optic 20, 294
palatine 94, 205, 212, 408, 425
petrosal 27, 200, 201, 210, 212, 262, 279, 281, 337–8
pterygoid canal 201, 211, 212
supraorbital 27, 373
supratrochlear 27
tongue 208–9
trigeminal 92, 131, 172, 294, 336–7
trochlear 294, 336
vagus 208, 209, 216, 217, 245, 261, 295, 337
vestibulocochlear 295, 337
zygomatic 94, 200, 408
neurocranium-viscerocranium-cervical spine balance 26
neurotransmitters/neuropeptides 95
nutritional defects 65

O

occipital bone
diagnosis 264–6
fascial dysfunctions 263
intraosseous dysfunctions 270–2
ligament dysfunctions 263
morphology 260
motion testing 266
muscular dysfunctions 262–3
osseous dysfunctions 261–2
overview 260
treatment 266–75
vascular disturbances 263–4
occipital squama technique 271
occiput-atlas release technique 146
occlusal splints 174–8
occlusion disturbances 66–72
oculomotricity 63
omohyoid 88
open bite 68, 169–70
oral cavity 198–200
oral cavity assessment 104–5
oral vestibule 199
orbital fascia 280
orofacial system
diagnostic investigations 227–9
exercise programs 249–56
overview 198
potential dysfunctions in 222–3
self-help techniques 249–56
treatment 232–56
oropharyngeal isthmus 213
oropharynx 214
ossification (synchronicity of) 41
osteoarthritis 167–8
otic ganglion 27, 28, 200, 200–1, 210
overbite 67, 68, 107
overjet 68

P

pain processing 92–4
pain visual analog scale (VAS) 101
palatine aponeurosis 280
palatine bones
clinical presentation of dysfunctions 424–5
diagnosis 425–7
mobilization of 428
motion testing 427
muscular dysfunctions 425
neural disturbances 425
osseous dysfunctions 424–5
palpation 426–7
sutural dysfunctions 429–30

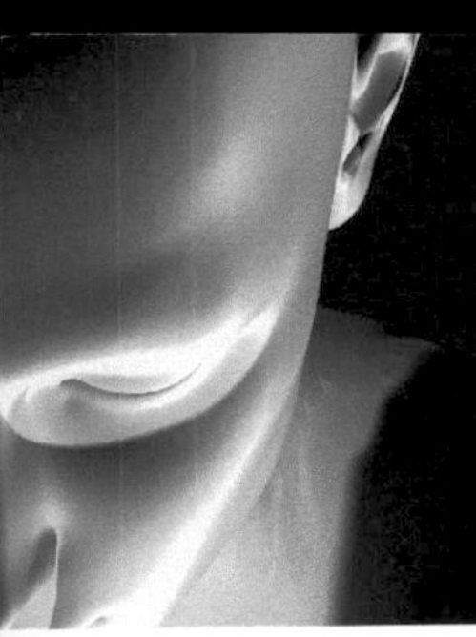

INDEX *continued*

palatine bones *cont.*
  treatment 428–30
  vascular disturbances 425
palatine tonsils 199, 218–9, 219, 249
palatoglossal arch 199
palatopharyngeal arch 199
palpation
  anterior dural fold 286
  atlanto-occipital joint 264
  carotid artery 158
  Chapman reflex points 231
  cranial dural sac 286
  ethnoid bone 305–7
  external and internal rotation motion 306–7
  flexion and extension motion 306
  floor of mouth 236
  frontal bone 374–5
  fronto-occipital 271–2
  lacrimal bones 445–7
  masseteric reflex 131
  masticatory muscles 120–5
  medial pterygoid muscle 139
  motion of TMJ 114–6
  for myofascial release 142–6
  nasal bones 442–3
  occipital bone 264
  osteopathic heart-focused 4
  palatine bones 426–7
  parietal bones 392–3
  resonance arising from 5–6
  sphenoid 282–3
  sphenomandibular ligament 119–20
  temporal bones 339, 339–41
  temporalis muscle 136
  trigeminal nerve exit points 131
  trigger points 123–7, 142
  vomer 322–4
  zygomatic bones 433–5
parasympathetic fibers 337–8
parietal bones
  clinical presentation of dysfunctions 390–2
  diagnosis 392–4
  dural techniques 396–8
  dysfunction in external rotation 394–6
  dysfunction in internal rotation 396
  dysfunctions of falx cerebri 391
  dysfunctions of tentorium cerebelli 391
  fascial dysfunctions 391
  intraosseous dysfunctions 394
  lift technique 396–8
  molding technique 394
  morphology of 390
  motion testing 394
  muscular dysfunction 391
  osseous dysfunctions 390–1
  palpation 392–3
  spread technique 394–6
  treatment 394–403
parietal lobe 391
parotid gland 29, 29–30, 200
parotid plexus 137
passive compression test 116
PBMT (point of balanced membranous tension) 6
pectoral girdle 82
perinatal trauma 65
periodontium 203
peripheral sensitization 92
perpendicular plate 314
petro-occipital fissure 261, 333, 354
petro-occipital synchondrosis 353, 353–65
petrosphenoidal fissure 362–3
pharyngeal plexus 216, 217
pharyngeal tonsil 219
pharyngeal wall 214–5
pharyngitis 232
pharynx 25, 207, 212–3, 212–20, 226, 227–9, 232, 239, 240, 241–2, 249
photographic analysis 108–10
phylogenesis (jaw development) 37
pivot
  condylosquamoso-mastoid pivot point (CSMP) 261, 333
  sphenosquamous 278, 334, 361
platybasia technique 270–1
posterior atlanto-occipital membrane 263
posterior attachment to temporal bone 33
posterior band 33
postural patterns 51–2
posture of the head
  functional triangles 49–51, 61–2
  Littlejohn model 45–8
  Samoian model 47–8
  theories 48–9
practitioner's positioning 9
premature contact (teeth) 67, 69–71
preserving the bite 174
pressure trajectories dysfunction 155–6
primary sensory cortex 95
PRM rhythm
  ethmoid bone 305–7
  frontal bone 374–5
  lacrimal bones 445–7
  maxillae 409–10
  nasal bones 442–3
  occipital bone 264–6
  palatine bones 426–7
  parietal bones 392–3
  sphenoid 282–3
  temporal bones 339–41
  vomer 322–4, 329
  zygomatic bones 433–5
protrusion 34–5
psychological-emotional factors 66
pterion 402–3
pterpterygoid processes 37
pterygo-temporo-mandibular aponeurosis 25, 26, 280
pterygoid branches 29
pterygoid canal 211
pterygoid process 211
pterygoid venous plexus 96, 248
pterygomandibular raphe 21, 26
pterygopalatine fossa 211
pterygopalatine ganglion 27, 86, 200, 205, 210, 211–2, 226, 228, 246, 295, 336, 408, 425
pterygotemporomandibular aponeurosis 91
pulp cavity 203
pussy-foot technique 368–9

R

ramus of mandible 20, 39
RBH-Index 228
recoil technique 7
reflex arm length test 111–4
relaxation exercises 162–4, 256
release techniques 142–6
Research Diagnostic Criteria for Temporomandibular Disorders (RDC/TMD) 98
resonance 5–6
retrusion 35
retrusive occlusion 169
rhagades at corner of mouth 170
rheumatic disorders 66
"Rideau stylien" 30
risorius 24
"roaring lion" 249–50
ruffini corpuscles 28

S

saliva 199–200
salivary glands 96, 200
salivary nucleus 200, 210
Samoian model 47–8
scalenus anterior 88
scalenus posterior 88
scales (testing using two) 57
scissorbite 168
self-help
  craniomandibular dysfunction (CMD) 161–7
  orofacial system 249–56
sinuses
  maxillary 20
  petrosal 338–9
  sagittal 392, 398
  sigmoid 338, 392
  superior sagittal 20, 374

techniques for 398
venous 338
six-legged table model 72–3
skull
growth 38–9
stress fibres 48
sleep disturbances 97–8
"small functional analysis" 98
soft palate 20, 199, 213, 219
spheno-occipital synchondrosis (SBS)
compression 293, 300–1
diagnosis/treatment 296–301
dysfunctions of 292–6
extension 292
flexion 292
flexion and extension 297
lateral flexion-rotation 292
lateral strain 293
metamorphosis of 290
overview 290
right and left lateral strain 299–300
right and left lateroflexion-rotation 298
right and left torsion 297–8
significance of 290–1
superior and inferior vertical strain 299
torsion 292
vertical strain 293
sphenobasilar synchondrosis 38, 77
sphenoid
diagnosis 281–3
dural techniques 286–7
dysfunctions of 278–81
fascial dysfunctions 280–1
fluid/electrodynamic techniques 285–6
intraosseous dysfunctions 283–5
ligamentous dysfunctions 280
morphology of 278
motion testing 283
muscular dysfunctions 280
osseous dysfunctions 278–80
overview 278
treatment 283–7
sphenopetrosal synchondrosis 279, 334, 362–3
spinal dura mater 293
splint correction 174–8
static dysfunctions 65
static occlusion 66
sternum 245
strengthening exercises 165–6
stretching exercises 162–4
stroking (effleurage) of connective tissue/fasciae 142
styloid process 209
subglottis 220
sublingual gland 200
submandibular ganglion 200, 201–2, 209
submandibular gland 200
supraglottis 220
Sutherland's cranial vault hold 282
Sutherland's technique 268–9
sutural dysfunctions 287, 327, 353–65, 381–8, 417–22, 429–30, 437–9
sutures
conchomaxillary 407
coronal 372, 383–4, 390
ethmoidoconchal 305
ethmoidolacrimal 305, 448
ethmoidomaxillary 305, 407
ethmoidonasal 305
ethmoidoseptal 305
frontoethmoidal 304, 304–5, 372
frontolacrimal 373, 387–8, 447
frontomaxillary 372, 385, 407, 419–20
frontonasal 372, 387, 444
frontozygomatic 372, 385–6, 433
incisive 407, 420
internasal 445
lacrimomaxillary 407, 448
lambdoid 261, 391, 400
median palatine 407, 422, 430
metopic 374–7
nasomaxillary 407, 444
occipitomastoid 261, 333, 355–8
palatoethmoidal 305
palatomaxillary 407, 418
parietomastoid 334, 358–9, 391
petrobasilar 261, 333, 353, 354–5
petrojugular 261, 333, 353–5, 354
sagittal 391, 400–1
sphenoethmoidal 279
sphenofrontal 279, 284, 372, 381–3
sphenopalatine 279, 424, 429
sphenoparietal 279, 391, 398–400
sphenosquamous 278–9, 334, 361
sphenovomerine 279, 327
sphenozygomatic 279, 432, 437–8
squamoparietal 359–60, 391
temporozygomatic 334, 363–4, 432–3, 439
transverse palatine 407, 417–8
vomeromaxillary 327, 407
zygomaticomaxillary 407, 421, 433
swallowing 218
swallowing disorders 222–3
swallowing exercises 253–4
swallowing tests 229–30
synchondroses of cranial base 76–7

T

technique
auditory ossicles 365
capsule 156
carotid artery 158–9, 246–7
circumlaryngeal 244
compression of fourth ventricle 272–4
compression of third ventricle 285–6
cranial nerves 161
ear pull technique 365–6
ethmoidal labyrinth 314–7
expansion of fourth ventricle 274–5
facial artery 246–7
falx cerebri/falx cerebelli 366–7
"Father Tom" reanimation technique 369–70
frontolacrimal suture 447
frontonasal suture 444
internasal suture 445
jugular foramen 161
jugular vein 159
lateral ligament 156
maxillary artery 246–7
nasomaxillary suture 444
omohyoid muscle 238
palatine artery 246
performing 9–10
pharynx 241–2
pterygoid muscles 139
pussy-foot technique 368–9
sphenomandibular ligament 157
sternum 245
stylomandibular ligament 157
suprahyoid muscles 237
thyroid artery 247–8
thyroid cartilage 243
teeth
dental nerves 204
dental structure 202–3
disturbances of occlusion 66–8
interactions with organs 204
malposition of 71–2
muscle force and development of 204–5
periodontal ligament 203–4
potential dysfunctions involving 225–6
treatment 235
visual assessment 105
teeth grinding 43, 64, 170–3
temporal bones
auditory ossicles 365
clinical presentation of dysfunctions 333–9
and CMD 76–7
diagnosis 339
dural techniques 365–6
dysfunction in anterior and posterior rotation, bilateral 351–2
dysfunction in anterior and posterior rotation, unilateral 350–1
dysfunction in external and internal rotation, bilateral 348–50
dysfunction in external and internal rotation, unilateral 345–8
fascial dysfunctions 336
fluid/electrodynamic techniques 368–70
Gehin's pivot technique 364–5

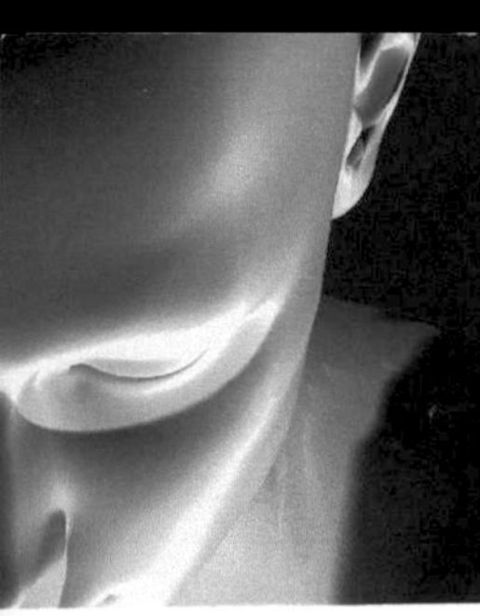

INDEX *continued*

temporal bones *cont.*
- in internal rotation 356–7, 359, 360
- intraosseous dysfunctions 335, 343–5
- lift technique 352
- ligamentous dysfunction 335–6
- in masticatory system 15
- molding technique 345
- morphology of 332–3
- motion testing 341
- muscular dysfunction 335
- opposite physiological motion 357–8
- osseous dysfunction 333–5
- petromastoid part/squamous part 344
- petromastoid part/tympanic part 343
- squamous part/tympanic part 344–5
- tentorium cerebelli 367
- testing external and internal rotation 241–2, 342–3
- treatment 343–70
- tympanic part 33

temporal fascia 26
temporal gyrus 95
temporal lobe 336
temporomandibular joint (TMJ)
- anatomy 12–29
- biomechanics 30–6
- and body posture 45
- compression and decompression of 146–8
- development of 37–42
- fasciae 26
- functional triangles and 49–51
- global treatment 148–9
- innervation 27–8
- manipulation (impulse technique) 150–1
- muscles 21–5
- often neglected 73
- osteoarthritis and degenerative processes 167–8
- overview 12
- relative position of upper/lower jaw 66
- resistant occlusal stress 167
- traumatic injury to 167
- treatment according to Blagrave 149–50
- treatment approaches for disturbances of 167–77
- *see also* craniomandibular dysfunction (CMD)

tendon of insertion 136
tension headache 43
tentorium cerebelli 293, 336, 367, 391
tests
- Barre's vertical alignment test 57–8
- cotton wool roll 104
- flexion test sitting 62
- Fukuda test 61
- isometric muscle test 123, 128–30
- Meersseman test 60–1
- motion of retrodiscal tissue 116, 117
- motion of TMJ 114–5
- mouth opening 106
- oculomotricity 63
- orofacial system 229–30
- passive compression test 116
- reflex arm length test 111–4
- singing/speaking 229–30
- three-finger metacarpal-joint test 105
- two scales 57
- Watt's test 107

thalamus 36, 95
thermoreceptors 36
three-finger metacarpal-joint test 105
thyroid cartilage 230, 243, 244
tinnitus 43, 64
tissue disposition 66
tongue
- anatomical relations 207
- consequences of incorrect position 224–5
- function 207
- muscles 24, 206–7, 208–11
- in orbital pyramid, ventral view 20
- position 207
- potential dysfunctions 223–4
- treatment 235–6
- "unwinding" the 236
- visual assessment 105

tongue training 250–3
tonsillitis 232
tonsils 218–20, 249
tooth extractions 65
trajectories of pull 156
trapezius 88
trigeminal ganglion 27, 92–3
trigeminal sensory nuclei 95
trigger points 123–7
trismus 78
tubular tonsil 219, 220

U

underbite 67
uvula 199, 213, 219

V

V-spread technique 308
vagus nerve 36
vascular disturbances 95–6, 296, 305
vascular retrodiscal pad 34
veins
- external jugular 96, 160
- inferior thyroid 248
- jugular 96, 159–60, 217, 263, 338
- maxillary 96
- meningeal 392
- occipital 96
- pharyngeal 217
- pterygoid venous plexus 96
- retromandibular 96
- submandibular 96
- superior and inferior labial 96

venolymphatic pharyngeal drainage 248
ventral pattern 51–4
visceral compartment 281
visceral dysfunctions 65
visual analog scale (VAS) 101
Voice Handicap Index (VHI) 228
vomer
- decompression 327–8
- diagnosis 322–4
- extension dysfunction 325–6
- flexion dysfunction 324–5
- lateral shear 326–7
- motion testing 323–4
- opposite physiological motion 329
- pump technique 328–9
- sutural dysfunctions 327
- testing motion of 323–4
- torsion dysfunction 326
- treatment 324–9

W

Waldeyer's lymphoid (tonsillar) ring 218, 219
Watt's test 107
whiplash injury 43

Z

zygomatic arch 20
zygomatic bone technique 320
zygomatic bones
- clinical presentation of dysfunctions 432–3
- decompression of 437
- diagnosis 433–6
- fascial dysfunctions 433
- morphology of 432
- motion testing 436
- osseous dysfunctions 432–3
- palpation 433–5
- rotation dysfunction 436–7
- sutural dysfunctions 437–9
- treatment 436–9